AF791438

Recent Strategies in High Risk Surgery

Joel Faintuch • Salomao Faintuch
Editors

Recent Strategies in High Risk Surgery

Springer

Editors
Joel Faintuch
Hospital das Clinicas
Sao Paulo, São Paulo, Brazil

Salomao Faintuch
Harvard Medical School
Beth Israel Deaconess Medical Center
BOSTON, MA, USA

ISBN 978-3-031-56269-3 ISBN 978-3-031-56270-9 (eBook)
https://doi.org/10.1007/978-3-031-56270-9

© The Editor(s) (if applicable) and The Author(s), under exclusive license to Springer Nature Switzerland AG 2024
This work is subject to copyright. All rights are solely and exclusively licensed by the Publisher, whether the whole or part of the material is concerned, specifically the rights of translation, reprinting, reuse of illustrations, recitation, broadcasting, reproduction on microfilms or in any other physical way, and transmission or information storage and retrieval, electronic adaptation, computer software, or by similar or dissimilar methodology now known or hereafter developed.
The use of general descriptive names, registered names, trademarks, service marks, etc. in this publication does not imply, even in the absence of a specific statement, that such names are exempt from the relevant protective laws and regulations and therefore free for general use.
The publisher, the authors and the editors are safe to assume that the advice and information in this book are believed to be true and accurate at the date of publication. Neither the publisher nor the authors or the editors give a warranty, expressed or implied, with respect to the material contained herein or for any errors or omissions that may have been made. The publisher remains neutral with regard to jurisdictional claims in published maps and institutional affiliations.

This Springer imprint is published by the registered company Springer Nature Switzerland AG
The registered company address is: Gewerbestrasse 11, 6330 Cham, Switzerland

If disposing of this product, please recycle the paper.

Preface

> Rather than reacting to every risk we hear and see, we should make an effort to discern which ones we can do something about.
> —Ben Carson, 2007 [1]

The first surgical operation (or should it be designated as a spiritual one?) was conducted on Adam (Genesis, Chap. 2). One of his ribs was extracted during sleep and converted into a whole woman, Eve. Theoretically it might, if viable stem cells were collected from bone marrow, fat, and other sources. They could then be grown in laboratory conditions and differentiated into all possible tissues. Yet establishing these myriads of cultures, converting them into full organs, assembling and harmonizing them into a living and functioning organism overnight would be a formidable task, definitely demanding a miraculous context.

Given enough time, if a recipient oocyte were used along with assisted reproduction techniques, a less mind-boggling nuclear transfer from Adam could perhaps do the trick. However, the book of Genesis provides no clue about a surrogate mother or a pregnancy preceding Eve's appearance. One way or another, both donor and recipient had a tranquil night. They were awake and in excellent shape the next morning, so the intervention could hardly qualify as high-risk surgery.

More dangerous were amputations performed during civilian life and particularly in military conditions, a rather recent and well-documented example being the Crimean War (1854–1856), often conducted on casualties suffering from severe injuries and shock. Indeed, amputations are deemed the oldest and most practiced major operation since Ancient Times, being documented even in the Prehistoric Era. Certainly not the safest procedures, as hemorrhage and infection were the rule. Due to lack of anesthesia, they had to be performed in minutes. It was not uncommon that a finger or two of the medical assistants holding the targeted limb were amputated as well depending on the haste, technical skill, and manual dexterity of the surgeon.

Reportedly, the most accomplished and humane of the professionals in the alluded to Eastern European clash was Nikolay Pirogov, Professor of Surgery at the Imperial Academy of Military Medicine in Saint Petersburg, Russia. Did he fulfill the requirements for a surgeon as defined in the Middle Ages by Guy de Chauliac (1300–1368): an eagle's eye, a lion's heart, a lady's hand? He is definitely credited with the invention of the first system of triage, classifying the injured Russian combatants into five modalities according to risk, as well as with the isolation of those bearing infected wounds in order to diminish cross contamination, insisting as well on thorough ventilation of the hospitals. Moreover, he established a group of volunteer nurses to take care of severely ill or disabled soldiers, one of the first such teams in the world.

By the way, the title of founder of modern nursing was conquered during the same Crimean War by a volunteer at the inimical British Army, namely Florence Nightingale, not only on account of her dauntless dedication to the wounded, but also because of her subsequent lucid and widespread publications, still cited today. Last but not least, it should be added to the merits of the previously mentioned Pirogov the pioneering introduction of anesthesia in the battlefield (with chloroform) [2].

What is currently the intraoperative complication surgeons abhorring most? All events that can be followed by sudden heart arrest, from anesthesia accidents to ventricular fibrillation to abrupt hypoxia are frightening; however, these are uncommon in general surgery. Less rarely, one encounters massive bleeding and hemorrhagic shock, particularly within the trauma context, which can run out of control. As a matter of fact, nowadays, the majority of the casualties die after the operation, not in the course of it, even though a few succumb on the spot. Epidemiological surveys confirm that uncontrolled bleeding is the most frequent cause of death in the surgical theater. Arrhythmias and heart arrest are also mentioned, whereas in the Intensive Care Unit infectious complications cannot be omitted.

Irreversible exsanguination has been particularly associated with certain subsets of trauma nominally liver bursting, crush injuries of the pelvis, rupture of the heart or major vessels, and post-transfusion coagulopathy. It represents an exorbitant challenge for the surgeon and should always be considered in high energy trauma requiring large volumes of blood, particularly in those with more ominous prognosis as indicated by the Injury Severity Score (ISS) or the regional Abbreviated Injury Scale (AIS).

Of course, the concept of high-risk surgical patients encompasses the whole perioperative period and all major organs and systems, not just the incision and the tissues temporarily under the scalpel blade. Book chapters are divided into preoperative and postoperative modalities for technical and didactic purposes only. Surgical risk is not a discrete measurement isolated from time, space, and context. On the contrary, its tools and resources such as clinical evaluation, validated indices and biomarkers, respiratory and circulatory dynamics, data collated from the operative field and other metrics need to be pieced together in a big and often changing meteorological map. Reflections and reinterpretations are mandatory until the patients is out of harm's way.

Are there surgical candidates of such a high risk that they are absolutely unfit for surgery? Even if they are not explicitly terminal or moribund? That's not an infrequent dilemma, potentialized by narrow-mindedly assessing indexes, scales, and scores. Currently, any operation with a probability of fatal outcome above 10% (some authorities set the cut-off point at 5%) is classified as a high-risk intervention. It goes beyond saying that these patients should be scrupulously reevaluated and discussed before any surgical decision is adopted.

What about operative repair of a ruptured abdominal aortic aneurysm, which incurs risks of up to 40–50% mortality? [3]. A legitimate argument in favor of the procedure is that no survival at all is the rule when nothing is done. Yet not many will consider this business as usual, or a stage for conventional indications and algorithm presets. Besides potentially beneficial alternatives like endovascular repair, seasoned and responsible professionals will walk the extra mile, meticulously addressing objective findings such as life expectancy along with functional, social, and cognitive status. From the point of view of ethics and human values, listening to the patient and his/her family is even more critical, with emphasis on their expectations and priorities regarding survival versus independence and quality of life.

According to the Aphorisms of Hippocrates (400 BCE), "He who would become a surgeon should join an army and follow it." Yet in less ancient times, it was emphasized that war was "the worst training for an immature surgeon and probably bad for a mature one" [4]. Historically, it has acted both ways. For most young medical professionals, draft evasion was the preferred route as recruitment meant career interruption, harsh life conditions, and the daily danger of death. At the same time, it was a magnet for a couple of others, ready to pay a high price for the chance of conducting anatomical studies and notably acquiring surgical experience, no matter how austere and chilling the environment is.

In Renaissance Italy (sixteenth century) Andreas Vesalius, known as the Father of Anatomy, was able to publish his masterpiece *De humani corporis fabrica*, on the basis of relatively undisturbed dissections. It is true that eventually the Catholic Inquisition decreed his death on account of such "profanations"; however, he was able to commute the sentence. Analogously Dr. Nicolaes Tulp, a renowned Amsterdam surgeon in the seventeenth century, could quite freely use human bodies collected from beggars or hanged criminals, for his surgical refinement and notably for teaching anatomy. There was no inquisition in the predominantly protestant Netherlands at that time, and one of his anatomy classes famously depicted by Rembrandt, ranks among the most reproduced paintings by the Old Master.

In Britain and the USA, there was no Tribunal of the Holy Office either, nonetheless use of cadavers for teaching or training was illegal or sharply limited till the middle 1800s, fostering the practice of bodysnatching. Around two centuries ago, medical students themselves sometimes engaged in graverobbing in the USA, so that their anatomical studies would not be compromised. Fortunately, along the twenty-first century legislation in virtually all countries regularized skeleton use for medical teaching. Yet in Britain supply was scarce leading to regular importations from Southeast Asia from the 1930s till the 1980s. Although little information is available, it is likely that these restrictions stimulated a few surgeons to forge ahead for professional advancement abroad, including armed conflicts.

Many landmark achievements in the handling of the seriously injured were effectively spearheaded by military personnel, such as the first mobile field hospitals in tents, as well as the first organized ambulance corps during the American Civil War of 1861–1865 (horse drawn wagons). Yet there is evidence in favor of Baron Dominique-Jean Larrey, renowned as the chief surgeon of Napoleon's army, for the invention of the *ambulances volantes* ("flying" ambulances) during the French Revolutionary Wars (1792–1799), more specifically in 1793. If simple carts and hammocks are considered, these were actually employed by fighting armies much earlier since ancient times.

Orthopedic care including fracture and nerve injury along with rehabilitation is believed to have started during World War I, blood transfusion and intravenous saline are inextricably linked to World War II (even though not widely available and thus sparingly used) [5], and helicopter transfer of critical cases to the Vietnam War (mostly during the last part of it, in the late 1960s and the 1970s). The last-mentioned conflict marked the advent of early mechanical ventilation for severe adult respiratory distress syndrome/ARDS. As soldiers were not as often succumbing to renal failure as during WWII, due to more abundant intravenous fluids and a better understanding of hemorrhagic shock, ARDS converted into a relatively early and irreversible mechanism of death. Forrest Bird, the inventor of the handy and ubiquitous mechanical ventilator, adapted the helicopters for apparatus use so more seriously injured casualties could be evacuated alive till the hospital [6].

At this point, one should not construe that civilian surgical life stood still. As early as 1505, the Royal College of Surgeons of Edinburgh was established. The French created the Académie Nationale de Chirurgie in 1731, to some extent emulated by the *Medical Surgical Society of Bologna, Italy* (*Societas Medica Chirurgica Bononiensis*) in 1802. A Collegium Chirurgicum Amstelaedamense had been organized in 1736 in Amsterdam (The Netherlands); however, it was more a professional guild than a scientific society. The USA joined the crowd much later. In 1879, an Academy of Surgery was established in Philadelphia, followed by the American Surgical Association (1880) and the American College of Surgeons (1913).

Such worthy trailblazers notwithstanding, the Extracorporeal Life Support Organization (ELSO) did not start before 1989, the Surviving Sepsis Campaign/SSC just in 2002, the Transplantation Society was born in 2003, the Enhanced Recovery After Surgery for Perioperative Care/ERAS Society in 2010, and the Surgical Data Science Initiative in 2016. It is not surprising that after such a relatively short life span concepts espoused by some of these organizations, particularly by SSC and ERAS, are still deemed as controversial.

Given that technical advances were not rarely marred by troublesome and costly backtracks, their implementation has been typically slow. Many active professionals who finished residency around the 80s and early 90s probably trained without surgical intensive care units, or at best with very simple and insufficiently equipped ones. Treatment protocols and guidelines for surgical emergencies were lacking or irregularly enforced, and monitoring devices were underused. Current concepts of fluid and electrolyte balance, sepsis, shock, mechanical ventilation, blood coagulation and thrombosis, nutritional and metabolic care, solid organ transplantation, therapeutic interventional radiology, endoscopic handling of complications, robotic surgery, not to speak of state-of-the-art antibiotics and anticoagulants, extracorporeal membrane oxygenation or mechanically assisted circulatory support, surfaced only in recent decades and are still evolving.

Within an environment so packed with challenges, uncertainties, and constraints, is it conceivable that personal attitudes of the surgeon enhance the problem ? In some circles, it is surmised that surgeons are intrinsically arrogant and narcissistic, carrying along a large ego. It is believed that they trust more their personal knowledge and accumulated experience than anything or anyone else [6]. Such frame of mind would not be conducive to careful patient evaluation, to consulting with or listening to colleagues and other healthcare professionals, and to a lifelong drive towards technically and scientifically updating oneself, which presuppose a hefty degree of humility and recognition of one's limitations.

From the point of view of patient care, excessive self-sufficiency could end up not only in ethical breaches but in sheer disaster, even in face of relatively common disease contexts [7]. However, there is an unquestionable exaggeration in these judgments. Ill prepared and overconfident surgeons definitely exist, as other healthcare and lay professionals, and their missteps lend themselves to deplorable situations such as the anecdote reproduced below, yet there is little ground for generalization.

One surgical resident after finishing his training program, settled in a faraway place. Years later, he revisited his *alma mater* and met his old mentors. He told them that he was quite happy in his city, where he had become a specialist in complicated cases. Who referred to him those complications? It is very simple, he answered. All patients that I operate on become complicated.

There is no question that high quality multidisciplinary teams handle even the most demanding redo operations cleanly and effectively, whereas for novices the tiniest deviation from the standard path could mean big trouble, whether the patient was previously classified as high risk or not. Major societies nominate centers of surgical excellence precisely for the guidance of residents and fellows, who search reputable places for training and professional update, in a range of clinical settings from the elective and straightforward till the most emergent and unpredictable ones. Of course, patients and health insurance companies are no less eager to engage with such centers, given their star performance, which enhances the stimulating atmosphere of such centers, and supports them so they can stay at the forefront of the specialty. However, even the most experienced and well-equipped units do not rest on their laurels and their phronesis. They prognostically investigate every single admission, very closely monitoring those in the higher echelons of risk.

If the fault does not squarely lie on the shoulders of the surgeons, at least not on the responsible and qualified ones, maybe surgical ambience and general atmosphere are flawed and biased, carrying part of the blame for inappropriate patient selection or matching intervention. Many generations of surgeons were trained to become lone heroes or commanding officers, something which translated into highly skilled and resolute technicians, not necessarily humanists and team workers. Some did consult whenever possible with clinical colleagues and with the anesthesiologist in case of serious comorbidities. The patient's feelings were also taken into consideration. However, the final decision in favor or against operation, as well as the choice of timing and extent of the intervention was unwaveringly personal and non-transferable. For many of them, it would be an intolerable loss of face, a "capitis diminutio" if others intervened in the process and they were instigated and coaxed to comply with, as the concept of multidisciplinarity was vague, misunderstood and underrated.

Only in recent decades have academic and a few nonacademic institutions established surgical committees composed of a variety of medical specialties, in charge of assessing candidates for elective high-risk surgery or organ transplantation, and of recommending the aptest operative treatment, if any. The surgeon's voice is respected: first and foremost, it is his or her procedure and ultimate responsibility. Nevertheless, the trend is always for the collective judgment to prevail, and indeed such becomes registered in hospital files. Although reluctant in the beginning surgeons now fully endorse such dialogue, as it leads to better tailored interventions with a safer postoperative period, more successful long-term outcomes, and much less overall morbidity and mortality. Potentially futile or poorly dimensioned procedures are openly discussed and appraised in this environment.

Incidentally, such initiatives also incentivize surgeons to expand the boundaries of the comfortable yet confined universe of their specialty, delving into and becoming familiar with the procedures, techniques, and therapies of internists, endoscopists, interventional radiologists, anesthesiologists, intensivists, and surgeons in competing domains, thus becoming able to robustly participate in the committee's deliberations. Of course, the opposite is analogously true, as other specialists will miss the point and fail to effectively contribute to the surgical committee, if they are not cognizant of all the tools, risks, and recent trends of the trade.

Do the abundant technical and scientific options and advances mean that a surgeon must convert into an omniscient, Olympic expert in all fields? A Renaissance style polymath at ease with all possible troubles, and a moving encyclopedia up to date till the very last article? Of course, these are tall orders demanding an artificial intelligence managed database, not a book, and a range of servers and data centers, not a human brain. Electronic libraries, surgical video repositories and scientific digital hubs exist of course, and a helpful selection is cited at the internet site item of the book. Ordinary chapters logically address more basic needs for bedside and general use. The crux of the endeavor is to assist the surgeon in an effective way and in the real world, not for grandiose performances in remote settings such as video conferences or surgical grand rounds. The prize is not for simply navigating the bewildering maze, but for safely arriving at the destination.

By the way the European Society for Vascular Surgery (ESVS), following the steps of a handful of other organizations, has recently implemented "Virtual Vascular—A living textbook with chapters published every month." The rationale is that the traditional vascular textbook (and by extension, any surgical book) is dead because "parts of even the latest textbooks are obsolete, as soon as they are published." Digital publishing in turn never should get old because it can promptly be amended, updated, or replaced. Moreover, it can be accessed with a variety of desk and portable devices from essentially anywhere.

One should not deride the praiseworthy approach. Nevertheless, what are review journals, electronic or in paper format, if not ongoing textbooks with new chapters all the time? Typical publications in other areas, however occasionally concerning surgery like CA-A Cancer Journal for Clinicians and Disease-A-Month, exist since respectively 1950 and 1954. More focused journals like *Surgery, Gynecology and Obstetrics* (now Journal of the American College of Surgeons/JACS) have been publishing reviews since the first half of last century, in early times of the narrative model and more recently as scoping, systematic, or umbrella modalities with or without meta-analysis.

It is unprecedented for standard books to be retracted or detracted as a consequence of such competition. There will always be room for virtual and printed material presented as journals, books, bulletins, internet sites, or electronic libraries. A galaxy of opportunities means that everyone can find his or her slot under the sun. The critical point is that all should be authoritative, pertinent, useful, well-referenced, and as up to date as feasible. Last minute electronic text and video guides, checklists, and technical sketches are not hard to come by, so missing or superseded information can and should be replaced and complemented.

According to renowned inventor Richard Buckminster Fuller (1895–1983), general human knowledge was estimated to duplicate every century until 1900. The interval dropped to a quarter of a century by 1945. Now doubling occurs after 12 h only [8]. Conflicting data is available for medical knowledge, yet still overpowering: it doubled every 50 years until 1950, then every 7 years in 1980, every 3–5 years by 2011, and the forecast for 2020 was 73 days [9]. Evidently, these figures are questionable and they oftentimes include pure trash. Regarding trustworthy and credible information, only a handful is directly or indirectly pertinent to surgery although still representing a data deluge.

Not even electronic chapters can be prepared every day or every few hours, like buns on the production line of a bakery, so as not to miss the very latest advances. If by chance they were, and this would require a Herculean commitment by both authors and readers, there would still exist fresher material waiting in the pipeline. It is not unlike the dog trying to catch its tail, or Aristotle's paradox of the hare chasing the slow tortoise. No matter how much success is accomplished or how punctiliously updated a text is, this will always be a job half done, a Sisyphean, never-ending task.

> To the best of our knowledge, this is the first book addressing a continuum of management, care, and strategies for high-risk surgical candidates, not just for conventional populations or encompassing routine therapeutic approaches. One that bypasses artificial dilemmas generated by a mega-data search of the literature, or improvised solutions which lack the indispensable groundwork, targeting instead tested and proven even though often innovative options and pathways. And despite multi-authorship from major universities in several continents, one with a streamlined presentation of conditions, tools and strategies, parsed and curated for ready implementation.

References

1. Carson B, Lewis G. Take the risk: learning to identify, choose and live with acceptable risk. Grand Rapids: Zondervan; 2007.
2. Barton CR, Beeson M. Anesthesia for trauma during wartime. CRNA. 1997;8(1):2–12.
3. Hoornweg LL, Storm-Versloot MN, Ubbink DT, Koelemay MJW, Legemate DA, Balm R. Meta analysis on mortality of ruptured abdominal aortic aneurysms. Eur J Vasc Endovasc Surg. 2008;35:558–70.
4. Gerbode F. A definition of surgery. Ann Surg. 1963;158(5):775–7.
5. Pierre NL, Yeo CJ, Tholey RM. What we owe the world wars: challenges that fueled surgical innovation. Am Surg. 2021;87(9):1525–28.
6. Forrest Bird. percussionaire.com/about/our-legacy. Accessed 22 Nov 2022.
7. Stanbouly D, Chuang SK. Humility will get you further than ego or pride in your career as a surgeon. J Stomatol Oral Maxillofac Surg. 2022;123(3):269–70.
8. Ray A. Human knowledge is doubling every 12 h. www.linkedin.com. Accessed 3 Jan 2023.
9. Anonymous. The importance of critical thinking skills at a time of exponential growth of medical knowledge. https://ifdhe.aha.org/education-events/importance-critical-thinking-skills-time-exponential-growth-medical-knowledge. Accessed 18 Feb 2023.

Sao Paulo, Brazil — Joel Faintuch
Boston, MA, USA — Salomao Faintuch

Contents

Part I
Preoperative Evaluation and Management

Chapter 1
Surgical Risk in Distressed or Underserved Populations

McKenzi Heide, Emma Johnson, and Christopher DuCoin

Introduction

Every surgical procedure comes with an associated risk of morbidity and mortality. However, there is large disparity in post-surgical outcomes between disadvantaged communities and their more privileged counterparts that is not explained simply by natural variability in inherent risk. For example, when a Black adult man is rolled in to an elective or emergent surgical procedure, he has as much as a 36% higher chance of death than his White counterpart [1]. In addition, ones' economic status can accurately predict their life expectancy [2, 9]. Although we persistently optimize surgical techniques, pre and postoperative management and standards of care, this gap in outcomes continues to elude us, likely signifying a systemic failure to address the true issue.

Medical care is estimated to account for roughly 20% of modifiable risk factors that contribute length and quality of life [3]. The remaining 80% are composed of modifiable risk factors that can be defined as social determinants of health (SDOH). The CDC describes these SDOH as "nonmedical factors that influence health outcomes … the conditions in which people are born, grow, work, live, and age, and the wider set of forces and systems shaping the conditions of daily life" [4].

Five key concepts of social determinants of health [4, 5]:

- *Healthcare access and quality*:
- Including geographic proximity to care, monetary access to care, and perceived discrimination by providers preventing care
- *Education access and quality:*

M. Heide (✉) · E. Johnson · C. DuCoin
Department of Surgery, University of South Florida Morsani College of Medicine, Tampa, FL, USA
e-mail: ejohnson229@usf.edu; cducoin@usf.edu

© The Author(s), under exclusive license to Springer Nature Switzerland AG 2024
J. Faintuch, S. Faintuch (eds.), *Recent Strategies in High Risk Surgery*,
https://doi.org/10.1007/978-3-031-56270-9_1

- Quality of free public schooling and access to higher education
- *Social and community context:*
- Social support from relationships and interactions with family, friends, co-workers, and community members as well as social stressors such as racism, marginalization, and bigotry
- *Economic stability:*
- Economic Stability refers to the stress of poverty, access to proper nutrition, and insurance etc. Economic stability is often used interchangeably with socioeconomic status (SES). In literature, SES is often assessed using the ADI index which is a composite measure of 17 census variables based on income, education, household characteristics, and housing [6]. Additionally, SES may also be described using geographic locations via the Social Vulnerability index (SVI) which also uses census data to rank locations on 16 social factors, including poverty, lack of vehicle access, and crowded housing, and minority status [7].
- *Neighborhood and built environment:*
- Neighborhood is the socioeconomic composition, crime, social cohesion, and support of the community as well as disorder such as trash, graffiti, abandoned or dilapidated buildings, and infrastructure [5].
- Built environment is the physical attributes of our surroundings that influence individual health behaviors. Examples include walkability and recreation; health amenities such as well stocked grocery stores and parks, and undesirable amenities such as fast-food restaurants and liquor stores [5].

It is well established that SDOH are associated with health outcomes in general and outcomes of surgical procedures. Despite this knowledge, the medical disparities seen along the lines of class, race, and location have not improved and continue to drastically affect the prognosis and outcomes of patients. One possible reason for this is that though these factors are often separated in literature for ease of organization and study, they will always be intertwined in reality. The systemic and confounding nature of SDOH makes them difficult to address as an individual practitioner. In the following chapter we will describe the outcomes of high-risk surgeries in economically and socially marginalized communities, with the ultimate goal being to identify specific variables seen in literature that may play a significant role in disparities and provide possible solutions for the individual surgeon in their practice.

Cardiothoracic and Vascular Surgeries

Cardiovascular disease (CVD) remains the leading cause of mortality in the United States. Thus, the effects of SDOH on CVD in particular have been more broadly studied than many other disease states. Regarding socioeconomic status, it is known that increasing social disadvantage is associated with more prevalent cardiovascular risk factors, inflammation, and incidental cardiovascular disease [8]. As for race, Black adults experience higher burden of cardiovascular risk factors such as hypertension and obesity and are more than twice as likely to die of CVD, relative to White adults [9]. When concerning neighborhood and built environment, those residing in high-vulnerability areas are less likely to receive care from high-volume hospitals and less likely to have stable primary care [9, 10]. Cardiothoracic and vascular surgeries are not immune to the effects of SDOH. When studied independently from chronic CVD, post-surgical outcomes in these fields are shown to be significantly linked to SDOH.

There is a clear racial divide between Black and White patients in surgical outcomes of many common high-risk cardiac surgeries. Wu et al. found Black race to be an independent risk factor for 30-day mortality following a carotid endarterectomy (CEA), with Black patients also showing a greater proportion of in-hospital death following a CEA procedure [11]. While studying race and coronary artery bypass graft (CABG) outcomes, Rangrass et al. found that non-white patients had 33% higher risk-adjusted mortality rates after the procedure than White patients (odds ratio [OR], 1.33; 95%CI, 1.23-1.45) [12]. Some of these gaps may be due to the quality of hospital and, when assessed independently, differences in hospital quality explained 35% of the observed disparity in mortality rates between races (OR, 1.22; 95%CI, 1.12-1.34). Overall Black patients are more likely to be in a low SES, present with greater disease burden, and receive care from lower volume surgeons and hospitals [9–12], all of which heavily impact surgical outcomes.

Low socioeconomic status, independent of race, is strongly associated with increased postoperative mortality and readmission following high-risk surgeries such as AAA repair, CABG and CEA [11– 15]. Impoverished patients are significantly more likely to present with ruptured AAA or symptomatic disease at initial carotid revascularizations, as well as more likely to undergo emergency rather than elective repair compared to patients of higher income class [11, 13]. Such differences in low-income populations may be attributed to decreased compliance with health screening, decreased access to primary care coverage, and increased use of low-volume surgeons [13]. It is logical to assume that the racial disparity is rooted in lower SES, as many of the same contributing SDOH are often cited when studying race and economic status, however SES does not fully explain outcome disparities as Black patients have worse outcomes following cardiac procedures than White patients of similar SES [15]. This suggests racism plays a fundamental role in disease or access to care and these healthcare disparities cannot be solely attributed to economic status. It is clear that while prior disease state affects surgical outcomes, there is no one sole contributor to risk. Rather, outcomes are affected by the complex interplay between socioeconomic status, access to health care, and the adverse effects (both generational and current) of stress and racism on overall health and wellbeing.

Surgical Oncology

Not surprisingly, the trend of health disparities is also seen in surgical oncology and those affected by these inequalities are disproportionately Black and Latinx. Despite NIH-funded research requiring inclusion of minorities since 1993, Stewart et al. found that racial and ethnic minorities and elderly patients are less likely to be involved in surgical oncology studies relative to the proportion of incident of cancer they bear when compared to the White and younger population [16]. They proposed several barriers to participation, including patient-physician interaction, and they found that Black patients not only refused surgical intervention more frequently, but also were offered surgical intervention less than their White counterparts. Additionally, SES plays a role in minority patients' ability to access oncological clinical trials further demonstrating the overarching relationship between low income and access to healthcare. Elderly patients are also less likely to be involved in surgical oncology trials although they disproportionately bear the burden of increased incidence of cancer diagnoses. Townsley C. et al. propose that geriatric patients' comorbidities contribute at least partially to their lesser enrollment [17].

When focusing on colorectal cancer surgical interventions, a study out of Scotland found that patients of a lower SES have worse overall and cancer-related survival after curative surgery [18]. "Deprived" in the context of this paper refers to the Scottish Index of Multiple Deprivation that measures relative differences in factors such as fewer resources, lower income, and less opportunity across area codes. These deprived patients had twice the risk of postop mortality (as an independent predictor) compared to the patients from the highest SES studied (odds ratio 2.26 95% CI 1.45-3.53). The 5-year survival rate was similarly disparate, with the lowest SES patients having a 25% increased risk of mortality from colorectal cancer (95% CI 1.03-1.51) when early mortality was included in the calculations. A study out of the UK found that similarly, "deprivation" was an independent predictor of curative resection as well as overall survival [19].

Race also plays a role in the disparities of surgical oncology. Tripathi et al. reported that Black patients had a significant diagnostic delay to definitive surgery for stages I-III melanoma when compared to their non-Hispanic White counterparts, which is associated with higher melanoma-specific deaths [20]. In breast cancer, patients with delays from diagnosis to surgery of only 6 weeks had decreased survival, with this effect on survival once again more prominent in Black patients, patients of lower SES, and patients without insurance/using public insurance [21]. Sheppard et al. found that the time to surgery for black patients was 47 days versus 33 days for white patients ($p < 0.01$), HR 0.58 (95% CI 0.44-0.78) [22]. When looking at survival in epithelial ovarian cancer, Chan J et al. found that race was an independent prognostic factor [23]. Their analysis showed that Black patients with stage I-II disease had fewer lymphadenectomies (23% vs. 27.1% in White patients, $P < 0.001$) and fewer nodes identified (5 vs. 7, $P < 0.001$). While prior findings had demonstrated lymphadenectomy's prognostic value in these patients, their analysis did not show a statistically significant survival difference in patients that had LN dissection.

High-risk surgery outcomes, such as those following pancreaticoduodenectomy, HCC, and esophagectomy also have disparities over race and ethnicity. Several studies have reported that there is a racial difference in patients who receive surgery for resectable pancreatic adenocarcinoma, which can only be partially accounted for as patient refusal [24]. When analyzing borderline-resectable pancreatic adenocarcinoma specifically, White patients had pancreaticoduodenectomies more than non-white patients (19.5% vs. 12.8%, $P < 0.001$) and RR 0.75 (CI 0.68-0.83, $P < 0.001$), with major influencing factors being insurance (Medicaid or lack of insurance), advanced patient age, and larger tumor size [25]. They did not find a significant difference in major non-curative surgeries between these two groups, which they propose is largely due to less access to care among Black patients. In a study that defines success of pancreaticoduodenectomy as TOO (Textbook Oncologic Outcome being resection, LN evaluation, normal hospital course, no mortality within 30 days, subsequent chemotherapy), several factors contributed to lower odds of achieving this success [26]. The failure to achieve TOO resulted in increased long-term mortality. These factors included having Medicaid (OR 0.85), being operated on at a community hospital (odds ratio 0.47), being Black (OR 0.79), and presenting at an advanced age (OR 0.97).

Similarly, with hepatocellular carcinoma, Black, Hispanic, and Native American/Alaskan patients had surgical treatment rates of 25–45% less than their White counterparts did, and these disparities were present even when adjusting for SES, geographic location, and tumor characteristics [27]. Patients were found to be 23% more likely to have surgery (resection with intention of removing all known cancer, ablation, or transplant) if their household income was over $45,510 ($P = 0.002$). For esophagectomies, there was a racial disparity in recommendation for surgery (odds ratio 3.03, CI 2.67-3.43, $p < 0.0001$), while lower SES was associated with worse overall survival [27, 28]. SES was measured with income quartiles, and there was a protective effect associated with higher incomes (hazard ratio 0.803, CI 0.742-0.867).

Trauma and Emergency General Surgery

As seen in previous sections of this chapter, SES is a known independent predictor of mortality following many major surgical procedures [31]. It is important to consider the comparison of circumstances of emergent surgery in trauma cases, versus planned or elective procedures and their disproportionately worse outcomes [32]. These emergent procedures may be even more prone to exacerbating SDOH. Unfortunately, there is less published on trauma surgery and race, age, gender, and geography than there is with other surgical subspecialties, but with the above in mind, similar conclusions may be drawn.

In trauma cases involving pediatric patients, LaPlant et al. found that Native American patients were 81% less likely than White patients to have emergency surgery after MVA [33]. In addition, Black patients were 23% less likely while Hispanic patients were 22% less likely. Rural patients also experience less frequent care from a Level I or II trauma center than their urban counterparts, at 3.32% vs. 11.83% and 2.63% vs. 9.67% respectively, and rural patients had a 14% higher risk of death after controlling for injury severity and type, age, sex, comorbidities, and region [34]. Cain et al. further discovered an increased mortality and complication rate in these high-risk surgeries directly associated with lower SES, stating that when compared to the highest SES, low-SES patients have a risk-adjusted mortality rate 29.9% higher [32]. They found that these risks were present with adjustment to other factors and were not mitigated despite the presence of hospital resources intended to help low SES patients.

Diaz, A et al. found that non-elective colon cancer and diverticulitis surgery was 20% more likely in counties with highest social vulnerability when compared to those with the lowest [31]. Similarly, these high-vulnerability counties are twice as likely to have emergent versus elective cholecystectomies. These poor outcomes have a myriad of attributing factors, such as lack of insurance, transportation and language barriers, and lack of a primary care providing them with their age-appropriate cancer screenings (specifically cervical, breast, and colorectal cancers) [3, 32]. In short, patients in these vulnerable communities have less access to healthcare thus making an emergency presentation more likely.

A 2023 study by McCrum et al. illustrated that patients with low access to hospitals and able to complete emergency surgical care had a higher in-hospital mortality than high-access patients [35]. In this case, "access" was defined by distance to the hospital, its capacity, and the population demand. Better geographic access was protective against in-hospital mortality (OR 0.95, CI 0.94-0.97), without a significant difference in morbidity. Notably, the patients who accounted for the "low-access" group were more likely to be White.

The Interplay Between Race, Neighborhood, and Socioeconomic Status

Low SES

As discussed in previous sections of this chapter, one's health is not just affected by individual circumstances, but by an intertwining root system of social determinants. Thus, to understand how our patients are affected by SDOH, we must understand how these determinants coexist.

Low socioeconomic status is the social determinant of health most broadly associated with poor post-surgical outcomes [15, 31]. It has been well described in literature that patients of lower SES experience higher operative mortality. This contrast may be due to higher comorbidities, more severe disease at time of presentation due to delayed care, unsafe discharge conditions, and decreased access to high-quality surgical care. An intuitive example of this is seen in those suffering from homelessness. Non-housed populations have an increased risk of postoperative readmission than housed patients, despite lower measured postoperative complication rates [36]. Additionally, non-housed patients' risk of readmission is more strongly correlated to their comorbidities than that of housed patients, suggesting that they are less able to mitigate potential complications due to these comorbidities [36]. While the non-housed population is an extreme example of low SES, any person's ability to afford healthy food, safe living conditions, medications, wound care supplies, and appropriate time for healing affects their health before and after surgery [9, 37]. From a broader view, the strong association between SES and health outcomes is likely aided by the interplay of the different SDOH. Often, lower income patients have several other social determinants of health such as living in highly vulnerable neighborhoods, non-white race, and decreased access to preventative health care, all of which lend themselves to worse health outcomes.

Neighborhood/Environment

Living in a disadvantaged or socially vulnerable neighborhood is independently associated with poorer post-surgical outcomes. One study found that the risk-adjusted probability of 30-day mortality was higher among patients from highly vulnerable counties after colectomy (OR 1.1 95%CI 1.1-1.3), CABG (OR 1.4, 95%CI 1.2-1.5) and lung resection (OR 1.4 [95%CI 1.1-1.8] [15]). Additionally, with these surgeries, patients who resided in highly vulnerable counties were 20–40% more likely to die and 10–20% more likely to experience a serious complication within 30-days of surgery [31].

Once again, the explanation for this disparity is likely multifactorial, as those residing in a highly vulnerable neighborhood are more likely to be socioeconomically disadvantaged, part of a minority ethnic group, or have more comorbidities [37]. Notably, independent of other factors, neighborhood is an important agent in one's personal health maintenance behaviors, that is, regular exercise or healthy diet. Highly vulnerable neighborhoods are less likely to have access to grocery stores with healthy food or safe recreational areas for exercise. This leads to worse baseline health and increased rate of comorbidities [9, 37]. These so-called food deserts are linked to poor health among all residents, but there is an even stronger association among individuals experiencing additional adverse SDOH such as economic instability [9]. Additionally, different neighborhoods may be more significantly affected by different SDOH. For example, predominantly non-white neighborhoods are more likely to exist in "pharmacy deserts," which are associated with worse medication adherence likely leading to worse treatment and prognosis.

Access

Access to care and access to high-quality care is also associated heavily with neighborhood, race, and SES. Those from highly vulnerable counties are more likely to present with advanced disease stage, more symptomatic disease, and need emergent surgery [11, 13, 15, 38]. This is likely largely due to decreased screening and access to primary care seen in low SES areas [9, 13, 39]. Simultaneously, despite more disease burden, low SES has also been associated with a decreased probability of receiving surgical care [15]. The exact cause of this is not well elucidated in literature, though access to insurance, geographic separation from quality care, and difference in referral patterns may play a role. Nonetheless, reduced access to timely, high-quality surgical care exacerbates already existing health disparities seen in these patients and affects surgical outcomes.

Independent of SES and geographic location, Black and minority patients are less likely to receive surgery [40]. What's more, minority and Black patients are more likely to refuse surgery when offered [41]. While the rate of patient refusal is not large enough to explain the racial gap in surgical care, it is an important addition to our understanding. Johnson et al. found that physicians were more verbally dominant and less patient-centered in their approach to Black patients [42]. In this study, physicians spoke twice as much during encounters with Black patients than White patients and showed a less positive effect. Both provider affect, described as tone of voice and body language, and patient-centered communication, such as greater patient input, have been associated with better treatment adherence, and health outcomes [42]. Thus, implicit biases and cultural exposure may guide a surgeon's approach to each patient and impact if a patient will undergo surgery at all. Altogether, this points to the relevance of cultural competence in determining appropriate access to care. This is especially important due to the synergistic nature of SDOH, as racial minorities are affected more strongly by determinants such as SES.

Hospital Quality and Volume

Hospital quality and Hospital or surgeon volume is a crucial factor in access to care. There is an established inverse relationship between hospital volume and surgical mortality. Within this, surgeon volume may account for a relatively large proportion of the apparent effect of hospital volume [43]. Patients in highly vulnerable communities, with low SES, or racial minorities are more likely to receive surgical care from both low-volume hospitals and low-volume surgeons [11, 15, 29, 41]. To solidify the importance of this relationship, it has been shown that surgery at a high-volume or high-quality hospital mitigates some of the risk associated between low economic status and postoperative morbidity and mortality [15]. One could assume that patients use low-quality hospitals out of the convenience or necessity of proximity, but hospital choice is not entirely due to geographic location. When examining several high-risk surgeries, Dimick J. et al. found that Black patients were almost twice as likely as White patients to live within five miles of a high-quality hospital [29]. Additionally, in a subset of patients living within five miles of a high-quality hospital, Black patients were 33%, 44%, 110% more likely than their White neighbors to go to a low-quality hospital for CABG, lung cancer resection, and AAA repair respectively. This disparity was stronger in highly segregated areas and completely disappeared when looking only at areas of low segregation. The mechanics of this are not well elucidated however, it may be explained by patient preference, as Black patients may feel unwelcome in hospitals with a low volume of Black patients, or by race-related differences in physician referral patterns [15].

Despite this, there is variable evidence of the volume-outcome relationship by specific surgery. An umbrella analysis by Hoshijima et al. showed that, when compared with several other oncologic, cardiac, and vascular high-risk surgeries, only pancreaticoduodenectomy fulfilled the criteria of class I and II evidence for both hospital and surgeon volume-mortality relationships, with a decrease in OR for hospital (0.42, 95% confidence interval [CI] [0.35–0.51]) and for surgeon (0.38, 95% CI [0.30–0.49]) [30]. Despite this, there is a clear association between SDOH and hospital choice and low-volume hospitals that largely serve marginalized and underfunded populations are consistently associated with worse outcomes. This may be linked to difficulty recruiting well-trained specialty surgeons or funding policies that have a disproportionally negative impact on low-volume/safety net hospitals. However, it is clear that the root cause of disparities in outcomes is complex and more research is needed before attempts at centralization can be made.

Race

Black race is a known risk marker for poor surgical outcomes. As seen throughout this chapter, Black patients are more likely to present later in the course of their disease, need emergent surgery, as well as seek treatment at lower-volume centers that often have worse quality of care [15, 29]. Again, research points largely to discrepancies in access to care being associated with factors such as SES or insurance status. But the clear gap in post-surgical mortality rates between Black and White patients cannot be attributed purely to this. Race continues to present as an independent risk factor even when adjusting for hospital quality and SES [12, 15, 44]. High SES does partially mitigate post-surgical risks of mortality and morbidity among Black patients. However, Black patients are more profoundly affected by SDOH than White patients are, and have worse surgical outcomes than White patients of the same SES [12, 15, 44]. Moreover, neighborhood-level racial/ethnic segregation is associated with increased risk of CVD in Black, compared with White patients [9]. This indicates that racism in the United States may play a fundamental part in underlying health and wellbeing.

Race as a Marker

It is important to consider the way in which we use race in the context of medical research. Race should not be framed as a "risk factor," as risk factor is defined as something with a causal role in disease development. Rather, it is racism that puts the burden of risk factors largely on certain groups of people. Assuming that race is a risk factor is a fallacy that ignores the generalization that not every Black, Latino, non-white patient has the same risk factors such as CAD, metabolic syndrome, SES, etc. [45]. It has been proposed that race should be thought of not as a risk factor but as a "risk marker" instead; a factor that is noncausal in its association to disease [46]. Additionally, race is not a biological entity, but a socially constructed one. It is often used in place of ethnicity or conflated with a genetic or biological cause for disease. Structural racism and generational trauma, as well as the healthcare inequalities that we've demonstrated in this chapter still exist today, continue to perpetuate health disparities [46]. This idea exemplifies the inherent difficulty of addressing SDOH confounding variables that are highly individualized to each patient. We must be careful not to use the massively oversimplified and incorrect implication of "race" as a risk factor to ease the logistics of our research and patient care. Instead, we must look at our patients as people with multifaceted risk markers that contribute to their health.

Addressing SDOH

Solutions at the Level of the Individual Surgeon

SDOH are often predetermined outside of the healthcare setting. This makes them difficult to address from the standpoint of the individual provider. Traditionally, the onus has been on the primary care physician to address chronic health issues, social issues, and lifestyle changes. When faced with the continued health disparities seen in this country, it is time to address a core idea that routine surgical care may not be sufficient. Though the individual provider is not responsible for changing a patients' social circumstances, surgical visits may be an untapped resource for the socially responsible surgeon to initiate risk factor reduction.

Ogden et al established a framework of sustained life change following la life crisis [47]. The authors found that most successful lifestyle changes were precipitated by a significant life crisis, be it health related or not. However, many people go through crisis and do not initiate sustaining changes. For example, a patient may not stop smoking until after their fourth MI. This study established that life crisis was an important trigger for change but became sustained when associated with three factors:

- *Disruption of function*: The unhealthy behavior served a function in a patient's life. For example, smoking was stress relief while in a bad romantic relationship. If a life crisis removes the function of the behavior, such as breaking up with the aforementioned significant other, sustained cessation is more likely.
- *Reduction of choice*: The precipitating life crisis creates a sense of decreased ability to choose to do the unhealthy behavior. For example, a patient may move into a social group where smoking is socially unacceptable, or a patient may be unable to eat certain foods after bariatric surgery.
- *Behavioral model of causes and solutions*: This is an internalized understanding that lifestyle choices are directly related to health consequences.

A life crisis gives patients an opportunity to create a new identity for themselves. Then subsequently, social or medical intervention decreases a need for the habit, medical intervention and education creates perceived decrease in choice to continue the habit, and education introduces a cause-and-effect behavioral model solidifying the foundation of healthy lifestyle choices as the core of ones' new self. Thus, a preoperative visit with a surgeon, particularly for a high-risk surgery as those discussed in this chapter, is the perfect opportunity to address lifestyle modification and other SDOH. It is in these moments that patients may be most willing to initiate change but it is unlikely that change will be sustained without proper support and education from their provider [48].

An example of this in practice is the program Strong for Surgery through the American College of Surgeons [49]. This campaign works to integrate preoperative checklists for elective operations to screen for potential risk factors that can lead to surgical complications, and to provide appropriate interventions to ensure better surgical outcomes. The checklists target eight areas known to be highly influential determinants of surgical outcomes: Nutrition, Glycemic Control, Medication Management, Smoking Cessation, Safe and Effective Pain Management after Surgery, Delirium, Prehabilitation, and Patient Directives. A purposeful initiative such as this enables change by providing clear health goals to both patients and surgeons. Additionally, a clear framework may aid in catching social determinants that actually can be addressed by individual providers.

Systemic Solutions

There is a need for improved data collection on SDOH. The current data collected on SDOH is often an indirect measure of true patient experience. Yet, to address determinants, researchers need to understand SDOH at a base level, such as through individual health behaviors, while also controlling for variables such as neighborhood and SES. Variables such as these have the ability to immensely modify the current data available on patient experience while simultaneously improving outcomes, making further investigation a necessity. Not only is SDOH data difficult to collect and time consuming for the individual provider, but there is also inconsistent use of standardized patient risk assessment protocols for screening, and a significant lack of diversity in research studies across all fields of medicine [50]. There needs to be a strong push from the surgical community for greater data collection. Emphasizing the importance of this increased data collection will inherently increase the *generalizability* of the work done and the applicability of this to the general population.

However, Individual surgeons are limited to the change they can make when addressing SDOH. The most enduring solution will come from systemic policy changes that would work to create a more equitable health care system and prioritize population health. Surgeons can and must play a role in championing change, which should begin through the advocacy of health equity in their own patients. It is indisputable that inequalities affect the health of both surgical and medical patients, thus health equity is everyone's responsibility. As a field, surgeons must accept the importance of SDOH, make a dedicated effort to identify disparities, and respond with advocacy.

References

1. Harris E. Older black men have higher mortality after elective surgery. JAMA. 2023;329(12):969. https://doi.org/10.1001/jama.2023.3197.
2. Fox M. Social determinants of health and surgery. An overview. The American College of Surgeons; 2021. https://bulletin.facs.org/2021/05/social-determinants-of-health-and-surgery-an-overview/. Accessed 6/30/23 2023.
3. Magnan S. Social determinants of health 101 for health care: five plus five. In: NAM perspectives. National Academy of medicine; 2017. https://nam.edu/social-determinants-of-health-101-for-health-care-five-plus-five/. Accessed 30 Jun 2023.
4. CDC. Social determinants of health at CDC. 2022. https://www.cdc.gov/(2022). Accessed 30 Jun 2023.
5. Gomez SL, Shariff-Marco S, DeRouen M, Keegan TH, Yen IH, Mujahid M, et al. The impact of neighborhood social and built environment factors across the cancer continuum: current research, methodological considerations, and future directions. Cancer. 2015;121(14):2314–30. https://doi.org/10.1002/cncr.29345.
6. Maroko ARDT, Arno PS, Hubel M, Yi S, Viola D. Integrating social determinants of health with treatment and prevention: a new tool to assess local area deprivation. Prev Chronic Dis. 2016;13:160221. https://doi.org/10.5888/pcd13.160221.
7. CDC. Agency for Toxic Substances and Disease Registry: CDC/ATSDR SVI Fact Sheet. 2022. https://www.atsdr.cdc.gov/placeandhealth/svi/fact_sheet/fact_sheet.html. Accessed 30 Jun 2023.
8. Acquah I, Hagan K, Javed Z, Taha MB, Valero-Elizondo J, Nwana N, et al. Social determinants of cardiovascular risk, subclinical cardiovascular disease, and cardiovascular events. J Am Heart Assoc. 2023;12(6):e025581. https://doi.org/10.1161/jaha.122.025581.
9. Javed Z, Haisum Maqsood M, Yahya T, Amin Z, Acquah I, Valero-Elizondo J, et al. Race, racism, and cardiovascular health: applying a social determinants of health framework to racial/ethnic disparities in cardiovascular disease. Circ Cardiovasc Qual Outcomes. 2022;15(1):e007917. https://doi.org/10.1161/circoutcomes.121.007917.
10. Khera R, Vaughan-Sarrazin M, Rosenthal GE, Girotra S. Racial disparities in outcomes after cardiac surgery: the role of hospital quality. Curr Cardiol Rep. 2015;17(5):29. https://doi.org/10.1007/s11886-015-0587-7.
11. Wu WW, Mota L, Marcaccio C, Liang P, Moreira CC, Hughes K, et al. Impact of neighborhood social disadvantage on carotid artery disease presentation, management, and discharge outcomes. J Vasc Surg. 2023;77(6):1700–9.e2. https://doi.org/10.1016/j.jvs.2023.01.204.
12. Rangrass G, Ghaferi AA, Dimick JB. Explaining racial disparities in outcomes after cardiac surgery: the role of hospital quality. JAMA Surg. 2014;149(3):223–7. https://doi.org/10.1001/jamasurg.2013.4041.
13. Perlstein MD, Gupta S, Ma X, Rong LQ, Askin G, White RS. Abdominal aortic aneurysm repair readmissions and disparities of socioeconomic status: a multistate analysis, 2007-2014. J Cardiothorac Vasc Anesth. 2019;33(10):2737–45. https://doi.org/10.1053/j.jvca.2019.03.020.
14. Al Adas Z, Nypaver TJ, Shepard AD, Weaver MR, Ryan JT, Huang J, et al. Survival after abdominal aortic aneurysm repair is affected by socioeconomic status. J Vasc Surg. 2019;69(5):1437–43. https://doi.org/10.1016/j.jvs.2018.07.084.
15. Diaz A, Pawlik TM. Social determinants of health and surgical care. Curr Probl Surg. 2023;60(4):101300. https://doi.org/10.1016/j.cpsurg.2023.101300.
16. Stewart JH, Bertoni AG, Staten JL, Levine EA, Gross CP. Participation in surgical oncology clinical trials: gender-, race/ethnicity-, and age-based disparities. Ann Surg Oncol. 2007;14(12):3328–34. https://doi.org/10.1245/s10434-007-9500-y.
17. Townsley C, Pond GR, Peloza B, Kok J, Naidoo K, Dale D, et al. Analysis of treatment practices for elderly cancer patients in Ontario. Canada J Clin Oncol. 2005;23(16):3802–10. https://doi.org/10.1200/jco.2005.06.742.

18. Oliphant R, Nicholson GA, Horgan PG, Molloy RG, McMillan DC, Morrison DS, et al. Deprivation and colorectal cancer Surgery: longer-term survival inequalities are due to differential postoperative mortality between socioeconomic groups. Ann Surg Oncol. 2013;20(7):2132–9. https://doi.org/10.1245/s10434-013-2959-9.
19. Bharathan B, Welfare M, Borowski DW, Mills SJ, Steen IN, Kelly SB, et al. Impact of deprivation on short- and long-term outcomes after colorectal cancer surgery. Br J Surg. 2011;98(6):854–65. https://doi.org/10.1002/bjs.7427.
20. Tripathi R, Archibald LK, Mazmudar RS, Conic RRZ, Rothermel LD, Scott JF, et al. Racial differences in time to treatment for melanoma. J Am Acad Dermatol. 2020;83(3):854–9. https://doi.org/10.1016/j.jaad.2020.03.094.
21. Smith EC, Ziogas A, Anton-Culver H. Delay in surgical treatment and survival after breast cancer diagnosis in young women by race/ethnicity. JAMA Surg. 2013;148(6):516–23. https://doi.org/10.1001/jamasurg.2013.1680.
22. Sheppard VB, Oppong BA, Hampton R, Snead F, Horton S, Hirpa F, et al. Disparities in breast cancer Surgery delay: the lingering effect of race. Ann Surg Oncol. 2015;22(9):2902–11. https://doi.org/10.1245/s10434-015-4397-3.
23. Chan JK, Zhang M, Hu JM, Shin JY, Osann K, Kapp DS. Racial disparities in surgical treatment and survival of epithelial ovarian cancer in United States. J Surg Oncol. 2008;97(2):103–7. https://doi.org/10.1002/jso.20932.
24. Tohme S, Kaltenmeier C, Bou-Samra P, Varley PR, Tsung A. Race and health disparities in patient refusal of Surgery for early-stage pancreatic cancer: an NCDB cohort study. Ann Surg Oncol. 2018;25(12):3427–35. https://doi.org/10.1245/s10434-018-6680-6.
25. Molina G, Clancy TE, Tsai TC, Lam M, Wang J. Racial disparity in Pancreatoduodenectomy for borderline Resectable pancreatic adenocarcinoma. Ann Surg Oncol. 2021;28(2):1088–96. https://doi.org/10.1245/s10434-020-08717-x.
26. Sweigert PJ, Eguia E, Baker MS, Paredes AZ, Tsilimigras DI, Dillhoff M, et al. Assessment of textbook oncologic outcomes following pancreaticoduodenectomy for pancreatic adenocarcinoma. J Surg Oncol. 2020;121(6):936–44. https://doi.org/10.1002/jso.25861.
27. Merritt RE, Abdel-Rasoul M, D'Souza DM, Kneuertz PJ. Racial disparities in provider recommendation for esophagectomy for esophageal carcinoma. J Surg Oncol. 2021;124(4):521–8. https://doi.org/10.1002/jso.26549.
28. Erhunmwunsee L, Gulack BC, Rushing C, Niedzwiecki D, Berry MF, Hartwig MG. Socioeconomic status, not race, is associated with reduced survival in Esophagectomy patients. Ann Thorac Surg. 2017;104(1):234–44. https://doi.org/10.1016/j.athoracsur.2017.01.049.
29. Dimick J, Ruhter J, Sarrazin MV, Birkmeyer JD. Black patients more likely than whites to undergo surgery at low quality hospitals in segregated regions. Health Aff (Millwood). 2013;32(6):1046–53. https://doi.org/10.1377/hlthaff.2011.1365.
30. Hoshijima H, Wajima Z, Nagasaka H, Shiga T. Association of hospital and surgeon volume with mortality following major surgical procedures: meta-analysis of meta-analyses of observational studies. Medicine (Baltimore). 2019;98(44):e17712. https://doi.org/10.1097/md.0000000000017712.
31. Diaz A, Hyer JM, Barmash E, Azap R, Paredes AZ, Pawlik TM. County-level social vulnerability is associated with worse surgical outcomes especially among minority patients. Ann Surg. 2021;274(6):881–91. https://doi.org/10.1097/sla.0000000000004691.
32. Cain BT, Horns JJ, Huang LC, McCrum ML. Socioeconomic disadvantage is associated with greater mortality after high-risk emergency general surgery. J Trauma Acute Care Surg. 2022;92(4):691–700. https://doi.org/10.1097/ta.0000000000003517.
33. LaPlant MB, Hess DJ. A review of racial/ethnic disparities in pediatric trauma care, treatment, and outcomes. J Trauma Acute Care Surg. 2019;86(3):540–50. https://doi.org/10.1097/ta.0000000000002160.
34. Jarman MP, Castillo RC, Carlini AR, Kodadek LM, Haider AH. Rural risk: geographic disparities in trauma mortality. Surgery. 2016;160(6):1551–9. https://doi.org/10.1016/j.surg.2016.06.020.

35. McCrum ML, Allen CM, Han J, Iantorno SE, Presson AP, Wan N. Greater spatial access to care is associated with lower mortality for emergency general surgery. J Trauma Acute Care Surg. 2023;94(2):264–72. https://doi.org/10.1097/ta.0000000000003837.
36. Titan A, Graham L, Rosen A, Itani K, Copeland LA, Mull HJ, et al. Homeless status, Postdischarge health care utilization, and readmission after Surgery. Med Care. 2018;56(6):460–9. https://doi.org/10.1097/mlr.0000000000000915.
37. Dugravot A, Fayosse A, Dumurgier J, Bouillon K, Rayana TB, Schnitzler A, et al. Social inequalities in multimorbidity, frailty, disability, and transitions to mortality: a 24-year follow-up of the Whitehall II cohort study. Lancet Public Health. 2020;5(1):e42–50. https://doi.org/10.1016/s2468-2667(19)30226-9.
38. Haider AH, Scott VK, Rehman KA, Velopulos C, Bentley JM, Cornwell EE 3rd, et al. Racial disparities in surgical care and outcomes in the United States: a comprehensive review of patient, provider, and systemic factors. J Am Coll Surg. 2013;216(3):482–92.e12. https://doi.org/10.1016/j.jamcollsurg.2012.11.014.
39. Kurani SS, McCoy RG, Lampman MA, Doubeni CA, Finney Rutten LJ, Inselman JW, et al. Association of Neighborhood Measures of social determinants of health with breast, cervical, and colorectal cancer screening rates in the US Midwest. JAMA Netw Open. 2020;3(3):e200618. https://doi.org/10.1001/jamanetworkopen.2020.0618.
40. Crawford S, Schold J. Association between geographic measures of socioeconomic status and deprivation and major surgical outcomes. Med Care. 2019;57(12):949–59. https://doi.org/10.1097/mlr.0000000000001214.
41. Delman AM, Ammann AM, Turner KM, Vaysburg DM, Van Haren RM. A narrative review of socioeconomic disparities in the treatment of esophageal cancer. J Thorac Dis. 2021;13(6):3801–8. https://doi.org/10.21037/jtd-20-3095.
42. Johnson RL, Roter D, Powe NR, Cooper LA. Patient race/ethnicity and quality of patient-physician communication during medical visits. Am J Public Health. 2004;94(12):2084–90. https://doi.org/10.2105/ajph.94.12.2084.
43. Birkmeyer JD, Stukel TA, Siewers AE, Goodney PP, Wennberg DE, Lucas FL. Surgeon volume and operative mortality in the United States. N Engl J Med. 2003;349(22):2117–27. https://doi.org/10.1056/NEJMsa035205.
44. Nathan H, Frederick W, Choti MA, Schulick RD, Pawlik TM. Racial disparity in surgical mortality after major hepatectomy. J Am Coll Surg. 2008;207(3):312–9. https://doi.org/10.1016/j.jamcollsurg.2008.04.015.
45. Nguyen LL, Henry AJ. Disparities in vascular surgery: is it biology or environment? J Vasc Surg. 2010;51(4 Suppl):36s–41s. https://doi.org/10.1016/j.jvs.2010.02.003.
46. Silverman-Lloyd LG, Bishop NS, Cerdeña JP. Race is not a risk factor: reframing discourse on racial health inequities in CVD prevention. Am J Prev Cardiol. 2021;6:100185. https://doi.org/10.1016/j.ajpc.2021.100185.
47. Ogden J, Hills L. Understanding sustained behavior change: the role of life crises and the process of reinvention. Health. 2008;12(4):419–37. https://doi.org/10.1177/1363459308094417.
48. Bamdad MC, Englesbe MJ. Surgery and population health-redesigning surgical quality for greater impact. JAMA Surg. 2020;155(9):799–800. https://doi.org/10.1001/jamasurg.2020.0808.
49. ACS. Strong for Surgery. 2023. https://www.facs.org/. Accessed 30 Jun 2023.
50. Mullangi S, Aviki EM, Hershman DL. Reexamining social determinants of health data collection in the COVID-19 era. JAMA Oncol. 2022;8(12):1736–8. https://doi.org/10.1001/jamaoncol.2022.4543.

Chapter 2
Implementation and Utilization of Checklists in Surgical Patient Safety

Michael Kochis, Nathan Turley, Mary Brindle, and Alex Haynes

Abbreviations

EPIS	Explore, Prepare, Implement, Sustain
HDI	Human Development Index
ICU	Intensive care unit
OR	Operating room
SSC	Surgical Safety Checklist
UK	United Kingdom
US	United States
VHA	Veterans Health Administration
WHO	World Health Organization

M. Kochis
Massachusetts General Hospital, Boston, MA, USA
e-mail: mkochis@mgh.harvard.edu

N. Turley
EQuIS Research, Department of Surgery, Cumming School of Medicine, The University of Calgary, Calgary, AB, Canada
e-mail: nturley@ucalgary.ca

M. Brindle
EQuIS Research, Department of Surgery, Cumming School of Medicine, The University of Calgary, Calgary, AB, Canada

Ariadne Labs, Boston, MA, USA
e-mail: mbrindle@ariadnelabs.org

A. Haynes (✉)
Department of Surgery and Perioperative Care, Dell Medical School, University of Texas at Austin, Austin, TX, USA
e-mail: Alex.Haynes@austin.utexas.edu

© The Author(s), under exclusive license to Springer Nature Switzerland AG 2024

J. Faintuch, S. Faintuch (eds.), *Recent Strategies in High Risk Surgery*,
https://doi.org/10.1007/978-3-031-56270-9_2

Introduction

Many people use checklists. Beyond routine applications like planning groceries or chores, checklists designed for teams are simple, low-cost, and effective tools for structuring communication and enhancing collaboration in high-stakes scenarios. They are used by airplane pilots (pre-flight, post-flight, and others), space agencies launching satellites, large businesses making financial decisions, and, in the case of many of our readers, surgical teams mitigating errors and complications [1].

Medicine has become increasingly complex, and multidisciplinary teams are common, especially in surgery. Within this environment, checklists help clinicians focus on relevant information at the most appropriate time. By understanding the history of surgical checklists and best practices in their implementation, you can better use them as a member of the perioperative team. It is not simply the existence of a checklist nor its declared use within an organization that effects change, but rather actual integration into routine practice. To achieve lasting change, integration requires resources, time, and cultural buy-in.

What Is a Checklist?

A checklist is a cognitive tool used to aid users' memories and guide actions. On a group level, it can provide a shared vision about how a process should progress or what situations should prompt discussion or intervention [1]. Depending on the exact circumstance, checklists can be used to help evaluate situations, confirm tasks have been completed, facilitate communication and decision-making, and guide step-by-step actions or considerations in real-time.

Checklists can take many forms, from a tangible instrument such as a paper or a poster, to an electronic application, to even being implied in the deliberate design of a kit of equipment. Weiser and Berry [1] posit there are two types of elements that commonly appear in checklists: "read-do" and "challenge-confirm." The former can be used as a log of items to consider or tasks to accomplish. A common example is a grocery list, in which an individual crosses off items as they are acquired. On the other hand, "challenge-confirm" checklist elements involve a closed-loop discussion between two users. One states an item on the list, and the other issues a response confirming a status or action. For example, before a plane takeoff, one pilot may read, "brake" to which the other replies, "released." The reality is that many industry checklists, including those used in medicine, combine elements of both formats.

As common as checklists may be, there is a growing science underpinning their design. When teams design checklists, they consider the items included on the checklist, the checklists' performance within the perioperative workflow, and, once the checklist is introduced, ways for ensuring its continued success.

Deliberate Design

Given the range of functions that checklists can achieve, teams must be deliberate in considering a specific checklist's content as it pertains to the task at hand and local context. For both aspects, attention to human factors is essential. A given checklist should arise from an identified concern and a thorough analysis of what contributes to it. Sometimes, introducing a degree of standardization into a process may be helpful in reducing errors [2].

Teams should be selective that the items they include in their checklist are well-grounded in data, meet local needs, and promote communication [3, 4]. Teams should be conservative in their approach and practice restraint: checklists should be concise and limited in items, as comprehensiveness sacrifices usability. After all, any change to a system may introduce new risks, and in healthcare, poorly designed checklists can reduce efficiency by distracting clinicians, complicating tasks, interrupting work flows, and ultimately hindering the delivery of high quality care [4].

Workflow Integration

Equally important to a checklist's content is its timing. If it is determined that a checklist is a worthwhile intervention, it should be carefully discussed how the checklist will be used and how it may fit into existing workflows [2]. Typically, checks are performed at natural pauses in a process, to ensure that all relevant materials are acquired, and elements are addressed to allow corrective actions before a non-reversible step forward. Checklists' progression in an anticipated sequence helps streamline use by ensuring consistency and minimizing disruptions, while identifying and correcting errors of omission or commission before consequences to the patient. While some checklists were designed for routine use in all circumstances, others were specifically designed for emergencies or uncommon situations beyond most people's familiarity. In the medical context, this ranges from routine pre-procedural time-outs or anesthesia machine set-up to "crisis checklists" which facilitate prompt, coordinated responses to events like venous air embolism, anaphylaxis, cardiac arrest, fire, or malignant hyperthermia, among others [5, 6].

Effectiveness

The process of checklist *design* is just one stage of the more-encompassing process of checklist *development* [2], which also includes the steps of trial and feedback, formal testing and evaluation, and modification [1].

A Role for Checklists in Surgery

Motives: Patient Safety

Surgical checklists originated in the patient safety movement [7]. While the scientific and technological advances of the mid-twentieth century fostered an immense growth in the healthcare industry's ability to treat many medical conditions, so too grew the frequency with which treatments, and particularly surgical interventions, caused inadvertent harm.

In the early 1990s, the "Harvard Medical Practice Study" by Brennan and colleagues examined outcomes from a year's worth of hospitalizations in New York State. Adverse events occurred in 3.7% of hospitalizations, of which 13.6% led to death [8]; 48% of these errors involved an operation [9]. Nearly a decade later, a similar analysis in Utah and Colorado found the rate of adverse events to be 2.9% of all hospitalizations [10]; among these, 66% were surgical [11]. These findings were replicated outside the United States (US), with adverse events occurring among 10.8% of hospitalized patients in the United Kingdom (UK) [12] and 7.5% of patients in Canada [13]; again, in both of these countries, surgical care was often the main contributor. In all these analyses, around half of the errors were considered to be preventable [11, 12, 14]. It became clear that action was necessary.

In 2000, the Institute of Medicine issued the landmark publication "To Err is Human." The publication not only defined the scope of medical errors as common causes of morbidity and mortality, but also examined how systems of care and human factors contribute to them. It served as a call to action to improve the care delivered by creating systems of safety in healthcare organizations [14]. "To Err is Human" spurred a proliferation of research examining the nature of the errors and, ultimately, how to prevent them.

Adverse Events in Surgery

Despite being called "never events" since they can have catastrophic results and are entirely preventable, wrong-site surgery still occurs in about 1 in 100,000 cases, and retained surgical items occur in 1 in 5000 to 10,000 cases [15]. Additional preventable complications common in the surgical context include infection, deep venous thrombosis, and pulmonary embolism [7]. Less dramatically but more commonly, surgical equipment failure, whether related to availability, configuration and settings, or direct malfunctioning, was found to occur a median 2.4 times per operation [16].

Given the diversity of negative outcomes, it should come as no surprise that there was great interest in determining their common features and root causes. While many classifications have been applied to this purpose, the human performance deficiency framework characterizes errors pertaining to planning or problem solving, execution, rules violation, communication, and teamwork. Among individual errors in problem solving and execution, cognitive bias and lack of recognition of important pieces of data are each just as frequent as technical errors [17].

Strikingly, 60–70% of sentinel events (serious safety events, registered by accredited hospitals) reported to the Joint Commission on Accreditation of Healthcare Organizations involved a failure of communication [18, 19]. In particular, the patterns of communication breakdowns resulting in injury to surgical patients often clustered around failure in verbal communication between a surgical attending and another caregiver, and ambiguity about responsibilities [18]. Such failures can relate to occasion, content, audience, or purpose: over a third of them affected patient safety by impacting efficiency, generating team tension, wasting resources, or resulting in procedural error [19]. The recognition of surgical errors and their relation to cognitive biases and communication failures sparked interest in interventions promoting systematic thinking and better interactions among operating room (OR) teams.

Antecedents for Checklist Interventions

In an ideal world, tasks would be sequential, predictable, and controllable. However, the real world has interruptions, concurrent tasks, changes in sequence, and unanticipated additions. These push us into situations where we try to multitask, which inevitably leads to important things being forgotten [20]. By providing an external reference, checklists compensate for the fallibility of human attention and memory under complex and stressful circumstances [4].

The aviation industry has used checklists for nearly a century, prompted by crashes of Boeing jets flown by experienced pilots in the 1930s. It was understood that some systems are simply too complex for even the most accomplished individual to manage alone. The airline industry is a useful parallel to medicine since both fields have unpredictable yet rare deviations, embedded role hierarchy, lengthy training requirements, and highly visible implications for everyone involved [21]. Another parallel field is the military, where checklists guide briefing and debriefing sessions to enhance safety by promoting discipline and eliminating errors of omission [22].

Central Line Infections

In 2001, anesthesiologist and critical care physician Dr. Peter Pronovost introduced a bundle of interventions pertaining to central line management at Johns Hopkins Hospital. These interventions included a checklist to reinforce adherence to infection-control practices during line insertion: handwashing, skin cleaning with chlorhexidine, sterile draping of the patient, wearing sterile equipment, and applying a sterile dressing. An initial study indicated the rate of catheter-related blood stream infections decreased dramatically, preventing multiple deaths and saving their hospital millions of dollars per year [23].

In October 2003, Pronovost's pilot was followed by a much larger initiative called the "Keystone ICU Project," which implemented the package at more than 100 intensive care units across Michigan. Over an 18-month study period, this intervention decreased the infection rate by 66% [24]. Though Pronovost's checklist was just one of several aspects to the Keystone ICU Project, his checklist's impact caught broad attention throughout the surgical space. It inspired surgeon and author Dr. Atul Gawande to muse, "If something so simple can transform intensive care, what else can it do?" [25].

Universal Protocol

Shortly after the Keystone ICU Project, the Joint Commission took decisive action to broadly implement checklists for tackling widespread surgical errors head-on. As such, by July 2004, all accredited organizations had to adhere to a "Universal Protocol for Preventing Wrong Site, Wrong Procedure, Wrong Person Surgery" [26]. This protocol involved verifying the patient, marking the surgical site, and performing a time-out before the procedure begins. While it is unclear whether the Universal Protocol achieved its goals in reducing the key avoidable surgical errors, it was a profound step toward institutions' incorporation and habituation of routine safety measures [15].

Additional Early Surgical Checklists

Also in 2003, while the Keystone ICU Project was happening in the US, a team from Canada developed and implemented a checklist focused on surgical teams and their communication [27]. Using a vascular surgery team as their participants, the researchers found that key communication functions were provision of adequate case-related information, confirmation of details, articulation of concerns, and team building. Practically speaking, the execution of this checklist took just a few minutes and, while it caused some inconveniences in terms of altered workflow, all participants felt the discussions were efficient. Thus, the Canadian study established that a team checklist could promote information exchange and facilitate team cohesion.

The Johns Hopkins OR Briefing checklist was another early tool which had three parts involving introducing members of the team, reviewing information about the procedure, and addressing anticipated hazards in the OR using call-and-response prompts [28].

Three years later, in 2006, the Veterans Health Administration (VHA) implemented a nationwide Medical Team Training program across more than 100 facilities. Following a 2-month preparation phase, training staff worked with implementation teams to assess problem areas and understand local contexts. The actual training session involved a day-long workshop where OR teams were trained to work together, challenge each other when they identified safety risks, and perform checklist-guided preoperative briefings and postoperative debriefings, among other elements. The initial implementation included quarterly check-ins to enhance transparency and aid in resolving issues. Facilities enrolled in the program witnessed notable reductions in mortality and morbidity, with longer implementation periods correlating with even greater decreases [29, 30].

The SURPASS Checklist

Based on the recognition that many, if not most, surgical errors occur outside the OR, the Surgical Patient Safety System (SURPASS) checklist was developed by a group of medical centers in the Netherlands to address the full scope of surgical patients' care from admission to discharge. Beyond participation from the surgeon, anesthesiologist, and operating assistant, the SURPASS checklist involves participation of the ward doctor and nurse with added components like hand-off of postoperative instructions and medication provision at discharge. While most surgical checklists' items take place within the OR, SURPASS contains 124 items collected across six time points and multiple potential locations.

The SURPASS checklist was studied from October 2007 to March 2009 in the Netherlands. While there was no change in the rate of complications in the control group before and after implementation, intervention hospitals saw a statistically significant decrease in postoperative complications from 27.3 to 16.7 per 100 patients and a reduction in mortality from 1.5% to 0.8%. Furthermore, when the results were stratified based on checklist compliance, patients for whom 80% or more of checklist items were completed had lower rates of complications than those for whom fewer items were completed [31]. While a benefit of the SURPASS checklist is that it is comprehensive and interdisciplinary, it is also complex to implement due to the involvement of multiple teams, time points, and locations, which often requires reorganization of care processes [32].

The World Health Organization Surgical Safety Checklist (SSC)

Development of the SSC

By the early 2000s, it was estimated that at least one million patients across the globe died after surgery annually, and seven million were injured from surgical complications [33]. This recognition led the WHO to launch the World Alliance for Patient Safety in October 2004. The Alliance framed their work under "Global Patient Safety Challenges" as a means of focusing and catalyzing global commitment to key risk areas. The first Challenge addressed healthcare-associated infections. The second Global Patient Safety Challenge, which began in January 2007, focused on safe surgery. Here, the WHO Patient Safety Programme convened focus groups of experts from around the globe to settle on four areas of opportunity for dramatic improvement: (1) surgical site infection prevention, (2) safe anesthesia, (3) safe surgical teams, and (4) measurement of surgical services. These discussions ultimately settled on ten safety standards that every surgical team in every setting should meet. Recognizing the simple power of previous checklist interventions in healthcare, the team tasked with the work chose a checklist as the tool to enact change.

Development of the checklist was guided by three principles: simplicity, wide applicability, and measurability. The content was selected based on a comprehensive review of safety practices with known benefits to surgical patients, with consideration of global settings with various resources [21]. In terms of timing, the team identified three points in the typical surgical workflow which were conducive to pauses for confirmation and action if needed: "Sign In" prior to induction of anesthesia: "Time Out" before skin incision, and "Sign Out" before the patient leaves the OR. The SSC was extensively trialed and iterated, whereby confusing actions and language were clarified and refined before being retested in new settings according to the Plan-Do-Study-Act model [21]. Through this iterative, consensus-based process, the initial standards were translated into a highly useable, one-page, 19-item checklist for use in ORs (Fig. 2.1) [33]. To successfully develop a surgical checklist, however, formal testing and evaluation are just as important as the initial creation of content, as will be discussed in subsequent sections.

Global SSC Adoption

The first stage of this work involved a global pilot. Eight international sites evaluated the WHO SSC between October 2007 and September 2008. After baseline data collection, local investigators were given information about site deficiencies and tasked with implementing the checklist based on an implementation manual that provided adaptable guidance. The implementation process was intensive and included translation into the local language and tailoring of the checklist and its use to fit local practices. This process was followed by written and in-person instruction of surgical teams to optimize buy-in and performance. Patients' death rate decreased from 1.5% to 0.8% following the SSC's introduction, and inpatient complication rate decreased from 11.0% to 7.0% [34]. It should be noted that while the sites represented a variety of economic circumstances and diverse patient populations, they were specifically chosen to maximize the chances of implementation success and were not necessarily representative of typical hospitals.

Shortly after that pilot study, the SSC proliferated. By March 2009, over 1000 hospitals around the world were using it; by January 2010, that number more than tripled [35]. Numerous health agencies endorsed the checklist and facilitated its

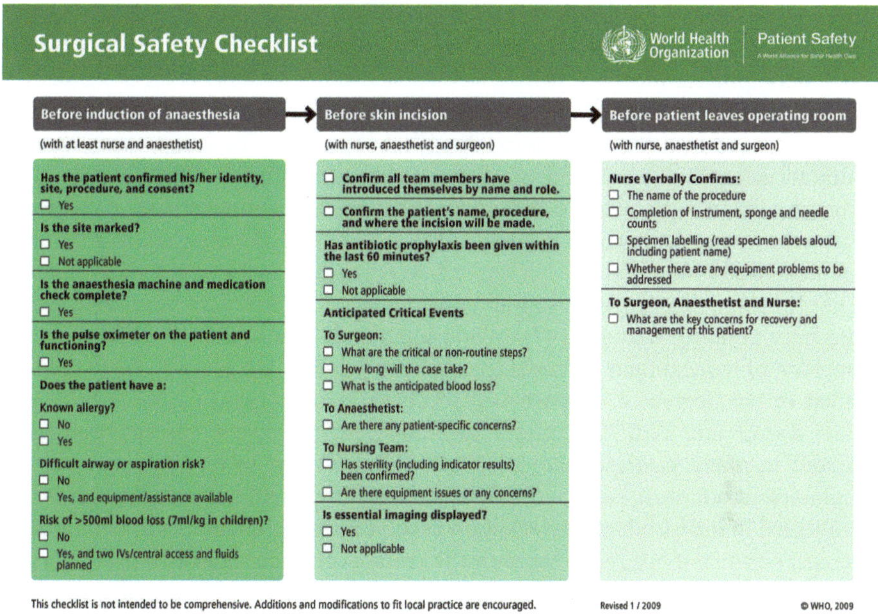

Surgical Safety Checklist

World Health Organization | Patient Safety

Before induction of anaesthesia

(with at least nurse and anaesthetist)

Has the patient confirmed his/her identity, site, procedure, and consent?
- ☐ Yes

Is the site marked?
- ☐ Yes
- ☐ Not applicable

Is the anaesthesia machine and medication check complete?
- ☐ Yes

Is the pulse oximeter on the patient and functioning?
- ☐ Yes

Does the patient have a:

Known allergy?
- ☐ No
- ☐ Yes

Difficult airway or aspiration risk?
- ☐ No
- ☐ Yes, and equipment/assistance available

Risk of >500ml blood loss (7ml/kg in children)?
- ☐ No
- ☐ Yes, and two IVs/central access and fluids planned

Before skin incision

(with nurse, anaesthetist and surgeon)

- ☐ **Confirm all team members have introduced themselves by name and role.**
- ☐ **Confirm the patient's name, procedure, and where the incision will be made.**

Has antibiotic prophylaxis been given within the last 60 minutes?
- ☐ Yes
- ☐ Not applicable

Anticipated Critical Events

To Surgeon:
- ☐ What are the critical or non-routine steps?
- ☐ How long will the case take?
- ☐ What is the anticipated blood loss?

To Anaesthetist:
- ☐ Are there any patient-specific concerns?

To Nursing Team:
- ☐ Has sterility (including indicator results) been confirmed?
- ☐ Are there equipment issues or any concerns?

Is essential imaging displayed?
- ☐ Yes
- ☐ Not applicable

Before patient leaves operating room

(with nurse, anaesthetist and surgeon)

Nurse Verbally Confirms:
- ☐ The name of the procedure
- ☐ Completion of instrument, sponge and needle counts
- ☐ Specimen labelling (read specimen labels aloud, including patient name)
- ☐ Whether there are any equipment problems to be addressed

To Surgeon, Anaesthetist and Nurse:
- ☐ What are the key concerns for recovery and management of this patient?

This checklist is not intended to be comprehensive. Additions and modifications to fit local practice are encouraged. Revised 1 / 2009 © WHO, 2009

Fig. 2.1 The World Health Organization/WHO Surgical safety checklist/SSC, initially developed in 2007 and containing 19 items across three perioperative stages. The complete list, reproduced by permission, is available in the chapter of Useful tables and internet sites

implementation in their jurisdictions. In some instances, the SSC was implemented along with a package of other patient safety interventions [36].

Checklist Outcomes in the Real World

SSC adoption is associated with decreased rates of complications and mortality across diverse global contexts [32, 37–39], even those with limited resources [40, 41]. Within the scope of research performed, there are some randomized controlled trials showing positive effects from the checklist, including ones in Norway [42] and India [40], but most studies were pre–/post-implementation designs without controls [32].

In January 2009, the United Kingdom's National Patient Safety Agency mandated that all National Health System organizations adopt the SSC within a year [43]. While most cases conducted at least one of the checklist's three panels, the entire checklist was completed only 62% of the time. Patients had a statistically significant reduced odds of experiencing a complication if all three elements were completed, but not if the checklist was only partially completed. Furthermore, there was a greater benefit for high-risk patients than low-risk patients [44].

In the Netherlands, the odds ratio for death within 30 days of surgery ranged from 0.44 for full implementation, to 1.09 for partial implementation, and up to 1.16 with noncompliance [45].

In July 2010, the Ontario (Canada) Ministry of Health and Long-Term Care mandated adherence to the SSC. Among the 101 hospitals in the study, there was no significant difference in risk of death during the hospital stay or within 30 days after discharge. There were also no differences in surgical complications, emergency department visits, or hospital readmissions in 3-month periods before and after implementation [46].

On reflection, the approach to implementation in Ontario may have contributed to the disappointing findings [47]. While almost all hospitals in Ontario reported some sort of educational intervention, it was unclear what these interventions entailed or the degree of support they received. Self-reported compliance across centers was greater than 92% during the study period. However, as has been demonstrated in many studies since, hospitals are motivated to report high levels of compliance in administrative auditing processes. These inflated numbers are often not reflected in independent observations, especially when compliance is financially rewarded or when it is a requirement for hospital accreditation [46].

In Ontario, it was observed that most hospitals did not modify the SSC for their local needs, raising concerns about whether the surgical teams were meaningfully engaged in implementation. Buy-in remains a critical piece of effective implementation, as people tend to embrace interventions they have a hand in designing [48]. Perhaps most importantly, one of the great lessons in these large scale interventions is that effective implementation takes time, and the 3-month follow-up period might not have been adequate to demonstrate meaningful change [49].

Implementation Matters

Building on early studies examining the impact of SSC effectiveness, a wave of research grounded in implementation science and quality improvement principles have explored the elements of successful implementation. Contrasting the former investigations' quantitative methods characterizing mortality or complication rates, these later investigations often relied on qualitative methods, employing practices from organizational psychology and medical sociology examining the human experience. In this field where the nuances of local circumstances are critical, case studies are particularly illustrative.

Behavioral Change

A follow-up study to the initial eight-site pilot trial with an intensive implementation strategy showed that checklist rollout was associated with a statistically significant increase in safety attitudes as measured by a validated questionnaire; the degree of improvement in safety scores correlated with a reduction in complication rate. Overall, 80% of respondents indicated the SSC was easy to use, 79% felt the program prevented errors, and 93% would want the checklist used if they were a patient [50]. Subsequent studies in many contexts delved deeper into exploring how checklist implementation impacted the culture and attitudes of the surgical teams and perceptions of surgical safety.

Case Study: South Carolina In the South Carolina experience, a state-wide implementation of the SSC was achieved through a partnership between the South Carolina Hospital Association and Ariadne Labs, a health systems research platform including many of the original developers of the WHO SSC at Harvard. These organizations co-developed a program of recommended practices to support and facilitate checklist implementation (Table 2.1). This process, although less intensive than the implementation of the initial WHO pilot, was performed over multiple years with significant financial and leadership investment. By design, it ensured a degree of rigor and commitment from the surgical teams involved in the checklist rollout.

As part of this process, surveys were performed that measured perceptions of perioperative safety practices. These surveys found that the process of checklist implementation was associated with improved perceptions of mutual respect, clinical leadership, and team coordination and communication; however,

Table 2.1 Barriers and Facilitators to Successful Checklist Implementation

Domain	Barriers	Facilitators
Checklist design	– Impractical layout – Confusing wording or content – Poor relevance – Ambiguity how to use (who, when)	– Straightforward format – Modification/adaptation
Culture	– Resistance to change – Skepticism about evidence – Anxiety of unfamiliarity Staff hierarchy – "Going through the motions" – Noncompliance	– Organizational priority – Demonstrable leadership – Local champions – Senior clinician buy-in – Support from hospital management
Workflow	– Increasing workload – Repetition, wasted time, delays – Unsuitable timing of checks	– Integration with existing processes
Execution	– Poor planning – Limited access to necessary resources (marking pens, antibiotics)	– Education/training on safety and improvement – Involving entire OR team – Starting small – Evident progress and execution of plans
Outcomes	– Unintended negative effects – Patient perceptions/anxiety	– Regular audits – Feedback on local data – Accountability for noncompliance

Adapted from [22, 39, 51, 52]

differences in perceptions based on professional role signified room for improvement [53].

These measures of improved perceptions of surgical safety and team culture were aligned with safety outcomes. Among the 14 hospitals that enrolled in the SSC program, there was a 22% decrease in 30-day mortality, but there was no such difference among control hospitals [54].

Best Practices for Implementation

The efficacy of a checklist depends on successful implementation, which is thoughtful and deliberate. While there are several frameworks available to teams, the Explore, Prepare, Implement, and Sustain (EPIS) framework is easy to understand and use across the pre-implementation, implementation, and post-implementation phases [55]. As a first step, teams should *Explore* their surgical context, its members, and their needs. Next, teams should *Prepare* a customized SSC by leveraging teams' experiences and contextual knowledge, so it aligns with their workflow and patient populations. The third step, *Implement*, entails the team introducing their customized SSC to the OR and working to engrain the new SSC into their processes. The last step of the EPIS framework, *Sustain*, involves teams evaluating their SSC's use and impact on their OR and finding ways to ensure teams' performance does not wane. This framework can also be applied to re-implementation if previous efforts have stalled [56].

The aspects of implementation described below reflect the robust theoretical frameworks relevant to effective implementation of the SSC. The findings and recommendations are based on studies with various methodologies ranging from a scoping review to a realist synthesis, which is an approach designed to consider what works for whom, under what circumstance, and why [57]. These insights will be just as relevant to other checklist interventions.

Pre-Implementation: Explore and Prepare

For the pre-implementation phase, which encompasses the Explore and Prepare steps, best practices include grounding the work within a theoretical framework, understanding barriers and facilitators, and analyzing the local safety culture [58].

Grounded in Theory

Two organizational behavior theories relevant to the SSC include the Normalization Process Theory and Response Regulation Theory. The former examines the cognitive and physical steps involved in embedding a practice into routine work patterns, while the latter describes how leaders use various methods to steer attitudes and behaviors [57].

Understanding the Local Context

In a systematic review of 33 studies, Treadwell et al. [39] summarized barriers into four categories: confusion regarding how to properly use the checklist, pragmatic challenges to efficient workflow, access to resources, and beliefs and attitudes of participating staff—particularly surgeons [39]. This latter finding was borne out in a qualitative study in the UK, which found the single most cited barrier to checklist implementation was active resistance or passive noncompliance among OR team members, with the vast majority being senior surgeons and/or anesthesiologists.

Even so, the study found the majority of reported barriers pertained to the checklist itself, either in terms of layout (e.g., no space to write answers) or content (e.g., confusing wording like "are there any unexpected steps?" since by definition they are not anticipated) [52]. Anticipating, identifying, and addressing barriers and optimizing facilitators is a key aspect of achieving initial success in SSC rollout as well as sustaining checklist use (Table 2.1).

To reference a real-world example, a strength of the aforementioned VHA checklist lies in the researchers' 2-month period dedicated to gathering information on safety barriers and understanding the local culture before implementing the team intervention [29].

Implementation

Here, strategies include customizing the SSC, empowering leaders, and providing support, awareness, and training. Gillespie and Marshall also found that active involvement of physicians and their adaptation of the checklist to their specific circumstances are critical aspects of this stage of implementation [57].

Customization

From the beginning, the WHO has encouraged teams to tailor the SSC based on their contextual needs. Modification of the SSC is associated with successful uptake, as a UK study found modification to be the most commonly cited implementation facilitator [52]. Making changes addresses surgical teams' needs in local contexts and helps create a sense of ownership. Additions should not introduce unnecessary burdens, and eliminations should not compromise opportunities for all team members to speak up; all changes should promote tool usage and teamwork [3]. In general, modifications may involve adding elements that the current checklist overlooks (e.g., surgical implants), or aspects of the procedure (e.g., robotic surgery) or patient (e.g., neonates) where additional processes need to be considered [3, 59].

As an example, adaptation of the checklist to ambulatory surgeries, where morbidity and especially mortality are so low, shifted the focus to reducing pain and preventing postoperative nausea/vomiting [60]. Checklists have been applied to many surgical subspecialties including Neurosurgery, Orthopedics, Cardiac Surgery, Urology, and Otolaryngology [61], each with their own adaptations. In Pediatric surgery, for example, a well-regarded practice is encouraging parental involvement in checklist activities [62].

However, adaptation should be viewed with caution due to potential downsides. First is diminished effectiveness, which can occur through either loss of important elements or addition of items that are irrelevant to regular use or make the tool too onerous, leading to disengagement or inefficiency. Second, modifications complicate comparability and aggregation which are necessary for benchmarking and research purposes. Such was a concern among researchers in Switzerland, who discovered significant variations in content, timing, and role definitions in checklists across the country [63].

Multi-Level Leadership

A study of SSC implementation at five hospitals in Washington State found leaders to be a strong factor for implementation success, since they can explain the reasoning behind checklist use and demonstrate how it is used in real life. When there was a lack of understanding on why or how the SSC works, it led to staff frustration, disinterest, and eventual abandonment [64]. Furthermore, the tone among high-level hospital or departmental decision-makers can have a profound influence on users' buy-in and acceptance of the SSC. As John Kotter, a thought leader on organizational change, once said, "Unless you win support for your ideas, from people at all levels of your organization, big ideas never seem to take hold or have the impact you want" [65]. Indeed, engagement of institutional stakeholders like hospital CEOs, and not just physicians and nurses, was believed to be a key element of the success of the South Carolina program [66].

Implementation Support

Finally, the last theme–providing support, awareness, and training–can again be illustrated through the South Carolina implementation (Table 2.1). Here, implementation success was associated with the completion of low- and high-touch activities: while inexpensive webinars and coaching phone calls were easy to implement and supported the process, more intensive activities like in-person meetings and teamwork skills trainings resulted in greater engagement and effectiveness [66]. It is likely that a combination of these approaches can address issues of feasibility and cost as well as efficacy.

Post-Implementation: Sustain

After evaluation, strategies that audit and improve the ongoing use of the SSC are critical so that its value can be sustained or augmented, and it can continue to address the changing needs of surgical teams. The key themes in this phase include ongoing monitoring in which data on the use of the checklist are documented, and feedback in which that data are shared with users for the sake of reinforcing positive behaviors or correcting problematic behaviors. While successful pre- and during-intervention initiatives are necessary for a checklist to achieve its best effect, demonstration of the benefits to the involved parties can enhance utilization and ensure that the outcomes are sustained in the long term. Locally collected data, observations, and anecdotes which are personally relevant are persuasive and should be fed back and discussed with teams frequently [52]. The Proctor framework introduces eight standard outcomes used to evaluate successful implementation of an intervention [67]; assessment of these outcomes helped demonstrate sustained nationwide checklist implementation in Benin [68].

After providing surgical teams with the knowledge and resources needed to implement the SSC, it is important to realize that change does not happen immediately. There is no standard implementation timeline, since acceptance of an intervention is idiosyncratic and multifactorial. The South Carolina program, for example, spanned 8 years, with additional hospitals joining the community as success became evident [66]. This underscores the notion that the act of translating knowledge into action should not be taken for granted.

Next Steps

SSC in Low and Middle-Income Countries

It is a common misperception that checklists' benefit is seen exclusively or primarily in low-resource settings. In reality, early studies demonstrated that the checklist could be effective in both high- and low-resource settings, the latter ranging from an under-resourced hospital in Moldova [41] to a large multi-specialty hospital in India [40]. However, low-resource settings face several barriers which hamper the efficacy of the SSC.

Slow Progress

The WHO sought nationwide implementation of the SSC in 15 African countries in 2011 by convening a group of one representative hospital from each country. By October 2012, 10 of the 15 hospitals reported successful implementation of the checklist, but none of them implemented it in all of their ORs, and no national efforts were underway [69]. While efforts since then have been limited, there have been some successes. For instance, the health ministries of Madagascar, Benin, and Guinea partnered with the non-profit Mercy Ships, which runs the world's largest civilian hospital ship [70]. Furthermore, several studies have examined successful implementation initiatives, identifying barriers and establishing best practices [68, 71].

Although SSC use does not rely on technology and is designed to be used in all settings, the competing demands, diminished infrastructure, and cultural barriers in low resource settings have resulted in poor adoption and sustainment of the SSC in these contexts. Ten years after introduction of the SSC, significant variability exists in terms of use of SSC, with decreased overall use in low Human Development Index (HDI) countries compared to those with very high HDI [72].

The Clean Cut Program

Developed by local surgical leaders both within and external to Lifebox, a non-profit organization focused on improving worldwide surgical care (lifebox.org), Clean Cut is an adaptive, multimodal checklist-based program that targets six areas: appropriate skin and hand antisepsis, maintenance of a sterile field, instrument sterilization, appropriate prophylactic antibiotic administration, routine gauze counting, and routine use of the SSC. Following program implementation in five hospitals in Ethiopia from August 2016 to October 2018, compliance with the six items increased, and the risk of infections decreased [73]. This program is currently being scaled throughout Ethiopia, and teams have begun to implement in several other African countries.

Beyond the WHO SSC

In many settings, it has been over a decade since the SSC's first implementation, with new users inheriting SSCs from a prior implementation period [3, 59]. In light of changing needs, organizations should periodically review and update their checklists, not only because it refreshes the items on their SSCs, but also because it galvanizes the team and recognizes new perspectives. Such a review should be comprehensive and systematic. While this process may seem daunting, there are various systems for changing teams' checklists and revitalizing their use. For example, in assessing SSC use at Singapore General Hospital, a team from Ariadne Labs developed a three-part evaluation plan involving assessing (1) quality of care via a review of surgical safety events, (2) safety culture through a validated survey and informal feedback, and (3) checklist performance through direct observations and a survey of staff. This allowed them to revise and re-implement the checklist in Singapore while also setting forth a framework for other organizations [56].

Technology Tools

The potential opportunities provided by visual displays, real data integration, and clinical decision support may result in further checklist evolution. One study used checklists displayed via an app on smart glasses. As compared to standard approaches such as a poster on the wall, the smart glasses group had improved completion rate and decreased time spent performing the checklists [74]. Another innovation involves a Digital Checklist Box, which projects the timeout information onto the patient's drapes and allows surgeons to navigate the interface with hand gestures [75].

References

1. Weiser TG, Berry WR. Review article: perioperative checklist methodologies. Can J Anaesth. 2013;60(2):136–42.
2. Burian BK, Clebone A, Dismukes K, Ruskin KJ. More than a tick box: medical checklist development, design, and use. Anesth Analg. 2018;126(1):223–32.
3. Solsky I, Berry W, Edmondson J, Lagoo J, Baugh J, Blair A, Singer S, Haynes AB. World Health Organization surgical safety checklist modification: do changes emphasize communication and teamwork? J Surg Res. 2020;246:614–22.
4. Winters BD, Gurses AP, Lehmann H, Sexton JB, Rampersad CJ, Pronovost PJ. Clinical review: checklists - translating evidence into practice. Crit Care. 2009;13(6):210.
5. Ariadne Labs. 2017. "Operating Room Crisis Checklists. ariadnelabs.org/wp-content/uploads/2017/11/OR-Crisis-Checklists-eVersion-042417-052217_CClicense-2.pdf. Accessed 16 Aug 2023.
6. Arriaga AF, Bader AM, Wong JM, Lipsitz SR, Berry WR, Ziewacz JE, Hepner DL, et al. Simulation-based trial of surgical-crisis checklists. NEJM. 2013;368(3):246–53.
7. Vats A, Nagpal K, Moorthy K. Surgery: a risky business. J Periop Pract. 2009;19(10):330–4.
8. Brennan TA, Leape LL, Laird NM, Hebert L, Localio AR, Lawthers AG, Newhouse JP, Weiler PC, Hiatt HH. Incidence of adverse events and negligence in hospitalized patients. Results of the Harvard medical practice study I. NEJM. 1991;324(6):370–6.
9. Leape LL, Brennan TA, Laird N, Lawthers AG, Localio AR, Barnes BA, Hebert L, Newhouse JP, Weiler PC, Hiatt H. The nature of adverse events in hospitalized patients. Results of the Harvard medical practice study II. NEJM. 1991;324(6):377–84.
10. Thomas EJ, Studdert DM, Burstin HR, Orav EJ, Zeena T, Williams EJ, Howard KM, Weiler PC, Brennan TA. Incidence and types of adverse events and negligent Care in Utah and Colorado. Med Care. 2000;38(3):261–71.
11. Gawande AA, Thomas EJ, Zinner MJ, Brennan TA. The incidence and nature of surgical adverse events in Colorado and Utah in 1992. Surgery. 1999;126(1):66–75.
12. Vincent CG, Neale G, Woloshynowych M. Adverse events in British hospitals: preliminary retrospective record review. BMJ. 2001;322(7285):517–9.
13. Ross Baker G, Norton PG, Flintoft V, Blais R, Brown A, Cox J, Etchells E, et al. The Canadian adverse events study: the incidence of adverse events among hospital patients in Canada. Can Med Assoc J. 2004;170(11):1678–86.
14. Institute of Medicine. To Err Is Human: Building a Safer Health System. 2000. pubmed.ncbi.nlm.nih.gov/25077248/. Accessed 16 Aug 2023.
15. Hempel S, Maggard-Gibbons M, Nguyen DK, Dawes AJ, Miake-Lye I, Beroes JM, Booth MJ, Miles JNV, Shanman R, Shekelle PG. Wrong-site surgery, retained surgical items, and surgical fires : a systematic review of surgical never events. JAMA Surg. 2015;150(8):796–805.

16. Weerakkody RA, Cheshire NJ, Riga C, Lear R, Hamady MS, Moorthy K, Darzi AW, Vincent C, Bicknell CD. Surgical technology and operating-room safety failures: a systematic review of quantitative studies. BMJ Qual Saf. 2013;22(9):710–8.
17. Suliburk JW, Buck QM, Pirko CJ, Massarweh NN, Barshes NR, Singh H, Rosengart TK. Analysis of human performance deficiencies associated with surgical adverse events. JAMA Netw Open. 2019;2(7):e198067.
18. Greenberg CC, Regenbogen SE, Studdert DM, Lipsitz SR, Rogers SO, Zinner MJ, Gawande AA. Patterns of communication breakdowns resulting in injury to surgical patients. J Am Col Surg. 2007;204(4):533–40.
19. Lingard L, Espin S, Whyte S, Regehr G, Baker GR, Reznick R, Bohnen J, Orser B, Doran D, Grober E. Communication failures in the operating room: an observational classification of recurrent types and effects. Qual Saf Health Care. 2004;13(5):330–4.
20. Loukopoulos LD, Dismukes RK, Barshi I. *The Multitasking Myth: Handling Complexity in Real-World Operations*. 2009. routledge.com/The-Multitasking-Myth-Handling-Complexity-in-Real-World-Operations/Loukopoulos-Dismukes-Barshi/p/book/9780754679974. Accessed 16 Aug 2023.
21. Weiser TG, Haynes AB, Lashoher A, Dziekan G, Boorman DJ, Berry WR, Gawande AA. Perspectives in quality: designing the WHO surgical safety checklist. Int J Qual Health Care. 2010;22(5):365–70.
22. Mahajan RP. The WHO surgical checklist. Clin Anaesthesiol. 2011;25(2):161–8.
23. Berenholtz SM, Pronovost PJ, Lipsett PA, Hobson D, Earsing K, Farley JE, Milanovich S, et al. Eliminating catheter-related bloodstream infections in the intensive care unit. Crit Care Med. 2004;32(10):2014–20.
24. Pronovost P, Needham D, Berenholtz S, Sinopoli D, Chu H, Cosgrove S, Sexton B, et al. An intervention to decrease catheter-related bloodstream infections in the ICU. NEJM. 2006;355(26):2725–32.
25. Gawande, A. A. 2007. "A Life-Saving Checklist." *The New Yorker*, 2007. newyorker.com/magazine/2007/12/10/the-checklist. Accessed 16 Aug 2023.
26. Saufl NM. Universal protocol for preventing wrong site, wrong procedure, wrong person surgery. J Perianesth Nurs. 2004;19(5):348–51.
27. Lingard L, Espin S, Rubin B, Whyte S, Colmenares M, Baker GR, Doran D, et al. Getting teams to talk: development and pilot implementation of a checklist to promote Interprofessional communication in the OR. Qual Saf Health Care. 2005;14(5):340–6.
28. Makary MA, Holzmueller CG, Thompson D, Rowen L, Heitmiller ES, Maley WR, Black JH, et al. Operating room briefings: working on the same page. Joint Com Res. 2006;32(6):351–5.
29. Neily J, Mills PD, Young-Xu Y, Carney BT, West P, Berger DH, Mazzia LM, Paull DE, Bagian JP. Association between implementation of a medical team training program and surgical mortality. JAMA. 2010;304(15):1693–700.
30. Young-Xu Y, Neily J, Mills PD, Carney BT, West P, Berger DH, Mazzia LM, Paull DE, Bagian JP. Association between implementation of a medical team training program and surgical morbidity. Arch Surg. 2011;146(12):1368–73.
31. de Vries EN, Prins HA, Crolla RMPH, den Outer AJ, van Andel G, van Helden SH, Schlack WS, et al. Effect of a comprehensive surgical safety system on patient outcomes. NEJM. 2010;363(20):1928–37.
32. Borchard A, Schwappach DLB, Barbir A, Bezzola P. A systematic review of the effectiveness, compliance, and critical factors for implementation of safety checklists in surgery. Ann Surg. 2012;256(6):925–33.
33. Safe Surgery Saves Lives. World Health Organization. 2008. apps.who.int/iris/bitstream/handle/10665/70080/WHO_IER_PSP_2008.07_eng.pdf;jsessionid=BC1B5640B5BA9EB0921993D6A3F28A4B?sequence=1. Accessed 16 Aug 2023.
34. Haynes AB, Weiser TG, Berry WR, Lipsitz SR, Breizat AHS, Dellinger EP, Herbosa T, et al. A surgical safety checklist to reduce morbidity and mortality in a global population. NEJM. 2009;360(5):491–9.

35. Harvard University. "Surgical safety web map." Center for geographic analysis. 2014. gis.harvard.edu/surgical-safety-web-map. Accessed 16 Aug 2023.
36. Ramsay G, Haynes AB, Lipsitz SR, Solsky I, Leitch J, Gawande AA, Kumar M. Reducing surgical mortality in Scotland by use of the WHO surgical safety checklist. Br J Surg. 2019;106(8):1005–11.
37. Bergs J, Hellings J, Cleemput I, Zurel O, De Troyer V, Van Hiel M, Demeere JL, Claeys D, Vandijck D. Systematic review and meta-analysis of the effect of the World Health Organization surgical safety checklist on postoperative complications. Br J Surg. 2014;101(3):150–8.
38. Sotto KT, Burian BK, Brindle ME. Impact of the WHO surgical safety checklist relative to its design and intended use: a systematic review and meta-meta-analysis. J Am Col Surg. 2021;233(6):794–809.e8.
39. Treadwell JR, Lucas S, Tsou AY. Surgical checklists: a systematic review of impacts and implementation. BMJ Qual Saf. 2014;23(4):299–318.
40. Chaudhary N, Varma V, Kapoor S, Mehta N, Kumaran V, Nundy S. Implementation of a surgical safety checklist and postoperative outcomes: a prospective randomized controlled study. J Gastroint Surg. 2015;19(5):935–42.
41. Kwok AC, Funk LM, Baltaga R, Lipsitz SR, Merry AF, Dziekan G, Ciobanu G, Berry WR, Gawande AA. Implementation of the World Health Organization surgical safety checklist, including introduction of pulse oximetry, in a resource-limited setting. Ann Surg. 2013;257(4):633–9.
42. Haugen AS, Søfteland E, Almeland SK, Sevdalis N, Vonen B, Eide GE, Nortvedt MW, Harthug S. Effect of the World Health Organization checklist on patient outcomes: a stepped wedge cluster randomized controlled trial. Ann Surg. 2015;261(5):821–8.
43. NHS National Patient Safety Agency. WHO Surgical Safety Checklist. 2009., cas.mhra.gov.uk/. Accessed 16 Aug 2023.
44. Mayer EK, Sevdalis N, Rout S, Caris J, Russ S, Mansell J, Davies R, et al. Surgical checklist implementation project: the impact of variable WHO checklist compliance on risk-adjusted clinical outcomes after National Implementation: a longitudinal study. Ann Surg. 2016;263(1):58–63.
45. van Klei WA, Hoff RG, van Aarnhem EEHL, Simmermacher RKJ, Regli LPE, Kappen TH, van Wolfswinkel L, Kalkman CJ, Buhre WF, Peelen LM. Effects of the introduction of the WHO 'surgical safety checklist' on in-hospital mortality: a cohort study. Ann Surg. 2012;255(1):44–9.
46. Urbach DR, Govindarajan A, Saskin R, Wilton AS, Baxter NN. Introduction of surgical safety checklists in Ontario, Canada. N Engl J Med. 2014;370(11):1029–38.
47. Reames BN, Krell RW, Campbell DA Jr, Dimick JB. A checklist-based intervention to improve surgical outcomes in Michigan: evaluation of the keystone surgery program. JAMA Surg. 2015;150(3):208–15.
48. Rosskam E. Using participatory action research methodology to improve worker health. In: Schnall P, Dobson M, Rosskam E, editors. Unhealthy work: causes, consequences, cures, vol. 369. Baywood Publishing Company; 2009. p. 211–29.
49. Leape LL. The checklist conundrum. NEJM 2014. 2014;370(11):1063–4.
50. Haynes AB, Weiser TG, Berry WR, Lipsitz SR, Breizat AHS, Dellinger EP, Dziekan G, et al. Changes in safety attitude and relationship to decreased postoperative morbidity and mortality following implementation of a checklist-based surgical safety intervention. BMJ Qual Saf. 2011;20(1):102–7.
51. Jain D, Sharma R, Reddy S. WHO safe surgery checklist: barriers to universal acceptance. J Anaesthesiol Clin Pharmacol. 2018;34(1):7–10.
52. Russ SJ, Sevdalis N, Moorthy K, Mayer EK, Rout S, Caris J, Mansell J, Davies R, Vincent C, Darzi A. A qualitative evaluation of the barriers and facilitators toward implementation of the WHO surgical safety checklist across hospitals in england: lessons from the 'surgical checklist implementation project. Ann Surg. 2015;261(1):81–91.

53. Molina G, Jiang W, Edmondson L, Gibbons L, Huang LC, Kiang MV, Haynes AB, Gawande AA, Berry WR, Singer SJ. Implementation of the surgical safety checklist in South Carolina hospitals is associated with improvement in perceived perioperative safety. J Am Col Surg. 2016;222(5):725–736.e5.
54. Haynes AB, Edmondson L, Lipsitz SR, Molina G, Neville BA, Singer SJ, Moonan AT, et al. Mortality trends after a voluntary checklist-based surgical safety collaborative. Ann Surg. 2017;266(6):923–9.
55. Moullin JC, Dickson KS, Stadnick NA, Rabin B, Aarons GA. Systematic review of the exploration, preparation, implementation, sustainment (EPIS) framework. Implement Sci: IS. 2019;14(1):1.
56. Moyal-Smith R, Etheridge JC, Lim SR, Sonnay Y, Tan HK, Yong TT, Havens JM, Brindle ME. Creating a high-performance surgical safety checklist: a multimodal evaluation plan to reinvigorate the checklist. J Eval Clin Pract. 2023;29(2):341–50.
57. Gillespie BM, Marshall A. Implementation of safety checklists in surgery: a realist synthesis of evidence. Implem Sci: IS. 2015;10:137.
58. Ramírez-Torres CA, Pedraz-Marcos A, Maciá-Soler ML, Rivera-Sanz F. A scoping review of strategies used to implement the surgical safety checklist. AORN J. 2021;113(6):610–9.
59. Turley N, Elam M, Brindle ME. International perspectives on modifications to the surgical safety checklist. JAMA Netw Open. 2023;6(6):e2317183.
60. Morgan PJ, Cunningham L, Mitra S, Wong N, Wu W, Noguera V, Li M, Semple J. Surgical safety checklist: implementation in an ambulatory surgical facility. Can J Anaesth. 2013;60(6):528–38.
61. Patel J, Ahmed K, Khan GKA, F, Marsh H, Khan MS, Dasgupta P. An overview of the use and implementation of checklists in surgical Specialities - a systematic review. Int J Surg. 2014;12(12):1317–23.
62. Corbally MT, Tierney E. Parental involvement in the preoperative surgical safety checklist is welcomed by both parents and staff. Int J Ped. 2014;2014:791490.
63. Fridrich A, Imhof A, Schwappach DLB. How much and what local adaptation is acceptable? A comparison of 24 surgical safety checklists in Switzerland. J Pat Saf. 2021;17(3):217–22.
64. Conley DM, Singer SJ, Edmondson L, Berry WR, Gawande AA. Effective surgical safety checklist implementation. J Am Col Surg. 2011;212(5):873–9.
65. James TA. Gaining leadership buy-in for organizational change in health care. 2020. postgraduateeducation.hms.harvard.edu/trends-medicine/gaining-leadership-buy-organizational-change-health-care. Accessed 16 Aug 2023.
66. Berry WR, Edmondson L, Gibbons LR, Childers AK, Haynes AB, Foster R, Singer SJ, Gawande AA. Scaling safety: the South Carolina surgical safety checklist experience. Health Aff. 2018;37(11):1779–86.
67. Proctor E, Silmere H, Raghavan R, Hovmand P, Aarons G, Bunger A, Griffey R, Hensley M. Outcomes for implementation research: conceptual distinctions, measurement challenges, and research agenda. Admin Pol Ment Health. 2011;38(2):65–76.
68. White MC, Randall K, NFE C-C, Sodogas F, Quenum S, Wright K, Close KL, Russ S, Sevdalis N, AJM L. Implementation and evaluation of Nationwide scale-up of the surgical safety checklist. Br J Surg. 2019;106(2):e91–102.
69. Kariyo PC, Hightower J, Ndihokubwayoii JB, Tumusiime P, Mwikisa C. Surgical safety checklist: a short experience in African countries. Afr Health Monit. 2013;16:36–9.
70. Buissonniere, Marine. "Checking in on the checklist." Lifebox, Ariadne Labs. 2020. lifebox.org/wp-content/uploads/2022/08/Checking-In-On-the-Checklist-web.pdf. Accessed 16 Aug 2023.
71. White MC, Peven K, Clancy O, Okonkwo I, Bakolis I, Russ S, Leather AJM, Sevdalis N. Implementation strategies and the uptake of the World Health Organization surgical safety checklist in low and middle income countries: a systematic review and meta-analysis. Ann Surg. 2021;273(6):e196–205.

72. Delisle M, Pradarelli JC, Panda N, Koritsanszky L, Sonnay Y, Lipsitz S, Pearse R, et al. Variation in global uptake of the surgical safety checklist. Br J Surg. 2020;107(2):e151–60.
73. Forrester JA, Starr N, Negussie T, Schaps D, Adem M, Alemu S, Amenu D, et al. Clean cut (adaptive, multimodal surgical infection prevention Programme) for low-resource settings: a prospective quality improvement study. Br J Surg. 2021;108(6):727–34.
74. Boillat T, Grantcharov P, Rivas H. Increasing completion rate and benefits of checklists: prospective evaluation of surgical safety checklists with smart glasses. JMIR Mhealth Uhealth. 2019;7(4):e13447.
75. Boillat T, Rivas H. It is in the box! Improving the usability and benefits of surgical safety checklists—a feasibility study. Int J Ind Erg. 2021;86:103217.

Chapter 3
Controversies in Antibiotic Prophylaxis in Orthopaedic Surgery

Elisha Krasin

Abbreviations

HIV	Human Immunodeficiency Virus
VRE	Vancomycin-resistant enterococci
MRSA	Methicillin-resistant staphylococcus aureus
MSSA	Methicillin-sensitive staphylococcus aureus
SSI	Surgical site infection
THA	Total hip arthroplasty
TKA	Total knee arthroplasty

Introduction

Surgical site infection is a highly concerning issue in the field of orthopaedic surgery. What starts as a simple injury that could be effectively treated with a standard procedure can quickly escalate into a chronic condition, necessitating prolonged hospitalisation, ongoing antibiotic therapy, and repeated surgeries. The complications associated with infection can result in treatment failure, disability, limb amputation, and even mortality. Given these implications, the prevention of infections in orthopaedics is of paramount importance.

E. Krasin (✉)
Maccabi Healthcare Services, Tel Aviv-Yafo, Israel

© The Author(s), under exclusive license to Springer Nature Switzerland AG 2024

J. Faintuch, S. Faintuch (eds.), *Recent Strategies in High Risk Surgery*,
https://doi.org/10.1007/978-3-031-56270-9_3

Early Experience

Once penicillin became available during World War II, it was used to prevent infections in orthopaedic surgery [1]. Controversy followed, when, in 1960, Pulaski and Taylor noted that most infecting organisms in orthopaedic surgery were resistant to the antibiotics commonly used for prophylaxis at the time. They also mentioned that infection rates were higher among patients who received antibiotics. Their conclusion was that "routine indiscriminate antibiotic prophylaxis for elective surgical conditions served no useful purpose" [2].

Burke pointed out in 1963 that "antibacterials can increase natural resistance when natural mechanisms are ineffective" [3]. The contemporary practice of perioperative antibiotic prophylaxis in orthopaedics is based on the work of Boyd and Burke, who in 1973 investigated ways to reduce the incidence of wound and soft tissue infections, as well as infections around orthopaedic implants [4]. Norden in 1976 still believed that antibiotic prophylaxis was a controversial issue [5] Originally, the decision to prescribe cephalosporins was mainly aimed at the prevalent *Staphylococcal* and *Streptococcal* infections. These bacteria were largely susceptible to methicillin as well as first and second generation cephalosporins.

The routine use of cephalosporins in orthopaedics has been proven by numerous clinical trials, which have convincingly demonstrated their effectiveness in reducing infection rates. Rosenfeld et al. concluded that "first-generation cephalosporins, such as cephalothin or cefazolin, are the best chemoprophylactic agents because of their excellent antistaphylococcal activity and lack of significant toxicity" [6].

Current Epidemiology and Microbiology

Most surgical site infections are obtained during the operation, with the most common source being the patient's skin as well as airborne micro-organisms from operating theatre staff [7]. In clean orthopaedic surgery, the reported wound infection rate is 5.1%, while the administration of preoperative antibiotics reduces it to 0.8%. In clean - contaminated surgery the rates are 10.1% and 1.3% respectively, and in contaminated surgery 21.9% and 10.2%, [8]. Administration of antibiotic prophylaxis in surgery of open fractures provided "a large, consistent reduction in infection risk" [9].

Present day developments in bacterial resistance and the increasing number of methicillin-resistant *staphylococci* may make the use of first- or second-generation cephalosporins in orthopaedics almost obsolete. This contrasts with their still fairly good acceptance in the field of general surgery. About 30% of infections after joint replacement are polymicrobial, meaning they are a combination of Gram-negative and Gram-positive bacteria. Of the monomicrobial infections,

43% are caused by *Staphylococcus aureus* (4% by methicillin-resistant bacteria) [10]. Coagulase-negative *Staphylococci* were found to be responsible for 30% of infections after knee replacement and 19% after hip replacement. Gram-negative bacteria were found in 17% of infections after hip and knee arthroplasty [10].

A Spanish study of total joint arthroplasties showed an increase in Gram-negative infections along the years, from 21% to 67%. *Staphylococcus aureus* remains the most common microorganism after fracture surgery, but resistance to methicillin is increasing and may even exceed susceptible species in some areas [10]. Coagulase-negative *staphylococci* are also common and 80–90% resistant to methicillin. The incidence of multidrug-resistant Gram-negative bacteria such as *Pseudomonas aeruginosa* and *Acinetobacter baumannii* is increasing, as is the incidence of gastrointestinal organisms such as *Escherichia coli*, *Enterobacter*, *Enterococcus*, *Klebsiella*, and *Proteus* [10, 11].

Our recent work demonstrated an increase in oxacillin resistance of *Staphylococci*, and high incidence of non-gastrointestinal Gram-negative bacteria and gastrointestinal bacteria [12]. Currently, *Staphylococcus aureus* resistance to vancomycin is rare, but could become a problem in the future. Intermediate vancomycin-resistant *Staphylococcus aureus* is already observed and is likely to become more of a problem in the near future [12].

Vancomycin-Resistant Enterococci

These are of major importance in orthopaedic surgery because of their potential to cause infections and complications that are difficult to treat. In addition, the presence of VRE in healthcare facilities raises concerns about the potential for transmission and outbreaks among patients, particularly those with compromised immune systems [13].

Cutibacterium acnes is considered a major pathogen in shoulder surgery and may exceed even *Staphylococci* in prevalence [7]. It shows good sensitivity to antibiotics commonly used for bone and joint infections, particularly beta-lactams, quinolones, and rifampicin. However, resistance to some antibiotics, in particular clindamycin, is emerging. Furthermore, *Cutibacterium acnes*, despite being an anaerobic bacterium, also shows natural resistance to metronidazole.

Fungal Infections

These occur in less than 1% of prosthetic joint infections, but should nevertheless be considered, if not in prophylaxis, in the diagnosis itself of the infection [14]. Precisely because of the low frequency, they tend to be overlooked and misdiagnosed, precipitating much tissue destruction and deleterious systemic effects.

General Recommendations

The optimal prophylactic antibiotic should include coverage for resistant Gram-positive as well as for common Gram-negative agents. Adequate bloodstream and tissue concentrations should be achieved along the entire procedure. Additionally, it is crucial that bacteria do not readily develop resistance to this antibiotic, considering its intended widespread utilisation.

Practical Guidelines

The simplest way to prevent postoperative infections is not to operate, whenever intervention is not mandatory. The indications for most orthopaedic operations are relative and in most cases, there is a conservative alternative. In patients with low functional requirements and increased risk for infection such as the elderly, the immunosuppressed and those with serious comorbidities, conservative non-surgical treatment should always be considered.

Preoperative screening and decolonisation of methicillin-resistant *Staphylococcus aureus* and methicillin-sensitive *Staphylococcus aureus* is a controversial issue, but most authorities recommend nasal swabs for screening in elective situations. If positive for *Staphylococcus aureus*, decolonisation by nasal application of mupirocin twice daily to both nares for 5 days should be considered [7]. Some recommend additional bathing with chlorhexidine daily before scheduled surgery for 5 days.

Current Practice

The adopted guidelines for perioperative antibiotic administration in orthopaedics are quite standard, and in my opinion, they will soon be obsolete. A preliminary distinction should be made between the prevention of infection in surgery of closed fractures and injuries as well as clean elective or semi-elective surgery, in comparison with open fractures and injuries.

Timing and Duration

These are somewhat controversial points as well. Most authors recommend administering the first dose about half an hour before the incision and no more than 2 h before. Administering the drug during or after the start of surgery renders treatment ineffective [15]. The ideal duration of postoperative antibiotic treatment is not yet clearly defined, although most reports suggest that there is no additional benefit from prophylactic antibiotic treatment more than 24 h after surgery [15].

A study of extended oral antibiotic prophylaxis in high-risk patients involved a 7-day antibiotic regimen (Cefadroxil 500 mg two times per day or Clindamycin 300 mg three times per day with Sulfamethoxazole and trimethoprim 800 mg/160 mg two times per day) in patients with a BMI ≥35, diabetes mellitus, smoking, chronic kidney disease, autoimmune disease or with nasal colonisation of MSSA or MRSA. Before the introduction of the extended antibiotic therapy protocol, the incidence of PJI in the primary THA and TKA in the high-risk subset were 4.3% and 2.1%, respectively. After the introduction of this protocol, the corresponding rates decreased to 1.1% and 0.4%, which is in line with the rates observed in patients without high risk receiving standard perioperative prophylaxis [16]. The American Academy of Orthopaedic Surgeons (AAOS) recommends prophylaxis for no more than 24 h, regardless of the use of drains or catheters [17].

Closed Fractures and Clean Elective or Semi-Elective Surgery

Cefazolin 2 g (or 3 g if >100 kg body weight) IV 30–60 min before skin incision, then cefazolin 2 g or 3 g IV every 8 h for 24 h is advised. In beta-lactam allergic patients the recommended protocol is vancomycin IV (15 mg/kg) or clindamycin 600–900 mg IV 60–90 min before skin incision, then vancomycin every 12 h or clindamycin 600–900 mg IV every 6 h for 24 h [8, 18].

Clostridioides Difficile

In the UK, cephalosporins are no longer first line prophylaxis in many centres, mainly due to concerns about *Clostridioides difficile* infection. Third-generation cephalosporins are strongly associated with such supervenient infection and prophylaxis with a single dose of cephalosporin is sufficient to cause the development of *Clostridioides difficile* colonisation. Flucloxacillin is a penicillinase-resistant penicillin with good coverage against Staphylococcus aureus (it is ineffective against MRSA and 90% of coagulase-negative staphylococci) and is commonly used in the UK as first-line treatment for *Staphylococcus aureus* infection [17].

Open Fractures

The Gustilo and Anderson classification is one of the most broadly used classifications for open fractures. The incidence of wound infection is directly correlated with the class of fracture, with 0–2% in grade I fractures, 2–7% in grade II fractures, 7–10% in grade IIIA fractures, 10–50% in grade IIIB fractures, and

25–50% in grade IIIC fractures [19]. The efficacy of prophylactic treatment for the types IIIB and IIIC is questionable, contrasting with types I-IIIA, for which the benefit is clear. In case of obesity of more than 100 kg, the doses should be doubled [20].

The duration of antibiotic therapy varies from one institution to another and the choice of drugs is not standardized. Penicillins, cephalosporins, aminoglycosides and fluoroquinolones are common options. Broader spectrum agents including monobactams and glycopeptides, have been used for additional coverage [21]. In general, antimicrobials are discontinued 24 h after surgery, but it may be appropriate to continue them for up to 72 h for heavily contaminated wounds. Antibiotics should not be given beyond 72 h unless a second surgery is performed within that time.

Here is an example of the protocol used by Garner et al. for open fractures:

- *For type I and II open fractures:* Cefazolin 2 g IV immediately and q8 hours, with three total doses.
  For penicillin allergic: Clindamycin 900 mg IV immediately and q8 hours (three total doses).
- *For type III open fractures:* Ceftriaxone 2 g IV immediately; Vancomycin 1 g IV immediately and after 12 h (two total doses).
  For penicillin allergic: Aztreonam 2 g IV immediately and q8 hours (three total doses); Vancomycin 1 g IV immediately and after 12 h (two total doses) [21].

Immunocompromised Patients

There is no conclusive evidence suggesting that HIV-positive patients experience a higher infection rate during elective surgery or trauma, and therefore, long-term antibiotic therapy is not warranted for these individuals. Despite the acknowledged heightened risk, there is insufficient evidence to justify deviations from standard antibiotic therapy for diabetic patients, or those with rheumatoid arthritis [17].

Local Antibiotics

High-quality evidence for combined local/ systemic prescription is scarce in orthopaedic surgery and particularly in surgery of the shoulder and elbow. The role of local wound antibiotics needs to be further established in future research [7].

The interest of combinations such as cefazolin and vancomycin in preventing periprosthetic knee infections remains uncertain, as strong prospective studies are lacking [22]. The risk of developing acute renal failure is a major drawback of this combination [23].

Future Developments

The task of creating a vaccine capable of preventing *Staphylococcus aureus* infection has proven to be formidable. This bacterium is a commensal organism found in the nasal mucosa and skin of humans, and it has developed a sophisticated arsenal specifically designed to evade the human immune system. However, the development of an effective vaccine holds the potential to address the escalating concerns of antibiotic resistance and the emergence of vancomycin-resistant *staphylococci*. Currently, there are at least five vaccines against *Staphylococcus aureus* that are undergoing various stages of clinical trials. Concurrently, research has also focused on bacteriophages, monoclonal antibodies, centyrins (monoclonal antibody mimetics), and novel types of antibiotics. Some of these approaches have shown promising results in human testing. Additionally, various strategies have been explored in preclinical settings to enhance the delivery of anti-staphylococcal drugs for specific infections, including skin and soft tissue infections, implant-associated osteomyelitis, and pneumonia [24].

Conclusion

First generation cephalosporins are still popular; second-generation cephalosporins offer greater protection against Gramnegative bacteria, but have reduced efficacy against staphylococci. Our recent results clearly indicate a worrying increase in resistance to clindamycin [12]. The choice of vancomycin for this task also presents a number of challenges [25]. Thus, a single regimen will hardly be ideal for all patients, and risk assessment should precede prophylactic prescriptions.

A shorter duration of antibiotic prophylaxis can be just as effective in preventing SSI as a longer duration, while reducing the risk of developing antibiotic resistance. A single dose of cefazolin administered 1 h before surgery was as effective as a three-dose regimen to prevent SSI in patients undergoing pure orthopaedic procedures, such as joint replacement [26]. In cases where there is a high prevalence of antibiotic-resistant bacteria, the use of alternative antibiotics or combinations thereof may be necessary to provide adequate prophylaxis.

References

1. Hampton OP. Reparative surgery of compound Battle fractures in the Mediterranean theater of operations. Ann Surg. 1945;122:289–332.
2. Pulaski EJ, Taylor LW. Pyogenic infections in orthopedic surgery—prevention and management. Calif Med. 1960;92:35–7.
3. Burke JF. Preoperative antibiotics. Surg Clin North Am. 1963;43:665–76. https://doi.org/10.1016/S0039-6109(16)36983-3.
4. Boyd RJ, Burke JF, Colton T. A double-blind clinical trial of prophylactic antibiotics in hip fractures. J Bone Joint Surg Am. 1973;55:1251–8.

5. Norden CW. Antibiotic prophylaxis in orthopedic surgery. Clin Orthop. 1976;114:203–6.
6. Rosenfeld MB, Campos J, Ratzan KR, Uredo I. Chemoprophylaxis with cefoxitin and cephalothin in orthopedic surgery: a comparison. Antimicrob Agents Chemother. 1981;19:826–30. https://doi.org/10.1128/AAC.19.5.826.
7. Boyle KK, Duquin TR. Antibiotic prophylaxis and prevention of surgical site infection in shoulder and elbow surgery. Orthop Clin North Am. 2018;49:241–56. https://doi.org/10.1016/j.ocl.2017.11.011.
8. Boyd J, Chmielewski R. Prevention of infection in foot and ankle surgery. Clin Podiatr Med Surg. 2019;36:37–58. https://doi.org/10.1016/j.cpm.2018.08.007.
9. Chang Y, Kennedy SA, Bhandari M, Lopes LC, Bergamaschi CC, de Silva MCDO, Bhatnagar N, Mousavi SM, Khurshid S, Petrisor B, Ren M, Sodhi SK, Mirza RD, Guyatt GH. Effects of antibiotic prophylaxis in patients with open fracture of the extremities: a systematic review of randomized controlled trials. JBJS Rev. 2015;3:e2. https://doi.org/10.2106/JBJS.RVW.N.00088.
10. Lamagni T, Elgohari S, Harrington P. Trends in surgical site infections following orthopaedic surgery. Curr Opin Infect Dis. 2015;28:125–32. https://doi.org/10.1097/QCO.0000000000000143.
11. Fang C, Wong T-M, Lau T-W, To KK, Wong SS, Leung F. Infection after fracture osteosynthesis—part I: pathogenesis, diagnosis and classification. J Orthop Surg. 2017;25:2309499017692712. https://doi.org/10.1177/2309499017692712.
12. Krasin E, Warschawski Y, Morgan S, Dekel M. Antibiotic prophylaxis in orthopedic surgery; has the time to reconsider the current practice arrived? J Orthop. 2022;32:68–71. https://doi.org/10.1016/j.jor.2022.05.008.
13. Peel T, Astbury S, Cheng AC, Paterson D, Buising K, Spelman T, Tran-Duy A, de Steiger RS, ASAP Trial Group. Multicentre randomised double-blind placebo controlled trial of combination vancomycin and cefazolin surgical antibiotic prophylaxis: the Australian surgical antibiotic prophylaxis (ASAP) trial. BMJ Open. 2019;9:e033718. https://doi.org/10.1136/bmjopen-2019-033718.
14. Beam E, Osmon D. Prosthetic joint infection update. Infect Dis Clin N Am. 2018;32:843–59. https://doi.org/10.1016/j.idc.2018.06.005.
15. Dhammi IK, Ul Haq R, Kumar S. Prophylactic antibiotics in orthopedic surgery: controversial issues in its use. Indian J Orthop. 2015;49:373–6. https://doi.org/10.4103/0019-5413.159556.
16. DeFrancesco CJ, Fu MC, Kahlenberg CA, Miller AO, Bostrom MP. Extended antibiotic prophylaxis may be linked to lower peri-prosthetic joint infection rates in high-risk patients: an evidence-based review. HSS J. 2019;15:297–301. https://doi.org/10.1007/s11420-019-09698-8.
17. Bryson DJ, Morris DLJ, Shivji FS, Rollins KR, Snape S, Ollivere BJ. Antibiotic prophylaxis in orthopaedic surgery: difficult decisions in an era of evolving antibiotic resistance. Bone Jt J. 2016;98-B:1014–9. https://doi.org/10.1302/0301-620X.98B8.37359.
18. Bratzler DW, Houck PM, Workgroup SIPGW. Antimicrobial prophylaxis for surgery: an advisory statement from the National Surgical Infection Prevention Project. Am J Surg. 2005;189:395–404. https://doi.org/10.1016/j.amjsurg.2005.01.015.
19. Isaac SM, Woods A, Danial IN, Mourkus H. Antibiotic prophylaxis in adults with open Tibial fractures: what is the evidence for duration of administration? A systematic review. J Foot Ankle Surg. 2016;55:146–50. https://doi.org/10.1053/j.jfas.2015.07.012.
20. Gaudias J. Antibiotic prophylaxis in orthopedics-traumatology. Orthop Traumatol Surg Res OTSR. 2021;107:102751. https://doi.org/10.1016/j.otsr.2020.102751.
21. Garner MR, Sethuraman SA, Schade MA, Boateng H. Antibiotic prophylaxis in open fractures: evidence, evolving issues, and recommendations. JAAOS - J Am Acad Orthop Surg. 2020;28:309. https://doi.org/10.5435/JAAOS-D-18-00193.
22. Villa JM, Pannu TS, Riesgo AM, Patel PD, Mont MA, Higuera-Rueda CA. Dual antibiotic prophylaxis in Total knee arthroplasty: where do we stand? J Knee Surg. 2020;33:100–5. https://doi.org/10.1055/s-0039-1695742.

23. Courtney MP, Melnic CM, Zimmer Z, Anari J, Lee G-C. Addition of vancomycin to cefazolin prophylaxis is associated with acute kidney injury after primary joint arthroplasty. Clin Orthop. 2015;473:2197–203. https://doi.org/10.1007/s11999-014-4062-3.
24. Clegg J, Soldaini E, McLoughlin RM, Rittenhouse S, Bagnoli F, Phogat S. *Staphylococcus aureus* vaccine Research and Development: the past, present and future, including novel therapeutic strategies. Front Immunol. 2021;12:705360.
25. Zastrow RK, Huang H, Galatz LM, Saunders-Hao P, Poeran J, Moucha CS. Characteristics of antibiotic prophylaxis and risk of surgical site infections in primary Total hip and knee arthroplasty. J Arthroplast. 2020;35:2581–9. https://doi.org/10.1016/j.arth.2020.04.025.
26. Berríos-Torres SI, Umscheid CA, Bratzler DW, Leas B, Stone EC, Kelz RR, Reinke CE, Morgan S, Solomkin JS, Mazuski JE, Dellinger EP, Itani KMF, Berbari EF, Segreti J, Parvizi J, Blanchard J, Allen G, Kluytmans JAJW, Donlan R, Schecter WP, Healthcare Infection Control Practices Advisory Committee. Centers for Disease Control and Prevention guideline for the prevention of surgical site infection, 2017. JAMA Surg. 2017;152:784–91. https://doi.org/10.1001/jamasurg.2017.0904.

Chapter 4
Perioperative Hemodynamic Monitoring for High Risk Surgical Patients

Raj Madhani, Jingyuan Biaesch, and Austin Puchany

Introduction

The administration of anesthesia leads to physiologic perturbations, including changes to hemodynamic regulation. These changes are primarily driven by loss of sympathetic drive leading to decreased vascular tone, blood pressure, and cardiac output [1–3]. This results in decreased perfusion and oxygenation of vital end organs including the brain, heart, and kidneys, leading to anesthesia-related morbidity and mortality. Mortality rates related to or directly caused by anesthesia are currently estimated to be 0.82 in 100,000 surgical in-patients [4]. This is a vast improvement since the 1940s when 100 in 100,000 (1 in 1000) healthy surgical patients died from anesthesia [5].

In one meta-analysis of over 3000 cases, optimizing hemodynamics reduced the number of major and minor postoperative gastrointestinal complications [6]. In another study, mean arterial pressures depressed by 30% led to an increased risk of postoperative stroke in non-cardiac and non-neurosurgical procedures [7]. Hypotension during non-cardiac surgeries has demonstrated an increased risk of postoperative myocardial infarction and acute kidney injury as well [8]. Clearly, hemodynamics guided patient management plays an essential role in achieving more positive outcomes, and in reducing poor perioperative courses. To that end, proper hemodynamic data acquisition and interpretation is required.

R. Madhani (✉) · J. Biaesch · A. Puchany
Department of Anesthesiology and Perioperative Medicine, University of Pittsburgh Medical Center, Pittsburgh, PA, USA
e-mail: rxm656@jefferson.edu; maj6@upmc.edu; puchanyaj@upmc.edu

© The Author(s), under exclusive license to Springer Nature Switzerland AG 2024

J. Faintuch, S. Faintuch (eds.), *Recent Strategies in High Risk Surgery*,
https://doi.org/10.1007/978-3-031-56270-9_4

Defining High-Risk Patients

With a wide array of hemodynamic monitoring tools available, deciding what resources to use can often become overwhelming, inefficient, and expensive. As with many aspects of medicine, a patient-specific approach can assist with these decisions; thus, it is important to consider each patient on a case-by-case basis to determine their monitoring needs. This starts with risk stratification by identifying the high-risk surgical patient. This subset of patients composes approximately 12% of all surgical patients but accounts for over 80% of surgical mortality [9].

Risk Index Calculators

Traditionally, high-risk surgical patients were those with a greater than 5% chance of mortality or twice the risk of mortality for a specific procedure when compared to the general population [10]. The problem with this assumption is the focus on mortality alone. As an aid to this narrow approach, a variety of risk index calculators has been created to assess for perioperative complications. Many scores for surgical use as well as for critical patients in general are available for online assessment at mdcalc.com along with other more specific platforms such as the American College of Surgeons—ACS-NSQIP.

American Society of Anesthesiologists Physical Status (ASA-PS)

The classic American Society of Anesthesiologists Physical Status (ASA-PS) is a six-level classification system that establishes and communicates a patient's pre-anesthesia medical comorbidities. While it does not explicitly calculate perioperative risk, it can be used in conjunction with other factors like type of surgery, age, and frailty to assess risk. Table 4.1 outlines this system [11]. The simplicity of this classification system is also its weakness. It has been shown to have moderate inter-rater reliability among anesthesiologists and lower inter-rater reliability among physicians of different specialties [12, 13]. When there is discordance among raters, a statistically significant increase in 30-day and 1-year mortality of the patient has been shown [13].

Numerous studies have demonstrated its utility despite the potential for discordance and the ASA's original purpose. Class I patients have a 0.1% mortality rate, while class V patients have a 93.3% mortality rate [10]. The classification system has also demonstrated its ability to predict the risk of readmission [14].

Table 4.1 American Society of Anesthesiologists Physical Status Classification [11]

ASA-PS Level	Definition
I	Normal healthy patient (non smoker, non drinker)
II	Patient with mild systemic disease (uncomplicated pregnancy, well controlled comorbidities)
III	Patient with severe systemic disease (poorly controlled chronic diseases, dialysis dependent renal failure)
IV	Patient with severe systemic disease that is a constant threat to life (severe cardiovascular event <3 months, shock, low ejection fraction)
V	Moribund patient not expected to survive without the surgery (ruptured aortic aneurysm, major intracranial bleed, ischemic bowel)
VI	Declared brain-dead

Revised Cardiac Risk Index (RCRI)

The Revised Cardiac Risk Index (RCRI) was created and validated in 1999 to assess the risk of major adverse cardiac complications in patients undergoing noncardiac surgery. These complications include myocardial infarction (MI), pulmonary edema, ventricular fibrillation or primary cardiac arrest, and complete heart block. This index uses six, independent factors namely, high-risk surgical procedure, history of ischemic heart disease, heart failure, cerebrovascular disease, preoperative treatment with insulin, and preoperative serum creatinine greater than 2.0 mg/dL [15]. Having at least two of these predictive factors leads to elevated risk. RCRI differentiates well between low and high-risk for noncardiac surgery. However, it has limited ability in vascular surgery and kidney transplant [16, 17].

American College of Surgeons National Surgical Quality Improvement Program (ACS-NSQIP)

The American College of Surgeons National Surgical Quality Improvement Program Universal Surgical Risk Calculator (ACS-NSQIP) was started in 2013 with data acquired from 393 hospitals and over 1.4 million patients, and is continuously improved. This tool considers 21 preoperative factors that cover demographics, comorbidities, and procedures [18]. Similar to a few other scores, ACS-NSQIP factors in ASA-PS which was previously discussed. Additionally, this vast calculator database factors in over 1500 unique Current Procedural Terminology codes when determining surgical risks. ACS-NSQIP uses patient-specific inputs and generates risk predictions for categories including cardiac complications such as cardiac arrest or myocardial infarction, pneumonia, surgical site infection, urinary tract infection, venous thromboembolism, renal failure, readmission, return to the operating room, death, discharge to an advanced care facility, sepsis, and predicted length of stay.

This risk stratification tool has the advantage of being comprehensive yet standardized. It considers a wide range of patient- and procedure-specific factors and relays risk stratification for a variety of complications. It is important to note that while ACS-NSQIP determines the risk of various cardiac complications, it does not specifically capture the risk associated with pulmonary edema and complete heart block [19]. Thus, it cannot completely replace RCRI but can be used in conjunction with it. Furthermore, the calculator was developed from patient databases acquired from 10% of hospitals in the United States that conduct 30% of the country's surgical procedures and has not been externally validated [18]. Despite these limitations, ACS-NSQIP provides useful risk stratification data that can allow for strategic perioperative surgical planning.

Physiological and Operative Severity Score for the Enumeration of Mortality and Morbidity (POSSUM)

The POSSUM system utilizes both preoperative and intraoperative conditions to determine postoperative morbidity and mortality [20]. Each category is scored 1–4 with a corresponding graded value. The summative score for the preoperative and intraoperative variables is inserted into a formula and then morbidity and mortality are calculated (Table 4.2).

The POSSUM score is a complex mathematical equation, yet available at mdcalc.com. It tends to overestimate morbidity and mortality in low-risk patients and underestimate in extreme age and in emergency surgical situations [19]. The Portsmouth-POSSUM (P-POSSUM) score is a modified equation of the original POSSUM score that appears to mitigate this overestimation [21]. Because this score cannot be calculated until the end of the procedure, its utility is limited to postoperative care. Though the score does not aid in the preoperative and intraoperative anticipation and preparation for hemodynamic monitoring, it does indicate which patients may need closer postoperative hemodynamic monitoring. It is also non-exclusive to any surgical specialty and has been validated in multiple continents [19].

Table 4.2 Physiological and Operative Severity Score for the Enumeration of Mortality and Morbidity (POSSUM score) [20]

Preoperative Variables	Intraoperative Variables
Age, chest X-ray, cardiac and pulmonary conditions, systolic blood pressure, pulse rate, Glasgow coma score, blood urea nitrogen, Na+, K+, hemoglobin, white blood cell count, electrocardiogram	Operative magnitude and urgency, operations within 30 days, blood loss, peritoneal contamination, malignancy

Surgical Apgar Score (SAS)

SAS calculates the 30-day postoperative risk of morbidity and mortality for general and vascular surgeries [22]. Each factor is given a graded score and the total sum is added to determine risk. It has been widely validated however appears to be less predictive in procedures where regional anesthesia is used [23]. Similar to ACS-NSQIP, SAS has been studied in combination with ASA-PS and found to augment postoperative risk prediction [24]. Analogous to POSSUM, it is calculated postoperatively and thus cannot help with preoperative preparation.

Functional Capacity Assessment

Functional capacity refers to the body's ability to uptake oxygen for use in aerobic metabolism to partake in activities of daily living [25]. Though it is mathematically defined by the maximal oxygen uptake based on cardiac output and arteriovenous oxygen difference at maximal exertion, it is typically represented as metabolic equivalents (MET). One MET is equivalent to basal energy usage, and can be thought of as the resting metabolic state within a given context. METs for activities of daily living are quantified, available electronically, and used to assess a patient's functional capacity [26].

Less than four METs are determined to be high-risk for perioperative complications and require further preoperative cardiac evaluation, such as cardiopulmonary exercise testing [27]. Subjective assessment of functional capacity involves asking patients about their ability to complete common activities of daily living. For example, four METs are the equivalent of climbing two flights of stairs. Subjective, patient-reported METs have demonstrated low sensitivity and thus cannot reliably exclude poor functional capacity [28].

The gold standard for determining functional capacity is cardiopulmonary exercise testing (CPET) [19]. This costly and time-consuming test does not represent a viable method for all patients undergoing surgery. An appropriate alternative would be to conduct an initial screening to determine who might need CPET. The Duke Activity Status Index (DASI) represents this alternative. DASI is a self-administered standardized questionnaire that has been validated as an accurate surrogate for functional capacity assessment [29]. Each question corresponds to a weighted value which is added together to determine functional status that positively correlates to METs. While it does not substitute for the accuracy of the CPET, it decreases the total number of patients who may need further testing.

Biomarkers

Most postoperative MIs are "silent" as patients do not display typical ischemic symptoms [30]. 30-day mortality rates are elevated in patients who experience a postoperative MI, with the majority occurring within 48 h of surgery. Thus, there is a need to identify those patients who are potentially at increased risk for cardiac morbidity and mortality. Natriuretic peptides, including B-type natriuretic peptide (BNP) and N-terminal-pro BNP (NTP-BNP), and cardiac troponin are two extensively studied biomarkers for perioperative risk stratification [19, 31]. Natriuretic peptides are released in response to ventricular dysfunction stemming from cardiac wall stretching. Troponins are released in response to cardiac ischemia and wall damage [3].

Both preoperative and postoperative BNP and NTP-BNP measurements have demonstrated significant predictability for 30- and 180-day mortality and cardiac morbidity in patients undergoing noncardiac surgery [32]. Threshold values for postoperative elevated risk include a BNP greater than 245 pg/mL and NTP-BNP greater than 718 pg/mL. The same concept holds true for perioperative troponin measurements. Both elevated preoperative and postoperative troponin measurements are independent predictors of 30-day mortality [31, 33]. Finally, these biomarkers have demonstrated augmentation of RCRI's ability to predict adverse cardiac events [34]. Current studies do not demonstrate how knowledge of these biomarkers can lead to directed therapeutics to improve outcomes [19]. One component of this solution will likely be to maintain comprehensive perioperative hemodynamic monitoring.

Standard ASA Monitors

The American Society of Anesthesiologists has created standards for basic anesthetic monitoring to be used in all procedures that utilize general, regional, or monitored anesthetic care, except for laboring obstetric patients and practice of pain management. The standard requirements include monitoring oxygenation, ventilation, circulation, and temperature [35]. These parameters are essential to the practice of anesthesiology. In higher-risk patients, a series of invasive and non-invasive devices can augment basic monitoring and should be utilized on a case-by-case basis.

Oxygenation

Monitoring oxygenation allows for adequate oxygen delivery to end organs and prevents anaerobic respiration with consequent end-organ damage secondary to hypoxemia. To monitor oxygenation, quantitative pulse oximetry should be used. Pulse oximeters measure blood oxygen saturation/SpO_2, a surrogate for oxygen saturation of arterial hemoglobin [36]. Light-emitting probes are placed on the fingertip, earlobe, or forehead; all are areas with high vascularity. SpO_2 is generated by differential absorption of red and near-infrared light as light passes through the artery overlying the light-emitting diode. This generates a percent saturation of arterial hemoglobin. When these devices were first designed, they were generated using healthy volunteers who had their arterial oxygen saturation altered from 70% to 100%, thus SpO_2 readings less than 70% are unlikely to be reliable. Additionally, these probes rely on adequate circulation through the body part the probe is analyzing. Patients with impaired peripheral circulation may have difficulty getting accurate readings.

Plethysmographic Waveform

This is another variable that can be collected with pulse oximeter and elucidates heart rate and rhythm as well as gives insight into the volume status of the patient [36, 37]. Volume status assessment by monitoring the pulse oximeter plethysmographic waveform amplitude (dPOP) allows for targeted volume resuscitation in fluid-responsive patients [38]. dPOP is a calculation of the variability seen in plethysmographs over the respiratory cycle and has been correlated with fluid responsiveness. However, it is not easily calculated from a bedside monitor. Pleth variability index (PVI), (Masimo Corp, Irvine, USA) is an accurate surrogate calculation for dPOP [38, 39]. It is a continuous, automatic calculation based on the plethysmographic waveform and is used in conjunction with pulse oximetry monitoring.

Ventilation

To assess for ventilation qualitative clinical signs, such as chest excursion and auscultation may be beneficial, but quantitative measurement is considered superior. This can be achieved through the measurement of end-tidal carbon dioxide via capnography and/or capnometry. These devices respectively provide waveforms and numerical measurements of end-tidal carbon dioxide, to evaluate the delivery of carbon dioxide back to the lungs via circulation [35, 40]. Thus, clinicians can glean information about a patient's hemodynamic status, including cardiac output, from ventilation assessment.

Circulation

Every patient receiving anesthesia should have continuous electrocardiogram (ECG) monitoring and arterial blood pressure measurements at least every 5 min [35]. Patients under general anesthesia should also have an additional mode of circulatory evaluation. This is most often done with plethysmographic waveform but can also be achieved with pulse palpation, cardiac auscultation, monitoring of arterial blood pressure tracing, or ultrasound of peripheral pulses.

ECG monitoring conveys information regarding the heart rate and rhythm, in addition to allowing for the detection of cardiac ischemia and electrolyte derangements [41]. Typically, five-electrode ECGs are used on patients in the operating room, allowing for monitoring of all limb leads and at least one precordial lead. Leads II and V5 are the most sensitive ones in detecting intraoperative myocardial ischemia and are typically displayed on the bedside monitor. Limitations to ECG analysis include improper lead placement and signal interference during electrocautery utilization.

Intraoperative hypotension increases the risk of postoperative morbidity and mortality. Thus, reliable and frequent blood pressure measurements are required during all surgeries. While the gold standard is arterial catheterization, cuff blood pressure measurements are more routinely used [1]. Cuffs measure blood pressure using oscillometry. This method relies on inflating the cuff to supra-systolic pressures, slowly deflating the cuff, and having a pressure transducer observe the oscillations produced as blood begins to flow within the artery [42]. The pressure at which maximum oscillations occur is the measured mean arterial pressure. Each cuff manufacturer has its own algorithm to calculate the systolic and diastolic pressures using the measured mean arterial pressure.

The cuff should be 80% of the length and 40% of the width of the extremity to be measured. Cuffs too small will result in pressure improperly elevated, and cuffs too large will result in pressure falsely low [43]. Measurements are typically done on the upper arm to record brachial artery pressures. For obese patients, finding an appropriately sized cuff may be challenging. Recently, it has been found that forearm cuff measurements may be more accurate than upper arm or lower leg cuff pressures in obese patients [44].

Temperature

Induction of anesthesia results in peripheral vasodilation and a reduction in core body temperature [45]. Patients can become hypothermic without appropriate warming and proper temperature monitoring. This can lead to complications including altered drug metabolism, prolonged recovery, and coagulopathy. Core temperature can be measured from the nasopharynx, mouth, esophagus, or bladder.

Pulse Contour Analysis Devices

The pulmonary artery catheter and the Swan Ganz catheter have been employed far less in recent decades due to high risks associated with placement and maintenance [46]. According to the Society of Cardiovascular Anesthesiologists, the pulmonary artery catheter was used by 68% of respondents 75% of the time, but that it is usually used with transesophageal echocardiography as an addition, and the decision is related to the geographical region and surgeon preference [47]. Pulmonary artery catheters have decreased in sales through the years while newer pulse contour analysis devices have become more popular [48]. These are minimally invasive by simply using a finger blood pressure cuff or thoracic electrical impedance. The system obtains a cardiac output value through calibration of heart rate multiplied by stroke volume. Stroke volume is obtained through the measurement of pressure, such that an estimated flow integrated over time is calculated to volume. The system provides cardiac output, stroke volume, stroke volume variation, systemic vascular resistance, and mean arterial pressure.

Customized Information

The system is enabled to receive specific demographic data to tailor the algorithm for specific patients, such as providing an estimated cardiac output goal. The hemodynamic values can be applied to intraoperative hypotension and large volume changes. They are relatively easy to use and monitor screens display easily interpreted trends. Well known products and manufacturers include FloTrac/Vigileo technology (Edwards LifeSciences, Irvine, CA, USA), ProAQT/PulsioFlex (Pulsion Medical Systems, Munich, Germany), LiDCOrapid system (Masimo Corp, Irvine, CA, USA), and pressure recording and analytic method MostCare Up (Vygon, Ecouen, France). ClearSight system (Edwards Lifesciences, Irvine, CA, USA) is comprised the ClearSight finger cuff and EV1000 clinical platform. These products often require an invasive arterial line, except for products similar to the ClearSight finger cuff [49].

Using indirect calculations to change pressure to volume, the data tends to contain errors, notably in patients with already low systemic vascular resistance. This combination would lead to even more inaccuracies in septic patients with depressed systemic vascular resistance. However better algorithms are constantly emerging, and the elimination of invasive access fosters the popularity of the pulse contour devices.

Cerebral Hemodynamics

In intracranial neurosurgical, cardiothoracic, and large intra-abdominal vascular cases, assessing cerebral autoregulation during surgery allows for not only immediate information during intraoperative maneuvers, but provide short to long term benefits, such as decreasing risk of stroke, postoperative delirium, and length of hospital stay [50]. These include somatosensory evoked potential (SSEP), transcranial Doppler ultrasonography, brain tissue oxygen monitor, intracranial pressure (ICP)—derived pressure reactivity index (PRx), brain tissue oxygen partial pressure (PbtO2), electroencephalography(EEG), and near-infrared spectroscopy (NIRS).

Most of these techniques require trained staff, are costly, and involve a lengthy set up. In order to be cost- effective, they should not be routinely employed, but indicated on a case by case basis [51].

NIRS measures the oxygenation of the cerebral cortex as it correlates to cerebral oxygenation. The cerebral oxygen supply can be added to regional blood flow and using other patient factors such as intraoperative surgical field events, hemoglobin values, pulse oximeter, mean arterial pressure, one can estimate cerebral oxygenation capacity [52].

Invasive Arterial Pressure

Common reasons to use an arterial line encompass induced hypotension, anticipated hypotension, hemodynamic instability, and precise beat-to-beat monitoring in patients with end organ disease. Other indications involve monitoring arterial waveforms for abnormal patterns, analyzing arterial pressure waveform to help predict fluid responsiveness, and obtaining arterial blood samples [53].

Contraindications list thrombus, infection, thrombocytopenia (<30,000 per microliter of blood) or distorted anatomy (aneurysm, congenital malformation, arteriovenous fistula, stent, vascular graft) at the puncture site. Concern for lack of collateral blood flow or vascular insufficiency (peripheral artery disease or Raynaud disease) deserves mention as well [54].

Complications include local or systemic infection, bruising, edema, vasospasm, bleeding, hematoma, thromboembolism, pseudoaneurysm of arteriovenous fistula formation at the site, air embolism, or damage to surrounding structures [53]. The shape of the arterial waveform is defined by the degree of upstroke which represents contractility, and the degree of downstroke which represents peripheral vascular resistance [53]. The shape of the waveform can provide insight into different hemodynamic variables and can be altered by different pathologies involving the heart, valves, surrounding vasculature and pericardium. The mean arterial pressure (MAP) is measured in every surgery to help ensure adequate organ perfusion.

Arterial pressure waveforms measured at the periphery have higher systolic blood pressures, steeper systolic upstroke, lower diastolic blood pressure, wider pulse pressures, and lower and later dicrotic notches [55]. The level of the pressure transducer position is critical. In most cases, the transducer should be placed even with the heart, which is either 5 cm behind the sternum or at the mid axillary line in a supine patient. If patient positioning is changed, the position of the transducer should be adjusted to make sure it continues level with the heart [56].

Arterial pressure waveform analysis can be used to assess various indices such as pulse pressure variation (PPV), systolic blood pressure variation (SPV) and stroke volume variation (SVV), to help determine fluid responsiveness [57].

Central Venous Pressure

Central Venous Pressure (CVP) is defined as the pressure that blood exerts on the walls of the inferior vena cava (IVC) near the entry to the right atrium. It reflects the amount of blood returning to the heart, and is used to estimate preload to the heart. The normal range for CVP is defined as 8–12 mmHg and can fluctuate with changes in intravascular volume or venous compliance [58]. Recent studies reveal that CVP is an unreliable predictor of fluid responsiveness [58, whereas arterial pulse pressure variation (PPV) evident in mechanically ventilated patients is a sensitive and specific marker of fluid responsiveness [59], yielding decreased postoperative complications and lengths of hospital stay [60]. Right atrial pressure and jugular venous pulse pressure could be alternative markers for poor systolic heart function and volume overload.

Systolic Pressure Variation (SPV)/Pulse Pressure Variation (PPV)

These are often documented variables in critically ill patients, and are endowed with prognostic value. Nevertheless, there are many pitfalls in their interpretation and bedside use [61, 62]. In mechanically ventilated patients, the degree of respiratory variation on stroke volume (SVV) can accurately predict fluid responsiveness [63].

PPV is most effective in patients on mechanical ventilation receiving a tidal volume of 6-8 mL/kg and who are not triggering spontaneous breaths, although spontaneous breathing activity might not interfere as much as previously thought [64] Also, the patients must be in sinus rhythm as arrhythmias can affect contractility and thus pulse pressure [65].

PPV has been shown to be more effective when compared to CVP [63]. Monitoring pulse pressure variation and minimizing the change in pulse pressure through fluid administration during high-risk surgical procedures has been found to improve postoperative outcomes and decrease hospital length of stay [66].

Stroke Volume Variation

Stroke Volume variation (SVV) is classified under the same physiological principles as PPV. It is usually measured through an arterial catheter that analyzes atrial compliance and systemic vascular resistance to create the arterial pressure waveform. SVV can be calculated from this waveform, as well as from devices that measure aortic blood flow velocity such as esophageal Doppler, bioimpedance, and bioreactance. Numerous studies have found that a SVV > 10% indicates fluid responsiveness [67].

$$SVV = 100 \times (SVmax - SVmin) / SVmean$$

SVV has the same limitations as PPV, plus some additional influential factors, such as patient position. One study showed that stroke volume (SV) is decreased in patients in prone and 30 degree head-up positions. This decrease in SV leads to an increase in SVV [68]. PPV may be preferred also because the transducer used to measure SVV is more expensive and may not always be available [69].

Pulmonary Capillary Wedge Pressure

Pulmonary capillary wedge pressure (PCWP) is often used to assess left atrial pressure. It is also related to left ventricle filling pressure, left ventricle end diastolic pressure (LVEDP) and mitral valve function. During heart relaxation in a patient without mitral stenosis, the left ventricle, left atrium, and pulmonary veins are in a continuous circuit therefore PCWP is indicative of LVEDP [70]. A normal pulmonary capillary wedge pressure is considered between 4-12 mmHg. Mitral stenosis and left ventricular failure can cause elevated PCWPs [71].

PCWP is useful in circumstances of mitral stenosis, as well as for diagnosing pulmonary hypertension. This last condition triggers increased perioperative morbidity and mortality. PCWP can be used to differentiate between cardiogenic and noncardiogenic pulmonary edema. Findings greater than 18 mmHg usually indicate increased cardiac pressures which back up through the pulmonary circulation causing elevated pulmonary capillary pressures and increase capillary permeability causing edema [72]. Given the invasiveness of pulmonary artery catheter (PAC) placement, its adoption is diminishing and other devices are preferred to assess hemodynamic status [72–74].

Mixed Venous Oxygen Saturation

Mixed venous oxygen saturation (SvO2) is believed to be endowed with prognostic abilities in seriously ill patients, as abnormal values are generally associated with tissue hypoxia and higher mortality [75]. Nevertheless precision and trending ability are low and only blood collected with a distally placed pulmonary artery catheter (ScvO2) permits reliable estimations [75–80].

Echocardiography

Transthoracic (TTE) and transesophageal (TEE) echocardiography (gehealthcare.com, philips.com and others) are valuable tools for bedside evaluation of a patient's cardiopulmonary conditions. Indications for TTE in a perioperative setting should generally be reserved for assessment of hemodynamic changes that are unresolving with standard care such as volume shifts, cardiac function, or pulmonary pathology, without the use of other imaging techniques that would require patient transportation. This includes invasive surgeries such as high risk cardiac and cardiothoracic procedures, certain liver resections, and major transplantations. The indication should be based on the patient's past medical conditions as well as on ongoing alterations in cardiac structure and function. TEE is much more invasive compared to the TTE with risk of esophageal injury, and requires a competent physician for interpretation. At the same time it provides a larger array of information including cardiac output, stroke volume and intra luminal pressures. It allows for evaluation and diagnosis of structural diseases relating to the heart chambers, valves or surrounding vessels. TEE can create three dimensional views of the heart, enabling diagnosis of structural diseases relating to the heart chambers, valves or surrounding vessels. Nevertheless TEE should be reserved to teams familiar with the technique, notably for operative decisions dependent on findings of TEE [81].

References

1. De Keijzer I, Scheeren T. Perioperative hemodynamic monitoring an overview of current methods. Anesthesiol Clin. 2021;39(3):441–56.
2. Secomb T. Hemodynamics. Compr Physiol. 2017;6(2):975–1003.
3. De Backer D, Aissaoui N, Cecconi M, et al. How can assessing hemodynamics help to assess volume status? Intensive Care Med. 2022;48(10):1482–94.
4. Guohua L, Warner M, Lang B, et al. Epidemiology of anesthesia-related mortality in the United States, 1999-2005. Anesthesiology. 2009;110(4):759–65.
5. Beecher H, Todd D. A study of the deaths associated with anesthesia and surgery: based on a study of 599,548 anesthesia in ten institutions 1948-1952, inclusive. Ann Surg. 1954;140(1):2–35.
6. Giglio M, Marucci M, Testini M, et al. Goal-directed Haemodynamic therapy and gastrointestinal complications in major surgery: a meta-analysis of randomized controlled trials. Br J Anaesth. 2009;103(5):636–46.
7. Bijker J, Persoon S, Peelen L, et al. Intraoperative hypotension and perioperative ischemic stroke after general surgery: a nested case-control study. Anesthesiology. 2012;116(3):658–64.
8. Salmasi V, Maheshwari K, Yang D, et al. Relationship between intraoperative hypotension, defined by either reduction from baseline or absolute thresholds, and acute kidney and myocardial injury after noncardiac surgery: a retrospective cohort analysis. Anesthesiology. 2017;126(1):47–65.
9. Pearse R, Harrison D, James P, et al. Identification and characterisation of the high-risk surgical population in the United Kingdom. Crit Care. 2006;10(3):R81.
10. Boyd O, Jackson N. How is risk defined in high-risk surgical patient management? Crit Care. 2005;9(4):390–6.
11. Committee on Economics. ASA physical status classification system. 2020. asahq.org/standards-and-guidelines/statement-on-asa-physical-status-classification-system. Accessed 17 May 2023.
12. Sankar A, Johnson S, Beattie W, et al. Reliability of the American Society of Anesthesiologists Physical Status Scale in clinical practice. Br J Anaesth. 2014;113(3):424–32.

13. Kwa C, Cui J, Lim D, et al. Discordant American Society of Anesthesiologists Physical Status Classification between anesthesiologists and surgeons and its correlation with adverse patient outcomes. Sci Rep. 2022;12(1):7110.
14. Tran A, Mai T, El-Haddad J, et al. Preinjury ASA score as an independent predictor of readmission after major traumatic injury. Trauma Surg Acute Care Open. 2017;2(1):e000128.
15. Lee T, Marcantonio E, Mangione C, et al. Derivation and prospective validation of a simple index for prediction of cardiac risk of major noncardiac surgery. Circulation. 1999;100(10):1043–9.
16. Ford M, Beattie S, Wijeysundera D. Systematic review: prediction of perioperative cardiac complications and mortality by the revised cardiac risk index. Ann Intern Med. 2010;152(1):26–35.
17. Olsen V, Borges F, Goldraich L, et al. Limited predictive role of the revised cardiac risk index in kidney transplant: single center evaluation and comparison with international literature. Curr Probl Cardiol. 2021;46(9):100908.
18. Bilimoria K, Liu Y, Paruch J, et al. Development and evaluation of the universal ACS NSQIP surgical risk calculator: a decision aide and informed consent tool for patients and surgeons. J Am Coll Surg. 2013;217(5):833–42.
19. Bose S, Talmor D. Who is a high-risk surgical patient? Curr Opin Crit Care. 2018;24(6):547–53.
20. Copeland G. The POSSUM system of surgical audit. JAMA Surg. 2002;137(1):15–9.
21. Prytherch D, Whiteley M, Higgins B, et al. POSSUM and Portsmouth POSSUM for predicting mortality. Physiological and operative severity score for the enumeration of mortality and morbidity. Br J Surg. 1998;85(9):1217–20.
22. Cagini L, Ceccarelli S, Bracale U, et al. Intraoperative risk factors for major complications after oesophagectomy: the surgical Apgar score. Interact Cardiovasc Thorac Surg. 2022;35(4):ivac111.
23. Nair A, Bharuka A, Rayani B. The reliability of surgical Apgar score in predicting immediate and late postoperative morbidity and mortality: a narrative review. Rambam Maimonides Med J. 2018;9(1):e0004.
24. Jering M, Marolen K, Shotwell M, et al. Combining the ASA physical classification system and continuous intraoperative surgical Apgar score measurement in predicting postoperative risk. J Med Syst. 2015;39(11):147.
25. Arena R, Myers J, Williams M, et al. Assessment of functional capacity in clinical and research settings. A scientific statement from the American Heart Association Committee on exercise, rehabilitation, and prevention of the council on clinical cardiology and the council on cardiovascular nursing. Circulation. 2007;116(3):329–43.
26. Jetté M, Sidney K, Blümchen G. Metabolic equivalents (METS) in exercise testing, exercise prescription, and evaluation of functional capacity. Clin Cardiol. 1990;13(8):555–65.
27. Fleisher L, Fleischmann K, Auerbach A, et al. 2014 ACC/AHA guideline on perioperative cardiovascular evaluation and Management of Patients Undergoing Noncardiac Surgery. A report of the American College of Cardiology/American Heart Association task force on practice guidelines. Circulation. 2014;130:e278–333.
28. Wijeysundera D, Pearse R, Shulman M, et al. Assessment of functional capacity before major non-cardiac surgery: an international prospective cohort study. Lancet. 2018;391(10140):2631–40.
29. Hlatky M, Boineau R, Higginbotham M, et al. A brief self-administered questionnaire to determine functional capacity (the Duke activity status index). Am J Cardiol. 1989;64(10):651–4.
30. Devereaux P, Xavier D, Pogue J, et al. Characteristics and short-term prognosis of perioperative myocardial infarction in patients undergoing noncardiac surgery. Ann Intern Med. 2011;154(8):523–8.
31. Biccard B, Devereaux P, Rodseth R. Cardiac biomarkers in the prediction of risk in the noncardiac surgery setting. Anaesthesia. 2014;69(5):484–93.
32. Rodseth R, Biccard B, Manach Y, et al. The prognostic value of pre-operative and postoperative B-type natriuretic peptides in patients undergoing noncardiac surgery: B-type natriuretic peptide and N-terminal fragment of pro-B-type natriuretic peptide: a systematic review and individual patient data meta-analysis. J Am Coll Cardiol. 2014;63(2):170–80.

33. Zhao B, Liu W, Deng Q, et al. Meta-analysis of preoperative high-sensitivity cardiac troponin measurement in non-cardiac surgical patients at risk of cardiovascular complications. Br J Surg. 2020;107(2):e81–90.
34. Vernooij L, van Klei W, Moons K, et al. The comparative and added prognostic value of biomarkers to the revised cardiac risk index for preoperative prediction of major adverse cardiac events and all-cause mortality in patients who undergo noncardiac surgery. Cochrane Database Syst Rev. 2021;12(12):CD013139.
35. Committee on Standards and Practice Parameters. Standards for Basic Anesthetic Monitoring. 2020. asahq.org/standards-and-guidelines/standards-for-basic-anesthetic-monitoring. Accessed 17 May 2023.
36. Chan E, Chan M, Chan M. Pulse oximetry: understanding its basic principles facilitates appreciation of its limitations. Respir Med. 2013;107(6):789–99.
37. Cannesson M, Talke P. Recent advances in pulse oximetry. F1000 Med Rep. 2009;1:66.
38. Cannesson M, Delannoy B, Morand A, et al. Does the Pleth variability index indicate the respiratory-induced variation in the Plethysmogram and arterial pressure waveforms? Anesth Analg. 2008;106(4):1189–94.
39. Cannesson M, Attof Y, Rosamel P, et al. Respiratory variations in pulse oximetry Plethysmographic waveform amplitude to predict fluid responsiveness in the operating room. Anesthesiology. 2007;106(6):1105–11.
40. Richardson M, Moulton K, Rabb D, et al. Capnography for monitoring end-tidal CO_2 in hospital and pre-hospital settings: a health technology assessment. Ottawa: CADTH; 2016.
41. John A, Fleisher L. Electrocardiography: the ECG. Anesthesiol Clin. 2006;24(4):697–715.
42. Roach J, Thiele R. Perioperative blood pressure monitoring. Best Pract Res Clin Anaesthesiol. 2019;33(2):127–38.
43. Sprafka J, Strickland D, Gomez-Marin O, et al. The effect of cuff size on blood pressure Management in Adults. Epidemiology. 1991;2(3):214–7.
44. Schumann R, Meidert A, Bonney I, et al. Intraoperative blood pressure monitoring in obese patients: arterial catheter, finger cuff, and Oscillometry. Anesthesiology. 2021;134:179–88.
45. Sessler D. Perioperative thermoregulation and heat balance. Lancet. 2016;387(10038):2655–64.
46. Bender JS, Smith-Meek MA, Jones CE. Routine pulmonary artery catheterization does not reduce morbidity and mortality of elective vascular surgery: results of a prospective, randomized trial. Ann Surg. 1997;226:229–36.
47. Judge O, Ji F, Fleming N, Liu H. Current use of the pulmonary artery catheter in cardiac surgery: a survey study. J Cardiothorac Vasc Anesth. 2015;29:69–75.
48. Staylor A. Recent trends in haemodynamic monitoring. USA: Medtech Insight; 2010.
49. Edwards Lifesciences Corporation. FloTrac sensor. 2023. https://www.edwards.com/healthcare-professionals/products-services/hemodynamic-monitoring/flotrac. Accessed 15 May 2023.
50. Zipser CM, Deuel J, Ernst J, et al. The predisposing and precipitating risk factors for delirium in neurosurgery: a prospective cohort study of 949 patients. Acta Neurochir. 2019;161:1307–15.
51. Arora D, Mehta Y. Recent trends on hemodynamic monitoring in cardiac surgery. Ann Card Anaesth. 2016;19(4):580–3. https://doi.org/10.4103/0971-9784.191557.
52. Rivera-Lara L, Geocadin R, Zorrilla-Vaca A, et al. Near-infrared spectroscopy derived cerebral autoregulation indices independently predict clinical outcome in acutely ill comatose patients. J Neurosurg Anesthesiol. 2020;32(3):234–41.
53. Butterworth J, Mackey D, Wasnick J. Cardiovascular monitoring. In: Morgan and Mikhail's clinical anesthesiology. 6th ed. New York: McGraw-Hill Education; 2018. p. 86–90.
54. AARC clinical practice guideline. Sampling for arterial blood gas analysis. American Association for Respiratory Care. Respir Care. 1992;37:913.
55. Weiss BM, Pasch T. Measurement of systemic arterial pressure. Curr Opin Anaesthesiol. 1997;10:459.
56. Gardner RM. Direct blood pressure measurement—dynamic response requirements. Anesthesiology. 1981;54:227.

57. Thiele RH, Bartels K, Gan TJ. Inter-device differences in monitoring for goal-directed fluid therapy. Can J Anaesth. 2015;62:169.
58. Russell PS, Hong J, Windsor JA, Itkin M, ARJ P. Renal lymphatics: anatomy, physiology, and clinical implications. Front Physiol. 2019;10:251.
59. Senthelal S, Maingi M. Physiology, jugular venous pulsation. In: StatPearls [internet]. Treasure Island (FL): StatPearls Publishing; 2022.
60. Michard F. Changes in arterial pressure during mechanical ventilation. Anesthesiology. 2005;103:419–28.
61. Stevens SL, Wood S, Koshiaris C, et al. Blood pressure variability and cardiovascular disease: systematic review and meta-analysis. BMJ. 2016;354:i4098.
62. Flick M, Sand U, Bergholz A, et al. Right ventricular and pulmonary artery pulse pressure variation and systolic pressure variation for the prediction of fluid responsiveness: an interventional study in coronary artery bypass surgery patients. J Clin Monit Comput. 2022;36(6):1817–25.
63. Marik PE, Cavallazzi R, Vasu T, Hirani A. Dynamic changes in arterial waveform derived variables and fluid responsiveness in mechanically ventilated patients: a systematic review of the literature. Crit Care Med. 2009;37:2642–7.
64. Grassi P, Lo Nigro L, Battaglia K, Barone M, Testa F, Berlot G. Pulse pressure variation as a predictor of fluid responsiveness in mechanically ventilated patients with spontaneous breathing activity: a pragmatic observational study. HSR Proc Intensive Care Cardiovasc Anesth. 2013;5(2):98–109.
65. Pinsky MR. Functional haemodynamic monitoring. Curr Opin Crit Care. 2014;20:288.
66. Lopes MR, Oliveira MA, Pereira VOS, et al. Goal-directed fluid management based on pulse pressure variation monitoring during high-risk surgery: a pilot randomized controlled trial. Crit Care. 2007;11:R100.
67. Pinsky MR. Functional hemodynamic monitoring. Curr Opin Crit Care. 2014;20:288.
68. Daihua Y, Wei C, Xude S, et al. The effect of body position changes on stroke volume variation in 66 mechanically ventilated patients with sepsis. J Crit Care. 2012;27:416.e7.
69. Rathore A, Singh S, Lamsal R, et al. Validity of pulse pressure variation (PPV) compared with stroke volume variation (SVV) in predicting fluid responsiveness. Turk J Anaesthesiol Reanim. 2017;45(4):210–7.
70. Pour-Ghaz I, Manolukas T, Foray N, et al. Accuracy of non-invasive and minimally invasive hemodynamic monitoring: where do we stand? Ann Transl Med. 2019, 2019, 7;(17):421.
71. Simmons J, Ventetuolo CE. Cardiopulmonary monitoring of shock. Curr Opin Crit Care. 2017;23(3):223–31.
72. Clark SB, Soos MP. Noncardiogenic pulmonary edema. Treasure Island (FL): StatPearls Publishing; 2022.
73. Oliveira RK, Ferreira EV, Ramos RP, et al. Usefulness of pulmonary capillary wedge pressure as a correlate of left ventricular filling pressures in pulmonary arterial hypertension. J Heart Lung Transplant. 2014;33(2):157–62.
74. Fortuni F, Tavazzi G, De Ferrari GM. Pulmonary Artery Catheter in Cardiogenic Shock: Will the Benefits Finally Outweigh the Costs and Complications? JACC Heart Fail. 2021;9(4):322–3.
75. Accuracy, Precision, and Trending Ability of Perioperative Lanning KM, Erkinaro TM, Ohtonen PP, et al. Central venous oxygen saturation compared to mixed venous oxygen saturation in unselected cardiac surgical patients. J Cardiothorac Vasc Anesth. 2022;36(7):1995–2001.
76. Kearney TJ, Shabot MM. Pulmonary artery rupture associated with the swan-Ganz catheter. Chest. 1995;108(5):1349–52.
77. Hartog C, Bloos F. Venous oxygen saturation. Best Pract Res Clin Anaesthesiol. 2014;28(4):419–28.
78. van Beest P, Wietasch G, Scheeren T, et al. Clinical review: use of venous oxygen saturations as a goal - a yet unfinished puzzle. Crit Care. 2011;15(5):232.

79. Evans L, Rhodes A, Alhazzani W, et al. international guidelines for management of severe sepsis and septic shock, 2021. Intensive Care Med. 2021;47(11):1181–247.
80. Cereuil A, Ronflé R, Culver A, et al. Septic shock: phenotypes and outcomes. Adv Ther. 2022;39(11):5058–71.
81. Efrimescu CI, Moorthy A, Griffin M. Rescue transesophageal echocardiography: a narrative review of current knowledge and practice. J Cardiothorac Vasc Anesth. 2023;37(4):584–600.

Part II
Lifestyle Interventions

Chapter 5
Prehabilitation for Gastrointestinal Cancer Surgery

Joel Lambert, Daren Subar, and Christopher Gaffney

Abbreviations

COPD	Chronic Obstructive Pulmonary Disease
COVID-19	Coronavirus disease 2019
CPET	Cardiopulmonary Exercise Test
ECG	Electrocardiography
ERAS	Enhanced Recovery After Surgery
ESPEN	European Society for Clinical Nutrition and Metabolism
GI	Gastrointestinal
MDT	Multi-Disciplinary Team
MUST	Malnutrition Universal Screening Tool
NHS	National Health Service
NIHR	National Institute of Health Research
RCT	Randomised Controlled Trial
SPECS	**S**tandard care versus **P**rehabilitation in patients undergoing **E**lective hepatopancreatobiliary and colorectal **C**ancer **S**urgery
WHO	World Health Organisation

J. Lambert · D. Subar
Lancaster Medical School, Lancaster University, Lancaster, UK

East Lancashire Hospitals NHS Trust, Blackburn, UK

BRIDGES Research Group, Department of General Surgery, Royal Blackburn Teaching Hospitals NHS Trust, Blackburn, UK
e-mail: j.lambert1@lancaster.ac.uk; Daren.Subar@elht.nhs.uk

C. Gaffney (✉)
Lancaster Medical School, Lancaster University, Lancaster, UK
e-mail: c.gaffney@lancaster.ac.uk

© The Author(s), under exclusive license to Springer Nature Switzerland AG 2024

J. Faintuch, S. Faintuch (eds.), *Recent Strategies in High Risk Surgery*,
https://doi.org/10.1007/978-3-031-56270-9_5

Prehabilitation: What Does It Mean in Healthcare Contexts?

"Prehabilitation" [1, 2] is a term used to capture interventions to prepare patients for healthcare treatment, typically surgery. Like a marathon, surgery is a huge stressor on the human body and training in the form of prehabilitation prepares the body for this challenge. Prehabilitation interventions typically comprise of exercise, nutrition, and psycho-social support [2] but are multi-factorial and even encompass the management of tobacco [3], alcohol [4], and other addictions.

Prehabilitation can improve cardiorespiratory fitness before cancer surgery [5], which improves functional capacity and reduces hospital length of stay [2], thus offering patient-centred and economic benefits. Indeed, prehabilitation has the potential to reduce the peri-operative risk profiles of patients who are deemed unfit for major operations. It is generally accepted that reducing complication rates and a quicker return to baseline functional capacity can accelerate the progression of cancer patients to chemotherapy. Reduced time to chemotherapy has been seen in some cancer cohorts to offer a survival benefit [6]. We have yet to identify a prehabilitation strategy that works for everyone; and like many exercise interventions [7], there is a heterogenous response to prehabilitation.

What Should Prehabilitation Comprise of?

Exercise

Programmes are designed to improve cardiovascular fitness and physiological reserve, to build muscle and improve strength, and augment well-being and psychological resilience. Most exercise programmes comprise of a combination of aerobic and strength training, delivered via a supervised or unsupervised format. This may involve a graded regime where patients complete a form of aerobic training at a percentage of their maximal heart rate, and increase this percentage every week to achieve a specified level of exertion (mild, moderate, or high intensity).

Published data suggests that bespoke supervised exercise interventions outperform unsupervised formats in achieving exertional intensity and compliance. Breathing exercises have also been suggested as a useful way of improving the function of the muscles of breathing and as a stress-reduction strategy [8].

Patients diagnosed with gastrointestinal (GI) malignancies often present with a series of clinical signs including tiredness, weight loss, anaemia, and jaundice. These signs often coincide with long periods of under-nutrition and deconditioning. The highest frequency of GI malignancy presentation is within the sixth to eighth decades, where sarcopenia may be another compounding factor. Several recent studies have alluded to poor muscle quality and function as an independent predictor of adjuvant chemotherapy toxicity, morbidity, and mortality in GI cancer surgery [9, 10].

Diminished Oxidative Stress

There is evidence to suggest that exercise may modulate the tumour micro-environment by reducing pro-inflammatory mediators associated with tumour spread [11]. Exercise may play an anti-inflammatory role by reducing oxidative stress [12], which may be important in patients undergoing concurrent chemotherapy and radiotherapy treatment. Although the psychological aspects of exercise within prehabilitation have not been extensively studied, there is evidence to suggest that exercise may improve psychological resilience peri-operatively [13]. This could be paramount in patients living with indolent or recurrent disease.

Within the clinical context, cardiopulmonary exercise testing (CPET), peak expiratory flow rates, and hand grip strength may be used to objectively measure improvements in fitness. However, outside clinical trials, these measures are rarely used for this purpose due to cancer target times, resourcing, and scheduling constraints. The challenge in designing exercise regimes revolves around a protocol that is acceptable in terms of ease of completion and scalability, while also being effective with high compliance and adherence.

Nutrition

The main goal of nutrition in prehabilitation is to first ensure that patients are eucaloric, then aiming to supplement macronutrients and micronutrients guided by a dietician within a multi-disciplinary team (MDT). This process often involves screening using the Malnutrition Universal Screening Tool (MUST), which is common in the UK settings but also used worldwide and based on the most recent European Society of Clinical Nutrition and Metabolism (ESPEN) guidelines . In addition, in patients with malignant biliary obstruction, pancreatic enzyme replacement therapy was associated with improved survival [14]. Within clinical practice, it would be beneficial to supplement patients as early as possible within their treatment pathways, and even prior to enrolment on a formal prehabilitation programme.

Although there is no specific nutrition regime that guarantees caloric goal achievement, carbohydrate, protein, fat, and micronutrient supplementation are commonplace. In GI cancer patients, there is often weight loss directly because of mechanical obstruction and/or malabsorption, and indirectly through tumour wasting effects or cachexia, often mediated through cytokine signalling pathways [15].

Commercial Supplements

Several regimes including whey protein [16, 17], fortified protein drinks [18], and amino acid-based compounds [19] have been used in controlled trial settings and more liberally based on hospital protocols. As a standalone measure, the impact of nutrition on outcomes has been difficult to quantify due to the integrated biological and physiological pathways through which nutrition may exert its effects. Details from prehabilitation trials involving supplementation suggest that timing of ingestion; usually just prior to or after exercise may be more beneficial as this relates to metabolism of substrates, especially regimes focused on building muscle.

The effect of nutrition may be best appreciated when employed within a multi-modal programme due to its synergy with exercise. Various delivery methods such as nasogastric, nasojejunal, and gastrostomy routes may be used in cases where there may be some anatomical anomaly, other gut dysfunction, or where feeding needs to be accelerated. Parenteral feeding is now indicated only in exceptional circumstances given its high costs, substantial morbidity, and inferior benefits.

Psycho-Social Support

Talking therapies and formal counselling, when integrated into multi-modal prehabilitation programmes, are associated with reduced levels of treatment related stress [20, 21]. As previously mentioned, there appears to be a positive association between exercise and improved well-being/psychological resilience. What is clear from other data concerning psychological challenges in cancer diagnoses in general, is that there may be several interrelated factors (biological, personal, and social) in the way patients perceive and manage illness [22]. Meaningful relationships, family support, baseline health, prior illnesses, and cancer diagnoses all contribute to the way patients may choose to deal with their illness, and their levels of engagement with cancer care teams.

Cessation of Smoking and Alcohol

It is now universal practice to support patients with nicotine and alcohol dependence by offering advice and interventions to facilitate cessation. These may take the form of pharmacological treatments such as nicotine replacement or psychosocial therapies. Smoking cessation may improve patients exercise tolerance and when considered within a prehabilitation exercise programme is likely to improve adherence. Likewise, alcohol dependence is often associated with macronutrient and micronutrient deficiencies that may impact on substrate utilisation and impede the positive adaptive effects following exercise.

While these interventions are likely to work alongside prehabilitation programmes, they are also important public health interventions that have long been established in the promotion of healthier lifestyles. The evidence suggests that smoking cessation for even relatively short durations preoperatively (2 weeks) [23] can reduce morbidity and complications in the peri-operative period.

Obesity Reduction

While prehabilitation may provide a platform for patients to adopt more healthy lifestyles postoperatively, in clinical practice, it is often unrealistic to expect considerable weight reduction within cancer operative timescales. For this reason, the success of prehabilitation programmes will inevitably depend on a community-based approach in promoting healthier lifestyles as part of a wider cancer risk reduction strategy.

Management of Other Medical Conditions and Pharmacological Treatments

Other important factors centred around peri-operative care include management of preoperative anaemia, blood glucose, rationalisation of medications, and optimising the treatment of any underlying chronic cardiorespiratory conditions such as atrial fibrillation, heart failure, and chronic obstructive pulmonary disease (COPD). Within healthcare systems, entire departments have evolved to adopt this important aspect of peri-operative optimisation. They are often given names such as 'Surgery School' to focus patients minds as to what they are likely to encounter when referred. In addition to giving procedure specific information, patients are also signposted to resources and support groups, and are given key-worker contact details. This aspect of care is often delivered by a multi-disciplinary team (MDT).

How Long Should Prehabilitation Be?

One of the greatest challenges of prehabilitation is the limited time available to intervene, particularly in circumstances of cancer. Unlike rehabilitation or enhanced recovery after surgery (ERAS) [24] where there are no time pressures, the National Health Service (NHS) in the UK and other world-healthcare bodies have timelines to start treatment, to maximise treatment outcomes. Indeed, prehabilitation should, where possible, not interfere with these timelines and rarely exceeds 31 days from a decision to treat. This timescale suggests that ideally one should start prehabilitation even before the point of diagnosis.

To manipulate changes in physiological function such as muscle metabolism or cardiorespiratory fitness, the minimum period to exert viable improvements is likely 2–4 weeks [21, 25]. Smoking and alcohol cessation are likely to complement and enhance the effectiveness of other strategies such as exercise and nutrition. Targets of cardiovascular fitness such as anaerobic threshold and peak oxygen consumption can be achieved on a 6-week high intensity exercise programme [26]. In turn, weight reduction in obese patients is likely to take much longer.

Cancer 4–6 Week Protocols

These are average routines, within a wider range. Patients undergoing long-course chemoradiotherapy for advanced rectal cancer have much longer times to participate in prehabilitation programmes, in some cases up to 9 weeks [27]. Within clinical trial environments, high motivation may influence the likelihood of completing prehabilitation regimes. In real life, chemo or radiotherapy side-effects preclude participation or completion of programmes, besides time constraints with cancer targets, personal patient factors, and surgery dates. Rather than offer a generic programme for a large cross-section of patients, resources may have to be targeted to the most 'at risk' groups, customised to their needs.

What Protocols are Typically Employed for Prehabilitation?

One author is currently involved in an NIHR study to map prehabilitation services across the UK (NIHR134282). Data collected to date show a wide spectrum of practice ranging from hospitals delivering no formal prehabilitation programmes to established, research-informed, multi-modal prehabilitation offers to most cancer patients. Those that offer prehabilitation programmes often fall into two groups (preoperative interventions versus pre- and postoperative interventions). In general, for gastrointestinal cancer surgery, the total time available before surgery is rarely over 9–12 weeks, with most being 4–6 weeks; this period is often dictated by the type of cancer and whether neoadjuvant therapy is required prior to surgery. Other factors such as correction of anaemia, biliary drainage, and pharmacological optimisation of chronic conditions may also extend the time before surgery and offer a longer window for prehabilitation.

Who Should Deliver Prehabilitation?

The world's population is ageing such that by 2050, the number of over-60 s will nearly double from 12% to 22% [28]. This will further stress healthcare systems across the globe and indeed, in the UK, waiting lists for elective surgery are currently the longest on record with 7.3 million people [29].

Prehabilitation is essential to optimise patient outcomes, but nonetheless, represents an additional burden on top of already stretched healthcare providers such as the NHS. Many prehabilitation programmes are delivered as part of the multi-disciplinary team (MDT) managing a patient's overall cancer care. The exercise interventions themselves can be delivered by local council gyms, private health clubs, and even football clubs in a local community, harnessing the power of existing infrastructure [30]. Nutrition advice can be delivered in these environments and also in local community settings such as you have for weight-loss clubs or similar.

Prehabilitation Clinics

These could be delivered by the private sector. They would need to include cardiopulmonary exercise testing (CPET), dietary analysis, and provision of dietary advice, and access to councillors or clinical psychologists, to ensure the psychological welfare of those undergoing prehabilitation. There is also the potential to empower patients to undertake prehabilitation themselves, seeking advice from both within and external to the MDT, perhaps including community support groups. This approach does, however, have potential risks. Cancer patients are clinically vulnerable and it's important that any intervention whether inpatient, outpatient or in the community is research informed, and those delivering any service are appropriately trained and resourced to deal with adverse events that are more likely in this than the general population.

How Could We Facilitate Remote Prehabilitation?

Remote prehabilitation removes any space or human resource requirement from healthcare providers, and it is scalable across a population at limited cost. However, adherence rates fall from >95% in hospital-based (supervised) prehabilitation interventions to 70% in remote unsupervised prehabilitation [31]. Compliance is a major determinant of the success, and the protocol should be similarly tailored to the patient's aerobic fitness, lifestyle, and personal preferences where appropriate [32]. It is also critical that some level of supervision is maintained throughout any intervention, to maximise adherence [32].

We can learn a lot from the space industry where exercise and nutrition interventions, and medical care, have been delivered remotely since 1971, onboard a space station, the Soviet Union's Salyut [33]. Two basic principles from spaceflight missions and telemedicine can be adopted for remote Prehabilitation: gastrointestinal cancer surgery: (1) health screening and (2) remote monitoring and communication.

Principles of Telehealth

High-risk participants may not be suitable for a remote intervention where medical help may not immediately be at hand. These might include cases with frailty who are at high risk of falls [34] but also cardiovascular abnormalities such as atrial fibrillation, where exercise might pose a threat of a significant adverse event, or those with a VO_2 peak (highest amount of oxygen consumed during exercise) $\leq$18 mL/min/kg [35]. Remote supervision can also be highly relevant. Depending on the patient and the intervention, this may need to be real-time monitoring of heart rate or ECG. It could encompass the delivery of exercise interventions over web-based video platforms, or online consultations with psychotherapists. A key tenet of remote interventions is that participants do not feel they are left to do things completely independently, as we know this negatively affects compliance with interventions and ultimately leads to high attrition rates [36].

The advent of new healthcare technologies (wearable devices) could be used to monitor the health of participants whilst exercising and advise the participant to adjust their effort accordingly.

How Can We Harness New Technologies to Facilitate Remote Prehabilitation?

The window between diagnosis and surgical treatment presents a unique opportunity where patients are more engaged and motivated for positive behaviour change, to maximise their health outcomes [37]. However, large scale implementation of prehabilitation is challenging due to the gap that currently exists between the resources and demands of healthcare services [38]. The use of digital technologies, so-called telehealth or telemedicine forms part of a solution to this problem, to deliver prehabilitation in a sustainable and efficient way [39]. Engagement in a patient's own treatment has been shown to improve patient outcomes [40] and home-based prehabilitation can be used to empower patients to play an active role in their treatment pre-surgery.

One of our own prehabilitation studies (SPECS, NCT04880772) employed a remote prehabilitation intervention as the study was started during the pandemic. The delivery of the exercise prehabilitation classes remotely over a web-based platform removed the need for patients (typically clinically vulnerable) to enter an environment with known coronavirus infections during the pandemic, thus reducing the risk of the prehabilitation offer. COVID-19 has accelerated the uptake of technology-based interventions and revolutionised patient care, certainly in primary care where 30% of appointments currently take place remotely, accounting for some 7.4 million appointments in the UK every year [41].

Limitations to Widespread Adoption of Prehabilitation

Such include patient access in remote areas, those of low socio-economic status who perhaps cannot afford frequent transport costs to and from a rehabilitation centre, and the finite time available with challenges of work, family-life, and other medical appointments in the run up towards surgery [42]. Technology-based prehabilitation can circumvent these limitations, thus increasing accessibility to prehabilitation and potentially reducing health inequalities.

Technologies can be app-based; web-based; video or game digital-based technology; and virtual reality [42]. Smart watches and mobile phone apps can be used both in the delivery of a prehabilitation intervention and in monitoring uptake and adherence of any intervention [43]. Evidence from a recent pilot study suggests that commercially available smart watches and associated apps can increase the volume of moderate and vigorous physical activity that patients undertake, and this results in an increase in functional capacity when measured by the 6-min walk test [43].

A major challenge to the implementation of any technology-based prehabilitation is the paucity of high-quality research on their efficacy. In a recent review of 11 RCTs, none measured complication rates, length of hospital stays, or readmission rates [39]. The psychosocial improvements of telehealth interventions appear the most well-documented, with increased return to work, reduction in pain catastrophising, and an improved perception of preparedness for surgery [39].

Should All Gastrointestinal Cancer Patients Be Enrolled?

From a biological disease point of view, we have not found any factors that preclude participation in prehabilitation, for any modality of gastrointestinal cancer. Time to cancer diagnosis and survivability have been viewed as quality measures of how well or poorly healthcare systems are functioning including the NHS (NHS England and NHS Improvement 2022). The concept of fast-track surgery is now commonplace in some units with highly selective patient criteria. This may present a challenge for prehabilitation services due to obvious time constraints.

Within the context of financial pressures the highest risk patients should be prioritized, in whom prehabilitation is likely to benefit the most. Strategically used available resources may seamlessly yield results provided that primary, secondary, social care systems can be integrated through better arrangements, data management, and use of healthcare technology. A useful starting point could be simply a reorganisation of patient treatment pathways where high-risk groups could be identified at primary care levels and referred to a prehabilitation service as a matter of course, like the way patients are referred as 2-week wait referrals for a new cancer diagnosis.

What are the Outcomes of Prehabilitation?

We have shown that there is a significant but modest reduction of length stay by 1.8 days in hepatobiliary, colorectal, and upper gastrointestinal cancer surgery [2]. Larger cohorts and longer follow ups may be needed. If morbidity and mortality are no different within a year of surgery, does this truly mean there is no effect longer-term?

Prehabilitation programmes are effective at improving exercise capacity both before and after gastrointestinal cancer surgery. A meta-analysis demonstrated that 6-min walking distance was improved by 33 m before surgery and 48 m 4–8 weeks after surgery [44]. However, no difference in Clavien-Dindo ≥ III complication rates was found. Additional studies have reported no effect on postoperative complications, hospital readmissions, mortality, and even hospital length of stay [45], though this latter result contrasts with our own [2].

References

1. Huang GH, Ismail H, Murnane A, et al. Structured exercise program prior to major cancer surgery improves cardiopulmonary fitness: a retrospective cohort study. Supp Care Cancer. 2016;24:2277–85.
2. Lambert JE, Hayes LD, Keegan TJ, et al. The impact of Prehabilitation on patient outcomes in hepatobiliary, colorectal, and upper gastrointestinal cancer surgery: a PRISMA-accordant meta-analysis. Ann Surg. 2021;274:70–7.
3. An D, Ayob F, Rajaleelan W, et al. Preoperative smoking cessation as part of surgical prehabilitation. Can J Anesth. 2019;66:476–9.
4. van Rooijen S, Carli F, Dalton SO, et al. Preoperative modifiable risk factors in colorectal surgery: an observational cohort study identifying the possible value of prehabilitation. Acta Oncol (Madr). 2017;56:329–34.
5. Minnella EM, Bousquet-Dion G, Awasthi R, et al. Multimodal prehabilitation improves functional capacity before and after colorectal surgery for cancer: a five-year research experience. Acta Oncol (Madr). 2017;56:295–300.
6. Hassinger TE, Mehaffey JH, Martin AN, et al. Implementation of an enhanced recovery protocol is associated with on-time initiation of adjuvant chemotherapy in colorectal cancer. Dis Colon Rectum. 2019;62:1305–15.
7. Timmons JA, Knudsen S, Rankinen T, et al. Using molecular classification to predict gains in maximal aerobic capacity following endurance exercise training in humans. J Appl Physiol. 2010;108:1487–96.
8. Carli F, Charlebois P, Stein B, et al. Randomized clinical trial of prehabilitation in colorectal surgery. Br J Surg. 2010;97:1187–97.
9. Vergara-Fernandez O, Trejo-Avila M, Salgado-Nesme N. Sarcopenia in patients with colorectal cancer: a comprehensive review. World J Clin Cases. 2020;8:1188–202.
10. Wang H, Yang R, Xu J, et al. Sarcopenia as a predictor of postoperative risk of complications, mortality and length of stay following gastrointestinal oncological surgery. Ann Roy Col Surg Eng. 2021;103:630–7.
11. Landskron G, De La Fuente M, Thuwajit P, et al. Chronic inflammation and cytokines in the tumor microenvironment. J Immunol Res. 2014;2014:149185.
12. Gleeson M, Bishop NC, Stensel DJ, et al. The anti-inflammatory effects of exercise: mechanisms and implications for the prevention and treatment of disease. Nat Rev Immunol. 2011;11:607–15.
13. Mandolesi L, Polverino A, Montuori S, et al. Effects of physical exercise on cognitive functioning and wellbeing: biological and psychological benefits. Front Psychol. 2018;9:509.
14. Roberts KJ, Schrem H, Hodson J, et al. Pancreas exocrine replacement therapy is associated with increased survival following pancreatoduodenectomy for periampullary malignancy. HPB. 2017;19:859–67.
15. Peterson SJ, Mozer M. Differentiating sarcopenia and cachexia among patients with cancer. Nutr Clin Pract. 2017;32(1):30–9.

16. Gillis C, Buhler K, Bresee L, et al. Effects of nutritional Prehabilitation, with and without exercise, on outcomes of patients who undergo colorectal surgery: a systematic review and meta-analysis. Gastroenterol. 2018;155:391–410.e4.
17. Minnella EM, Awasthi R, Loiselle SE, et al. Effect of exercise and nutrition Prehabilitation on functional capacity in Esophagogastric cancer surgery: a randomized clinical trial. JAMA Surg. 2018;153:1081–9.
18. Mazzola M, Bertoglio C, Boniardi M, et al. Frailty in major oncologic surgery of upper gastrointestinal tract: how to improve postoperative outcomes. Eur J Surg Oncol. 2017;43:1566–71.
19. Nakajima H, Yokoyama Y, Inoue T, et al. Clinical benefit of preoperative exercise and nutritional therapy for patients undergoing Hepato-Pancreato-biliary surgeries for malignancy. Ann Surg Oncol. 2019;26:264–72.
20. Bousquet-Dion G, Awasthi R, Loiselle SÈ, et al. Evaluation of supervised multimodal prehabilitation programme in cancer patients undergoing colorectal resection: a randomized control trial. Acta Oncol. 2018;57:849–59.
21. Chen BP, Awasthi R, Sweet SN, et al. Four-week prehabilitation program is sufficient to modify exercise behaviors and improve preoperative functional walking capacity in patients with colorectal cancer. Supp Care Cancer. 2017;25:33–40.
22. Seiler A, Jenewein J. Resilience in Cancer Patients. Front. Psychiatry. 2019;10:208.
23. Jung KH, Kim SM, Choi MG, et al. Preoperative smoking cessation can reduce postoperative complications in gastric cancer surgery. Gastric Cancer. 2015;18:683–90.
24. Lambert J, Mair T, Arujunan K, et al. The effect of the enhanced recovery programme on long-term survival following liver resection for colorectal liver metastases. Langenbeck's Arch Surg. 2023;408:239.
25. Faithfull S, Turner L, Poole K, et al. Prehabilitation for adults diagnosed with cancer: a systematic review of long-term physical function, nutrition and patient-reported outcomes. Eur J Cancer Care. 2019;28:e13023.
26. Dunne DFJ, Jack S, Jones RP, et al. Randomized clinical trial of prehabilitation before planned liver resection. Br J Surg. 2016;103:504–12.
27. Loughney L, West MA, Kemp GJ, et al. The effects of neoadjuvant chemoradiotherapy and an in-hospital exercise training programme on physical fitness and quality of life in locally advanced rectal cancer patients (the EMPOWER trial): study protocol for a randomised controlled trial. Trials. 2016;17:24.
28. WHO. Ageing and health. 2022. who.int/news-room/fact-sheets/detail/ageing-and-health. Accessed 28 Jun 2023.
29. Royal College of Surgeons of England. NHS waiting list at record high of over 7.3 million. 2023. rcseng.ac.uk/news-and-events/media-centre/press-releases/rtt-waiting-times-march-2023. Accessed 28 Jun 2023.
30. Moore J, Merchant Z, Rowlinson K, et al. Implementing a system-wide cancer prehabilitation programme: The journey of greater Manchester's 'Prehab4cancer'. Eur J Surg Oncol. 2021;47:524–32.
31. Thomas G, Tahir MR, Bongers BC, et al. Prehabilitation before major intra-abdominal cancer surgery: a systematic review of randomised controlled trials. Eur J Anaesthesiol. 2019;36(12):933–45.
32. Beck A, Vind Thaysen H, Hasselholt Soegaard C, et al. What matters to you? An investigation of patients' perspectives on and acceptability of prehabilitation in major cancer surgery. Eur J Cancer Care (Engl). 2021;30:e13475.
33. Gaffney CJ, Etheridge T, Szewczyk NJ. Minimizing muscle atrophy. In: Shayler DJ, Seedhouse E, editors. Handbook of life support Systems for Spacecraft and Extraterrestrial Habitats. Heidelberg: Springer; 2020. p. 1–27.
34. Michalik C, Maciukiewicz P, Drewa T, et al. Frailty, geriatric assessment and prehabilitation in elderly patients undergoing urological surgery—is there a need for change of the daily clinical practice? Synthesis of the available literature. Cent European J Urol. 2020;73:220–5.

35. Franssen RFW, Bongers BC, Vogelaar FJ, Janssen-Heijnen MLG. Feasibility of a tele-prehabilitation program in high-risk patients with colon or rectal cancer undergoing elective surgery: a feasibility study. Periop Med. 2022;11:28.
36. Ferreira V, Agnihotram RV, Bergdahl A, et al. Maximizing patient adherence to Prehabilitation: gastrointestinal cancer surgery: what do the patients say? Supp Care Cancer. 2018;26:2717–23.
37. McDonald S, Yates D, Durrand JW, et al. Exploring patient attitudes to behaviour change before surgery to reduce peri-operative risk: preferences for short- vs. long-term behaviour change. Anaesthesia. 2019;74:1580–8.
38. Barberan-Garcia A, Cano I, Bongers BC, et al. Digital support to multimodal community-based Prehabilitation: gastrointestinal cancer surgery: looking for optimization of health value generation. Front Oncol. 2021;11:662013.
39. Blumenau Pedersen M, Saxton J, Birch S, et al. The use of digital technologies to support home-based prehabilitation prior to major surgery: a systematic review. Surgeon. 2023;S1479-666X(23):00060–4.
40. Schierbeck G. Prehabilitation as novel paradigm shift in cancer care. Semin Oncol Nurs. 2022;38:151327.
41. NHS. Appointments in general practice. 2023. england.nhs.uk/cancer/faster-diagnosis/. Accessed 28 Jun 2023.
42. Steffens D, Delbaere K, Young J, et al. Evidence on technology-driven preoperative exercise interventions: are we there yet? Br J Anaesth. 2020;125:646–9.
43. Waller E, Sutton P, Rahman S, et al. Prehabilitation with wearables versus standard of care before major abdominal cancer surgery: a randomised controlled pilot study. Surg Endosc. 2022;36:1008–17.
44. Lau CSM, Chamberlain RS. Prehabilitation programs improve exercise capacity before and after surgery in gastrointestinal cancer surgery patients: a meta-analysis. J Gastroint Surg. 2020;24:2829–37.
45. Mareschal J, Hemmer A, Douissard J, et al. Surgical Prehabilitation in patients with gastrointestinal cancers: impact of unimodal and multimodal programs on postoperative outcomes and prospects for new therapeutic strategies-a systematic review. Cancers (Basel). 2023;15(6):1881.

Chapter 6
Efficacy of Prehabilitation in Abdominal Cancer Surgery

Lara Edbrooke, Shaza Abo, and Linda Denehy

Introduction

Colorectal cancer is the third most common form of cancer and the second leading cause of cancer-related death globally [1]. Major surgical resection, with or without neoadjuvant treatment (chemo/radiotherapy), is the only curative treatment option. However, surgery is not without risk. Despite its excellent survival benefit, this treatment carries a significant burden to patients and the health care system, as many surgical patients develop short—and/or long-term complications [2]. Death within 30 days after surgery is the third leading cause of death worldwide [3], and one-quarter of patients suffer major postoperative complications such as respiratory infections [4]. This risk is predominantly driven by a subgroup of high-risk patients (as detailed below), where approximately 12% of patients and 12% of surgical procedures (predominantly major abdominal surgery) account for more than 80% of postoperative complications [5].

L. Edbrooke (✉)
Department of Physiotherapy, The University of Melbourne, Melbourne, VIC, Australia
e-mail: larae@unimelb.edu.au

L. Denehy
Department of Physiotherapy, The University of Melbourne, Melbourne, VIC, Australia

Department of Health Services Research, The Peter MacCallum Cancer Centre, Melbourne, VIC, Australia
e-mail: l.denehy@unimelb.edu.au

S. Abo
Department of Physiotherapy, The University of Melbourne, Melbourne, VIC, Australia

Department of Physiotherapy, The Peter MacCallum Cancer Centre, Melbourne, VIC, Australia
e-mail: shaza.abo@unimelb.edu.au

© The Author(s), under exclusive license to Springer Nature Switzerland AG 2024

J. Faintuch, S. Faintuch (eds.), *Recent Strategies in High Risk Surgery*, https://doi.org/10.1007/978-3-031-56270-9_6

It is anticipated that the number of patients with increased surgical risk will increase three-fold over the next 30 years, due to a rising number of patients over 50 years receiving surgery, adversely impacting healthcare budgets. This is driven by an ageing global population, with associated increased co-morbid disease, and the prevalent use of neoadjuvant therapy (chemotherapy/radiotherapy before surgery) that deconditions patients before cancer surgery [6].

Whole Body Prehabilitation

Prehabilitation modifies the preoperative deconditioned state by improving the physiologic capacity of patients to withstand the stressor of major surgery. Prehabilitation is commonly delivered as a multimodal intervention bundle tailored to the individual and comprising medical optimisation for example, assessment of haematinics and treatment including iron infusions (as appropriate), smoking cessation, patient education delivered by the multidisciplinary team (including pain management, the importance of early mobilisation), exercise, nutrition and psychological support [7]. Enhanced recovery after surgery (ERAS) protocols are multimodal perioperative care pathways designed to achieve early recovery after surgical procedures [8]. Even though they have a different structure they usually include preoperative counselling, preoperative nutrition (including avoidance of strict perioperative fasting, and carbohydrate loading up to 2 h preoperatively), standardised anaesthetic and analgesic regimens (epidural and nonopioid analgesia) and early mobilisation. Often, both are included in the care package of ERAS Plus.

Randomised Trials

In a multicentre trial in colorectal cancer surgery ($n = 251$), participants were randomised to receive 4 weeks of supervised, multimodal prehabilitation or standard care (ERAS pathway with no additional nutrition, exercise or psychological counselling). Prehabilitation included exercise, nutrition, psychosocial support, and smoking cessation (if required). The number of severe complications was significantly lower (OR 0.47 [95%CI 0.26–0.87]; $p = 0.02$), along with fewer medical complications (e.g., respiratory) compared with standard care (OR 0.48 [95%CI 0.26–0.89]; $p = 0.02$). Between-group 6-min walk test distance, 4 weeks postoperatively, was not significantly different. Unfortunately, the trial was ceased early due to the COVID-19 pandemic and did not reach its powered sample size [9].

Systematic reviews and meta-analyses [10–18] similarly support multidisciplinary prehabilitation to reduce operative risks and improve postoperative patient outcomes, although not all aspects of patient recovery have been found to be significant. Given the large number of trials in prehabilitation in the past 10 years McIsaac et al. performed an overview of systematic reviews which included 55 reviews examining the efficacy of prehabilitation [19]. Moderate-certainty evidence (GRADE) favouring prehabilitation (either uni—or multimodal) to improve functional recovery was reported the 6-min walk test (6MWT). However, evidence certainty in favor of prehabilitation over standard care for the outcomes of complications, discharge destination and hospital length of stay was graded low to very low certainty.

Respiratory Prehabilitation

Depending on postoperative pulmonary complications (PPC) definition, incidence can range from 10 to 60% [4, 20]. PPCs are associated with worse postoperative outcomes including prolonged length of hospital stay [4], hospital readmissions [21], and worse quality of life [22]. As occurs with prehabilitation in general, respiratory education and training should be provided prior to surgery to target prevention of PPC [23]. Nearly 50% of all PPCs develop within the first two postoperative days, with many developing on the first day [24]. Deep breathing exercises, coughing instruction and the reasons these are important can be explained to patients in the preoperative period.

Boden et al. compared usual care with one 30-min face to face education session prior to surgery delivered within existing preadmission clinics. The patient education session included an explanation of surgical impact on the lungs, deep breathing instruction, and practise. This randomised trial of 440 patients reported a halving of PPC after major abdominal surgery (adjusted hazard ratio 0.48, 95% confidence interval 0.30 to 0.75, $p = 0.001$), reduced 12-month mortality in patients who did not develop a PPC and found the intervention cost effective [25, 26]. These results are supported in a meta-analysis ($n = 1345$) that provides moderate certainty evidence for respiratory physiotherapy in reducing PPC [27].

Inspiratory Muscle Training (IMT)

Inspiratory muscle training (IMT) is strength training specifically targeting the skeletal muscles responsible for inspiration. A load on the inspiratory muscles is generated through a mouth-held device [28]. The efficacy of IMT [29] as a breathing technique taught preoperatively is supported for patients undergoing cardiac and thoracic surgery [10] but to date no trials have reported efficacy in the colorectal surgical population. In patients with oesophageal cancers IMT is recommended pre-operatively due to the demonstrated benefits in improving pulmonary function [30].

Who Needs Prehabilitation?

Modifiable risk factors (deconditioning, malnutrition, psychological distress) impact surgical outcomes. *Deconditioning:* Physical fitness predicts complications after major cancer surgery [31, 32]. Neoadjuvant therapy, chemo—and/or radiotherapy prior to major surgery, further impairs functional capacity, and importantly this may be offset with exercise-based prehabilitation [33]. *Malnutrition:* About 26% of hospitalised patients are malnourished, and a greater proportions (39%) of patients are nutritionally at-risk. In abdominal cancer surgery, 44% of patients are malnourished, with associated increased hospital length of stay complications or death after surgery [34].

The "Higher-Risk" Surgical Patient

These patients are typically older, have multiple comorbidities and functional limitations including deconditioning, malnutrition and sarcopenia (muscle wasting), and may be frail [35]. Frailty is a multidimensional clinical syndrome characterised by reduced physiological reserve against stressors due to age-related disability. However, a common definition (and measurement) of frailty is lacking. Frailty is associated with poor treatment tolerance, adverse postoperative outcomes, and higher risk of mortality; and these factors worsen with more severe frailty. The role of prehabilitation in frail individuals has not been extensively studied but in general the current evidence is supportive of prehabilitation to improve function in this patient group. Frail patients may need more prolonged intervention (more than 4–5 weeks) to experience functional gains [36].

The Impact of Neo-Adjuvant Cancer Treatments

Patients receiving neo-adjuvant treatments may also be at higher risk. Chemo/radiotherapy related side effects including nausea, vomiting, diarrhoea and fatigue are common and impact nutrition, weight, body composition, and functional status [37, 38]. These contribute further to the development of adverse events and inordinately high cost of care [39]. In the EMPOWER trial participants were randomised to receive either hospital-based exercise or routine care, post-neoadjuvant treatment and prior to surgery. Adherence was high with participants attending 91% of scheduled sessions. Exercise capacity improved significantly following the intervention (between-group mean difference (95% CI) for the change in oxygen uptake (VO_2) at anaerobic threshold (AT) = 2.9 mL/kg/min (0.8 to 5.1), $p = 0.011$) [40]. Pilot studies demonstrate safety, feasibility, and trends towards positive outcomes favouring prehabilitation in rectal cancer surgery [41]; however, further high-quality research is required regarding the efficacy of prehabilitation during neoadjuvant therapies prior to abdominal cancer surgery.

Stepped Care

Escalating interventions can be individualised to the severity of risk and to the patient's response. Current recommendations are to provide stepped, individualised interventions based on risk assessment (Fig. 6.1, adapted from Macmillan Cancer Support) [42]. Not all centres use this stepped approach and it may need modification depending on the demographics of the population referred for prehabilitation.

This model of prehabilitation care shows three levels of stepped multimodal prehabilitation: Universal, Targeted and Specialised prehabilitation and was developed by an international working group for the Macmillan Cancer Support group in partnership with the Royal College of Anaesthetists and the National Institute of Health Research (UK) [42]. Universal prehabilitation targets all patients and focuses on educating patients and improving patient self-efficacy and empowerment before surgery. Patients (with a family member or friend) may receive education from content experts, with presentations on their surgical pathway, the importance of exercise, physical activity, nutrition, stress reduction, pain management and oral and respiratory care. This may be delivered face to face or by webinar

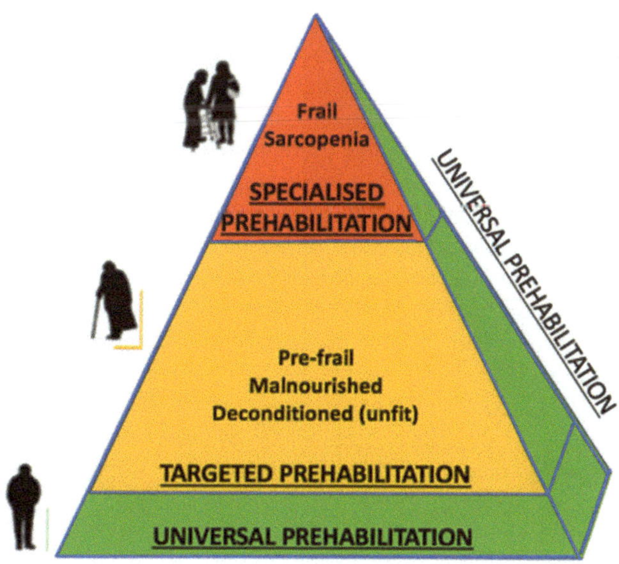

Fig. 6.1 Prehabilitation model of care (adapted from Macmillan Cancer Support)

or videos supported with written educational materials. Patients may also be taught the principles of ERAS and encouraged to participate in their care journey. Risk factor triggers can identify patients requiring Targeted or Specialised Care levels of prehabilitation, centred on exercise, nutritional and psychological support. Research to assess outcomes from the Universal component of prehabilitation has not yet been undertaken.

Patients receiving Targeted prehabilitation are commonly prescribed an individual exercise programme, consisting of aerobic exercise and strength training. Exercise prescription and progression follow the American College of Sports Medicine guidelines and FITT (Frequency, Intensity, Type and Time) principles to achieve progressive overload and maximise gains [43]. Aerobic exercise is performed as continuous or interval training—commonly using a treadmill or stationary cycling. Resistance training involves upper and lower limb exercises of the major muscle groups using machines, resistance bands, body weight, or free-weights. This is often prescribed at moderate intensity initially, with the aim to progress towards higher intensities. Intensity may be prescribed and exercise progressed based on findings from the patient's cardiopulmonary exercise test (CPET) using maximal heart rate at the point of peak oxygen uptake (HR max at $VO_{2\ peak}$), or using the Borg scale (aiming to start at 3–4/10 'somewhat hard' level) [44].

It is recommended that exercise sessions include behaviour change strategies, including setting of personalised goals. Patients are commonly also prescribed a home exercise programme, aiming to work towards the guidelines of achieving 150 min of moderate-intensity physical activity per week [45]. Individualised dietary advice is given dependent on the patient's anthropometric and nutritional assessment findings and this advice can include education to optimise nutrition to achieve adequate energy and protein intake, oral protein supplementation, and enteral or parenteral nutrition, if required. Immunonutrition, providing nutrients in larger amounts than required to regulate immune activities, is not used consistently but is shown to reduce postoperative complications (infections, anastomotic leak) and hospital length of stay following gastrointestinal cancer surgery [46]. Psychological support during prehabilitation is aimed at helping patients prepare for surgery and addresses any factors which may impact on the ability to engage with additional aspects of the prehabilitation programme. Psychological interventions may include psycho-education, stress management, problem solving, motivational therapy, and cognitive behavioural approaches [47]. Screening and risk assessment are needed to use this model wisely and to direct resources to those most in need of prehabilitation. Table 6.1 describes commonly used screening and assessment measures to risk stratify patients to receive Universal, Targeted or Specialized prehabilitation.

Table 6.1 Commonly used screening and assessment tools

Surgical Risk	Tool	Interpretation
Postoperative complications	Clavien-Dindo classification [57] Postoperative morbidity survey (POMS) [58] Days alive and at home up to 30 days after surgery [59]	Graded I-V (death). Major complications ≥ III POMS—9 domains of morbidity (presence/absence)
Exercise capacity	Cardiopulmonary exercise test (gold standard) [60] 6-min walk test [61] Incremental shuttle walk test [61] Patient-reported—Duke Activity Status Index [32]	Greater complications are associated with peak oxygen uptake (VO_2 peak) <15 mL/kg/min or anaerobic threshold <11 mL/kg/min [62] < 400 m greater risk [63] Range 0—58.2 (≤ 34 greater complication risk)
Physical activity (exercise is a sub-category [64])	Accelerometry International Physical Activity Questionnaire-Short Form [65]	3 days × 8 h/day wear time is valid [66] Meeting guidelines yes/no and continuous variable (weekly metabolic equivalent of task minutes)
Performance status	Australia-modified Karnofsky Performance Status [67]	0–100 (higher scores indicate better function)
Physical function	Sit-to-stand (STS)—30 [68] or 60 s, 5 times chair stand (5-CTS) [69]	30 s STS <12 (females) <14 (males) is below average for 60–64 y and associated with higher falls risk [70]; 5-CTS > 15 s = at risk/ probable sarcopenia [71]
Skeletal muscle	Handgrip strength (HGS), quadriceps dynamometry [72]	HGS <27 kg males <16 kg females = at risk/probable sarcopenia [71]
Malnutrition	Malnutrition Screening Tool [73] Patient-Generated Subjective Global Assessment [74]	0–1 = low risk, 2 = moderate risk, 3–5 = high risk Typical range 0–35; A = well-nourished; B = moderate/ suspected; C = severe malnutrition
Sarcopenia (muscle loss)	SARC-F: Strength, assistance walking, rise from chair, climb stairs, falls history [75] Bioimpedance appendicular lean mass (ALM) [71, 76] CT scan (muscle mass third lumbar vertebra)	Score 0–10 (higher score = increased probability of sarcopenia) ALM <20 kg male <15 kg female at risk/probable sarcopenia Local standards sarcopenia
Frailty	Clinical Frailty Scale [77] Fried's Frailty Phenotype [78]	1 (very fit) to 9 (terminally ill) ≥ 5 indicate frailty
Anxiety and depression	Generalised anxiety disorder (GAD-7 item) [79] Patient health questionnaire (PHQ-9) [80] Hospital Anxiety and Depression Scale [81]	0–21: 0–4 minimal, 5–9 mild, 10–14 moderate, 15–21 severe 0–27: 0–4 minimal, 5–9 mild, 10–14 moderate, 15–19 moderately severe, 20–27 severe 0–21:0–7 no, 8–10 mild, 11–14 moderate, 15–21 severe

Table 6.1 (continued)

Surgical Risk	Tool	Interpretation
PROMS		
Health-related quality of life	European Organisation for Research and Treatment of Cancer Quality of Life Questionnaire-Core 30 [82]/ EuroQoL (EQ-5D-5L) [83]	0–100 (higher scores represent higher physical function, quality of life or symptoms, according to respective scales)
Fatigue	Functional Assessment of Chronic Illness Therapy-Fatigue [84]	0–52 (<30 indicates severe fatigue)
PREMS	NHS National Cancer Patient Experience Survey [85]	Local standards patient experience

Risks are assessed and managed in conjunction with medical optimisation, pain management, smoking cessation (if required); *PREMS* patient-reported experience measures, *PROMS* patient-reported outcome measures, *Euro-Qol* European organisation for research and treatment of cancer quality of life questionnaire;

Controversies in Prehabilitation

While prehabilitation as a 'package of care' is shown to improve patient outcomes, the components included vary between centres. The definition of prehabilitation also varies, for example the inclusion of the medical optimisation of anaemia and smoking cessation could be considered to be standard medical care but are often included in the prehabilitation package. In the McIsaac overview, only four reviews (7%) delineated how prehabilitation was defined to inform review inclusion eligibility [19]. Risk stratification is important before surgery but many different tools are used to assess risk such as the National Surgical Quality Improvement Program (NSQIP) calculator, American Society of Anesethesiologists' (ASA) classification, and the Assess Respiratory Risk in Surgical Patients in Catalonia (ARISCAT) risk index. However, these tools do not take into account the social determinants of health which are shown to impact recovery outcomes [48].

In colorectal cancer the length of prehabilitation interventions requires additional research. What is the minimum period preoperatively needed to be effective? The prehabilitation intervention time needed to enhance patient fitness is debated in the literature with variations between a minimum of 2 weeks or 4 weeks of intervention remaining a controversy [37]. This may be dependent on the patient preoperative condition and the cancer surgery planned. For example, the more frail and deconditioned patients may need a longer prehabilitation intervention.

Whilst most research involves combined aerobic and resistance exercise interventions there is a need for further research regarding optimal exercise intervention types, according to individual needs and surgery type, which are feasible to deliver during the prehabilitation period. The most common components included in prehabilitation are aerobic, resistance and respiratory training with nutrition intervention commonly added [37]. With a focus on pre-operative aerobic fitness, a comparative review of prehabilitation prior to abdominal cancer surgery found three out of four included studies reported significant increases in VO_2 at AT or $VO_{2\ peak}$ following high-intensity interval training interventions. In contrast, neither study of moderate-intensity exercise training reported significant changes in aerobic fitness [49]. However, others report significant outcomes for moderate intensity activity. One study compared high to moderate intensity interval training in 42 patients before surgery for colorectal cancer and found both improved short term $VO_{2\ peak}$ [50].

Prehabilitation publications also vary regarding the setting of interventions, home or hospital based, supervised or unsupervised. The consensus regarding supervised exercise interventions is that they are superior to unsupervised in impact on both adherence to exercise and outcomes of fitness and/or strength [51]. Home based exercises can be supervised using video conferencing or web based real time methods [52].

Finally, the reporting of interventions and measurement of specific outcomes is variable. In the McIsaac overview, only thirty-five (64%) reviews reported the duration of prehabilitation [19]. Guidelines regarding reporting are needed to improve comparisons between trials and a core set of outcomes that are measured will allow greater combinations of trials in future meta-analyses.

Case Reports

These cases were accessed from our centre where prehabilitation is included as usual care in abdominal cancer surgery. Each case detailed below attended 'surgery school' as part of the Universal approach to prehabilitation. This online education session, including question and answer time, from the multidisciplinary team included topics what to expect; pain management; optimising muscle and nutrition; the role of exercise and the importance of respiratory care and early mobilisation; and preparing psychologically for surgery. Education followed respiratory prehabilitation principles to reduce the risk of postoperative complications (covering **a**ctive deep breathing, **c**ough, **o**ral care, **u**nderstanding your surgery and recovery, **g**etting out of bed and **h**ead of bed elevation; aCOUGH). Both patients were educated about the importance of performing Active Cycle of Breathing Techniques (ACBT) in the pre—and early postoperative periods.

Case 1—Mr. D

Mr. D is a 72-year-old man with a non-English speaking background who lives with his wife. An ex-smoker, he had previously worked as a gardener and enjoys 3–4 standard alcoholic drinks per day. His past history includes mild osteoarthritis in both hips and hypertension.

Following reporting to his GP some swallowing difficulties and a sensation of pressure in his chest, Mr. D underwent investigations and was diagnosed with an oesophageal squamous cell carcinoma. He was scheduled for high-risk surgery, an oesophagectomy, following 6 weeks of neoadjuvant chemoradiotherapy. Key points along Mr. D's prehabilitation pathway are summarised in Fig. 6.2. As part of his surgical consultation, he was referred to prehabilitation by his surgical team, due to the high risk of the planned procedure. His Duke Activity Status Index (DASI) score

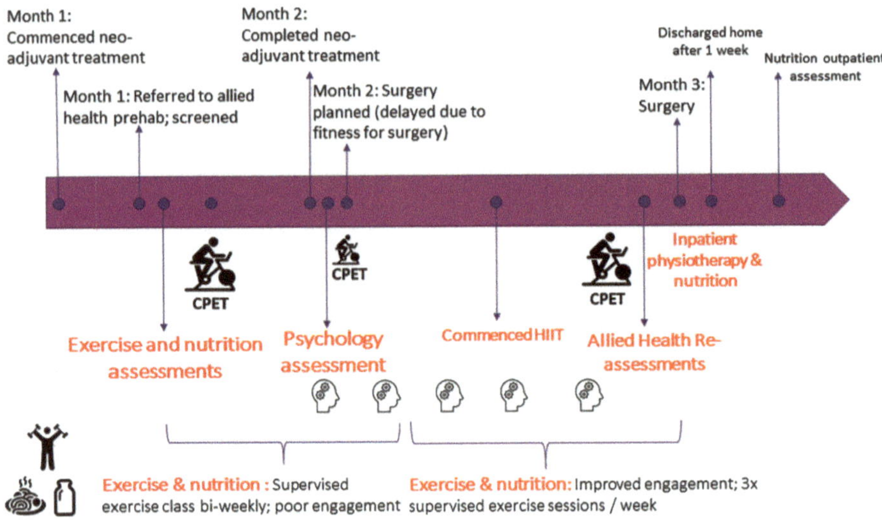

Fig. 6.2 Case 1 summary timeline

of 30/58 indicated reduced exercise capacity. At the prehabilitation consultation the perioperative physician (anaesthetist) initiated referrals to the allied health prehabilitation team and for a cardiopulmonary exercise test (CPET) to further assess his exercise capacity and risk of postoperative complications. The prehabilitation team provide holistic and co-ordinated care with regular multidisciplinary team meetings including clinicians from anaesthetics, surgery, nursing and allied health. The aim of these meetings is to ensure consistent messaging, common goals and a clear understanding of progress.

Allied health screening and initial assessment findings, outlined in detail in Table 6.2, included reduced physical function and adequate nutrition. Mr. D initially met criteria for referral to exercise and nutrition services, due to the high-risk surgical procedure planned with neoadjuvant treatment. Using the International Physical Activity Questionnaire —Short Form (IPAQ-SF), Mr. D self-reported being physically inactive and highly sedentary since retiring. He struggled to set goals and engage in prehabilitation treatment sessions during this period. Mr. D reported the main barriers to participation were nausea and dizziness, which were side effects of the neoadjuvant treatment he was receiving. He was offered daily, supervised, centre-based exercise sessions (aerobic and resistance training), but often failed to attend scheduled exercise and nutrition appointments.

Mr. D performed his initial CPET a 2 weeks later during neoadjuvant treatment. Due to his low body weight CPET $VO_{2\ peak}$ and AT were not reflective of his true exercise capacity (Table 6.2). After adjusting for body surface area, CPET performance indicated Mr. D was at high risk of postoperative pulmonary complications. Following completion of neoadjuvant treatment repeat CPET findings indicated that Mr. D was not fit for surgery, he was deconditioned and was losing weight. The

Table 6.2 Mr. D's screening and assessment findings, treatment, and progress

<table>
<tr><td colspan="4">Screening Measures and Findings</td></tr>
<tr><td>Exercise</td><td colspan="3">AKPS 70/100 (cares for self, unable to carry on normal activity or do active work); IPAQ-SF—not meeting PA guidelines</td></tr>
<tr><td>Nutrition (MST)</td><td colspan="3">1/5 (not at risk of malnutrition)</td></tr>
<tr><td>Psychology (PHQ-4)</td><td>Baseline
2/12 (not experiencing anxiety or depression)</td><td colspan="2">Post-neoadjuvant Rx
7/12 (moderate), clinical notes documented anxiety</td></tr>
<tr><td colspan="4">Assessment measures and findings</td></tr>
<tr><td>CPET</td><td>During-neoadjuvant Rx (initial)
$VO_{2\ peak}$ = 18.3 mL/kg/min
AT = 14.7 mL/kg/min
$VO_{2\ peak}$/ BSA = 585 mL (normative 750)</td><td colspan="2">Post-prehab
$VO_{2\ peak}$ = 20.3 mL/kg/min
AT = 14.0 mL/kg/min
$VO_{2\ peak}$/ BSA = 643 mL (normative 750)</td></tr>
<tr><td>Exercise</td><td>During-neoadjuvant Rx (initial)
6MWT (metres) = 447
30 s STS (chair stands) = 16
handgrip strength (kg) = 25 (right), 20 (left)</td><td colspan="2">Post-prehab
6MWT (metres) = 560
30 s STS (chair stands) = 19 handgrip strength (kg) = unchanged</td></tr>
<tr><td>Nutrition</td><td>During-neoadjuvant Rx (initial)
PG-SGA = 6A (adequately nourished)
Weight (kg) = 52.0
Nutrition = poor appetite, mild nausea, mild oesophagitis</td><td>Post-neoadjuvant Rx
PG-SGA = 10A
Weight (kg) = 46.0</td><td>Post-prehab
PG-SGA = 6A
weight (kg) = 51.5</td></tr>
<tr><td>Psychology</td><td>Post-neoadjuvant Rx (initial)
FTA due to inpatient admission
1/52 later: PHQ-9 = 9/27 (mild)
GAD-7 = 14/21 (moderate).
Fear of dying, anxious about surgical risks and potential for prolonged recovery. Sleep improved with medication.</td><td colspan="2">Post-prehab
PHQ-9 = 3/27 (minimal)
GAD-7 = 7/21 (mild)</td></tr>
<tr><td colspan="4">Treatment and progress</td></tr>
<tr><td>Exercise</td><td>2 months post-neoadjuvant Rx (initial)
F: 2–3/week, supervised
I: Moderate-intensity (aerobic: 70% Watts of initial CPET AT; resistance: 80% of 10RM, 8 reps × 2 sets)
T: Aerobic: 30 s intervals (stationary cycle); resistance: UL/LL free weights, body weight
Aerobic:2 × 5 min;resistance:10 min
Home walking: x2/week, 10 min, moderate (Borg 3/10)</td><td colspan="2">Progression (1-month later)
F: 2–3/week, supervised
I: High-intensity (aerobic: 85% Watts most recent CPET AT; resistance: 80% most recent 10RM, 12 reps × 3 sets)
T: Aerobic: 90 s interval (stationary cycle); resistance:
UL/LL free weight, body weight
Aerobic: 3 × 5 min;resist.:10 min
Home walking: x4/week, 20 min, moderate (Borg 4/10)</td></tr>
</table>

Table 6.2 (continued)

Nutrition	*2 months post-neoadjuvant Rx (initial)* Education protein/ energy needs, nutrition impact symptoms (dietary modifications and medication)	*Progress* Fortnightly/weekly reviews (increased frequency as NIS worsened)—Oral supplements, NGT feeding for poor intake
Psychology	*Five sessions over 3.5 months* Relaxation training (breathing exercises) Activating supports and identification of barriers to this Behavioural activation and avoidance of distress; goal setting; Discussion regarding physical barriers to exercise (pain and continence) Education about exercise (that it will increase fatigue) Anxiety management and psycho-education in context of fears Education regarding further support postoperatively if required	

AKPS Australia-modified Karnofsky performance status, *AT* anaerobic threshold, *BSA* body surface area, *CPET* cardiopulmonary exercise test, Exercise (*F* frequency, *I* intensity, *T* type, *T* time); *FTA* failed to attend, *GAD-7* generalised anxiety disorder-7 item, *IPAQ-SF* international physical activity questionnaire-short form, *LL* lower limb, *NIS* nutrition impact symptoms, *NGT* naso-gastric tube, *PG-SGA* patient generated-subjective global assessment, *PHQ-9* patient health questionnaire-9 item, *RM* repetition maximum, *Rx* treatment, *UL* upper limb, $VO_{2\,peak}$ peak oxygen uptake, *6MWT* 6-min walk test, *30 s STS* 30-s sit-to-stand

perioperative physician recommended a further 6 weeks of prehabilitation aiming to improve his nutritional and functional status. Mr. D was referred and commenced treatment with the prehabilitation psychologist and commenced engaging during nutrition sessions. With care from the multidisciplinary team Mr. D's symptoms improved. Over several weeks of treatment and with regular communication at multidisciplinary team meetings, the psychologist was able to unpack motivational issues and highlight the burden his symptoms were having. He worked with the dietician on strategies to improve his nausea. As his symptom burden lessened, Mr. D was able to attend the centre for supervised face to face exercise three times a week. Following prehabilitation his weight had increased and CPET and 6MWT results indicated significant and clinically important improvements in his exercise capacity (Table 6.2).

Three-months post diagnosis Mr. D underwent the planned surgery (oesophagectomy), his postoperative course was uncomplicated and followed the standard ERAS postoperative pathway which included enteral feeding via a jejunostomy on days 3–6 and respiratory physiotherapy and early mobilisation which commenced on the day of surgery [53]. Mr. D was discharged home after 7 days. Follow-up, short-term outpatient review with the dietician was planned due to expected swallowing difficulties associated with the surgical procedure.

Case 2—Ms. S

Ms. S is a 75-year-old woman who works part time in human resources for an educational organisation. Her past medical history includes osteoporosis, hypertension, and removal of bilateral cataracts. Although living alone, Ms. S has a supportive partner. She has not been active or able to eat well over the last few months due to fatigue, more frequent bowel, diarrhoea-like movements (causing anal discomfort)

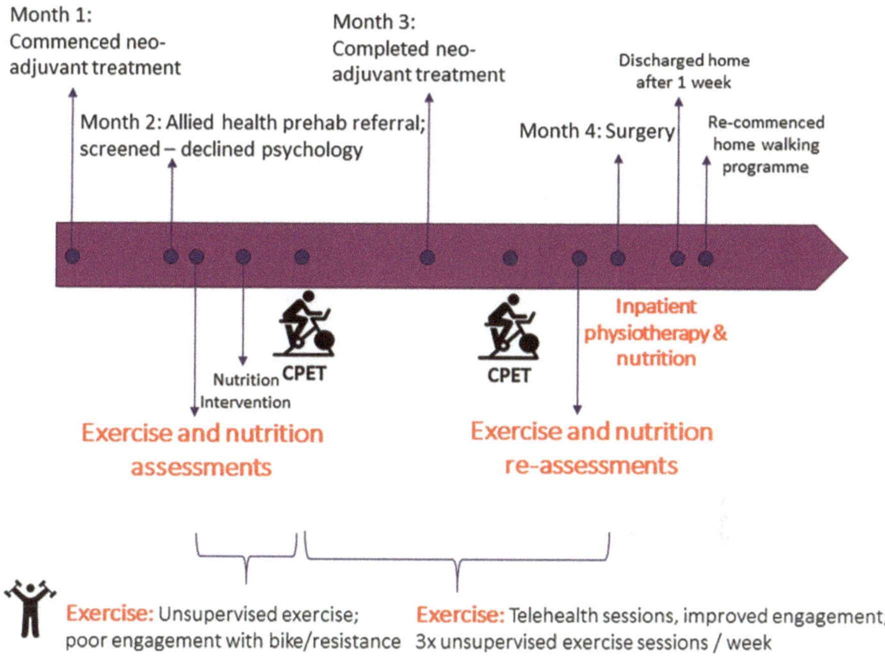

Fig. 6.3 Case 2 summary timeline

and abdominal discomfort, but prior to that she enjoyed bushwalking and cycling and did this for 30 min 2–3 times per week.

Ms. S was referred for investigation due to her symptoms and an MRI scan and biopsy provided a diagnosis of stage II rectal cancer. Following surgical consultation and discussion at a multidisciplinary team meeting, Ms. S's treatment plan was to commence neoadjuvant chemotherapy, fluorouracil, with radiation prior to abdominoperineal resection (APR). Ms. S was referred to the allied health team for prehabilitation. Her prehabilitation timeline is shown in Fig. 6.3. Ms. S was screened 3 days after referral and booked in for allied health assessments the following week. Due to the high-risk procedure, Ms. S was eligible to be assessed by exercise, nutrition, and psychology disciplines. She declined a psychology assessment stating that she felt she was managing well currently and had a good network of social supports. Details of screening and assessment are provided in Table 6.3. During screening her clinician-rated Clinical Frailty Scale (CFS) score was 3 'managing well'. This is defined as patients whose medical problems are well controlled but who are not active regularly beyond walking to complete daily tasks.

Ms. S's nutrition assessment indicated that she was at risk of malnutrition and she was given education regarding how to achieve a diet that was high in protein and energy. Given her previous enjoyment of cycling, the goal she set during her initial exercise assessment was to commence unsupervised aerobic training on her home exercise bike. She was also prescribed resistance training exercises to maintain her

Table 6.3 Ms. S's screening and assessment findings, treatment, and progress

Screening Measures and Findings		
[Exercise]	AKPS 90/100; DASI 34.95	
Nutrition	MST = 3/5 (at risk malnutrition) Weight 65 kg; weight loss 5 kg (7.1%) previous 6/12 months	
Psychology	PHQ-4 baseline = 0/12	
Assessment measures and findings		
	During-neoadjuvant Rx	*Post-prehab*
CPET	$VO_{2\,peak}$ = 19.8 mL/kg/min AT = 12.5 mL/kg/min $VO_{2\,peak}$/ BSA = 731 mL	$VO_{2\,peak}$ = 19.8 mL/kg/min AT = 16.0 mLl/kg/min $VO_{2\,peak}$/BSA = 743 mL
Exercise	6MWT (metres) = 530 30 s STS (chair stands) = 14 handgrip (kg) = 18 (right), 18 (left); CFS =3 IPAQ—Below PA guidelines	6MWT (metres) = 567 30 s STS (chair stands) = 16 handgrip (kg) = 20 (right), 18(left); CFS =1 IPAQ—Meeting PA guidelines
Nutrition	PG-SGA = 15B (malnourished) poor appetite; weight = 65.0 kg	PG-SGA = 7A (adequate) Poor appetite, mild nausea, oesophagitis; weight = 59.0
Treatment and progress		
Exercise	*Initial (during neoadjuvant Rx)* Education (effects exercise, treatment vs. exercise capacity, safe exercising) Goal setting Home exercise: Aerobic—Stationary cycle, walking 20 min × 7 days; moderate intensity (Borg 3) Resistance × 3 days/week (step up, squats, calf raise, bicep curl, shoulder raise, kickback); from 10RM, 2 sets × 10 reps with 4 kg; Borg 3	*Progression* Fortnightly telehealth reviews—Compliant with home walking, minimal bike or RT initially, then improved. Was educated, self-progressed resistance exercises maintaining Borg 3–4 (3 sets × 12 reps with 8 kg on discharge)
Nutrition	Single in-person session following initial assessment, set goals to muscle mass/ weight maintenance –high energy-high protein diet, and oral nutrition supplements pre-op	

Abbreviations: *AKPS* Australia-modified Karnofsky Performance Status, *AT* anaerobic threshold, *SA* body surface area, *CPET* cardiopulmonary exercise test, *DASI* duke activity status index, *IPAQ-SF* international physical activity questionnaire-short form, *PG-SGA* patient generated-subjective global assessment, *RM* repetition maximum, *RT* resistance training, *Rx* treatment, $VO_{2\,peak}$ peak oxygen uptake, *6MWT* 6-min walk test; *30 s STS* 30-s sit-to-stand

skeletal muscle mass and a home-walking programme. Ms. S was reviewed by her physiotherapist fortnightly via telehealth. She completed three cycles of chemotherapy prior to surgery and reported moderate levels of fatigue and mild nausea as the main side effects. She found walking outside was the most effective strategy to control her symptoms. Because of this, she was initially adherent only to her prescribed walking programme. Some discomfort associated with sitting on the exercise bike and boredom with resistance training impacted her adherence. Behaviour change techniques utilised during telehealth sessions included action planning, barrier identification/problem solving, and social support [54]. The physiotherapist provided further education to Ms. S regarding the importance of resistance training, not only for maintaining function, but also for her ability to recover post-surgery and re-commence chemotherapy. Ms. S's partner modified her exercise bike seat to improve comfort. With greater adherence, Ms. S began to notice improvements in her strength which made her more motivated to continue her exercise sessions.

Eight weeks after referral Ms. S was admitted to hospital and underwent an abdominoperineal resection. Her postoperative management followed ERAS guidelines including respiratory physiotherapy and early mobilisation and return to a high-protein diet (supported with oral nutrition supplements) within 24 h of surgery [55, 56]. She was discharged home after 8 days, returning for a further three cycles of chemotherapy. Since discharge, she has continued with her strength training exercises twice a week and has gradually built up her home walking programme with support from her partner. She is scheduled to commence an outpatient rehabilitation programme in 2 weeks' time to help her return to her previous level of fitness and commence a graduated return to work plan.

Conclusions and Future Directions

Despite the growing research outputs and gradual implementation of prehabilitation in abdominal surgery, there are many different avenues of research still needed to improve efficacy and implementation to influence patient outcomes. Prehabilitation guidelines are required in the next 2 years to standardise interventions and outcome variables further. Figure 6.4 summarises areas for future research in prehabilitation for colorectal and other surgical patient populations. There are many groups internationally currently working on these research priorities.

Acknowledgements The authors would like to thank Dr. Christina Prickett, Ms. Jess Crowe and Ms. Anna Beaumont for their assistance with the development of the first case study.

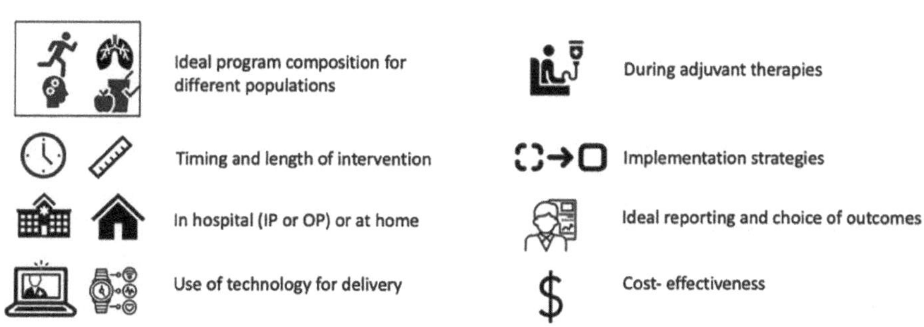

Fig. 6.4 Diagrammatic representation of the areas for future research in prehabilitation

References

1. Xi Y, Xu P. Global colorectal cancer burden in 2020 and projections to 2040. Transl Oncol. 2021;14(10):101174.
2. Brown KGM, Solomon MJ, Mahon K, O'Shannassy S. Management of colorectal cancer. BMJ (Clinical research ed). 2019;366:l4561.
3. Nepogodiev D, Martin J, Biccard B, Makupe A, Bhangu A. Global burden of postoperative death. Lancet. 2019;393(10170):401.
4. Fernandez-Bustamante A, Frendl G, Sprung J, Kor DJ, Subramaniam B, Martinez Ruiz R, Lee JW, Henderson WG, Moss A, Mehdiratta N, Colwell MM, Bartels K, Kolodzie K, Giquel J, Vidal Melo MF. Postoperative pulmonary complications, early mortality, and hospital stay following noncardiothoracic surgery: A multicenter study by the perioperative research network investigators. JAMA Surg. 2017;152(2):157–66.
5. Pearse RM, Harrison DA, James P, Watson D, Hinds C, Rhodes A, Grounds RM, Bennett ED. Identification and characterisation of the high-risk surgical population in the United Kingdom. Crit Care. 2006;10(3):R81.
6. Ludbrook G. Hidden pandemic of postoperative complications-time to turn our focus to health systems analysis. Br J Anaesth. 2018;121(6):1190–2.
7. Schier R, Levett D, Riedel B. Prehabilitation: the next challenge for anaesthesia teams. Eur J Anaesthesiol. 2020;37(4):259–62.
8. Brindle M, Nelson G, Lobo DN, Ljungqvist O, Gustafsson UO. Recommendations from the ERAS® society for standards for the development of enhanced recovery after surgery guidelines. BJS Open. 2020;4(1):157–63.
9. Molenaar CJL, Minnella EM, Coca-Martinez M, Ten Cate DWG, Regis M, Awasthi R, Martínez-Palli G, López-Baamonde M, Sebio-Garcia R, Feo CV, van Rooijen SJ, Schreinemakers JMJ, Bojesen RD, Gögenur I, van den Heuvel ER, Carli F, Slooter GD. Effect of multimodal Prehabilitation on reducing postoperative complications and enhancing functional capacity following colorectal cancer surgery: the PREHAB randomized clinical trial. JAMA Surg. 2023;158(6):572–81.
10. Assouline B, Cools E, Schorer R, Kayser B, Elia N, Licker M. Preoperative exercise training to prevent postoperative pulmonary complications in adults undergoing major surgery: A systematic review and meta-analysis with trial sequential analysis. Ann Am Thorac Soc. 2020;18(4):678–88.
11. Duro-Ocana P, Zambolin F, Jones AW, Bryan A, Moore J, Quraishi-Akhtar T, McPhee J, Degens H, Bagley L. Efficacy of supervised exercise prehabilitation programs to improve major abdominal surgery outcomes: A systematic review and meta-analysis. J Clin Anesth. 2023;86:111053.
12. Kamarajah SK, Bundred J, Weblin J, Tan BHL. Critical appraisal on the impact of preoperative rehabilitation and outcomes after major abdominal and cardiothoracic surgery: A systematic review and meta-analysis. Surgery. 2020;167(3):540–9.
13. Lau CSM, Chamberlain RS. Prehabilitation programs improve exercise capacity before and after surgery in gastrointestinal cancer surgery patients: A meta-analysis. J Gastrointest Surg. 2020;24(12):2829–37.
14. Mareschal J, Hemmer A, Douissard J, Dupertuis YM, Collet TH, Koessler T, Toso C, Ris F, Genton L. Surgical Prehabilitation in patients with gastrointestinal cancers: impact of unimodal and multimodal programs on postoperative outcomes and prospects for new therapeutic strategies-A systematic review. Cancers. 2023;15(6):21.
15. Perry R, Herbert G, Atkinson C, England C, Northstone K, Baos S, Brush T, Chong A, Ness A, Harris J, Haase A, Shah S, Pufulete M. Pre-admission interventions (prehabilitation) to improve outcome after major elective surgery: a systematic review and meta-analysis. BMJ Open. 2021;11(9):e050806.
16. Piraux E, Reychler G, de Noordhout LM, Forget P, Deswysen Y, Caty G. What are the impact and the optimal design of a physical prehabilitation program in patients with esophagogastric cancer awaiting surgery? A systematic review. BMC Sports Sci Med Rehabil. 2021;13(1):33.

17. Steffens D, Beckenkamp PR, Hancock M, Solomon M, Young J. Preoperative exercise halves the postoperative complication rate in patients with lung cancer: a systematic review of the effect of exercise on complications, length of stay and quality of life in patients with cancer. Br J Sports Med. 2018;52(5):344.
18. Waterland JL, McCourt O, Edbrooke L, Granger CL, Ismail H, Riedel B, Denehy L. Efficacy of Prehabilitation including exercise on postoperative outcomes following abdominal cancer surgery: A systematic review and meta-analysis. Front Surg. 2021;8:628848.
19. McIsaac DI, Gill M, Boland L, Hutton B, Branje K, Shaw J, Grudzinski AL, Barone N, Gillis C. Prehabilitation in adult patients undergoing surgery: an umbrella review of systematic reviews. Br J Anaesth. 2022;128(2):244–57.
20. Abbott TEF, Fowler AJ, Pelosi P, Gama de Abreu M, Møller AM, Canet J, Creagh-Brown B, Mythen M, Gin T, Lalu MM, Futier E, Grocott MP, Schultz MJ, Pearse RM. A systematic review and consensus definitions for standardised end-points in perioperative medicine: pulmonary complications. Br J Anaesth. 2018;120(5):1066–79.
21. Kassin MT, Owen RM, Perez SD, Leeds I, Cox JC, Schnier K, Sadiraj V, Sweeney JF. Risk factors for 30-day hospital readmission among general surgery patients. J Am Coll Surg. 2012;215(3):322–30.
22. Brown SR, Mathew R, Keding A, Marshall HC, Brown JM, Jayne DG. The impact of postoperative complications on long-term quality of life after curative colorectal cancer surgery. Ann Surg. 2014;259(5):916–23.
23. Schwartz J, Parsey D, Mundangepfupfu T, Tsang S, Pranaat R, Wilson J, Papadakos P. Preoperative patient optimization to prevent postoperative pulmonary complications-insights and roles for the respiratory therapist: A narrative review. Can J Respir Ther. 2020;56:79–85.
24. Serpa Neto A, Hemmes SN, Barbas CS, Beiderlinden M, Fernandez-Bustamante A, Futier E, Hollmann MW, Jaber S, Kozian A, Licker M, Lin WQ, Moine P, Scavonetto F, Schilling T, Selmo G, Severgnini P, Sprung J, Treschan T, Unzueta C, Weingarten TN, Wolthuis EK, Wrigge H, Gama de Abreu M, Pelosi P, Schultz MJ. Incidence of mortality and morbidity related to postoperative lung injury in patients who have undergone abdominal or thoracic surgery: a systematic review and meta-analysis. Lancet. Respir Med. 2014;2(12):1007–15.
25. Boden I, Robertson IK, Neil A, Reeve J, Palmer AJ, Skinner EH, Browning L, Anderson L, Hill C, Story D, Denehy L. Preoperative physiotherapy is cost-effective for preventing pulmonary complications after major abdominal surgery: a health economic analysis of a multicentre randomised trial. J Physiother. 2020;66(3):180–7.
26. Boden I, Skinner EH, Browning L, Reeve J, Anderson L, Hill C, Robertson IK, Story D, Denehy L. Preoperative physiotherapy for the prevention of respiratory complications after upper abdominal surgery: pragmatic, double blinded, multicentre randomised controlled trial. BMJ. 2018;360:j5916.
27. Odor PM, Bampoe S, Gilhooly D, Creagh-Brown B, Moonesinghe SR. Perioperative interventions for prevention of postoperative pulmonary complications: systematic review and meta-analysis. BMJ. 2020;368:m540.
28. Boden I, Denehy L. Respiratory Prehabilitation for the prevention of postoperative pulmonary complications after major surgery. Curr Anesthesiol Rep. 2022;12(1):44–58.
29. Kendall F, Oliveira J, Peleteiro B, Pinho P, Bastos PT. Inspiratory muscle training is effective to reduce postoperative pulmonary complications and length of hospital stay: a systematic review and meta-analysis. Disabil Rehabil. 2018;40(8):864–82.
30. Tórtola-Navarro A, Gallardo-Gómez D, Álvarez-Barbosa F, Salazar-Martínez E. Cancer survivor inspiratory muscle training: systematic review and Bayesian meta-analysis. BMJ Support Palliat Care. 2024;13(e3):e561–9.
31. Snowden CP, Prentis JM, Anderson HL, Roberts DR, Randles D, Renton M, Manas DM. Submaximal cardiopulmonary exercise testing predicts complications and hospital length of stay in patients undergoing major elective surgery. Ann Surg. 2010;251(3):535–41.
32. Wijeysundera DN, Pearse RM, Shulman MA, Abbott TEF, Torres E, Ambosta A, Croal BL, Granton JT, Thorpe KE, Grocott MPW, Farrington C, Myles PS, Cuthbertson BH. Assessment of functional capacity before major non-cardiac surgery: an international, prospective cohort study. Lancet. 2018;391(10140):2631–40.

33. West MA, Loughney L, Lythgoe D, Barben CP, Sripadam R, Kemp GJ, Grocott MP, Jack S. Effect of prehabilitation on objectively measured physical fitness after neoadjuvant treatment in preoperative rectal cancer patients: a blinded interventional pilot study. Br J Anaesth. 2015;114(2):244–51.
34. Pirlich M, Schütz T, Norman K, Gastell S, Lübke HJ, Bischoff SC, Bolder U, Frieling T, Güldenzoph H, Hahn K, Jauch KW, Schindler K, Stein J, Volkert D, Weimann A, Werner H, Wolf C, Zürcher G, Bauer P, Lochs H. The German hospital malnutrition study. Clin Nutr. 2006;25(4):563–72.
35. Story DA, Leslie K, Myles PS, Fink M, Poustie SJ, Forbes A, Yap S, Beavis V, Kerridge R. Complications and mortality in older surgical patients in Australia and New Zealand (the REASON study): a multicentre, prospective, observational study. Anaesthesia. 2010;65(10):1022–30.
36. Sadlonova M, Katz NB, Jurayj JS, Flores L, Celano CM, von Arnim CAF, Silver JK. Surgical prehabilitation in older and frail individuals: a scoping review. Int Anesthesiol Clin. 2023;61(2):34–46.
37. Steffens D, Denehy L. Prehabilitation exercise programs for patients undergoing cancer surgery, does one size fit all? Eur J Surg Oncol. 2023;49(2):303–5.
38. Trestini I, Cintoni M, Rinninella E, Grassi F, Paiella S, Salvia R, Bria E, Pozzo C, Alfieri S, Gasbarrini A, Tortora G, Milella M, Mele MC. Neoadjuvant treatment: A window of opportunity for nutritional prehabilitation in patients with pancreatic ductal adenocarcinoma. World J Gastroint Surg. 2021;13(9):885–903.
39. Lim R, Ellett LMK, Semple S, Roughead EE. The extent of medication-related hospital admissions in Australia: A review from 1988 to 2021. Drug Saf. 2022;45(3):249–57.
40. Loughney L, West MA, Moyses H, Bates A, Kemp GJ, Hawkins L, Varkonyi-Sepp J, Burke S, Barben CP, Calverley PM, Cox T, Palmer DH, Mythen MG, Grocott MPW, Jack S. The effects of neoadjuvant chemoradiotherapy and an in-hospital exercise training programme on physical fitness and quality of life in locally advanced rectal cancer patients: a randomised controlled trial (the EMPOWER trial). Perioper Med. 2021;10(1):23.
41. Moug SJ, Barry SJE, Maguire S, Johns N, Dolan D, Steele RJC, Buchan C, Mackay G, Anderson AS, Mutrie N. Does prehabilitation modify muscle mass in patients with rectal cancer undergoing neoadjuvant therapy? A subanalysis from the REx randomised controlled trial. Tech Coloproctol. 2020;24(9):959–64.
42. Macmillan Cancer Support. Prehabilitation for people with cancer. 2019. macmillan.org.uk/assets/prehabilitation-guidance-for-people-with-cancer.pdf. Accessed 2 Aug 2023.
43. American College of Sports Medicine. ACSM's guidelines for exercise testing and prescription. 11th ed. Philadelphia: Wolters Kluwer; 2022. acsm.org/education-resources/books/guidelines-exercise-testing-prescription. Accessed 2 Aug 2023.
44. Borg G. Ratings of perceived exertion and heart rates during short-term cycle exercise and their use in a new cycling strength test. Int J Sports Med. 1982;3(3):153–8.
45. Campbell KL, Winters-Stone KM, Wiskemann J, May AM, Schwartz AL, Courneya KS, Zucker DS, Matthews CE, Ligibel JA, Gerber LH, Morris GS, Patel AV, Hue TF, Perna FM, Schmitz KH. Exercise guidelines for cancer survivors: consensus statement from international multidisciplinary roundtable. Med Sci Sports Exerc. 2019;51(11):2375–90.
46. Khan A, Wong J, Riedel B, Laing E, Beaumont A, Kong J, Warrier S, Heriot A. The impact of Peri-operative enteral Immunonutrition on post-operative complications in gastrointestinal cancer surgery: A meta-analysis. Ann Surg Oncol. 2023;30(6):3619–31.
47. Grimmett C, Heneka N, Chambers S. Psychological interventions prior to cancer surgery: a review of reviews. Curr Anesthesiol Rep. 2022;12(1):78–87.
48. Jerath A, Austin PC, Ko DT, Wijeysundera HC, Fremes S, McCormack D, Wijeysundera DN. Socioeconomic status and days alive and out of hospital after major elective noncardiac surgery: A population-based cohort study. Anesthesiology. 2020;132(4):713–22.
49. Franssen RFW, Janssen-Heijnen MLG, Barberan-Garcia A, Vogelaar FJ, Van Meeteren NLU, Bongers BC. Moderate-intensity exercise training or high-intensity interval training to improve aerobic fitness during exercise prehabilitation in patients planned for elective abdominal cancer surgery? Eur J Surg Oncol. 2022;48(1):3–13.

50. Minnella EM, Ferreira V, Awasthi R, Charlebois P, Stein B, Liberman AS, Scheede-Bergdahl C, Morais JA, Carli F. Effect of two different pre-operative exercise training regimens before colorectal surgery on functional capacity: A randomised controlled trial. Eur J Anaesthesiol. 2020;37(11):969–78.
51. Buffart LM, Kalter J, Sweegers MG, Courneya KS, Newton RU, Aaronson NK, Jacobsen PB, May AM, Galvao DA, Chinapaw MJ, Steindorf K, Irwin ML, Stuiver MM, Hayes S, Griffith KA, Lucia A, Mesters I, van Weert E, Knoop H, Goedendorp MM, Mutrie N, Daley AJ, McConnachie A, Bohus M, Thorsen L, Schulz KH, Short CE, James EL, Plotnikoff RC, Arbane G, Schmidt ME, Potthoff K, van Beurden M, Oldenburg HS, Sonke GS, van Harten WH, Garrod R, Schmitz KH, Winters-Stone KM, Velthuis MJ, Taaffe DR, van Mechelen W, Kersten MJ, Nollet F, Wenzel J, Wiskemann J, Verdonck-de Leeuw IM, Brug J. Effects and moderators of exercise on quality of life and physical function in patients with cancer: an individual patient data meta-analysis of 34 RCTs. Cancer Treat Rev. 2017;52:91–104.
52. Denehy L, Edbrooke L. The role of exercise before cancer treatment. Semin Oncol Nurs. 2022;38(5):151330.
53. Low DE, Allum W, De Manzoni G, Ferri L, Immanuel A, Kuppusamy M, Law S, Lindblad M, Maynard N, Neal J, Pramesh CS, Scott M, Mark Smithers B, Addor V, Ljungqvist O. Guidelines for perioperative Care in Esophagectomy: enhanced recovery after surgery (ERAS(®)) society recommendations. World J Surg. 2019;43(2):299–330.
54. Michie S, Ashford S, Sniehotta FF, Dombrowski SU, Bishop A, French DP. A refined taxonomy of behaviour change techniques to help people change their physical activity and healthy eating behaviours: the CALO-RE taxonomy. Psychol Health. 2011;26(11):1479–98.
55. Gustafsson UO, Scott MJ, Hubner M, Nygren J, Demartines N, Francis N, Rockall TA, Young-Fadok TM, Hill AG, Soop M, de Boer HD, Urman RD, Chang GJ, Fichera A, Kessler H, Grass F, Whang EE, Fawcett WJ, Carli F, Lobo DN, Rollins KE, Balfour A, Baldini G, Riedel B, Ljungqvist O. Guidelines for perioperative Care in Elective Colorectal Surgery: enhanced recovery after surgery (ERAS(®)) society recommendations: 2018. World J Surg. 2019;43(3):659–95.
56. Hasil L, Fenton TR, Ljungqvist O, Gillis C. From clinical guidelines to practice: the nutrition elements for enhancing recovery after colorectal surgery. Nutr Clin Pract. 2022;37(2):300–15.
57. Dindo D, Demartines N, Clavien PA. Classification of surgical complications: a new proposal with evaluation in a cohort of 6336 patients and results of a survey. Ann Surg. 2004;240(2):205–13.
58. Grocott MP, Browne JP, Van der Meulen J, Matejowsky C, Mutch M, Hamilton MA, Levett DZ, Emberton M, Haddad FS, Mythen MG. The postoperative morbidity survey was validated and used to describe morbidity after major surgery. J Clin Epidemiol. 2007;60(9):919–28.
59. Myles PS. More than just morbidity and mortality - quality of recovery and long-term functional recovery after surgery. Anaesthesia. 2020;75(Suppl 1):e143–e50.
60. Levett DZH, Jack S, Swart M, Carlisle J, Wilson J, Snowden C, Riley M, Danjoux G, Ward SA, Older P, Grocott MPW. Perioperative cardiopulmonary exercise testing (CPET): consensus clinical guidelines on indications, organization, conduct, and physiological interpretation. Br J Anaesth. 2018;120(3):484–500.
61. Holland AE, Spruit MA, Troosters T, Puhan MA, Pepin V, Saey D, McCormack MC, Carlin BW, Sciurba FC, Pitta F, Wanger J, MacIntyre N, Kaminsky DA, Culver BH, Revill SM, Hernandes NA, Andrianopoulos V, Camillo CA, Mitchell KE, Lee AL, Hill CJ, Singh SJ. An official European Respiratory Society/American Thoracic Society technical standard: field walking tests in chronic respiratory disease. Eur Respir J. 2014;44(6):1428–46.
62. Lee CHA, Kong JC, Ismail H, Riedel B, Heriot A. Systematic review and meta-analysis of objective assessment of physical fitness in patients undergoing colorectal cancer surgery. Dis Colon Rectum. 2018;61(3):400–9.
63. Gillis C, Fenton TR, Gramlich L, Sajobi TT, Culos-Reed SN, Bousquet-Dion G, Elsherbini N, Fiore JF Jr, Minnella EM, Awasthi R, Liberman AS, Boutros M, Carli F. Older frail prehabilitated patients who cannot attain a 400 m 6-min walking distance before colorectal surgery suffer more postoperative complications. Eur J Surg Oncol. 2021;47(4):874–81.

64. Caspersen CJ, Powell KE, Christenson GM. Physical activity, exercise, and physical fitness: definitions and distinctions for health-related research. Public Health Rep. 1985;100(2):126–31.
65. Craig CL, Marshall AL, Sjostrom M, Bauman AE, Booth ML, Ainsworth BE. International physical activity questionnaire: 12-country reliability and validity. Med Sci Sports Exerc. 2003;35(8):1381–95.
66. Western B, Demmelmaier I, Vistad I, Hansen BH, Stenling A, Henriksen HB, Nordin K, Blomhoff R, Berntsen S. How many days of continuous physical activity monitoring reliably represent time in different intensities in cancer survivors. PLoS One. 2023;18(4):e0284881.
67. Abernethy AP, Shelby-James T, Fazekas BS, Woods D, Currow DC. The Australia-modified Karnofsky performance status (AKPS) scale: a revised scale for contemporary palliative care clinical practice [ISRCTN81117481]. BMC Palliat Care. 2005;4:7.
68. Jones CJ, Rikli RE, Beam WC. A 30-s chair-stand test as a measure of lower body strength in community-residing older adults. Res Q Exerc Sport. 1999;70(2):113–9.
69. Muñoz-Bermejo L, Adsuar JC, Mendoza-Muñoz M, Barrios-Fernández S, Garcia-Gordillo MA, Pérez-Gómez J, Carlos-Vivas J. Test-retest reliability of five times sit to stand test (FTSST) in adults: A systematic review and meta-analysis. Biology. 2021;10(6):510.
70. Rikli RE, Jones CJ. Functional fitness normative scores for community-residing Older adults, ages 60-94. J Ageing Phys Act. 1999;7(2):162–81.
71. Cruz-Jentoft AJ, Bahat G, Bauer J, Boirie Y, Bruyère O, Cederholm T, Cooper C, Landi F, Rolland Y, Sayer AA, Schneider SM, Sieber CC, Topinkova E, Vandewoude M, Visser M, Zamboni M. Sarcopenia: revised European consensus on definition and diagnosis. Age Ageing. 2019;48(1):16–31.
72. Trutschnigg B, Kilgour RD, Reinglas J, Rosenthall L, Hornby L, Morais JA, Vigano A. Precision and reliability of strength (Jamar vs. Biodex handgrip) and body composition (dual-energy X-ray absorptiometry vs. bioimpedance analysis) measurements in advanced cancer patients. Appl Physiol Nutr Metab. 2008;33(6):1232–9.
73. Ferguson ML, Bauer J, Gallagher B, Capra S, Christie DR, Mason BR. Validation of a malnutrition screening tool for patients receiving radiotherapy. Australas Radiol. 1999;43(3):325–7.
74. Bauer J, Capra S, Ferguson M. Use of the scored patient-generated subjective global assessment (PG-SGA) as a nutrition assessment tool in patients with cancer. Eur J Clin Nutr. 2002;56(8):779–85.
75. Miller J, Wells L, Nwulu U, Currow D, Johnson MJ, Skipworth RJE. Validated screening tools for the assessment of cachexia, sarcopenia, and malnutrition: a systematic review. Am J Clin Nutr. 2018;108(6):1196–208.
76. Price KL, Earthman CP. Update on body composition tools in clinical settings: computed tomography, ultrasound, and bioimpedance applications for assessment and monitoring. Eur J Clin Nutr. 2019;73(2):187–93.
77. Rockwood K, Song X, MacKnight C, Bergman H, Hogan DB, McDowell I, Mitnitski A. A global clinical measure of fitness and frailty in elderly people. Can Med Assoc J. 2005;173(5):489–95.
78. Decoster L, Liposits G, Dumontier C. Frailty screening and comprehensive geriatric assessment. In: Gomes F, editor. Frailty in Older adults with cancer. Springer; 2022. p. 41–56. link.springer.com/book/10.1007/978-3-030-89162-6; Accessed 2 Aug 2023.
79. Esser P, Hartung TJ, Friedrich M, Johansen C, Wittchen HU, Faller H, Koch U, Harter M, Keller M, Schulz H, Wegscheider K, Weis J, Mehnert A. The generalized anxiety disorder screener (GAD-7) and the anxiety module of the hospital and depression scale (HADS-A) as screening tools for generalized anxiety disorder among cancer patients. Psycho-Oncology. 2018;27(6):1509–16.
80. Hinz A, Mehnert A, Kocalevent RD, Brahler E, Forkmann T, Singer S, Schulte T. Assessment of depression severity with the PHQ-9 in cancer patients and in the general population. BMC Psychiatr. 2016;16:22.
81. Zigmond AS, Snaith RP. The hospital anxiety and depression scale. Acta Psychiatr Scand. 1983;67(6):361–70.

82. Aaronson NK, Ahmedzai S, Bergman B, Bullinger M, Cull A, Duez NJ, Filiberti A, Flechtner H, Fleishman SB, de Haes JC, et al. The European Organization for Research and Treatment of cancer QLQ-C30: a quality-of-life instrument for use in international clinical trials in oncology. J Nat Canc Inst. 1993;85(5):365–76.
83. Herdman M, Gudex C, Lloyd A, Janssen M, Kind P, Parkin D, Bonsel G, Badia X. Development and preliminary testing of the new five-level version of EQ-5D (EQ-5D-5L). Qual Life Res. 2011;20(10):1727–36.
84. Cella D, Lai JS, Chang CH, Peterman A, Slavin M. Fatigue in cancer patients compared with fatigue in the general United States population. Cancer. 2002;94(2):528–38.
85. National Health Service. National cancer patient experience survey 2023. ncpes.co.uk/interactive-results/. Accessed 2 Aug 2023.

Chapter 7
Elective Surgery for Patients with Substance Use Disorder or Recent Substance Misuse

Talia Scott and Ethan O. Bryson

Abbreviations

AUD	Alcohol use disorder
AUDIT	Alcohol use disorders identification test
COPD	Chronic obstructive pulmonary disease
CUD	Cannabis use disorder
MI	Myocardial infarction
NIDA	National institute on drug abuse
NMDA	N-methyl-D-aspartate
NSDUH	National survey on drug use and health
OUD	Opioid use disorder
PCA	Patient-controlled analgesia
SAMHSA	Substance abuse and mental health services administration
SUD	Substance use disorder
THC	tetrahydrocannabinol
US	United States
TSA	Total shoulder arthroplasty
WHO	World Health Organization

T. Scott
Department of Anesthesiology, Perioperative and Pain medicine, Icahn School of Medicine at Mount Sinai, New York, NY, USA
e-mail: talia.scott@mountsinai.org

E. O. Bryson (✉)
Department of Anesthesiology and Psychiatry, Icahn School of Medicine at Mount Sinai, New York, NY, USA
e-mail: ethan.bryson@mountsinai.org

© The Author(s), under exclusive license to Springer Nature Switzerland AG 2024

J. Faintuch, S. Faintuch (eds.), *Recent Strategies in High Risk Surgery*,
https://doi.org/10.1007/978-3-031-56270-9_7

Introduction

Substance use disorder (SUD), including alcohol use disorder (AUD), affects a significant percentage of the population worldwide, and up to 16.5% of the United States (U.S.) population alone, which includes persons above the age of 12, are affected [1]. So prevalent is the issue of recreational substance use that one recent study suggests that up to 40% of patients undergoing elective surgery present with a history of recent substance use preoperatively [2]. Substance use is an independent risk factor for increased complications, cost, and length of stay, and should therefore be taken into consideration when planning for elective surgery [3]. These complications can include higher risk of hemorrhage, sepsis, stroke, respiratory issues, renal failure, and issues with wound or graft healing [3]. Patients with a history of substance use are also more likely to have other serious medical conditions, such as liver disease, chronic obstructive pulmonary disease (COPD), and human immunodeficiency virus (HIV) infection [3].

Detecting a substance use disorder perioperatively can be a challenging task. These diagnoses are commonly missed, whether as a result of absent inquiry or an unwillingness on the part of the patient to admit use, either due to the stigma attached to substance use or ignorance of its potential effects during the perioperative period [4]. Patients may not understand the implications of recent substance use on perioperative outcomes, thinking it is only a concern if they are acutely intoxicated. Because of this, it is essential to explain to patients that disclosing substance use prior to elective surgery will not be reported to authorities, is protected by the doctor-patient relationship, is essential for safe administration of anesthesia, and has significant implications for the success of and recovery from surgery. It should be emphasized that asking these types of questions does not imply judgment but are only asked to gain knowledge that is essential to keep the patient safe during the perioperative period and do not necessarily preclude proceeding with the procedure. Clearly, if, on the day of surgery, the patient appears acutely intoxicated, concerns about the ability to fully understand the informed consent process should be evaluated and the elective surgery should be rescheduled.

There is considerable evidence that patients with a current or recent history of drug use or misuse are at a significantly higher risk for experiencing any number of perioperative complications associated with elective surgery. When it comes to patients with underlying medical conditions, the risk for complications increases substantially, often leading to increased morbidity, longer hospital stays and higher risk for perioperative mortality [3]. According to this recent report, current or recent drug misuse also has the potential to increase the length of hospital stay resulting in higher costs, regardless of the patient's age or medical comorbidities [3].

Consumption Screening

It can be very challenging to identify these patients in the perioperative period as recreational substance misuse if often not disclosed, reported or previously diagnosed when they present for elective surgery [4]. Despite this, it is estimated that up to 40% of patients presenting for elective surgery do so with a history of recent or current substance misuse which has the potential to increase their risks for perioperative complications [2]. In the following sections we will discuss the identification, implications, and management of the patient who presents for elective surgery with recent or current substance use.

Commonly Misused Substances

Alcohol

Alcohol is ubiquitous and in many countries social drinking is considered acceptable substance use. That being said, there is a fine line between alcohol use and misuse, with the definition of alcohol misuse varying between cultures, religions and geographical areas. In general, alcohol misuse includes heavy or binge drinking which is beyond the accepted norms for the population, but even regular acceptable consumption has implications for patients presenting for elective surgery. Alcohol use disorder (AUD) encompasses both alcohol misuse and dependence, and involves negative consequences related to use [5]. AUD is a highly prevalent disorder which affects 237 million men and 46 million women worldwide [6]. In the United States alone, AUD affects 13.2% of adult men and 9.5% of adult women [7]. Patients who present for elective surgery should be questioned regarding their specific daily intake as this has significant implications for anesthesia and post-surgical recovery success.

Identification

While many patients will occasionally drink alcohol, the stigma attached with perceived excessive alcohol consumption varies from culture to culture. From the standpoint of the anesthesiologist or surgeon, no judgment is made regarding individual use, but the quantity and frequency of use must be identified. The Alcohol Use Disorders Identification Test (AUDIT-C) tool consists of three questions that can be used to screen for AUD [8]. The AUDIT-C is scored on a scale of 0–12 (a score of 0 reflects no alcohol use).

Implications for Surgery

Intraoperatively, chronic alcohol use can create tolerance, leading to higher anesthetic requirements, while on the other hand, acute intoxication lowers the anesthetic requirement [9]. Obviously the patient who presents for elective surgery either acutely intoxicated or who reports same day alcohol use should be rescheduled and encouraged not to drink prior to surgery, but it is more often that the patient who regularly uses or misuses alcohol will under-report their actual consumption.

There appears to be a dose-dependent relationship between alcohol consumption and surgical complications, with one study finding that the complication rate was 50% higher with consumption of three to four drinks daily but climbed to 200–400% higher in those who consumed five or more drinks a day. These complications included postoperative infection, cardiopulmonary events, and increased bleeding [10].

Alcohol Use Disorder is associated with increased length of hospital stay and cost across surgical fields [11–13]. These risks are particularly notable in colectomy patients. Colectomies are already one of the most expensive surgeries, costing up to $25,000 [14]. Patients undergoing colectomy with a history of AUD have increased hospital cost from an already high baseline. Even more concerning is that, patients with AUD who undergo this procedure are at increased risk for in-hospital mortality [11].

A history of AUD is also significant in patients undergoing orthopedic surgery. An association has been demonstrated between alcohol use and decreased bone remodeling in animal models, so it follows that poor post-orthopedic surgery recovery in this population [15]. In arthroplasty patients, those with AUD had higher risks of dislocation and readmission [12]. According to the Hospital Readmissions Reduction Program (HRRP), a value-based purchasing program run by the Center for Medicare and Medicaid services (U.S.) designed to reduce avoidable readmissions, increases in readmission could lead to financial repercussions for the hospital [12].

Management Strategies

Preoperative abstinence can have beneficial effects. One study found that patients who were abstinent from alcohol for 1 month preoperatively had less postoperative arrhythmia, hypoxemia, and myocardial ischemia than those who continued drinking [16]. A meta-analysis agreed that 1–2 months of abstinence preoperatively was associated with fewer complications, although the effect on mortality was unclear [17]. Cessation of alcohol use should be guided by specialists who will be able to wean the patient from alcohol while limiting risk of withdrawal and also providing psychosocial support.

Tobacco

According to the World Health Organization (WHO), as of 2022, 22.3% of the global population used tobacco (36.7% men and 7.8% women) [18]. While cigarette smoking is the most common form of tobacco use worldwide, tobacco products also include waterpipe tobacco, commonly referred to as hookahs, which have cultural significance in many populations and are symbolic of friendship, trust, and respect, as the pipes are shared with physically connected inhalation tubes. The tobacco smoked in this manner is inhaled unfiltered and regular users are often exposed to increased levels of nicotine and other products of combustion which have significant implications for patients during the perioperative period.

Smokeless tobacco products, such as "vapes," "e-cigarettes," or other electronic nicotine delivery devices, chewing tobacco, nicotine gum and patches reduce exposure to many of the toxic chemicals associated with the inhalation of cigarette smoke but still provide the user with nicotine, which also has significant implications for the perioperative patient. Although designed as a replacement for cigarettes, the popularity of e-cigarette use has risen dramatically among young people, and by 2022 4.5% of middle school students and 16% of high school students in the U.S. had used an e-cigarette in the past 30 days compared to approximately 3.7% of adults [19, 20]. In one survey of preoperative patients it was found that 13.9% of those who used e-cigarettes had used them in the last week [21].

Identification

The easiest way to identify patients who use tobacco products is to ask direct questions during the preoperative interview. Unlike alcohol, which patients may minimize their actual use, or illicit drugs, which they may deny using altogether, patients who smoke are usually forthcoming when asked. Preoperatively, patients should be screened for both tobacco and nicotine-containing e-cigarette use. Of note, those who use e-cigarettes commonly do not believe the term "smoking" includes e-cigarette use [21]. Patients can then be counseled on smoking cessation and given the appropriate tools, support, and resources to quit successfully.

Implications for Surgery

Individuals who smoke heavily for several years are more prone to developing complications in their lungs after surgery, but even those who smoke occasionally or in small quantities may face an elevated risk. Smoking causes airway hyper-reactivity, contributing to pulmonary complications during anesthesia such as laryngospasm, bronchospasm, reintubation, and hypoxemia even in the absence of reactive airway disease. Age and body habitus are also important, with a 6.3x increased risk of pulmonary complications in obese young smokers compared to 2.3x in young smokers and 1.8x in all smokers [22]. Given these pulmonary risks, it follows that smokers are more likely to be admitted to the ICU postoperatively [23]. In one study the relative risk for any of these pulmonary complications was 1.8 for all smokers but significantly higher in patients aged 16–39 years (2.3) and jumped to 6.3 if these patients were also obese [22]. In the same study, young smokers with chronic bronchitis were 25.7 times more likely to experience bronchospasm in the perioperative setting.

In colorectal surgery, current smokers had increased risk of major complications such as infection, cardiac events, and sepsis as well as increased mortality risk. Overall, within 30 days of surgery, smokers had a 30% increased risk of sustaining either a major complication or mortality [24]. In total hip arthroplasties, there was a higher rate of revision in patients who smoke [25].

Wound healing is well-known to be impaired in cigarette smokers [26]. Nicotine is thought to directly cause injury to the vascular intima, leading to atherosclerosis. This can be especially detrimental in plastic surgery and surgery involving grafts, as cutaneous tissue beds are most susceptible to decreased blood flow. Particularly in the case of elective surgery, poor wound healing can detrimentally impact the desired outcome [27].

Although e-cigarettes avoid inhalation of combustible material, their use is still associated with pulmonary toxicity including airway hyperreactivity [28]. The nicotine contained in e-cigarettes stimulates catecholamine release affecting the cardiovascular system, which in turn can make the effects of anesthetics less predictable [29]. E-cigarette use in total joint arthroplasty patients was associated with longer operative time, hospital length of stay, and readmission [30]. In plastic surgery, those who used e-cigarettes had similar rates of flap necrosis to cigarette smokers, implying that nicotine is the substance toxic to flap survival [31]. E-cigarettes may be a helpful tool in smoking cessation, but their use should be considered when proceeding with elective surgery.

Management Strategies

Smokers who stop at least 6–8 weeks prior to elective surgery have been shown to reduce their risk for intraoperative and postoperative complications [32]. Surgery may provide good incentive to quit smoking and may be a good time to quit. One review found that 8% of those who quit do so because of surgery [33]. Additionally, in one study, 28 subjects (46.7%) who were able to stop smoking prior to surgery remained abstinent at follow-up 1 year after intervention [34].

The detrimental effects of smoking on surgical outcomes decrease the longer the period between smoking cessation and surgery and each week of cessation can increase the magnitude of this effect by up to 19% [35]. Cessation of greater than 4 weeks was associated with a 20% decreased risk of complications compared to cessation of less than 4 weeks [36]. The benefits of a longer time frame are explained by the weeks to months it can take for the pulmonary cilia to heal and pulmonary function to return, making 8 weeks of abstinence before elective surgery ideal [37].

At a minimum, from an anesthesia standpoint, the patient should not smoke for at least 12 h preoperatively so that levels of nicotine and carboxyhemoglobin can decline. Carboxyhemoglobin can significantly decrease the bioavailability of oxygen, which can be catastrophic in patients with a history of coronary artery disease. If a patient with coronary history reports smoking the day of elective surgery, it may be reasonable to postpone the case [38].

Marijuana

According to the United States Substance Abuse and Mental Health Services Administration (SAMHSA) National Survey on Drug Use and Health (NSDUH), 52.5 million people aged 12 or older (18.8% of the population) reportedly used marijuana in 2020 [1]. With an increasing move toward decriminalization and legalization in many areas, these numbers will undoubtedly increase, either to come in line with true numbers as the stigma of marijuana use is lessened by the elimination of legal consequences or as new users begin to adopt the habit.

Identification

Signs of acute marijuana intoxication include anxiety, tachycardia, decreased short-term memory (the individual may not be able to adequately participate in the preoperative interview), Dry mouth, conjunctival injection, impaired perception, and motor skills. In chronic users who have not recently used and are not currently under the influence these findings are not common. Simply asking about regular marijuana use, however, usually elicits an honest response. In patients who are hesitant it is important to emphasize that questions about regular use are not intended to judge but to obtain information important to keep the patient safe during the procedure.

Signs such as a "green tinge" on the tongue (related to inhaling chlorophyll, or artificial green dye which is sometimes added to vaping preparations) has been reported, though these signs are non-specific and rare [39].

Screening tests for marijuana use are, as of this writing, only reliable in chronic users and require regular use over a period of 30 or more days to produce a consistently positive result. After the initial use, one-third of the major psychoactive component of marijuana which is tested for, tetrahydrocannabinol (THC), is excreted in the urine. After a single use, THC may be detected on a urine drug screen for 2–3 days, though this is not consistently reliable. With chronic use, however, and depending on the test used, the length of time after the last ingestion during which THC can be detected in the urine increases to 1–4 weeks [40]. False positive drug screen results have been reported in patients who have been taking over the counter medications such as ibuprofen and naproxen [41].

Implications for Surgery

In 2020 a retrospective cohort analysis published by Goel et al. provided significant evidence that patients with active cannabis use disorder (CUD) who underwent elective surgery were at increased perioperative risk of myocardial infarction (MI) [42]. In this cohort of 27,206 patients the odds of postoperative MI was 1.88 times higher for patients with a reported active cannabis use disorder, as defined by the International Classification of Diseases, Ninth Edition, Clinical Modification (ICD-9-CM) diagnostic codes for cannabis dependence and cannabis abuse. Prior to this, most evidence in the literature regarding recent or chronic marijuana use as related to surgical implications were, in part, extrapolated from studies performed on patients who reported tobacco smoking, and focused on wound healing [43]. While the route of ingestion of cannabis products is important to consider when looking at outcomes such as wound healing related to decreased vascular perfusion related to vasoconstriction and tissue ischemia, the potential for physiological withdrawal symptoms during the perioperative period, when access to cannabis may be limited, is important to consider as a potential etiology for postoperative MI, especially in the chronic user who presents for elective surgery.

Similar to patients who are chronic tobacco smokers, patients who regularly smoke marijuana are subject to the same pulmonary risks outlined above [38]. Additionally, case reports of uvulitis or uvular edema leading to airway obstruction, laryngospasm and bronchospasm while under anesthesia in patients who regularly smoke marijuana highlight the increased risk for these patients who present for elective surgery [44–46]. Anecdotal evidence suggests that, much in the same way patients with AUD present with increased tolerance for anesthetic agents, patients with CUD also have increased intraoperative anesthetic requirements and are, as a result, at increased risk for complications related to a lighter plane of anesthesia, including awareness.

The route of ingestion preferred by the user is important to consider. Much like the hookah, commercially available marijuana is not, as of this writing, produced in the form of filtered cigarettes. Due to the absence of filters significantly more products of combustion such as tar and other carcinogens are inhaled than with commercially available filtered tobacco cigarettes [47]. The carboxyhemoglobin level in the blood of a marijuana smoker can be up to five times higher than that of a tobacco smoker, primarily due to the practice of deep inhalation, holding the smoke in lungs longer [48]. Patients who use marijuana in different forms, other than smoking, are still subject to the effects of the drug. Edibles, tinctures, and other forms of non-inhaled cannabis will still increase in heart rate, produce ectopy, and in patients with underlying coronary vascular disease, can result in reversible ST or T segment abnormalities visible on the perioperative electrocardiogram (ECG). These factors alone can make the safe induction of anesthesia challenging, increase the risk for perioperative MI, and require higher doses of anesthesia to achieve a depth adequate for elective surgery [38, 49].

Management Strategies

For chronic marijuana users, regardless of the route of ingestion, use within 72 h of elective surgery should be discouraged [43]. Patients who cannot or will not abstain prior to surgery should be counseled as to the risks involved with continued use during the perioperative period. For the patient who presents with recent use, informed consent should be obtained at least 2 h after the last ingestion and in the absence of signs of impairment.

Inhalants

Nitrous Oxide

Inhalants represent a very small portion of the commonly misused drugs worldwide, but deserve mention as they are most often used by the younger, healthier patients who would seem, without knowing this history, to fall into the very-low risk category for elective surgery. Nitrous oxide (N_2O) or laughing gas specifically has long been established as a very commonly misused drug, especially in the United Kingdom (UK), the United States (US), and Australia (38.6% and 29.4% lifetime prevalence) [50]. In this study, the eighth most commonly misused substance was N_2O. Intoxication with this substance is achieved through inhalation of the gas, often in the absence of supplemental oxygen, which generates auditory and visual hallucinations, euphoria, and total body insensitivity to pain. As a result of this inability to feel pain, accidental injury sometimes severe is not uncommon. Misuse of N_2O represents a significant problem because of the difficulty involved with identification, as we will see below, and the toxicity associated with chronic misuse [51].

Paint Solvents

So called huffing or the inhalation of the volatile agents present in paints (particularly spray paints), paint thinner, and industrial solvents, induce a state of euphoria, similar to that which is achieved by the inhalation of N_2O. Unlike N_2O, however, the effects are longer lasting and are more likely to be associated with dependence, tolerance, irritability, anxiety, and cravings. Commonly available household items including air freshener, nail polish remover, and model glue have documented misuse potential [52]. Due to the low cost and high availability of these agents these are most commonly misused by adolescents, including those of low income countries [53].

Anesthetic Gases

The misuse of the volatile hydrocarbon anesthetics, most commonly sevoflurane, has also been reported, especially among people with access to these agents such as physicians, nurses, and even hospital employees as these drugs are not controlled in the same way that opioids and other scheduled drugs are.

Identification

With the exception of the patient who presents for elective surgery with a history of neurological complications related to chronic N_2O misuse or who admits to this misuse in the preoperative interview, identification of chronic use is difficult. The effects of the drug are transient and, while there is the potential for addiction, the stigmata of N_2O misuse, even in the most severe cases, is often absent. Nitrous oxide misuse is not detected by any available screening tools due to its short half-life and rapid elimination through the lungs [54]. Intoxication lasts for a brief period, measured in seconds or minutes, and there is no evidence that even chronic N_2O use has any residual effects on the sensorium. Absent laboratory confirmation, the interview is the best opportunity to elicit this information.

Identification of the patient who chronically misuses commercially available industrial solvents is difficult. On routine pre-op laboratory examination, the presence of anemia or leukopenia may indicate chronic misuse and should be further evaluated [55]. Physical signs include the residue of paint or adhesive around the oropharynx, commonly associated with the practice of "bagging" whereby the agent is placed in a paper bag and ingested via hyperventilation, or by the neurologic deficits associated with chronic misuse. There are currently no commercially available laboratory tests which can identify the chronic user, so an increased index of suspicion is essential during the preoperative interview. The misuse of the volatile anesthetic agents is even more difficult to identify, as chronic use of these agents is much less likely to result in neurologic sequelae.

Implications for Surgery

Chronic exposure to N_2O is thought to put the user at risk for the development of a hypercoagulable state, increasing the risk for deep venous thrombosis (DVT) and potential pulmonary embolism (PE) during elective surgery. Several case reports of thromboembolisms, especially in young, otherwise healthy individuals, point to the increased risk when these patients opt to undergo elective surgery in this setting [56–58].

The effects of chronic N_2O and volatile agent misuse are similar regardless of chemical structure, and depend primarily on the degree to which the agent has been used, including length of use and total dose. During use, peripheral vasodilation occurs, resulting in compensatory tachycardia, but decreased myocardial contractility often causes orthostatic hypotension. It is unclear if these physiological phenomena occur in the chronic user who presents for elective surgery while not under the influence, but this should be a concern, as tachycardia combined with decreased myocardial contractility resulting in hypotension have been reported. With acute intoxication, bradycardia, decreased cardiac output, and "sudden sniff death syndrome" may occur, most likely related to the development of a malignant dysrhythmia [59].

Management Strategies

Patients with chronic inhalation misuse are at increased risk for nausea and vomiting, which can lead to aspiration, and reactive airway disease, even in the absence of asthma, which increases the risk for bronchospasm and laryngospasm. These volatile agents are known hepatotoxins and chronic users are also at risk for undiagnosed liver disease, which has the potential to affect many of the anesthetic agents used during elective surgery. Renal injury, specifically chronic renal tubular acidosis, has also been reported and should be evaluated prior to elective surgery. Chronic use can also lead to vitamin B12 deficiency, commonly manifesting as peripheral neuropathy [60].

CNS Depressants

Opioids

Opioids are a broad class of drugs that interact with opioid receptors and cause pain relief and euphoria. The term "opioid" includes all drugs in this class. The term "opiate" refers to natural opioid compounds such as heroin, morphine, and codeine. Semi-synthetic and synthetic opioids are commonly prescribed for postoperative pain management and include the popular fentanyl and its derivatives.

It has been well-established that opioid misuse is a pressing public health issue. Over the past few decades, there has been a dramatic increase in opioid prescriptions with a parallel increase in opioid misuse, abuse, and overdose. The opioid crisis has become so severe that it has been declared a public health emergency by the U.S. government, with the CDC citing 44 deaths daily from opioid overdose [61]. 3.7% of the United States population has misused opioids in the past year, the most common substance being prescription pain relievers [62]. Approximately 25% of preoperative patients will be using opioids [63].

It is important to note that not all patients who chronically use opioids are misusing them or have opioid use disorder (OUD). Some patients may present for surgery who are using prescribed opioids appropriately for chronic pain conditions. After a few weeks of consistent opioid use however, patients will become "dependent," meaning they will experience withdrawal symptoms if they stop taking the medication. Physical dependence can exist without addiction or a use disorder. If a patient is addicted to opioids or has OUD, there is physical dependence as well as cravings and inability to control drug use.

Identification

Opioids can be taken by a variety of routes, including oral, inhaled, and injected. In those who inject, marks may be seen on the skin. Signs of acute opioid intoxication include slowed respiratory rate, pinpoint pupils, nausea and vomiting, and confusion or delirium. The usual urine drug screen is able to detect heroin, but is not sensitive for synthetic opioids such as oxycodone, hydrocodone, methadone, or fentanyl. These drugs can be tested with specific immunoassay panels [39].

Implications for Surgery

Those who chronically use opioids will have a higher tolerance for the drug class, which can make pain management intraoperatively and postoperatively challenging. Patients may be admitted to the hospital for pain management who would have otherwise been able to be discharged from the PACU. Studies across surgical fields have found that having OUD is associated with longer hospital stay by approximately 2 days [64, 65]. In orthopedic surgery, OUD was associated with increased mortality and morbidity such as respiratory failure, myocardial infarction, and surgical site infection [66]. Patients who use opioids intravenously, such as heroin, have even more risk. Due to the route of administration, they are at risk for endocarditis, pulmonary infection, infected deep venous thrombosis, and sepsis [67].

Management Strategies

Preoperatively, it is important to distinguish if the patient has an OUD or uses opioids chronically for pain. Those with OUD should be referred to appropriate resources where they can be weaned from opioids safely before surgery takes place [4]. In contrast, those who use prescribed opioids for pain conditions should continue their medications. They should take their usual pain medication the morning of surgery, especially if they take any long-acting opioids such as methadone [68].

Pain may be difficult to control in patients who have a tolerance to opioids. There are no formal guidelines for pain management, but most recommend a multimodal approach [69]. Instead of higher doses of a single medication type, lower doses of a variety of medications with different mechanisms of action are used [70]. Acetaminophen, ketorolac, and lidocaine patches are mainstays of treatment. Regional anesthesia can be useful, including nerve blocks, peripheral nerve catheters, and epidural catheters. In patients with refractory pain, ketamine infusion can be considered [71]. Patient-controlled analgesia (PCA) pumps administering opioids are a great tool for hospitalized patients [72].

Opioid maintenance therapy is used for patients with OUD and includes three main medication options: buprenorphine, methadone, and naltrexone [73]. Buprenorphine is a partial mu agonist and full kappa antagonist with weak analgesic effect. Importantly, it has a ceiling effect on respiratory depression which makes overdose less likely [74]. Because it blocks the binding of any additional opioids to pain receptors, it can make the treatment of pain difficult [75]. A multimodal pain approach is recommended, and additional buprenorphine can be given [76]. As acute cessation can precipitate withdrawal symptoms, it is recommended to continue through surgery [77]. Methadone is a full mu agonist with more analgesic effect than buprenorphine. It is long acting with a biphasic elimination. It can also be taken preoperatively including the day of surgery. Those who take methadone may need higher doses of opioid medications to adequately treat pain. The QTc can be prolonged by methadone and should be monitored. These two drugs are not interchangeable; in patients treated with methadone, treating with a partial agonist such as buprenorphine will precipitate withdrawal [78]. Naltrexone is an opioid antagonist that prevents the binding of opioids to pain receptors [79]. It follows that patients taking naltrexone can have postoperative pain that is extremely difficult to control, and that naltrexone should be discontinued preoperatively. Oral naltrexone should be discontinued for 2–3 days and injectable naltrexone for 28 days before elective surgery [80]. Because chronic naltrexone use leads to an upregulation of opioid receptors, patients are at an increased risk of overdose once naltrexone is discontinued (Table 7.1) [81].

All opioid-dependent patients who are admitted to the hospital postoperatively are at risk for withdrawal. Acute withdrawal can cause central excitability such as insomnia and anxiety, and autonomic hyperactivity such as tachycardia, hypertension, sweating, and hyperthermia [4]. Other classic signs include piloerection, lacrimation, nausea and vomiting, and pupillary dilation. Withdrawal can be

Table 7.1 Perioperative opioid maintenance therapy

Drug	Type	Preoperative management	Postoperative considerations
Buprenorphine	Partial mu agonist, full kappa antagonist	Continue, take day of surgery	• Inhibits additional opioids from binding to receptors, making them less effective at treating pain • Multimodal pain approach is beneficial
Methadone	Full mu agonist	Continue, take day of surgery	• Those taking methadone may require higher doses of opioids • Can prolong QTc
Naltrexone	Competitive mu antagonist, partial kappa agonist	PO: Stop 2–3 days preoperatively IM: Stop 28 days preoperatively	• Patients are more sensitive to opioids, increased risk of overdose

life-threatening, and so any patients who present with opioid use preoperatively should be carefully monitored in the postoperative period.

CNS Stimulants

Cocaine and Methamphetamines

In the United States in the past year, 1.7% of the population has used cocaine [82]. Cocaine is involved in one in five overdose deaths. The rate of patients who present for elective surgery and are found to be positive for cocaine on drug testing likely varies regionally, though one center reports a rate of 1% [83]. Cocaine can be used as a powder which is inhaled nasally, used orally, or dissolved and injected intravenously. Crack cocaine is a form with a quicker euphoric effect that is smoked. Recently, there has been a rise in cocaine contaminated with fentanyl and fentanyl analogues, which should be kept in mind with any reported history of cocaine use [84].

Identification

Signs of acute cocaine intoxication include tachycardia, hypertension, pupillary dilation, diaphoresis, tremor, restlessness, and agitation. Chronic misuse can cause seizure, stroke, and cognitive impairment [85, 86]. Physical exam findings concerning for cocaine misuse include nasal/septal/palatal defects, gingivitis, and pulmonary symptoms in crack cocaine users. A urine drug screen is positive after acute use for 2–3 days and for several weeks with chronic use [39].

The signs of acute intoxication with methamphetamines are similar to acute cocaine intoxication and include akathisia, hypervigilance, volatile or violent behavior, psychosis, dilated and minimally reactive pupils, tachycardia, hypertension, hyperthermia, and diaphoresis [87]. Chronic misuse is evident in most users by the presence of so-called meth mouth which is characterized by severe tooth decay and loss caused by associated corrosive chemicals, xerostomia, impaired gingival and tooth perfusion, and poor diet. There may be the odor of ammonia on the breath, and the presence of 'meth mites' or 'meth bugs' caused by intense localized pruritus which chronic users commonly scratch until open wounds are created [39].

Of note, while methamphetamines are commonly included in most urine toxicology drug screens, false positive results have been reported in those taking brompheniramine (an antihistamine), phenylpropanolamine (a nasal decongestant), bupropion and trazodone (common antidepressants), chlorpromazine and promethazine (common antipsychotics), and ranitidine (an H_2 blocker) [41].

Implications for Surgery

Cocaine has been shown to induce thrombocytopenia [88]. This may cause some anesthesiologists to not perform neuraxial techniques or regional blocks due to risk of hematoma in nerve spaces. Surgically, this can increase risk of operative bleeding. Cocaine use can also cause pseudovasculitis and may impair wound healing [39].

There are concerns about the deleterious effects of cocaine use on organ systems during general anesthesia. Cocaine use is a known risk factor for cardiovascular events including severe hypertension, dysrhythmias, MI, and aortic dissection [49]. Case reports have reported severe cardiac events in chronic cocaine users in the absence of acute intoxication [89]. Cocaine use can also cause spontaneous pneumothorax [90].

The risks for the patient who chronically misuses methamphetamines are similar and include uncontrolled hypertension, perioperative MI, and coronary artery spasm. Chronic users may have developed cardiomyopathy and pulmonary hypertension and are at risk for aortic dissection [91]. In one study, patients who tested positive for methamphetamines within 24 h of surgery were 31.4% more likely to experience hemodynamic instability during the first hour of general anesthesia as compared to 26.1% who tested positive between 2–7 days prior to surgery and only 6.3% of controls [92].

Management Strategies

Elective surgery in a patient who is acutely intoxicated should be postponed. There is debate about the best management strategy for a patient who is not acutely intoxicated, but presents for elective surgery with a positive drug screen. The conservative approach is to wait 1 week after cessation or for a negative drug screen [89]. Cancelation of cases leads to increased cost, and some studies suggest that general anesthesia is safe in a non-acutely intoxicated patient [83, 93]. For these reasons, it may also be appropriate to observe the patient for 8 h (the time it would take for any active cocaine to be metabolized), and if asymptomatic, proceed with surgery [94]. Overall, the decision to proceed with elective surgery should take into consideration the patient history, acuity of the surgery, discussion between the surgeon and anesthesiologist, and discussion between the surgical team and the patient. Postponing surgery up to 7 days somewhat decreases the risks associated with methamphetamine use, but not to the levels of patients who do not use methamphetamines [92].

Hallucinogens

Lysergic Acid Diethylamide (LSD), Psilocybin, and Phencyclidine

First synthesized by Swiss Chemist Albert Hofmann from ergot derivatives in an attempt to find a drug capable of reducing postpartum hemorrhage, lysergic acid diethylamide (LSD) has recently seen a resurgence in use as a treatment for anxiety, depression, psychosomatic disorders and addiction [95]. While its use today remains primarily as a recreational hallucinogen, LSD has a long history of medical application, particularly within the psychiatric community, as a means to facilitate remission of psychiatric symptoms. With the recent move toward decriminalization and legalization of psychoactive drugs, LSD should be considered, along with other hallucinogens, as a potential agent which will complicate the perioperative management of the patient presenting for elective surgery.

Identification

LSD, as with other "classical hallucinogens" such as psilocybin and dimethyltryptamine, alters perception and creates an altered state of consciousness. Alterations include distortions in the perception of time, depth, the size and shape of objects, movement, color, sounds, touch and are associated with delusions which have led to unintentional self-harm or harm to others [96]. When acutely intoxicated, patients may appear to be psychotic, exhibiting symptoms of anxiety, dysphoria and confusion. Increases in heart rate and blood pressure are often accompanied by mydriasis, almost to the point of elimination of the iris, mild hyper or hypothermia, piloerection, and hyperglycemia. Use is not associated with physical dependence nor is there a withdrawal syndrome, though tolerance for the effects of LSD has been reported [97].

Implications for Surgery

It is likely that LSD works as an agonist at the serotonin 2A receptor (5-HT2A), and there is evidence that HT2A antagonists can attenuate and perhaps reverse the main effects of these substances [98]. If a patient presents for elective surgery under the influence of LSD, the procedure should be rescheduled. Recent use does not preclude elective surgery, though use of other recreational pharmaceuticals should be investigated through discussion prior to proceeding.

Management Strategies

Patients who present for elective surgery not currently under the influence of LSD do not require any specific management strategies directly related to recent use. It should be noted, however, that recent or chronic use has been associated with "flashbacks", in which the individual experiences the effects of the hallucinogen even though they are no longer under its influence [99]. These events can be triggered by the stress of surgery, fatigue, or by the concomitant administration of other medications during the perioperative period, and should the patient experience symptoms as described above, this should be considered as part of the differential diagnosis. Supportive care is indicated and the patient may benefit from anxiolytics and, in extreme cases, psychiatric consultation.

Conclusion

Surgery should take into consideration the recency and extent of use, the surgical and anesthetic risks, and the necessity of the surgery. Programmed discussion of substance misuse with surgical candidates is fundamental as it allows time to refrain from the substance preoperatively, but also may provide a motivation to quit that did not exist earlier.

There are always new drugs with misuse potential being synthesized, and it would behoove the surgeon to stay up-to-date with novel substances that may be prevalent in their community. For example, xylazine ("Tranq") has recently become epidemic to certain cities in the USA, with overdose deaths increasing 1127% from 2020 to 2021 in the South [100]. Patients may not disclose drug use if not specifically asked, so by knowing the common names of drugs of misuse a more accurate history may be obtained (Table 7.2).

Table 7.2 Implications for surgery and preoperative management for commonly misused substances

Substance	Implications for surgery	Preoperative management
Alcohol	• Increased risk of cardiopulmonary events, bleeding, and infection • Increased length of hospital stay and cost	• Ideally abstain for 1 month preoperatively • Can proceed if not acutely intoxicated
Tobacco	• Increased risk of pulmonary complications (laryngospasm, bronchospasm, reintubation), ICU admission, infection, cardiac events • Poor wound healing	• Ideally abstain for 6–8 weeks preoperatively • For patients with coronary disease: At a minimum abstain for 12 h preoperatively, if not may postpone • If recent use, may discuss risks with patient and obtain informed consent

(continued)

Table 7.2 (continued)

Substance	Implications for surgery	Preoperative management
Marijuana	• Increased risk of MI, ectopy, airway obstruction, laryngospasm, bronchospasm, awareness under anesthesia	• Ideally abstain for 72 h preoperatively • If recent use, may discuss risks with patient and obtain informed consent at least 2 h after ingestion in absence of signs of impairment
Nitrous oxide	• Increased risk of DVT, PE, tachycardia and hypotension, dysrhythmia, aspiration, laryngospasm, bronchospasm	• In chronic users evaluate for reactive airway disease, hepatic and renal disease, vitamin B12 deficiency • If not acutely intoxicated, no contraindication to proceeding with surgery
Opioids	• Challenging pain management • Increased risk of respiratory failure, MI, surgical site infection	• OUD: Wean off opioids before elective surgery • maintenance therapy: See Table 7.1 • Chronic pain: Continue regimen up to day of surgery
Cocaine	• Increased risk of thrombocytopenia, cardiovascular event (aortic dissection, MI, hypertension, dysrhythmias), spontaneous pneumothorax	• Postpone for 7 days after last use • If case is more urgent, can observe for 8 h and proceed if asymptomatic
Methamphetamine	• Increased risk of coronary artery spasm, aortic dissection, MI, hypertension	• Postpone for 7 days after last use
Lysergic acid diethylamide (LSD)	• HT2A antagonists (ex. trazodone) can attenuate and perhaps reverse the main effects of the drug	• If not acutely intoxicated, no contraindication to proceeding with surgery

References

1. SAMHSA. Announces National Survey on Drug Use and Health (NSDUH) Results Detailing Mental Illness and Substance Use Levels in 2021. U.S. Department of Health and Human Services' (HHS) Substance Abuse and Mental Health Services Administration; 2021. https://www.hhs.gov/about/news/2023/01/04/samhsa-announces-national-survey-drug-use-health-results-detailing-mental-illness-substance-use-levels-2021.html.
2. Fernandez AC, Waljee JF, Gunaseelan V, Brummett CM, Englesbe MJ, Bicket MC. Prevalence of unhealthy substance use and associated characteristics among patients presenting for surgery. Ann Surg. 2022;278(4):e740–4. https://doi.org/10.1097/SLA.0000000000005767.
3. Dakour-Aridi H, Arora M, Nejim B, Locham S, Malas MB. Association between drug use and in-hospital outcomes after Infrainguinal bypass for peripheral arterial occlusive disease. Ann Vasc Surg. 2019 Jul;58:122–133.e4.
4. Anitescu M. The patient with substance use disorder. Curr Opin Anaesthesiol. 2019 Jun;32(3):427–37.
5. Understanding alcohol use disorder. National Institute on Alcohol Abuse and Alcoholism. https://www.niaaa.nih.gov/publications/brochures-and-fact-sheets/understanding-alcohol-use-disorder.

6. Global status report on alcohol and health 2018. World Health Organization; 2018. https://www.who.int/substance_abuse/publications/global_alcohol_report/en/. Accessed 20 Apr 2023.
7. 2021 National Survey on Drug Use and Health. Table 5.6A—Alcohol use disorder in past year: among people aged 12 or older; by age group and demographic characteristics, numbers in thousands, 2021. SAMHSA, Center for Behavioral Health Statistics and Quality. 2021. https://www.samhsa.gov/data/sites/default/files/reports/rpt39441/NSDUHDetailedTabs2021/NSDUHDetailedTabs2021/NSDUHDetTabsSect5pe2021.htm#tab5.6a.
8. Reinert DF, Allen JP. The alcohol use disorders identification test: an update of research findings. Alcohol Clin Exp Res. 2007;31:185–99. https://doi.org/10.1111/j.1530-0277.2006.00295.x.
9. Wolfson B, Freed B. Influence of alcohol on anesthetic requirements and acute toxicity. Anesth Analg. 1980;59(11):826–30.
10. Tønnesen H. Alcohol abuse and postoperative morbidity. Dan Med Bull. 2003;50(2):139–60.
11. Rolfzen ML, Mikulich-Gilbertson SK, Natvig C, Carrico JA, Lobato RL, Krause M, Bartels K. Association between alcohol use disorder and hospital outcomes in colectomy patients - a retrospective cohort study. J Clin Anesth. 2022 Jun;78:110674.
12. White CA, Quinones A, Tang JE, Butler LR, Duey AH, Kim JS, Cho SK, Cagle PJ. A national analysis of the effect alcohol use disorder has on short-term complications and readmissions following total shoulder arthroplasty. J Orthop. 2022 Oct;27(35):13–7.
13. Ponce BA, Oladeji LO, Raley JA, Menendez ME. Analysis of perioperative morbidity and mortality in shoulder arthroplasty patients with preexisting alcohol use disorders. J Shoulder Elb Surg. 2015;24(2):167–73.
14. HCUP. Most common operations during inpatient stays. Agency for healthcare research and quality. 2021. https://www.hcup-us.ahrq.gov/.
15. Gaddini GW, Turner RT, Grant KA, Iwaniec UT. Alcohol: a simple nutrient with complex actions on bone in the adult skeleton. Alcohol Clin Exp Res. 2016;40(4):657–71.
16. Tønnesen H, Rosenberg J, Nielsen HJ, et al. Effect of preoperative abstinence on poor postoperative outcome in alcohol misusers: randomised controlled trial. BMJ. 1999;318(7194):1311–6.
17. Egholm JW, Pedersen B, Møller AM, Adami J, Juhl CB, Tønnesen H. Perioperative alcohol cessation intervention for postoperative complications. Cochrane Database Syst Rev. 2018;11(11):CD008343. https://doi.org/10.1002/14651858.CD008343.pub3.
18. Tobacco. World Health Organization; 2022. https://www.who.int/news-room/fact-sheets/detail/tobacco.
19. Park Lee E, Ren C, Cooper M, Cornelius M, Jamal A, Cullen KA. Tobacco product use among middle and high school students—United States, 2022. Morb Mortal Wkly Rep. 2022;71:45.
20. Cornelius ME, Loretan CG, Wang TW, Jamal A, Homa DM. Tobacco product use among adults — United States, 2020. MMWR Morb Mortal Wkly Rep. 2022;71:397–405.
21. Feinstein MM, Schlosberg I, Israilov S, Sison M, Katz D. A survey assessing the vaping habits of patients undergoing surgery. Respir Care. 2022;67(10):1332–4. https://doi.org/10.4187/respcare.09830.
22. Schwilk B, Bothner U, Schraag S, Georgieff M. Perioperative respiratory events in smokers and nonsmokers undergoing general anaesthesia. Acta Anaesthesiol Scand. 1997;41(3):348–55.
23. Møller AM, Maaløe R, Pedersen T. Postoperative intensive care admittance: the role of tobacco smoking. Acta Anaesthesiol Scand. 2001;45(3):345–8. https://doi.org/10.1034/j.1399-6576.2001.045003345.x.
24. Sharma A, Deeb AP, Iannuzzi JC, Rickles AS, Monson JR, Fleming FJ. Tobacco smoking and postoperative outcomes after colorectal surgery. Ann Surg. 2013;258(2):296–300. https://doi.org/10.1097/SLA.0b013e3182708cc5.
25. Kapadia BH, Issa K, Pivec R, Bonutti PM, Mont MA. Tobacco use may be associated with increased revision and complication rates following total hip arthroplasty. J Arthroplast. 2014;29(4):777–80. https://doi.org/10.1016/j.arth.2013.08.023.
26. Frick WG, Seals RR Jr. Smoking and wound healing: a review. Tex Dent J. 1994;111(6):21–3.

27. Krueger J, Rohrich R. Clearing the smoke: the scientific rationale for tobacco abstention with plastic surgery. Plast Reconstr Surg. 2001;108:1063.
28. Chun LF, Moazed F, Calfee CS, Matthay MA, Gotts JE. Pulmonary toxicity of e-cigarettes. Am J Physiol Lung Cell Mol Physiol. 2017;313(2):L193–206. https://doi.org/10.1152/ajplung.00071.2017.
29. Roberts M, Davies M. Dangers of using e-cigarettes before anaesthesia. BMJ. 2014;348:g1310.
30. Bieganowski T, Singh V, Kugelman DN, Rozell JC, Schwarzkopf R, Lajam CM. Vaping trends and outcomes in primary Total joint arthroplasty patients: an analysis of 21,341 patients. J Am Acad Orthop Surg Glob Res Rev. 2023;7(1):e22.00110.
31. Rau AS, Reinikovaite V, Schmidt EP, Taraseviciene-Stewart L, Deleyiannis FW. Electronic cigarettes are as toxic to skin flap survival as tobacco cigarettes. Ann Plast Surg. 2017;79(1):86–91. https://doi.org/10.1097/SAP.0000000000000998.
32. Møller AM, Villebro N, Pedersen T, Tønnesen H. Effect of preoperative smoking intervention on postoperative complications: a randomised clinical trial. Lancet. 2002;359(9301):114–7.
33. Shi Y, Warner DO. Surgery as a teachable moment for smoking cessation. Anesthesiology. 2010;112:102–7.
34. Rao BM, Moylan DD, Sochacki KR, Kollmorgen RC, Atwal L, Ellis TJ. Mandatory nicotine cessation for elective orthopedic hip procedures results in reduction in postoperative nicotine use. Cureus. 2020;12(12):e12158.
35. Mason DP, Subramanian S, Nowicki ER, et al. Impact of smoking cessation before resection of lung cancer: a Society of Thoracic Surgeons general thoracic surgery database study. Ann Thorac Surg. 2009;88(2):362–71. https://doi.org/10.1016/j.athoracsur.2009.04.035.
36. Mills E, Eyawo O, Lockhart I, Kelly S, Wu P, Ebbert JO. Smoking cessation reduces postoperative complications: a systematic review and meta-analysis. Am J Med. 2011;124(2):144–154.e8. https://doi.org/10.1016/j.amjmed.2010.09.013.
37. Warner MA, Diverti MR, Tinker JH, et al. Preoperative cessation of smoking and pulmonary complications in coronary artery bypass patients. Anesthesiology. 1984;60:380–3.
38. Bryson EO, Frost EA. The perioperative implications of tobacco, marijuana, and other inhaled toxins. Int Anesthesiol Clin. 2011 Winter;49(1):103–18.
39. Selvaggi G, Spagnolo AG, Elander A. A review of illicit psychoactive drug use in elective surgery patients: detection, effects, and policy. Int J Surg. 2017 Dec;48:160–5.
40. Weaver MF, Hopper JA, Gunderson EW. Designer drugs 2015: assessment and management. Addict Sci Clin Pract. 2015;10:8.
41. Brahm NC, Yeager LL, Fox MD, Farmer KC, Palmer TA. Commonly prescribed medications and potential false-positive urine drug screens. Am J Health Syst Pharm. 2010;67(16):1344–50.
42. Goel A, McGuinness B, Jivraj NK, Wijeysundera DN, Mittleman MA, Bateman BT, Clarke H, Kotra LP, Ladha KS. Cannabis use disorder and perioperative outcomes in major elective surgeries: a retrospective cohort analysis. Anesthesiology. 2020 Apr;132(4):625–35.
43. Huson HB, Granados TM, Rasko Y. Surgical considerations of marijuana use in elective procedures. Heliyon. 2018;4(9):e00779.
44. Guarisco JL, Cheney ML, LeJeune FE Jr, Reed HT. Isolated uvulitis secondary to marijuana use. Laryngoscope. 1988;98(12):1309–12.
45. Mallat A, Roberson J, Brock-Utne JG. Preoperative marijuana inhalation--an airway concern. Can J Anaesth. 1996;43(7):691–3.
46. White SM. Cannabis abuse and laryngospasm. Anaesthesia. 2002;57(6):622–3.
47. Tashkin DP, Coulson AH, Clark VA, et al. Respiratory symptoms and lung function in habitual heavy smokers of marijuana alone, smokers of marijuana and tobacco, smokers of tobacco alone, and nonsmokers. Am Rev Respir Dis. 1987;135(1):209–16.
48. Benson M, Bentley AM. Lung disease induced by drug addiction. Thorax. 1995;50:1125–7.
49. Hernandez M, Birnbach DJ, Van Zundert AA. Anesthetic management of the illicit-substance-using patient. Curr Opin Anaesthesiol. 2005;18(3):315–24.

50. Kaar SJ, Ferris J, Waldron J, Devaney M, Ramsey J, Winstock AR. Up: the rise of nitrous oxide abuse. An international survey of contemporary nitrous oxide use. J Psychopharmacol. 2016;30(4):395–401. https://doi.org/10.1177/0269881116632375.
51. Garakani A, Jaffe RJ, Savla D, et al. Neurologic, psychiatric, and other medical manifestations of nitrous oxide abuse: a systematic review of the case literature. Am J Addict. 2016;25(5):358–69. https://doi.org/10.1111/ajad.12372.
52. Kong JT, Schmiesing C. Concealed mothball abuse prior to anesthesia: mothballs, inhalants, and their management. Acta Anaesthesiol Scand. 2005;49:113–6.
53. Kurtzman TL, Otsuka KN, Wahl RA. Inhalant abuse by adolescents. J Adolesc Health. 2001;28:170–80.
54. Therapeutic Drug Management and Toxicology Division: Nitrous Oxide. American Association for Clinical Chemistry. https://www.aacc.org/community/divisions/tdm-and-toxicology/toxin-library/nitrous-oxide.
55. Broussard LA. The role of the laboratory in detecting inhalant abuse. Clin Lab Sci. 2000;13:205–9.
56. Caris MG, Kuipers RS, Kiestra BE, et al. Nitrous oxide abuse leading to extreme homocysteine levels and thrombosis in young adults: a case series. J Thromb Haemost. 2023;21(2):276–83. https://doi.org/10.1016/j.jtha.2022.10.002.
57. den Uil SH, Vermeulen EGJ, Metz R, Rijbroek A, de Vries M. Aortic arch thrombus caused by nitrous oxide abuse. J Vasc Surg Cases Innov Tech. 2018;4(2):80–2. https://doi.org/10.1016/j.jvscit.2018.01.001.
58. Vollenbrock SE, Fokkema TM, Leijdekkers VJ, Vahl AC, Konings R, van Nieuwenhuizen RC. Nitrous oxide abuse associated with severe thromboembolic complications. Eur J Vasc Endovasc Surg. 2021;62(4):656–7. https://doi.org/10.1016/j.ejvs.2021.05.041.
59. Bass M. Sudden sniffing death. JAMA. 1970;212:2075–9.
60. Campdesuner V, Teklie Y, Alkayali T, Pierce D, George J. Nitrous oxide-induced vitamin B12 deficiency resulting in myelopathy. Cureus. 2020;12(7):e9088. https://doi.org/10.7759/cureus.9088.
61. Centers for Disease Control and Prevention. Wide-ranging online data for epidemiologic research (WONDER). Atlanta, GA: CDC, National Center for Health Statistics; 2021. http://wonder.cdc.gov
62. Key substance use and mental health indicators in the United States: Results from the 2019 National Survey on Drug Use and Health (HHS Publication No. PEP20–07–01-001, NSDUH Series H-55). Center for Behavioral Health Statistics and Quality, Substance Abuse and Mental Health Services Administration; 2020. https://www.samhsa.gov/data/.
63. Henshaw DS, Turner JD, Khanna AK. Opioid abuse and perioperative care: a new medical disease. Curr Opin Anaesthesiol. 2022;35(3):401–8. https://doi.org/10.1097/ACO.0000000000001121.
64. Shah RM, Hirji SA, Percy E, Landino S, Yazdchi F, Bellavia A, Pelletier MP, Shekar PS, Kaneko T. Cardiac surgery in patients with opioid use disorder: an analysis of 1.7 million surgeries. Ann Thorac Surg. 2020 Apr;109(4):1194–201.
65. Arora S, Bronkema C, Majdalany SE, Corsi N, Rakic I, Piontkowski A, Sood A, Davis MJ, Modonutti D, Novara G, Rogers CG, Abdollah F. Impact of preexisting opioid dependence on morbidity, length of stay, and inpatient cost of urological oncological surgery. World J Urol. 2023;41(4):1025–31. https://doi.org/10.1007/s00345-023-04306-1.
66. Menendez ME, Ring D, Bateman BT. Preoperative Opioid Misuse is Associated With Increased Morbidity and Mortality After Elective Orthopaedic Surgery. Clin Orthop Relat Res. 2015;473(7):2402–12. https://doi.org/10.1007/s11999-015-4173-5.
67. Lavender TW, McCarron B. Acute infections in intravenous drug users. Clin Med (Lond). 2013 Oct;13(5):511–3. https://doi.org/10.7861/clinmedicine.13-5-511.
68. Fisher RB, Johnson QL, Reeves-Viets JL, Pain management mini-series. Part II. Chronic opioid drug therapy: implications for perioperative anesthesia and pain management. Mo Med. 2013;110(3):231–5.

69. Thomas DA, Boominathan P, Goswami J, et al. Perioperative management of patients with addiction to opioid and nonopioid medications. Cur Pain Headache Rep. 2018;22:52.
70. Shah S, Kapoor S, Durkin B. Analgesic management of acute pain in opioid tolerant patients: a growing challenge. Curr Opin Anaesthesiol. 2015;28:398–402.
71. Schwenk S, Viscusi ER, Buvanendran A, et al. Consensus guidelines on the use of intravenous ketamine infusions for acute pain management from the American Society of Regional Anesthesia and Pain Medicine, the American Academy of Pain medicine, and the American Society of Anesthesiologists. Reg Anesth Pain Med. 2018;43(5):456–66.
72. McNicol ED, Ferguson MC, Hudcova J. Patient controlled opioid analgesia versus non-patient controlled opioid analgesia for postoperative pain. Cochrane Database Syst Rev. 2015;2015(6):CD003348.
73. Harrison TK, Kornfeld H, Aggarwal AK, Lembke A. Perioperative considerations for the patient with opioid use disorder on buprenorphine, methadone or naltrexone maintenance therapy. Anesthesiol Clin. 2018;36:345–59.
74. Exclusivity Data. Orange book: approved drug products with therapeutic equivalence evaluations. 37th ed. US Dept. of Health and Human services, Food and Drug Administration, Center for Drug Evaluation and Research, Office of Pharmaceutical Science, Office of Generic Drugs; 2017.
75. Kornfeld H, Manfredi L. Effectiveness of full agonist opioids in patients stabilized on buprenorphine undergoing major surgery: a case series. Am J Ther. 2010;17:523–8.
76. Childers JW, Arnold RM. Treatment of pain in patients taking buprenorphine for opioid addiction #221. J Palliat Med. 2012;15:613–4.
77. Anderson TA, Quaye AN, Ward N, et al. To stop or not to stop, that is the question-acute pain management for the patient on chronic buprenorphine. Anesth Analg. 2017;126:1180–6.
78. McCance-Katz EF, Sullivan LE, Nallani S. Drug interactions of clinical importance among opioids, methadone and buprenorphine, and other frequently prescribed medications: a review. Am J Addict. 2010;19:4–16.
79. Sudakin D. Naltrexone: not just for opioids anymore. J Med Toxicol. 2016;12(71–75):21.
80. Bryson EO. The perioperative management of patients maintained on medication used to manage opioid addiction. Curr Opin Anesthesiol. 2014;27:359–64.
81. Sordo L, Bario G, Bravo MJ, et al. Mortality risk during and after opioid substitution treatment: systematic review and meta-analysis of cohort studies. BMJ. 2017;357:j1550.
82. What is the scope of cocaine use in the United States? NIDA; 2023. https://nida.nih.gov/publications/research-reports/cocaine/what-scope-cocaine-use-in-united-states. Accessed 9 May 2023.
83. Hill GE, Ogunnaike BO, Johnson ER. General anaesthesia for the cocaine abusing patient. Is it safe? Br J Anaesth. 2006 Nov;97(5):654–7. https://doi.org/10.1093/bja/ael221.
84. O'Donnell J, Gladden RM, Mattson CL, Kariisa M. Notes from the field: overdose deaths with Carfentanil and other fentanyl analogs detected—10 states, July 2016-June 2017. MMWR Morb Mortal Wkly Rep. 2018;67(27):767–8.
85. Brust JC. Neurologic complications of illicit drug abuse. Continuum (Minneap Minn). 2014;20(3 Neurology of Systemic Disease):642–56.
86. Levent A, Davelaar EJ. Illegal drug use and prospective memory: a systematic review. Drug Alcohol Depend. 2019;204:107478.
87. Derlet RW, Rice P, Horowitz BZ, Lord RV. Amphetamine toxicity: experience with 127 cases. J Emerg Med. 1989;7(2):157–61.
88. Burday MJ, Martin SE. Cocaine-associated thrombocytopenia. Am J Med. 1991;91(6):656–60.
89. Vagts DA, Boklage C, Galli C. Intraoperative ventricular fibrillation in a patient with chronic cocaine abuse—a case report [in German]. Anaesthesiol Reanim. 2004;29:19–24.
90. Ciriaco P, Rossetti F, Carretta A, Sant'Angelo M, Arrigoni G, Negri G. Spontaneous pneumothorax in cocaine users. QJM. 2019;112(7):519–22. https://doi.org/10.1093/qjmed/hcz070.
91. Paratz ED, Cunningham NJ, MacIsaac AI. The cardiac complications of methamphetamines. Heart Lung Circ. 2016;25(4):325–32.

92. Safdari KM, Converse C, Dong F, et al. Hemodynamic Effects of Methamphetamine and General Anesthesia. Anesthesiol Res Pract. 2022;2022:7542311.
93. Moon TS, Pak TJ, Kim A, Gonzales MX, Volnov Y, Wright E, Vu KQ, Lu RD, Sharifi A, Minhajuddin A, Chen JL, Fox PE, Gasanova I, Fox AA, Stewart J, Ogunnaike B. A positive cocaine urine toxicology test and the effect on intraoperative hemodynamics under general anesthesia. Anesth Analg. 2021;132(2):308–16. https://doi.org/10.1213/ANE.0000000000004808.
94. Granite EL, Farber NJ, Adler P. Parameters for treatment of cocaine-positive patients. J Oral Maxillofac Surg. 2007;65(10):1984–9.
95. José FJ, Francina F, Matilde E, Magí F, Marta T. Therapeutic use of LSD in psychiatry: a systematic review of randomized-controlled clinical trials. Front Psychiatry. 2020;10:943.
96. Liester MB. A review of lysergic acid diethylamide (LSD) in the treatment of addictions: historical perspectives and future prospects. Curr Drug Abuse Rev. 2014;7:146.
97. Bogenschutz MP, Johnson MW. Classic hallucinogens in the treatment of addictions. Prog Neuro-Psychopharmacol Biol Psychiatry. 2016;64:250–8.
98. Kometer M, Schmidt A, Jancke L, Vollenweider FX. Activation of serotonin 2A receptors underlies the psilocybin-induced effects on oscillations, N170 visual-evoked potentials, and visual hallucinations. J Neurosci. 2013;33:10544–1.
99. Hwang KAJ, Saadabadi A. Lysergic Acid Diethylamide (LSD). In: StatPearls [internet]. Treasure Island (FL): StatPearls Publishing; 2023. ncbi.nlm.nih.gov/books/NBK482407/.
100. The growing threat of Xylazine and its mixture with illicit drugs. DEA Joint Intelligence Report, 2022. www.dea.gov/sites/default/files/2022-12/The%20Growing%20Threat%20of%20Xylazine%20and%20its%20Mixture%20with%20Illicit%20Drugs.pdf.

Chapter 8
Illicit Drugs and Candidates for Endoscopy and Surgery

John P. Gallagher, Patrick A. Twohig, Agnes Crnic, and Fedja A. Rochling

Abbreviations

HIV	Human immunodeficiency virus
IDU	Illicit drug use
THC	Tetrahydrocannabinol
UDS	Urine drug screen

Introduction

Scope of the Problem

Illicit drug use (IDU) encompasses a broad spectrum of substances and patterns of use, and it is a common occurrence in the healthcare system. Patients with IDU are frequently encountered during preprocedural evaluation in outpatient and emergent settings. IDU is projected to rise as drug legalization continues to expand [1, 2]. These patients are at increased risk for complications from anesthesia and intraoperative complications related to recent drug use. When encountering patients with IDU, providers must decide whether to cancel the procedure or proceed while managing

J. P. Gallagher
Department of Internal Medicine, University of Nebraska Medical Center, Omaha, NE, USA
e-mail: john.gallagher@unmc.edu

P. A. Twohig (✉) · F. A. Rochling
Division of Gastroenterology and Hepatology, The University of Nebraska Medical Center, Omaha, NE, USA
e-mail: frochling@unmc.edu

A. Crnic
Department of Anesthesiology and Pain Medicine, University of Ottawa, The Ottawa Hospital, Ottawa, ON, Canada
e-mail: acrni047@uottawa.ca

© The Author(s), under exclusive license to Springer Nature Switzerland AG 2024

J. Faintuch, S. Faintuch (eds.), *Recent Strategies in High Risk Surgery*,
https://doi.org/10.1007/978-3-031-56270-9_8

potential complications. Careful consideration must be taken to prevent anesthetic interactions with commonly used drugs, as it can be challenging to ascertain the recency of use, the severity of intoxication, and the potential for interactions with anesthesia. Procedural delays are associated with significant negative impacts on both patients and the healthcare system. They should not be used universally in patients with positive UDS, especially those who may appear non-toxic at presentation [3].

Delays or cancelations in elective procedures can create a significant burden to both patients and the healthcare system. It results in increased costs, care delays, and decreased trust in the medical community [4, 5]. In addition, IDU is associated with socioeconomically disadvantaged populations with greater comorbidity and limited healthcare utilization [5]. Procedural delays may risk further marginalizing this population and preventing access to care. It is critical to examine each patient individually to determine procedural candidacy.

Current Practices

The management of elective procedures in cases with IDU varies significantly across institutions [1, 6, 7]. The absence of standardized guidelines often leads physicians to rely on individual practices and expert recommendations when dealing with such cases, despite a clear desire by practitioners for additional guidance [1].

Current practice patterns often delay elective procedures by up to 7 days since the last use as determined by urine or serum testing [8]. The majority of established guidelines for administering anesthesia to patients with IDU focus on emergency cases and managing the effects of acute intoxication [9, 10]. In such cases, specific measures are required to mitigate potential interactions with anesthetics. Patients who undergo emergency surgery have been found to require higher levels of sedation and exhibit an association with increased perioperative morbidity. There is also an association between patients presenting for emergency surgery and increased rates of the human immunodeficiency virus (HIV) and Syphilis, which can complicate perioperative care [11]. However, multiple studies have demonstrated comparable 30-day clinical outcomes to the general population for patients who test positive for illicit drugs in urine drug screen (UDS) but are non-toxic [6, 12–14]. Most literature also examines cases with general anesthesia rather than the lighter sedation used for endoscopy. Here we discuss the systemic effects of frequently encountered illicit drugs and procedural management considerations.

Anesthetic Considerations

The impact of IDU depends on the type of sedation being used. In the United States, most endoscopies are performed using conscious sedation [15–17]. Notably, endoscopic procedures use significantly lower doses of anesthetics when compared to general anesthesia, and it is unknown what degree of procedural risk exists in this clinical setting [17].

Cannabis

Physiologic Effects and Pharmacodynamics

Cannabis is the most used illicit drug in the United States. It targets the cannabinoid receptors, CB1 and CB2, located throughout the body and acting as G-protein-coupled receptors [18, 19]. It is a psychoactive agent that can act as a depressant, stimulant, or hallucinogen in different settings. It is available in various forms, but delta-9 tetrahydrocannabinol (THC) is the most psychoactive compound. The effects of acute intoxication are highly variable and related to dose, formulation, route of ingestion, and frequency of use. Physiologic manifestations of acute intoxication may include hypertension, tachypnea, tachycardia, euphoria, increased appetite, and conjunctival injection (Table 8.1). The onset of action for acute intoxication is approximately 15 min when inhaled and up to 1–2 h when ingested [19]. Duration is 3–4 h when inhaled and up to 12 h if ingested. It is highly lipid soluble and can be detected on urine drug testing for up to 30 days after use [20].

Table 8.1 Duration of Urine drug screen positivity and anesthetic complications associated with commonly encountered drugs. All values included in the table serve as estimates for general use (Adapted with permission from "Illicit drug use and endoscopy: when do we say no?")

Drug	Duration of intoxication (hours)	Duration of urine positivity	Anesthetic complications with acute toxicity
Marijuana	Inhaled: Up to 4 Ingested: Up to 12	3–30 days with chronic use	Airway irritability, hypotension, increased anesthetic requirements
Cocaine	Intravenous: 0.5–1 Intranasal: 1–2 Inhaled: 0.5–1 Ingested: Indeterminate	1–8 days in most cases, up to 22 days reported with high-dose, chronic use (30 g/d inhaled)	Tachyarrhythmias, bronchospasm, hemodynamic instability, agitation
Methamphetamines	Indeterminate, ranges from 4 h to 48 h with residual psychologic changes	1–7 days, longer in chronic use	Hemodynamic instability, myocardial ischemia, tachyarrhythmias
Heroin	0.5, up to 4–5 for active metabolites (6-monoacetylmorphine)	24–48 h	Respiratory depression, hypotension, increased sedation requirements
Ecstasy	Ingested: 4–6	48 h	Tachycardia, hypertension, hyperthermia, hyperglycemia
Phencyclidine (PCP)	Intravenous: 1–2 Intranasal: Indeterminate Inhaled: 1–2 Ingestion: 1–3 May experience prolonged intoxication with delayed release from adipose tissue	>1 week	Pulmonary hypertension, tachycardia, psychosis, cerebral hemorrhage

Procedural Considerations

Patients with coronary artery disease are at increased risk of coronary spasms, which are associated with myocardial ischemia, as well as arrhythmias, including atrial fibrillation and ventricular fibrillation [21, 22].

When inhaled, cannabis use is associated with an increased risk for reactive airway disease, bronchospasm, laryngospasm, vocal cord dysfunction, uvular inflammation, and airway edema. These risks can result in significant intraoperative complications, including hypoxemia when undergoing airway manipulation and intubation and a higher risk of obstruction with airway instrumentation [21]. There is limited data regarding the duration of increased risk after smoke exposure, but it appears to be highest within 1–2 h of use [21, 23]. Lastly, patients should be treated with the same precautions as tobacco users, as there has been a similar risk profile demonstrated with chronic cannabis use. Additional associations include increased risk for cerebrovascular events, psychosis, hypothermia, and venous thromboembolism [24].

Anesthetic Interactions

Patients using cannabis have been shown to have inconsistent responses to various forms of anesthesia and a need for increased analgesia postoperatively. Patients with chronic use note more refractory pain and may require increased doses of as-needed pain medication postoperatively compared to controls [21, 24]. In addition, patients require more anesthesia to achieve sedation for both general anesthesia, deep sedation, and conscious sedation [24–26]. Due to the potential for tachycardia with acute intoxication, drugs with chronotropic stimulation should be avoided, including ketamine, pancuronium, and atropine [27].

Perioperative Recommendations

The American Society of Regional Anesthesia and Pain Medicine released a 2023 consensus guidelines statement addressing periprocedural management of cannabis use [28]. These included universal screening for THC prior to surgery, postponing elective procedures in patients with signs of acute intoxication by at least 2 h, and counseling cannabis users on potential negative effects on postoperative pain control. It was also recommended to counsel pregnant patients on the fetal/neonatal risks of cannabis use. Preprocedural UDS was not recommended due to inconsistencies and the inability to predict recency of use.

Due to the risk of increased anesthesia requirements and risk for withdrawal, patients should be counseled on abstaining from cannabis use for up to 7 days

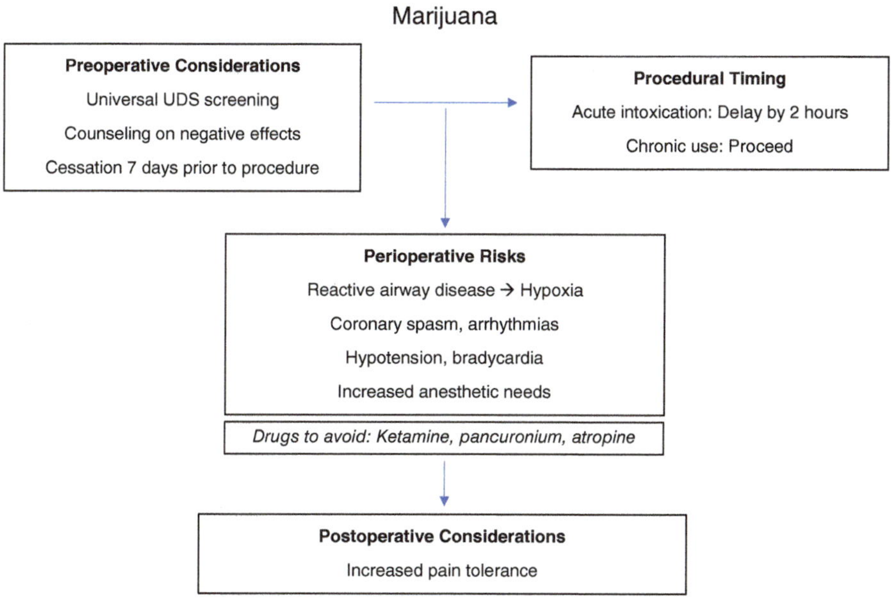

Fig. 8.1 Procedural guidance with recent Marijuana use. *UDS* Urine drug screen

prior to planned procedures. It is reasonable to delay cases in the setting of acute intoxication by at least 2 h, but non-toxic patients with recent use should be allowed to proceed with procedures on a case-by-case basis. Special considerations must be taken intraoperatively and with pain management in the postoperative setting to avoid adverse outcomes in this population. In emergent cases where the surgery will occur in less than 1 day, it is important to note that patients with acute intoxication may require increased sedation and have variable hemodynamic responses to anesthesia with an increased risk of hypotension and bradycardia at high doses [9, 29]. In patients with chronic use, weaning or cessation is not recommended due to the risk of cannabis withdrawal and/or increased anxiety or pain (Fig. 8.1) [23].

Cocaine

Physiologic Effects and Pharmacodynamics

Cocaine is a stimulant and can be used in multiple formulations, including inhalation, intranasal, intravenous, and less commonly ingestion. The onset of action is rapid and less than 5 min, and the duration is between 60 min to 2 h [30]. Cocaine blocks catecholamine uptake in the central nervous system and peripheral tissues, which leads to vasoconstrictive effects, as well as endorphin release. The drug also blocks sodium channels, resulting in local anesthesia and up-regulation of stimulating amino acids [31, 32]. This can cause a sympathomimetic symptom storm in acute intoxication, with symptoms including hypertension, psychomotor agitation, tachycardia, mydriasis, and pupillary dilation.

Procedural Considerations

Acute intoxication can result in extreme blood pressure lability, which is compounded by anesthetic interactions. With severe variations in intraoperative blood pressure, acutely intoxicated patients have higher rates of complications such as cardiac arrhythmias, myocardial infarction, and intracranial hemorrhage [33, 34]. Hyperthermia and seizures can occur from CNS activation. There are multiple pulmonary effects from chronic use, including bronchospasms, venous thromboembolisms, pneumothorax, diffuse alveolar hemorrhage, and eosinophilic pneumonia [35–38].

Upon cessation of use, withdrawal symptoms include hyper-somnolence, depression, and profound fatigue. Some patients may also experience significant agitation in the withdrawal phase, which presents a challenge for those who remain admitted postoperatively in emergency settings. Withdrawal can last between 2 and 4 weeks, and more severe or prolonged symptoms are suggestive of increased use [39].

Anesthetic Interactions

Ketamine and halothane should be avoided, given the increased risk of cardiac arrhythmias and increased systemic vascular resistance [9, 27]. Etomidate administration is also associated with an increased risk of myoclonus, seizures, and hyperreflexia and should be avoided, with propofol and thiopental generally considered preferred agents for induction [27].

Extreme hypertension has been reported intraoperatively in patients with cocaine use, which is thought to be related to anesthetic interactions as well as systemic activation during surgery.

On the contrary, chronic use can result in the depletion of catecholamines, and patients will rarely develop profound hypotension during procedures, requiring vasopressor support to maintain perfusion [23, 40, 41]. Patients with chronic use are also at higher risk of developing agitation and psychomotor instability that can require escalating doses of anesthetic to achieve adequate sedation [35, 40].

Perioperative Recommendations

Current guidance on preoperative screening for cocaine use is based on expert opinion. Recommendations include avoiding general anesthesia in patients with signs of acute intoxication due to CNS stimulation and risk for interactions with common anesthetics, especially for elective procedures. However, the half-life of cocaine is relatively short at 60–90 min, and the drug should be eliminated by 8 h in most cases [3, 42, 43]. However, UDS testing can remain positive for up to 7 days and cannot reliably guide procedural timing in non-toxic patients. Studies have shown that non-toxic patients with positive UDS have similar outcomes to their non-using counterparts [3, 43, 44].

In the absence of clear guidelines for procedural management, cases must be managed individually with close monitoring in the postoperative setting to prevent and manage possible hemodynamic instability, especially in cases of acute withdrawal [42]. It is reasonable to proceed with anesthesia in non-toxic patients who present after 8 h of ingestion with hemodynamic stability and without acute abnormalities on ECG or with CNS examination [9, 42].

In cases of trauma and emergent procedures in acutely intoxicated patients, caution should be exercised when prescribing beta-blockers, as this can precipitate unopposed alpha-receptor stimulation. In cases with chronic use, patients may experience hypotension due to catecholamine depletion, which can require vasopressor support if refractory to intravenous fluids (Fig. 8.2).

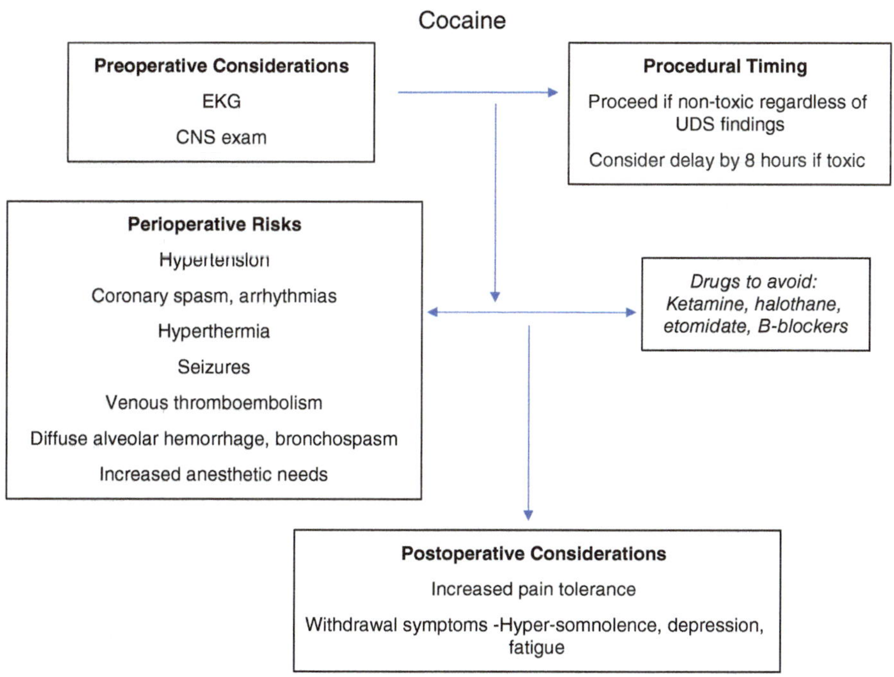

Fig. 8.2 Procedural guidance with recent Cocaine use

Methamphetamines

Physiologic Effects and Pharmacodynamics

Methamphetamines are stimulants that can be used via inhalation, intravenous, intranasal, or ingestion. They primarily promote norepinephrine release as an indirect agonist but can also target dopamine and serotonin receptors [45]. Onset and duration vary depending on the route of use. Timing to peak effect is less than 15 min with intravenous and intranasal use and up to 3 h when ingested [46–48]. Duration of intoxication can be up to 9–12 h for all formulations, although typically longest when ingested orally. However, it can be detected much longer with UDS, with up to 7–9 days depending on the dose, route, and chronicity of use [48, 49].

Intoxication is associated with a variety of CNS and peripheral effects. At lower doses, intoxication causes increased attention, hyperfocus, and improved motor coordination related to the effects of dopaminergic signaling [50, 51]. At increased doses, patients can experience anxiety and paranoia, with up to 10% progressing to acute psychosis when an overdose occurs [48, 52, 53]. With norepinephrine release at higher doses, hemodynamic changes include tachycardia, tachypnea, and significant hypertension [48]. Potential adverse events related to this include malignant hypertension, risk of cardiac arrhythmias, and a significant increase in non-ischemic cardiomyopathy with chronic use. Patients are also at elevated risk of hemorrhagic stroke due to hypertension [54–56]. Withdrawal symptoms can include fatigue, impaired concentration, depression, and irritability. While the most significant symptoms occur in the first 48–72 h, up to 25% of patients can have persistent symptoms of depression for months after use [48].

Procedural Considerations

Results have been mixed in the operative setting regarding outcomes for patients with a history of methamphetamine use who receive general anesthesia. Trauma patients appear to have higher rates of perioperative cardiovascular complications, higher incidence of ICU admissions requiring laparotomy, and higher rates of rhabdomyolysis [57]. They are also more likely to have intraoperative hypotension and vasopressor requirements in a time-dependent manner where risk remains at 7 days from last use [58, 59]. However, these effects do not persist, and there appear to be similar rates of mortality and hospitalization length in patients with prior use [60].

In addition, for UDS-positive patients requiring emergent surgeries, it appears that drug use plays a much smaller role in hemodynamic instability than factors such as age and intravascular depletion [61].

Anesthetic Interactions

Similar to cocaine, methamphetamines are stimulating agents, and acute intoxication can be associated with labile blood pressure and refractory intraoperative hyper or hypotension. It is recommended to avoid anesthetics that can worsen tachycardia and adrenergic stimulation.

Perioperative Recommendations

Current data suggests that patients who are acutely intoxicated with methamphetamines are at higher risk of significant hypotension, as well as increased anesthetic requirements [61, 62]. They are also at increased risk for cardiac complications in the perioperative and postoperative setting. Due to these risks, it is reasonable to postpone surgeries for up to 48 h in elective cases where patients present acutely intoxicated. However, these assessments must be made clinically, as UDS does not appear to be a reliable screening tool for acute intoxication. In patients who are non-toxic with a positive UDS and > 48 h from most recent use, they may tolerate proceeding with general anesthesia on a case-by-case basis. Patients demonstrating signs of acute withdrawal postoperatively should be managed in an inpatient setting.

If a patient presents with acute intoxication and surgery cannot be delayed, there are several intraoperative considerations. Providers should avoid physical restraints due to the risk of agitation, muscle contractions, and risk of rhabdomyolysis or cardiovascular complications [57]. Chemical restraints with benzodiazepines can be used, as well as first-generation antipsychotics if agitation persists. Patients are initially at elevated risk for refractory hypertension, which may then progress to significant hypotension as catecholamine depletion develops. These patients may require treatment with vasopressor support [61]. There is also an increased risk of coronary spasm with beta-blocker use, and they are not recommended in cases with acute intoxication [63].

Finally, induction with succinylcholine can induce rhabdomyolysis and should be avoided (Fig. 8.3) [64, 65].

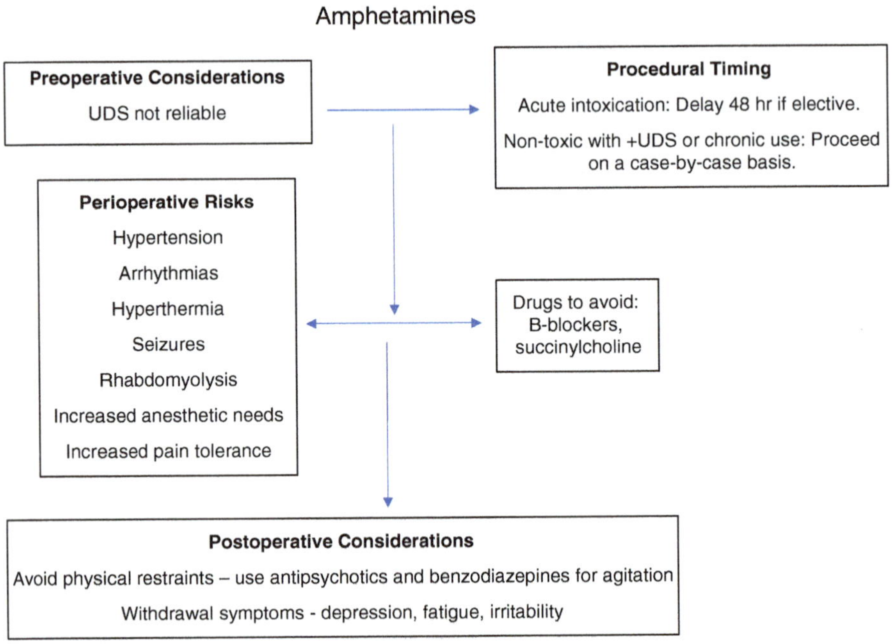

Fig. 8.3 Procedural guidance with recent Amphetamine use

Opioids

Physiologic Effects and Pharmacodynamics

Opioid analgesics act on multiple different opioid receptors in the central and peripheral nervous system and range from medications with misuse potential, including natural (morphine) and synthetic (fentanyl) compounds, to illicit drugs (heroin). Potency varies significantly by the compound, with heroin being 3–5 times more potent than morphine and fentanyl up to 50–100 times more potent [66]. Opioids can be taken via intravenous, subcutaneous, ingestion, and inhalational routes. The onset of action and duration of acute intoxication is dependent on the formulation and route of ingestion and is difficult to generalize. Effects are derived from targeting three opioid receptors (mu, kappa, delta), primarily in the central and peripheral nervous system and the gastrointestinal tract [67].

Opiates primarily act as depressants, and symptoms of acute intoxication include analgesia, euphoria, and delayed mentation. Withdrawal symptoms last up to 1 week and typically peak at 36–48 h [68]. Symptoms can include severe nausea/vomiting, anxiety, diaphoresis, rhinorrhea, malaise, and insomnia [69].

Procedural Considerations

Patients may demonstrate miosis, slowed gastrointestinal motility, and respiratory depression, which is the primary adverse outcome of overdose and can be fatal [70]. Patients are also commonly treated with a concomitant medication for opioid use disorder, such as methadone, naloxone, or buprenorphine, and these must be managed during admission. Due to opioid tolerance with chronic use, patients may also require increased doses of analgesia postoperatively, which can worsen outcomes and increase the risk of worsening opioid use disorder [71–73]. Patients are also more likely to be chronically ill, which also increases morbidity and mortality from emergent or elective procedures [71].

Anesthetic Considerations

Patients with chronic opioid use have an increased association with spinal and epidural infections, likely related to bacterial seeding with intravenous use [74]. Chronic use can also result in cross-tolerance with other depressants and anesthetics due to receptor down-regulation. Patients may also experience an exaggerated pain response postoperatively, requiring increased analgesia [9, 27].

Perioperative Recommendations

Patients using opioids must first be assessed for chronicity of use and opioid prescriptions. Those with acute intoxication should be evaluated for respiratory depression and hemodynamic instability. Patients with lethargy or hypoventilation require emergent intervention and procedural delay. Chronic use requires considerations for likely increased sedation needs intraoperatively, as well as increased postprocedural analgesia compared to opioid naïve patients. These cases are best managed with the assistance of pain specialists to incorporate multimodal approaches with opioid and non-opioid pain management strategies. These can include local anesthetic blocks, ketamine infusions, and non-pharmacologic support [75]. They may also benefit from opioid agonist therapy or weaning opioid doses to prevent withdrawal while admitted [73]. In patients with acute intoxication requiring emergent intervention, patients are at elevated risk for pulmonary edema, hypoxia, and aspiration due to delayed gastric emptying (Fig. 8.4) [9].

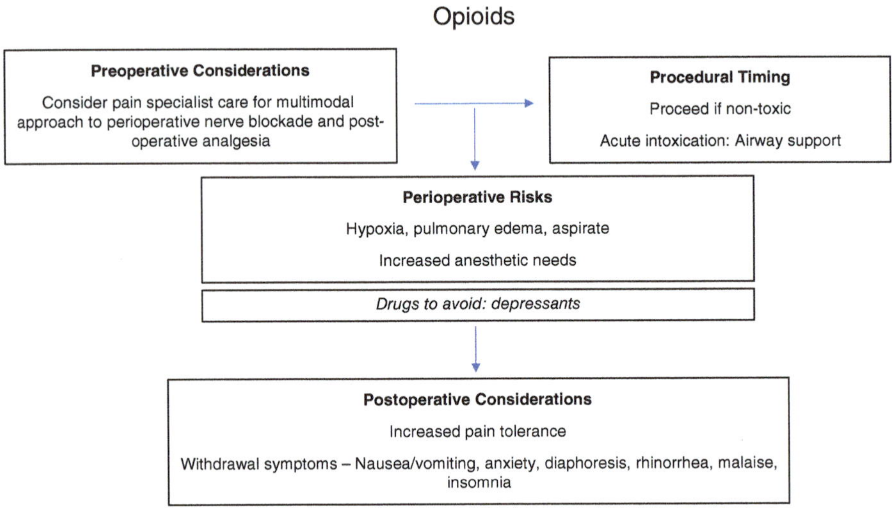

Fig. 8.4 Procedural guidance with recent Opioid use

Alcohol

Physiologic Effects and Pharmacodynamics

Alcohol misuse is a leading cause of preventable death worldwide [72]. Alcohol is a depressant and acts on multiple receptors, primarily by disrupting the inhibitory neurotransmitter GABA and its counter-enzyme, glutamate. It is ingested orally, and the onset of action is within 15–30 min in a dose-dependent manner [76]. Symptoms of acute intoxication include decreased awareness, disinhibited behaviors, slurred speech, and somnolence. Chronic use can lead to increased tolerance and decreased effects of acute intoxication despite elevated blood alcohol levels on serum testing. These patients are also at elevated risk of alcohol withdrawal syndrome, which can be fatal [76].

Procedural Considerations

Acute intoxication is associated with multiple periprocedural risks, including aspiration, agitation, and increased anesthetic requirements for sedation. Chronic alcohol use also has significant complications on multiple organ systems, which can affect perioperative management. Patients are at risk of developing cardiomyopathy, chronic liver disease, and profound electrolyte and nutritional abnormalities. In addition, patients must be monitored for alcohol withdrawal postoperatively, as this can progress to seizures and delirium tremens in patients with chronic use. Symptoms begin at approximately 24 h from the last consumption with anxiety, tremors, and psychomotor agitation, and they peak at 48–72 h. If possible, patients should be monitored in a setting with a standardized protocol for the treatment of withdrawal [77].

Anesthetic Considerations

Alcohol has multiple sedating effects and acts via a similar mechanism as many anesthetics, including opioids, propofol, and thiopentone [78]. Patients may require lower doses of anesthetics to achieve adequate sedation in patients with recent or chronic alcohol use.

Perioperative Recommendations

Patients with acute intoxication are at elevated risk for poor outcomes and intraoperative complications, specifically related to anesthetic interactions, risk of aspiration and airway compromise, and risk of significant hemodynamic instability during procedures. They may also present with symptoms of confusion, decreased mental functioning, and aggression. In these cases, it is reasonable to delay procedures until acute effects have resolved [79, 80]. Serum alcohol testing is generally considered a reliable marker for acute intoxication, although it is difficult to standardize, as patient symptoms partially depend on chronicity of use rather than the quantitative value of the test.

Patients with a history of chronic use but who do not appear acutely intoxicated should be screened for recency of use and history of withdrawal symptoms. In those who are at high risk of withdrawal, cases should be delayed at least 72 h, and patients should be monitored in a controlled setting with a standardized program for managing withdrawal symptoms. Chronic misuse and dependence are associated with pathologies that can complicate procedural care, such as cirrhosis and cardiomyopathy. Cases in which the patient has a history of significant chronic use should involve screening for sequelae of liver disease, such as esophageal varices, renal injury, and coagulopathy [77]. This evaluation is critical, even in urgent or emergent cases, to prevent complications from surgery. Patients may also be treated prophylactically for withdrawal with benzodiazepines in emergent cases associated with acute intoxication to prevent seizures and delirium tremens (Fig. 8.5).

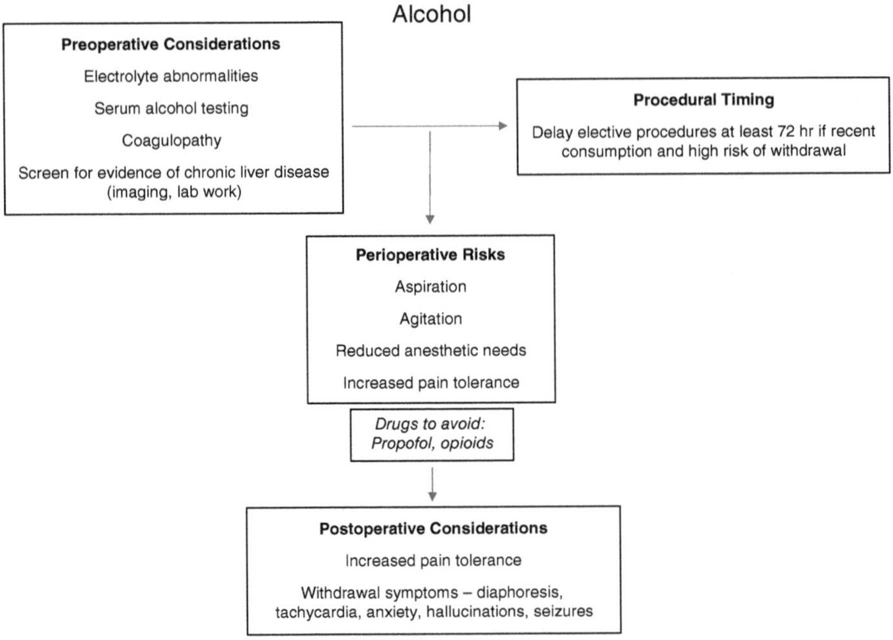

Fig. 8.5 Procedural guidance with recent Alcohol use

Disclosures The authors have no grants or financial support to acknowledge or disclose in the development of this chapter.

References

1. Elkassabany N, Speck RM, Oslin D, et al. Preoperative screening and case cancellation in cocaine-abusing veterans scheduled for elective surgery. Anesthesiol Res Pract. 2013;2013:149892. https://doi.org/10.1155/2013/149892.
2. Desai PM, Yap J, Yu J, Kotwal V, Attar BM. 573 safety of esophagogastroduodenoscopy in patients with active cocaine use: a pilot study. Am J Gastroenterol. 2019;114(1):S329–30. https://doi.org/10.14309/01.ajg.0000591824.64246.22.
3. Bartels K, Schacht JP. Cocaine-positive patients undergoing elective surgery—from avoiding case cancellations to treating substance use disorders. Anesth Analg. 2021;132(2):305–7. https://doi.org/10.1213/ANE.0000000000004969.
4. Alboraie M, Piscoya A, Tran QT, et al. The global impact of COVID-19 on gastrointestinal endoscopy units: an international survey of endoscopists. Arab Journal of Gastroenterology. 2020;21(3):156–61. https://doi.org/10.1016/j.ajg.2020.08.008.
5. de Jager E, Levine AA, Udyavar NR, et al. Disparities in surgical access: a systematic literature review, conceptual model, and evidence map. J Am Coll Surg. 2019;228(3):276–98. https://doi.org/10.1016/j.jamcollsurg.2018.12.028.
6. Granite EL, Farber NJ, Adler P. Parameters for treatment of cocaine-positive patients. J Oral Maxillofac Surg. 2007;65(10):1984–9. https://doi.org/10.1016/j.joms.2006.11.037.

7. Melendez I. Analgesia and anesthesia for the substance use disorder patient. In: American Association of Nurse Anesthesiology; 2019. p. 1–16.
8. Gallagher JP, Twohig PA, Crnic A, Rochling FA. Illicit drug use and endoscopy: when do we say no? Dig Dis Sci. 2022;67(12):5371–81. https://doi.org/10.1007/s10620-022-07619-0.
9. Moran S, Isa J, Steinemann S. Perioperative Management in the Patient with substance abuse. Surg Clin N Am. 2015;95(2):417–28. https://doi.org/10.1016/j.suc.2014.11.001.
10. Lewellen D. Should we proceed? Implications of marijuana use for GI endoscopy procedures. Gastroenterol Nurs. 2020;43(6):480–2. https://doi.org/10.1097/SGA.0000000000000568.
11. Li J, Ma H, Liao R, Huang Y, Chen G. Preoperative screening for illicit drug use in patients undergoing emergency surgery: a prospective observational study. Sci Rep. 2018;8:7405. https://doi.org/10.1038/s41598-018-25829-3.
12. Fischer SP, Schmiesing CA, Guta CG, Brock-Utne JG. General anesthesia and chronic amphetamine use: should the drug be stopped preoperatively? Anesth Analg. 2006;103(1):203–6. https://doi.org/10.1213/01.ane.0000221451.24482.11.
13. Ryb GE, Cooper C. Outcomes of cocaine-positive trauma patients undergoing surgery on the first day after admission. J Trauma. 2008;65(4):809–12. https://doi.org/10.1097/TA.0b013e318187803f.
14. Moon TS, Pak TJ, Kim A, et al. A positive cocaine urine toxicology test and the effect on intraoperative hemodynamics under general anesthesia. Anesth Analg. 2021;132(2):308–16. https://doi.org/10.1213/ANE.0000000000004808.
15. Lin OS. Sedation for routine gastrointestinal endoscopic procedures: a review on efficacy, safety, efficiency, cost and satisfaction. Intest Res. 2017;15(4):456–66. https://doi.org/10.5217/ir.2017.15.4.456.
16. Cohen LB, Wecsler JS, Gaetano JN, et al. Endoscopic sedation in the United States: results from a nationwide survey. Am J Gastroenterol. 2006;101(5):967–74. https://doi.org/10.1111/j.1572-0241.2006.00500.x.
17. Zeneca Pharmaceuticals. DIPRIVAN® (propofol) injectable emulsion for IV administration. https://www.accessdata.fda.gov/drugsatfda_docs/label/2014/019627s062lbl.pdf. Accessed 24 Jan 2022.
18. Adams IB, Martin BR. Cannabis: pharmacology and toxicology in animals and humans. Addiction. 1996;91(11):1585–614.
19. Ashton CH. Pharmacology and effects of cannabis: a brief review. Br J Psychiatry. 2001;178(2):101–6. https://doi.org/10.1192/bjp.178.2.101.
20. Huestis MA, Mitchell JM, Cone EJ. Urinary excretion profiles of 11-Nor-9-Carboxy-ag-Tetrahydrocannabinolin humans after single smoked doses of marijuana. J Anal Toxicol. 1996;20:12.
21. Huson HB, Granados TM, Rasko Y. Surgical considerations of marijuana use in elective procedures. Heliyon. 2018;4(9):e00779. https://doi.org/10.1016/j.heliyon.2018.e00779.
22. Alexander JC, Joshi GP. A review of the anesthetic implications of marijuana use. Baylor Univ Med Cent Proc. 2019;32(3):364–71. https://doi.org/10.1080/08998280.2019.1603034.
23. Ladha KS, McLaren-Blades A, Goel A, et al. Perioperative pain and addiction interdisciplinary network (PAIN): consensus recommendations for perioperative management of cannabis and cannabinoid-based medicine users by a modified Delphi process. Br J Anaesth. 2021;126(1):304–18. https://doi.org/10.1016/j.bja.2020.09.026.
24. Echeverria-Villalobos M, Todeschini AB, Stoicea N, Fiorda-Diaz J, Weaver T, Bergese SD. Perioperative care of cannabis users: a comprehensive review of pharmacological and anesthetic considerations. J Clin Anesth. 2019;57:41–9. https://doi.org/10.1016/j.jclinane.2019.03.011.
25. Richtig G, Bosse G, Arlt F, Von HC. Cannabis consumption before surgery may be associated with increased tolerance of anesthetic drugs: a case report. IJCRI. 2015;6(7):436. https://doi.org/10.5348/ijcri-201573-CR-10534.
26. Donvito G, Nass SR, Wilkerson JL, et al. The endogenous cannabinoid system: a budding source of targets for treating inflammatory and neuropathic pain. Neuropsychopharmacology. 2018;43(1):52–79. https://doi.org/10.1038/npp.2017.204.

27. Hernandez M, Birnbach DJ, Van Zundert AA. Anesthetic management of the illicit-substance-using patient. Curr Opin Anesthesiol. 2005;18(3):315. https://doi.org/10.1097/01.aco.0000169241.21680.0b.
28. Shah S, Schwenk ES, Sondekoppam RV, et al. ASRA pain medicine consensus guidelines on the management of the perioperative patient on cannabis and cannabinoids. Reg Anesth Pain Med. 2023;3:97–117. https://doi.org/10.1136/rapm-2022-104013.
29. Recreational drug misuse: issues for the cardiologist|Heart. https://heart.bmj.com/content/83/6/627. Accessed 19 Jun 2023.
30. Drake LR, Scott PJH. DARK classics in chemical neuroscience: cocaine. ACS Chem Neurosci. 2018;9(10):2358–72. https://doi.org/10.1021/acschemneuro.8b00117.
31. Tella SR, Schindler CW, Goldberg SR. Cocaine: cardiovascular effects in relation to inhibition of peripheral neuronal monoamine uptake and central stimulation of the sympathoadrenal system. J Pharmacol Exp Ther. 1993;267(1):153–62.
32. Smith JA, Mo Q, Guo H, Kunko PM, Robinson SE. Cocaine increases extraneuronal levels of aspartate and glutamate in the nucleus accumbens. Brain Res. 1995;683(2):264–9. https://doi.org/10.1016/0006-8993(95)00383-2.
33. Kuczkowski KM. The cocaine abusing parturient: a review of anesthetic considerations. Can J Anesth. 2004;51(2):145.
34. Luft A, Mendes FF. Anestesia no paciente usuário de cocaína. Rev Bras Anestesiol. 2007;57(3):307–14. https://doi.org/10.1590/S0034-70942007000300009.
35. Ramachandaran S, Khan AU, Dadaparvar S, Sherman MS. Inhalation of Crack Cocaine Can Mimic Pulmonary Embolism. Clin Nucl Med. 2004;29(11):756–7. https://doi.org/10.1097/00003072-200411000-00028.
36. Devlin RJ, Henry JA. Clinical review: major consequences of illicit drug consumption. Crit Care. 2008;12(1):202. https://doi.org/10.1186/cc6166.
37. Oh PI, Balter MS. Cocaine induced eosinophilic lung disease. Thorax. 1992;47(6):478–9.
38. Alnas M, Altayeh A, Zaman M. Clinical course and outcome of cocaine-induced pneumomediastinum. Am J Med Sci. 2010;339(1):65–7. https://doi.org/10.1097/MAJ.0b013e3181c371da.
39. Sofuoglu M, Dudish-Poulsen S, Poling J, Mooney M, Hatsukami DK. The effect of individual cocaine withdrawal symptoms on outcomes in cocaine users. Addict Behav. 2005;30(6):1125–34. https://doi.org/10.1016/j.addbeh.2004.10.010.
40. Bernards CM, Teijeiro A. Illicit cocaine ingestion during anesthesia. Anesthesiology. 1996;84(1):218–20. https://doi.org/10.1097/00000542-199601000-00025.
41. O'Donnell K, Boyle S, Abdulrahman S, O'Leary E. Unexpected intraoperative hypotension in a chronic cocaine user. Anaesth Rep. 2022;10(2):e12177. https://doi.org/10.1002/anr3.12177.
42. Saggese NP, Chang C, Cardo VA. Perioperative Management for the Cocaine-Positive Patient Undergoing Elective Surgery under General Anesthesia. J Oral Maxillofac Surg. 2019;77(5):894–5. https://doi.org/10.1016/j.joms.2019.01.016.
43. Moon TS, Gonzales MX, Sun JJ, et al. Recent cocaine use and the incidence of hemodynamic events during general anesthesia: a retrospective cohort study. J Clin Anesth. 2019;55:146–50. https://doi.org/10.1016/j.jclinane.2018.12.028.
44. Liyen Cartelle A, Nguyen A, Desai PM, et al. Safety of upper endoscopy in patients with active cocaine use. World J Gastrointest Endosc. 2021;13(10):510–7. https://doi.org/10.4253/wjge.v13.i10.510.
45. Rothman RB, Baumann MH, Dersch CM, et al. Amphetamine-type central nervous system stimulants release norepinephrine more potently than they release dopamine and serotonin. Synapse. 2001;39(1):32–41. https://doi.org/10.1002/1098-2396(20010101)39:1<32::AID-SYN5>3.0.CO;2-3.
46. Harris D. The bioavailability of intranasal and smoked methamphetamine. Clin Pharmacol Ther. 2003;74(5):475–86. https://doi.org/10.1016/j.clpt.2003.08.002.
47. Perez-Reyes M, White WR, McDonald SA, et al. Clinical effects of daily methamphetamine administration. Clin Neuropharmacol. 1991;14(4):352–8. https://doi.org/10.1097/00002826-199108000-00007.

48. Cruickshank CC, Dyer KR. A review of the clinical pharmacology of methamphetamine. Addiction. 2009;104(7):1085–99. https://doi.org/10.1111/j.1360-0443.2009.02564.x.
49. Vandevenne M, Vandenbussche H, Verstraete A. Detection time of drugs of abuse in urine. Acta Clin Belg. 2000;55(6):323–33. https://doi.org/10.1080/17843286.2000.11754319.
50. Shappell SA, Kearns GL, Valentine JL, Neri DF, DeJohn CA. Chronopharmacokinetics and Chronopharmacodynamics of Dextromethamphetamine in man. J Clin Pharmacol. 1996;36(11):1051–63. https://doi.org/10.1177/009127009603601109.
51. Ramos BP, Arnsten AFT. Adrenergic pharmacology and cognition: focus on the prefrontal cortex. Pharmacol Ther. 2007;113(3):523–36. https://doi.org/10.1016/j.pharmthera.2006.11.006.
52. Derlet RW, Rice P, Zane Horowitz B, Lord RV. Amphetamine toxicity: experience with 127 cases. J Emerg Med. 1989;7(2):157–61. https://doi.org/10.1016/0736-4679(89)90263-1.
53. Gray SD, Fatovich DM, McCoubrie DL, Daly FF. Amphetamine-related presentations to an inner-city tertiary emergency department: a prospective evaluation. Med J Aust. 2007;186(7):336–9. https://doi.org/10.5694/j.1326-5377.2007.tb00932.x.
54. Jacobs LJ. Reversible dilated cardiomyopathy induced by methamphetamine. Clin Cardiol. 1989;12(12):725–7. https://doi.org/10.1002/clc.4960121211.
55. Yeo KK, Wijetunga M, Ito H, et al. The Association of Methamphetamine use and Cardiomyopathy in young patients. Am J Med. 2007;120(2):165–71. https://doi.org/10.1016/j.amjmed.2006.01.024.
56. Westover AN, McBride S, Haley RW. Stroke in young adults who abuse amphetamines or cocaine: a population-based study of hospitalized patients. Arch Gen Psychiatry. 2007;64(4):495. https://doi.org/10.1001/archpsyc.64.4.495.
57. Krogh J, Lanzillotta-Rangeley J, Paratz E, et al. Practice considerations for the anesthesia professional for methamphetamine substance use disorder patients. Anesthesia Patient Safety Foundation. 2021;36(2):67–70.
58. Safdari KM, Converse C, Dong F, et al. Hemodynamic effects of methamphetamine and general anesthesia. Anesthesiol Res Pract. 2022;2022:7542311. https://doi.org/10.1155/2022/7542311.
59. Githens T, DeBaun MR, Campbell ST, et al. Rates of perioperative complications among patients undergoing orthopedic trauma surgery despite having positive results for methamphetamine. Orthopedics. 2019;42(4):192–6. https://doi.org/10.3928/01477447-20190523-01.
60. Hadjizacharia P, Green DJ, Plurad D, et al. Methamphetamines in trauma: effect on injury patterns and outcome. J Trauma Acute Care Surg. 2009;66(3):895. https://doi.org/10.1097/TA.0b013e318164d085.
61. Edwards AM, Johnson EG, Bernard AC. Intraoperative vasopressor use during emergency surgery on injured meth users. Trauma Surg Acute Care Open. 2020;5(1):e000553. https://doi.org/10.1136/tsaco-2020-000553.
62. Cornwell DQ, Thompson AR, Ivie RM, Working ZM, Friess DM, Meeker JE. Methamphetamine in Orthopaedics: considerations of an at-risk population. JBJS Reviews. 2021;9(6):e20. https://doi.org/10.2106/JBJS.RVW.20.00229.
63. Amsterdam EA, Wenger NK, Brindis RG, et al. 2014 AHA/ACC guideline for the Management of Patients with non-ST-elevation acute coronary syndromes: a report of the American College of Cardiology/American Heart Association task force on practice guidelines. J Am Coll Cardiol. 2014;64(24):e139–228. https://doi.org/10.1016/j.jacc.2014.09.017.
64. Eilert RJ, Kliewer ML. Methamphetamine-induced rhabdomyolysis. Int Anesthesiol Clin. 2011;49(2):52. https://doi.org/10.1097/AIA.0b013e3181ffc0e5.
65. Murray EP, Mansy L, Lackey JT, et al. Methamphetamine intoxication and perioperative complications following Orthopaedic surgical procedures. Cureus. 2021;13(10):e19082. https://doi.org/10.7759/cureus.19082.
66. Drewes AM, Jensen RD, Nielsen LM, et al. Differences between opioids: pharmacological, experimental, clinical and economical perspectives. Br J Clin Pharmacol. 2013;75(1):60–78. https://doi.org/10.1111/j.1365-2125.2012.04317.x.
67. Feng Y, He X, Yang Y, Chao D, Lazarus LH, Xia Y. Current research on opioid receptor function. Curr Drug Targets. 2012;13(2):230–46.

68. Schumacher MA, Basbaum AI, Naidu RK. Opioid Agonists & Antagonists. In: Katzung BG, editor. Basic & clinical pharmacology. 14th ed. McGraw-Hill Education; 2017. accessmedicine.mhmedical.com/content.aspx?aid=1148437600. Accessed 20 Jan 2022.
69. Opiate and opioid withdrawal: MedlinePlus medical encyclopedia. https://medlineplus.gov/ency/article/000949.htm. Accessed 20 Jan 2022.
70. Sporer KA. Acute Heroin Overdose. Ann Intern Med. 1999;130(7):584–90. https://doi.org/10.7326/0003-4819-130-7-199904060-00019.
71. Hser YI, Mooney LJ, Saxon AJ, et al. High mortality among patients with opioid use disorder in a large healthcare system. J Addict Med. 2017;11(4):315–9. https://doi.org/10.1097/ADM.0000000000000312.
72. Colvin LA, Bull F, Hales TG. Perioperative opioid analgesia—when is enough too much? A review of opioid-induced tolerance and hyperalgesia. Lancet. 2019;393(10180):1558–68. https://doi.org/10.1016/S0140-6736(19)30430-1.
73. Ward EN, Quaye ANA, Wilens TE. Opioid use disorders: perioperative Management of a Special Population. Anesth Analg. 2018;127(2):539–47. https://doi.org/10.1213/ANE.0000000000003477.
74. Koppel BS, Tuchman AJ, Mangiardi JR, Daras M, Weitzner I. Epidural spinal infection in intravenous drug abusers. Arch Neurol. 1988;45(12):1331–7. https://doi.org/10.1001/archneur.1988.00520360049011.
75. Harrison TK, Kornfeld H, Aggarwal AK, Lembke A. Perioperative considerations for the patient with opioid use disorder on buprenorphine, methadone, or naltrexone maintenance therapy. Anesthesiol Clin. 2018;36(3):345–59. https://doi.org/10.1016/j.anclin.2018.04.002.
76. Liang J, Olsen RW. Alcohol use disorders and current pharmacological therapies: the role of GABAA receptors. Acta Pharmacol Sin. 2014;35(8):981–93. https://doi.org/10.1038/aps.2014.50.
77. Ungur AL, Neumann T, Borchers F, Spies C. Perioperative Management of Alcohol Withdrawal Syndrome. Visc Med. 2020;36(3):160–6. https://doi.org/10.1159/000507595.
78. dfwanes. Anesthesia and Alcohol Use - DFW Anesthesia Professionals. 2019. https://anesthesiologydfw.com/anesthesia-and-alcohol-use/, https://anesthesiologydfw.com/anesthesia-and-alcohol-use/. Accessed 26 June 2023.
79. Chapman R, Plaat F. Alcohol and anaesthesia. Continuing Education in Anaesthesia Critical Care & Pain. 2009;9(1):10–3. https://doi.org/10.1093/bjaceaccp/mkn045.
80. Lipari RN. Key substance use and mental health indicators in the United States: results from the 2019 national survey on drug use and health; 2019. p. 114.

Chapter 9
Nutritional Care in Gastrointestinal Surgery

Maria Wobith and Arved Weimann

Abbreviations

BIA	Bioelectrical impedance analysis
BMI	Body mass index
CT	Computertomography
DXA	Dual-X-absorptiometry
ERAS	Enhanced Recovery after Surgery
ESPEN	European Society for Clinical Nutrition and Metabolism
GCP	Good clinical practice
GLIM	Global Leadership Initiative on Malnutrition
MRI	Magnitude resonance imaging
NRS	Nutritional risk score
ONS	Oral nutrition supplement
PG-SGA	Patient-Generated Subjective Global Assessment
SGA	Subjective Global Assessment
SMI	Skeletal muscle index
6 MWD	6-Minute Walking Distance
CCI	Comprehensive Complication Index
95% CI	95% Confidence interval
OR	Odds ratio
NCJ	Needle catheter jejunostomy
NJ	Nasojejunal tube
ICU	Intensive care unit

M. Wobith · A. Weimann (✉)
Department for General, Visceral and Oncological Surgery, St. George Hospital, Leipzig, Germany
e-mail: Maria.Wobith@sanktgeorg.de; Arved.Weimann@sanktgeorg.de

© The Author(s), under exclusive license to Springer Nature Switzerland AG 2024

J. Faintuch, S. Faintuch (eds.), *Recent Strategies in High Risk Surgery*,
https://doi.org/10.1007/978-3-031-56270-9_9

Introduction

In an overweight population, the "metabolic risk" is often underestimated, with special regard to sarcopenic obesity [1–5]. The impact of malnutrition and sarcopenia for the risk of postoperative complications and the length of hospital stay has been shown very often [2–5]. Nutritional conditioning or "prehabilitation" should be considered for those exhibiting significant metabolic risk, in accordance with ERAS protocols [6–10].

Malnutrition, Sarcopenia, Sarcopenic Obesity

Malnutrition often goes along with sarcopenia. While sarcopenia means a decrease in muscle mass and function, malnutrition is characterized by a global decrease of body cell mass. Especially in geriatric patients, sarcopenia can be present without malnutrition [11, 12]. Diagnosing sarcopenia is not easy in obese patients [13], and in seriously ill older populations, up to 83% can be affected [14].

Prognostic Implications

Preoperatively impaired functionality along with impaired nutritional status is crucial for postoperative mobilization and pulmonary function [15, 16]. In gastric cancer, preoperative sarcopenia has been shown to be associated with overall survival [17].

Sarcopenic obesity is a separate risk factor, where an increased amount of fat may hide a decrease in muscle mass [13, 18, 19].

Metabolic Risk

A well validated tool is the Nutritional Risk Score (NRS-2002) [20]. NRS ≥3 indicates a risk for malnutrition, and assessment should then be initiated. Parameters of the NRS are body mass index (BMI), unintended weight loss, reduced food intake, and severity of disease. Furthermore, serum albumin can be used as preoperative predictor for the underlying risk for postoperative complications [5] in line with the Joint Consensus Statement on Nutritional Screening and Therapy within a Surgical Enhanced Recovery Pathway of the American Society for Enhanced Recovery and Perioperative Quality Initiative [21]. A high metabolic risk is defined by the ESPEN guidelines if one of the following criteria is fulfilled: [5]:

- BMI less than 18.5 kg/m^2
- Involuntary weight loss of more than 10–15% within 6 months
- SGA grade C, NRS ≥5
- Serum albumin <30 g/L (no liver/renal disease, no trauma/surgery)

Malnutrition According to GLIM Criteria

Muscle mass measurement has been incorporated into the Global Leadership Initiative on Malnutrition (GLIM) criteria with (1) phenotypic criteria (low body mass index (BMI), reduced muscle mass, non-volitional weight loss and (2) etiological criteria (reduced food intake or assimilation, disease burden/inflammatory condition) [12]. One variable from each category confirms the suspicion of malnutrition.

Measurement of Muscle Mass

As patients undergoing surgery for gastrointestinal cancer always undergo computer tomography/CT for cancer staging, CT can also be exploited to determine muscle quantity and quality. Skeletal muscle index (SMI) is highly regarded as a marker of muscle mass by GLIM criteria. In the axial scan at lumbar level 3 skeletal muscle area and density can be calculated [16, 22–25].

So far, no specific GLIM cut-off values have been anticipated, however proposals should soon emerge. GLIM criteria could be also appropriate to predict postoperative complications, in many cancer and non-cancer settings [26–30].

For patients undergoing colorectal cancer surgery, it has been suggested that low risk or no need for intensive nutritional therapy would correspond to high SMI, excluding patients with BMI ≥35 kg/m^2. High-risk subjects would be in the opposite category: low SMI plus those with BMI ≥35 kg/m^2 [31].

Sarcopenic Obesity

This condition features high body fat and reduced muscle mass. Clinical, functional, and imaging diagnostic methods are available and are strongly recommended for surgical services, as postoperative complications and slow recovery are likely. Stage I is not associated with comorbidities, stage II displaying metabolic, functional, or cardiopulmonary dysfunction [32].

Nutritional Assessment in the Preoperative Period

Evaluation of CT scan (preferably utilizing existing images, without new expenses and X-ray exposure), bioelectrical impedance analysis (BIA), and handgrip strength can be performed very easily, and cut-off points have been defined for such variables. In case body composition from CT or BIA is not available, severe metabolic risk may be defined according to the ESPEN guideline [5].

Indication for Nutrition Therapy

Nutritional counseling should be offered to patients undergoing gastrointestinal cancer surgery. Ideally, the perioperative trajectory will be accompanied by an experienced dietician, or by the Nutrition Support Team if available [33]. It should not be waited until overt malnutrition is present. A risk for malnutrition or an underlying metabolic derangement could underlie the start of nutrition therapy.

ESPEN guidelines [5] advise nutritional support in case of malnutrition or nutritional risk, when dietary intake is likely for more than 5 days before operation, or when <50% of the necessary requirements will be consumed more than 7 days.

For severe nutritional risk 7–14 days assistance is indicated, if necessary postponing surgical intervention [5, 7]. Parenteral nutrition is nowadays an exception, reserved for intolerance of the gastrointestinal tract [5] (Table 9.1).

Immune Enhancement

Benefits regarding infectious complications have been established [35–37]. Rather similar outcomes were documented within an ERAS protocol [38]. According to ESPEN, ONS is recommended for 5–7 days before surgery when risky interventions are programmed, and immunomodulating supplements are suggested [5].

Prehabilitation

This technique is increasingly used in many parts of the world, notably for elderly, unfit, and inadequately nourished individuals. ERAS directives endorse nutritional therapy combined with exercise (physical training) and psychological support for 4–6 weeks [8, 9, 39, 40]. If severe malnutrition is diagnosed there must be an interdisciplinary decision, if and for how long the surgical procedure may be delayed for sufficient conditioning of the patient [40].

Table 9.1 Postoperative enteral and parenteral supplementation related to anticipated oral intake [34]

Oral intake (% caloric requirement) >5 days	Feeding
None	Enteral
<30–50%	Enteral (possible combination with parenteral)
>50%	Monitoring of oral intake

In a recently published multicentric trial targeting non-metastasized colorectal cancer patients who underwent a 4 weeks hospital based trimodal prehabilitation versus standard care, the nutritional intervention was dietary advice aiming a protein intake of 1.5 g/kg body weight. Furthermore, patients were encouraged to take a whey protein supplement (30 g) 1 h after in-hospital training and 1 h before sleeping daily. A multivitamine supplement including vitamin D was also provided. In the intervention group the rate of severe and medical complications was significantly reduced, a result that coincides with other reports, however divergent results have been published as well [41, 42].

Specific evidence-based recommendations concerning nutritional therapy are lacking [8, 9, 43–45]. Most randomized studies have been performed for a duration of 7–14 days, and there is no data for a period of 4–6 weeks. Preoperative immunonutrition and synbiotics may be discussed and are supported in some circumstances [35, 46].

Perioperative Nutrition Therapy

In general, even after upper gastrointestinal resections, oral intake can be started on the first day after surgery [5]. NRS ≥3 tends to be a predictor for low compliance to ERAS protocol and for longer stay in hospital [47]. Compliance to ERAS of less than 70% signals a higher rate of postoperative complications. Nevertheless, outcomes concerning recovery time or complications are heterogeneous [48, 49]. A scheme for clinical practice is shown in Fig. 9.1 [34].

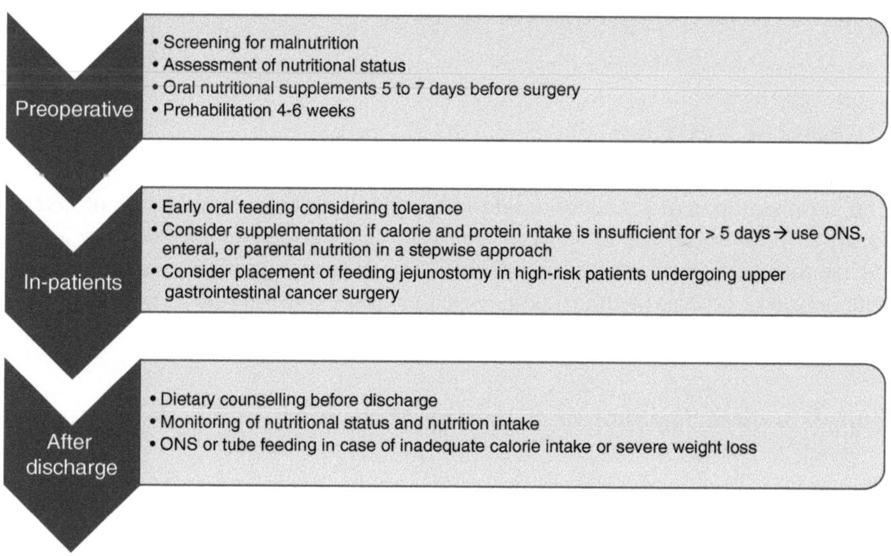

Fig. 9.1 Nutrition therapy for gastrointestinal cancer patients during the trajectory (after discharge ***)

Enteral Feeding—Jejunostomy and Nasojejunal Tube

A "bariatric effect" of upper GI operations for cancer including ghrelin deficiency has been advocated. Typically these patients lose 10% or more of their body weight in the first 6 months after the procedure, with parallel muscle wasting, a condition that adversely affects tolerance and response to cancer adjuvant treatments.

Nasojejunal feeding, and needle catheter jejunostomy when a longer period is considered, are classic recommendations in such circumstances. The tubes can be placed during surgery, whenever oral alimentation is impaired or malabsorption is anticipated, as a consequence of extensive anatomical changes induced by the operation [5, 50–59].

Gastrointestinal Complaints

Limited gastrointestinal tolerance should be always kept in mind [60, 61]. Diarrhea has been a serious problem during long term enteral alimentation in the past. Currently with less risk of contamination of ready-to-use liquid diets, and a variety of protein and calorie compositions to choose from, depending on individual tolerance and absorptive function, this has become a much less troubling condition.

Vomiting, gastroesophageal reflux and abdominal distension can still precipitate aspiration pneumonitis, and are one of the reasons some prefer jejunostomy instead of nasoenteral tube, in high-risk patients.

Parenteral Nutrition

The peripheral parenteral route is safe [60] and allows complementation of enteral feeding, for those unable to achieve >50% of their caloric needs more than 7 days [5] via the oral/enteral route. Nevertheless, this may be a cumbersome but reasonable option in patients with inadequate oral/enteral intake on pod 3 [61].

Supplemented Parenteral Nutrition Mixtures

Glutamine and omega-3 fatty acids have been extensively used to enrich intravenous dietary mixtures. However, their use remains mostly optional, as long term outcomes are not clearly improved [5, 62, 63]. Whenever possible, enteral feeding should be adopted, even if only partially, as a more complete and affordable source of a balanced diet.

Complicated Course/Intensive Care Unit

Measured body weight (BMI ≤30 kg/m^2), or corrected body weight (BMI >30 kg/m^2) corresponding to BMI of 22 kg/m^2 only, have been advised to guide routine dietary prescriptions. Indirect calorimetry is a reliable tool and should be employed especially in critically ill cases [64, 65].

Late Postoperative Period, After Discharge

After undergoing extensive cancer surgery prolonged loss of 10% or 20% of previous body weight is frequently seen and can interfere not only with functional status, but also with response to chemotherapy. This reinforces the importance enteral support in the subsequent months as prophylaxis, for those classified as high risk [66, 67].

Therefore, dietary counseling and follow-up may be mandatory. If appropriate additionally oral nutritional supplements (ONS) may be helpful [68].

With special regard to patients with upper gastrointestinal resections, several studies have pointed out home enteral nutrition as superior to ONS. Counseling can be employed as well, however home enteral nutrition is still endowed with more predictable outcomes, generally including body mass index and skeletal muscle mass index (SMI) [68–72]. Another more simple alternative to attenuate weight loss during the first year could be ONS providing up to 400 kcal/day, but compliance of the patients may be often limited [73].

The Bariatric Effect

Pharmacologic treatment may become more important in the future. In a recent randomized trial ghrelin was postoperatively administered in patients undergoing esophagectomy. A dosage dependent beneficial effect of ghrelin infusion was observed on *erector spinae*, a marker of muscle loss [74].

Based on the available positive data, a randomized nutritional trial may be debatable from an ethical point of view. Patient reported outcomes (PROMS) will provide a measure for shared decision making regarding post-discharge enteral nutrition. Overall, nutritional care may be considered an essential item of perioperative management in gastrointestinal cancer patients. While changes may often be "marginal", underestimated cumulative effects will impact postoperative outcome [75].

Conflict of Interest Arved Weimann: Lecture fees: Abbott, B. Braun, Fresenius Kabi, Falk Foundation. Research grant: B. Braun, Mucos. Maria Wobith: Lecture fees: Fresenius Kabi. Research grant: B Braun.

References

1. Williams DGA, Molinger J, Wischmeyer PE. The malnourished surgery patient: a silent epidemic in perioperative outcome? Curr Opin Anesthesiol. 2019;32:405–11.
2. Simonsen C, de Heer P, Bjerre ED, Suetta C, Hojman P, Pedersen BK, Svendsen LB, Christensen JF. Sarcopenia and postoperative complication risk in gastrointestinal surgical oncology: a meta-analysis. Ann Surg. 2018;268:58–69.
3. Cao Y, Han D, Zhou X, Han Y, Zhang Y, Li H. Effects of preoperative nutrition on postoperative outcomes in esophageal cancer: a systematic review and meta-analysis. Dis Esophagus. 2022;35(3):doab028.
4. Kenny E, Samavat H, Touger-Decker R, Parrott JS, Byham-Gray L, August DA. Adverse perioperative outcomes among patients undergoing gastrointestinal cancer surgery: quantifying attributable risk from malnutrition. JPEN J Parenter Enteral Nutr. 2022;46(3):517–25.
5. Weimann A, Braga M, Carli F, Higashiguchi T, Hübner M, Klek S, Laviano A, Ljungqvist O, Lobo DN, Martindale R, Waitzberg DL, Bischoff SC, Singer P. ESPEN guideline: clinical nutrition in surgery. Clin Nutr. 2017;36(3):623–50.
6. Ljungqvist O, de Boer HD, Balfour A, Fawcett WJ, Lobo DN, Nelson G, Scott MJ, Wainwright TW, Demartines N. Opportunities and challenges for the next phase of enhanced recovery after surgery: a review. JAMA Surg. 2021;156(8):775–84.
7. Gustafsson UO, Scott MJ, Hübner M, Nygren J, Demartines N, Francis N, Rockall TA, Young-Fadol TW, Hill AG, Soop M, de Boer HD, Urman RD, Chang GJ, Fichera A, Kessler H, Grass F, Whang EE, Fawcett WJ, Carli F, Lobo DN, Rollins KE, Balfour A, Baldini G, Riedel B, Ljungqvist O. Guidelines for perioperative care in elective colorectal surgery: Enhanced Recovery after Surgery (ERAS) Society Recommendations 2018. World J Surg. 2019;43:659–95.
8. Berkel AEM, Bongers BC, Kotte H, Weltevreden P, de Jongh FHC, Eijsvogel MMM, Wymenga M, Bigirwamungu-Bargeman M, van der Palen J, van Det MJ, van Meeteren NLU, Klaase JM. Effects of community-based exercise prehabilitation for patients scheduled for colorectal surgery with high risk for postoperative complications: results of a randomized clinical trial. Ann Surg. 2022;275(2):e299–306.
9. Carli F, Bousquet-Dion G, Awasthi R, Elsherbini N, Liberman S, Boutros M, Stein B, Charlebois P, Ghitulescu G, Morin N, Jagoe T, Scheede-Bergdahl C, Minnella EM, Fiore JF Jr. Effect of multimodal prehabilitation vs postoperative rehabilitation on 30-day postoperative complications for frail patients undergoing resection of colorectal cancer: a randomized clinical trial. JAMA Surg. 2020;155(3):233–42.
10. Weimann A, Braga M, Carli F, Higashiguchi T, Hübner M, Klek S, Laviano A, Ljungqvist O, Lobo DN, Martindale RG, Waitzberg D, Bischoff SC, Singer P. ESPEN practical guideline: clinical nutrition in surgery. Clin Nutr. 2021;40(7):4745–61.
11. Muscaritoli M, Arends J, Bachmann P, Baracos V, Barthelemy N, Bertz H, Bozzetti F, Hütterer E, Isenring E, Kaasa S, Krznaric Z, Laird B, Larsson M, Laviano A, Mühlebach S, Oldervoll L, Ravasco P, Solheim TS, Strasser F, de van der Schueren M, Preiser JC, Bischoff SC. ESPEN practical guideline: clinical nutrition in cancer. Clin Nutr. 2021;40(5):2898–913.
12. Cederholm T, Jensen GL, Correia MITD, Gonzalez MC, Fukushima R, Higashiguchi T, Baptista G, Barazzoni R, Blaauw R, Coats A, Crivelli A, Evans DC, Gramlich L, Fuchs-Tarlovsky V, Keller H, Llido L, Malone A, Mogensen KM, Morley JE, Muscaritoli M, Nyulasi I, Pirlich M, Pisprasert V, de van der Schueren MAE, Siltharm S, Singer P, Tappenden K, Velasco N, Waitzberg D, Yamwong P, Yu J, Van Gossum A, Compher C, GLIM Core Leadership Committee; GLIM Working Group. GLIM criteria for the diagnosis of malnutrition—a consensus report from the global clinical nutrition community. Clin Nutr. 2019;38(1):1–9.
13. Barazzoni R, Jensen GL, Correia MITD, Gonzalez MC, Higashiguchi T, Shi HP, Bischoff SC, Boirie Y, Carrasco F, Cruz-Jentoft A, et al. Guidance for assessment of the muscle mass phenotypic criterion for the Global Leadership Initiative on Malnutrition (GLIM) diagnosis of malnutrition. Clin Nutr. 2022;41(6):1425–33.

14. Caillet P, Liuu E, Raynaud Simon A, Bonnefoy M, Guerin O, Berrut G, Lesourd B, Jeandel C, Ferry M, Rolland Y, Paillaud E. Association between cachexia, chemotherapy and outcomes in older cancer patients: a systematic review. Clin Nutr. 2017;36(6):1473–82.
15. Wang P-Y, Chen X-K, Liu Q, Yu Y-K, Xu L, Liu X-B, Zhang R-X, Wang Z-F, Li Y. Highlighting sarcopenia management for promoting surgical outcomes in esophageal cancers: evidence from a prospective cohort study. Int J Surg. 2020;83:206–15.
16. Ishida T, Makino T, Yamasaki M, Yamashita K, Tanaka K, Saito T, Yamamoto K, Takahashi T, Kurokawa Y, Motoori M, Kimura Y, Nakajima K, Eguchi H, Doki Y. Quantity and quality of skeletal muscle as an important predictor of clinical outcomes in patients with esophageal cancer undergoing esophagectomy after neoadjuvant chemotherapy. Ann Surg Oncol. 2021;28(12):7185–95.
17. Kuwada K, Kikuchi S, Kuroda S, Yoshida R, Takagi K, Noma K, Nishizaki M, Kagawa S, Umeda Y, Fujiwara T. Survival impact of postoperative skeletal muscle loss in gastric cancer patients who underwent gastrectomy. Anticancer Res. 2023;43(1):223–30.
18. Gruber ES, Jomrich G, Tamandl D, Gnant M, Schindl M, Sahora K. Sarcopenia and sarcopenic obesity are independent adverse prognostic factors in resectable pancreatic ductal adenocarcinoma. PLoS One. 2019;14(5):e0215915.
19. Barazzoni R, Gortan CG. Double burden of malnutrition in persons with obesity. Rev Endocr Metab Disord. 2020;21(3):307–13.
20. Kondrup J, Allison SP, Elia M, Vellas B, Plauth M, Educational and Clinical Practice Committee, European Society of Parenteral and Enteral Nutrition (ESPEN). ESPEN guidelines for nutrition screening 2002. Clin Nutr. 2003;22(4):415–21.
21. Wischmeyer PE, Carli F, Evans DC, Guilbert S, Kozar R, Pryor A, Thiele RH, Everett S, Grocott M, Gan TJ, Shaw AD, Thacker JKM, Miller TE, Hedrick TL, McEvoy MD, Mythen MG, Bergamaschi R, Gupta R, Holubar SD, Senagore AJ, Abola RE, Bennett-Guerrero E, Kent ML, Feldman LS, Fiore JF Jr, Perioperative Quality Initiative (POQI) 2 Workgroup. American Society for Enhanced Recovery and Perioperative quality initiative joint consensus statement on nutrition screening and therapy within a surgical enhanced recovery pathway. Anesth Analg. 2018;126(6):1883–95.
22. Mayanagi S, Tsubosa Y, Omae K, Niihara M, Uchida T, Tsushima T, Yokota T, Sato H, Naito T, Yasui H. Negative impact of skeletal muscle wasting after neoadjuvant chemotherapy followed by surgery on survival for patients with thoracic esophageal cancer. Ann Surg Oncol. 2017;24(12):3741–7.
23. Martin L, Gioulbasanis I, Senesse P, Baracos VE. Cancer-associated malnutrition and CT-defined sarcopenia and myosteatosis are endemic in overweight and obese patients. JPEN J Parenter Enteral Nutr. 2020;44(2):227–38.
24. Wobith M, Herbst C, Lurz M, Haberzettl D, Fischer M, Weimann A. Evaluation of malnutrition in patients undergoing major abdominal surgery using GLIM criteria and comparing CT and BIA for muscle mass measurement. Clin Nutr ESPEN. 2022;50:148–54.
25. Gomez-Perez SL, Haus JM, Sheean P, Patel B, Mar W, Chaudhry V, McKeever L, Braunschweig C. Measuring abdominal circumference and skeletal muscle from a single cross-sectional computed tomography image: a step-by-step guide for clinicians using National Institutes of Health ImageJ [Erratum in: JPEN J Parenter Enteral Nutr 2016; 40(5): 742-3.]. JPEN J Parenter Enteral Nutr. 2016;40(3):308–18.
26. Yin L, Cheng N, Chen P, Zhang M, Li N, Lin X, He X, Wang Y, Xu H, Guo W, Liu J. Association of Malnutrition, as defined by the PG-SGA, ESPEN 2015, and GLIM criteria, with complications in esophageal cancer patients after esophagectomy. Front Nutr. 2021;8:632546.
27. Kakavas S, Karayiannis D, Bouloubasi Z, Poulia KA, Kompogiorgas S, Konstantinou D, Vougas V. Global leadership initiative on malnutrition criteria predict pulmonary complications and 90-day mortality after major abdominal surgery in cancer patients. Nutrients. 2020;12(12):1–11.
28. Skeie E, Tangvik RJ, Nymo LS, Harthug S, Lassen K, Viste A. Weight loss and BMI criteria in GLIM's definition of malnutrition is associated with postoperative complications

following abdominal resections—results from a National Quality Registry. Clin Nutr 2020. 2019;39(5):1593–9.
29. Clark AB, Reijnierse EM, Lim WK, Maier AB. Prevalence of malnutrition comparing the GLIM criteria, ESPEN definition and MST malnutrition risk in geriatric rehabilitation patients: RESORT. Clin Nutr. 2020;39(11):3504–11.
30. Sanchez-Rodriguez D, Locquet M, Reginster JY, Cavalier E, Bruyère O, Beaudart C. Mortality in malnourished older adults diagnosed by ESPEN and GLIM criteria in the SarcoPhAge study. J Cachexia Sarcopenia Muscle. 2020;11(5):1200–11.
31. López-Rodríguez-Arias F, Sánchez-Guillén L, Lillo-García C, Aranaz-Ostáriz V, Alcaide MJ, Soler-Silva Á, Soriano-Irigaray L, Barber X, Arroyo A. Assessment of body composition as an indicator of early peripheral parenteral nutrition therapy in patients undergoing colorectal cancer surgery in an enhanced recovery program. Nutrients. 2021;13(9):3245.
32. Donini LM, Busetto L, Bischoff SC, Cederholm T, Ballesteros-Pomar MD, Batsis JA, Bauer JM, Boirie Y, Cruz-Jentoft AJ, Dicker D, Frara S, Frühbeck G, Genton L, Gepner Y, Giustina A, Gonzalez MC, Han HS, Heymsfield SB, Higashiguchi T, Barazzoni R. Definition and diagnostic criteria for Sarcopenic obesity: ESPEN and EASO consensus statement. Obes Facts. 2022;15(3):321–35.
33. Ligthart-Melis GC, Weijs PJ, te Boveldt ND, Buskermolen S, Earthman CP, Verheul HM, de Lange-de Klerk ES, van Weyenberg SJ, van der Peet DL. Dietician-delivered intensive nutritional support is associated with a decrease in severe postoperative complications after surgery in patients with esophageal cancer. Dis Esophagus. 2013;26(6):587–93.
34. Wobith M, Weimann A. Postoperative nutrition management—who needs what? Visc Med. 2022;38(5):354–62.
35. Slim K, Badon F, Vacheron CH, Occean BV, Dziri C, Chambrier C. Umbrella review of the efficacy of perioperative immunonutrition in visceral surgery. Clin Nutr ESPEN. 2022;48:99–108.
36. Adiamah A, Skořepa P, Weimann A, Lobo DN. The impact of preoperative immune modulating nutrition on outcomes in patients undergoing surgery for gastrointestinal cancer. Ann Surg. 2019;270(2):247–56.
37. Cao Y, Han D, Yang S, Shi Y, Zhao S, Jin Q, Li J, Li C, Zhang Y, Shen W, He J, Wang M, Ji G, Li Z, He Y, Chen Q, Wei W, Chen C, Gong X, Wang J, Tan L, Wang H, Li H. Effects of pre-operative enteral immunonutrition for esophageal cancer patients treated with neoadjuvant chemoradiotherapy: protocol for a multicenter randomized controlled trial (point trial, pre-operative immunonutrition therapy). BMC Cancer. 2022;22(1):650.
38. Moya P, Soriano-Irigaray L, Ramirez JM, Garcea A, Blasco O, Blanco FJ, Brugiotti C, Miranda E, Arroyo A. Perioperative standard oral nutrition supplements versus immunonutrition in patients undergoing colorectal resection in an enhanced recovery (ERAS) protocol: a multicenter randomized clinical trial (SONVI study). Medicine (Baltimore). 2016;95(21):e3704.
39. Ligthart-Melis GC, Luiking YC, Kakourou A, Cederholm T, Maier AB, de van der Schueren MAE. Frailty, sarcopenia, and malnutrition frequently (co-)occur in hospitalized older adults: a systematic review and meta-analysis. J Am Med Dir Assoc. 2020;21(9):1216–28.
40. Davies SJ, West MA, Rahman SA, Underwood TJ, Marino LV. Oesophageal cancer: the effect of early nutrition support on clinical outcomes. Clin Nutr ESPEN. 2021;42:117–23.
41. McIsaac DI, Gill M, Boland L, Hutton B, Branje K, Shaw J, Grudzinski AL, Barone N, Gillis C, Akhtar S, Atkins M, Aucoin S, Auer R, Basualdo-Hammond C, et al. Prehabilitation in adult patients undergoing surgery: an umbrella review of systematic reviews. Br J Anaesth. 2022;128(2):244–57.
42. Molenaar CJL, Minnella EM, Coca-Martinez M, Ten Cate DWG, Regis M, Awasthi R, Martínez-Palli G, López-Baamonde M, Sebio-Garcia R, Feo CV, van Rooijen SJ, Schreinemakers JMJ, Bojesen RD, Gögenur I, van den Heuvel ER, Carli F, Slooter GD, PREHAB Study Group. Effect of multimodal prehabilitation on reducing postoperative complications and enhancing functional capacity following colorectal cancer surgery: the PREHAB randomized clinical trial. JAMA Surg. 2023;58(6):572–81.
43. Daniels SL, Lee MJ, George J, Kerr K, Moug S, Wilson TR, Brown SR, Wyld L. Prehabilitation in elective abdominal cancer surgery in older patients: systematic review and meta-analysis. BJS Open. 2020;4(6):1022–41.

44. Gillis C, Buhler K, Bresee L, Carli F, Gramlich L, Culos-Reed N, Sajobi TT, Fenton TR. Effects of nutritional prehabilitation, with and without exercise, on outcomes of patients who undergo colorectal surgery: a systematic review and meta-analysis. Gastroenterology. 2018;155(2):391–410.e4.
45. Hughes MJ, Hackney RJ, Lamb PJ, Wigmore SJ, Christopher Deans DA, Skipworth RJE. Prehabilitation before major abdominal surgery: a systematic review and meta-analysis. World J Surg. 2019;43(7):1661–8.
46. Chowdhury AH, Adiamah A, Kushairi A, Varadhan KK, Krznaric Z, Kulkarni AD, Neal KR, Lobo DN. Perioperative probiotics or synbiotics in adults undergoing elective abdominal surgery: a systematic review and meta-analysis of randomized controlled trials. Ann Surg. 2020;271(6):1036–47.
47. Martin L, Gillis C, Atkins M, Gillam M, Sheppard C, Buhler S, Hammond CB, Nelson G, Gramlich L. Implementation of an enhanced recovery after surgery program can change nutrition care practice: a multicenter experience in elective colorectal surgery. JPEN J Parenter Enteral Nutr. 2019;43(2):206–19.
48. Berkelmans GHK, Fransen LFC, Dolmans-Zwartjes ACP, Kouwenhoven EA, van Det MJ, Nilsson M, Nieuwenhuijzen GAP, Luyer MDP. Direct oral feeding following minimally invasive esophagectomy (NUTRIENT II trial): an international, multicenter, open-label randomized controlled trial. Ann Surg. 2020;271(1):41–7.
49. Zhang B, Najarali Z, Ruo L, Alhusaini A, Solis N, Valencia M, Sanchez MIP, Serrano PE. Effect of perioperative nutritional supplementation on postoperative complications-systematic review and meta-analysis. J Gastrointest Surg. 2019;23(8):1682–93.
50. Baker M, Halliday V, Williams RN, Bowrey DJ. A systematic review of the nutritional consequences of esophagectomy. Clin Nutr. 2016;35(5):987–94.
51. Wobith M, Wehle L, Haberzettl D, Acikgöz A, Weimann A. Needle catheter jejunostomy in patients undergoing surgery for upper gastrointestinal and pancreato-biliary cancer—impact on nutritional and clinical outcome in the early and late postoperative period. Nutrients. 2020;12:2564.
52. Koterazawa Y, Oshikiri T, Takiguchi G, Urakawa N, Hasegawa H, Yamamoto M, Kanaji S, Yamashita K, Matsuda T, Nakamura T, Suzuki S, Kakeji Y. Severe weight loss after minimally invasive oesophagectomy is associated with poor survival in patients with oesophageal cancer at 5 years. BMC Gastroenterol. 2020;20(1):1–9.
53. Aoyama T, Yoshikawa T, Maezawa Y, Kano K, Numata M, Hara K, Komori K, Yamada T, Hayashi T, Sato T, Tamagawa H, Yukawa N, Rino Y, Masuda M, Ogata T, Cho H, Oshima T. The postoperative lean body mass loss at one month leads to a poor survival in patients with locally advanced gastric cancer. J Cancer. 2019;10(11):2450–6.
54. Aoyama T, Kawabe T, Fujikawa H, Hayashi T, Yamada T, Tsuchida K, Yukawa N, Oshima T, Rino Y, Masuda M, Ogata T, Cho H, Yoshikawa T. Loss of lean body mass as an independent risk factor for continuation of s-1 adjuvant chemotherapy for gastric cancer. Ann Surg Oncol. 2015;22(8):2560–6.
55. Weijs TJ, van Eden HWJ, Ruurda JP, Luyer MP, Stenhagen E, Nieuwenhuijzen GAP, van Hilgersberg R. Routine jejunostomy tube feeding following esophagectomy. J Thorac Dis. 2017;9:S851–60.
56. Zhuang W, Wu H, Liu H, Huang S, Wu Y, Deng C, Tian D, Zhou Z, Shi R, Chen G, Piessen G, Khaitan PG, Koyanagi K, Ozawa S, Qiao G. Utility of feeding jejunostomy in patients with esophageal cancer undergoing esophagectomy with a high risk of anastomotic leakage. J Gastrointest Oncol. 2021;12(2):433–45.
57. Li HN, Chen Y, Dai L, Wang Y-Y, Chen M-W, Mei L-X. A meta-analysis of jejunostomy versus nasoenteral tube for enteral nutrition following esophagectomy. J Surg Res. 2021;264:553–61.
58. Holmén A, Hayami M, Szabo E, Rouvelas I, Agustsson T, Klevebro F. Nutritional jejunostomy in esophagectomy for cancer, a national register-based cohort study of associations with postoperative outcomes and survival. Langenbecks Arch Surg. 2020;406(5):1415–23.
59. Shen X, Zhuo Z-G, Li G, Alai G-H, Song T-N, Xu Z-J, Yao P, Lin Y-D. Is the routine placement of a feeding jejunostomy during esophagectomy worthwhile? A systematic review and meta-analysis. Ann Palliat Med. 2021;10:4232–41.

60. Durán-Poveda M, Bonavina L, Reith B, Caruso R, Klek S, Senkal M. Nutrition practices with a focus on parenteral nutrition in the context of enhanced recovery programs: an exploratory survey of gastrointestinal surgeons. Clin Nutr ESPEN. 2022;50:138–47.
61. Gao X, Liu Y, Zhang L, Zhou D, Tian F, Gao T, Tian H, Hu H, Gong F, Guo D, Zhou J, Gu Y, Lian B, Xue Z, Jia Z, Chen Z, Wang Y, Jin G, Wang K, Zhou Y, Chi Q, Yang H, Li M, Yu J, Qin H, Tang Y, Wu X, Li G, Li N, Li J, Pichard C, Wang X. Effect of early vs late supplemental parenteral nutrition in patients undergoing abdominal surgery: a randomized clinical trial. JAMA Surg. 2022;157(5):384–93.
62. Pradelli L, Mayer K, Klek S, Omar Alsaleh AJ, Clark RAC, Rosenthal MD, Heller AR, Muscaritoli M. ω-3 Fatty-acid enriched parenteral nutrition in hospitalized patients: systematic review with meta-analysis and trial sequential analysis. JPEN J Parenter Enteral Nutr. 2020;44(1):44–57.
63. Ziegler TR, May AK, Hebbar G, Easley KA, Griffith DP, Dave N, Collier BR, Cotsonis GA, Hao L, Leong T, Manatunga AK, Rosenberg ES, Jones DP, Martin GS, Jensen GL, Sax HC, Kudsk KA, Galloway JR, Blumberg HM, Evans ME, Wischmeyer PE. Efficacy and safety of glutamine-supplemented parenteral nutrition in surgical ICU patients: an American multicenter randomized controlled trial. Ann Surg. 2016;263(4):646–55.
64. Elke G, Hartl WH, Kreymann KG, Adolph M, Felbinger TW, Graf T, de Heer G, Heller AR, Kampa U, Mayer K, Muhl E, Niemann B, Rümelin A, Steiner S, Stoppe C, Weimann A, Bischoff SC. Clinical nutrition in critical care medicine—guideline of the German Society for Nutritional Medicine (DGEM). Clin Nutr ESPEN. 2019;33:220–75.
65. Ridley EJ, Parke RL, Davies AR, Bailey M, Hodgson C, Deane AM, McGuinness S, Cooper DJ. What happens to nutrition intake in the post-intensive care unit hospitalization period? An observational cohort study in critically ill adults. JPEN J Parenter Enteral Nutr. 2019;43:88–95.
66. Heneghan HM, Zaborowski A, Fanning M, McHugh A, Doyle S, Moore J, Ravi N, Reynolds JV. Prospective study of malabsorption and malnutrition after esophageal and gastric cancer surgery. Ann Surg. 2015;262(5):803–7.
67. Wobith M, Weimann A. Oral nutritional supplements and enteral nutrition in patients with gastrointestinal surgery. Nutrients. 2021;13(8):2655.
68. Meng Q, Tan S, Jiang Y, Han J, Xi Q, Zhuang Q, Wu G. Post-discharge oral nutritional supplements with dietary advice in patients at nutritional risk after surgery for gastric cancer: a randomized clinical trial. Clin Nutr. 2021;40:40–6.
69. Chen X, Zhao G, Zhu L. Home enteral nutrition for postoperative elderly patients with esophageal cancer. Ann Palliat Med. 2021;10(1):278–84.
70. Xueting H, Li L, Meng Y, Yuqing C, Yutong H, Lihong Q, June Z. Home enteral nutrition and oral nutritional supplements in postoperative patients with upper gastrointestinal malignancy: a systematic review and meta-analysis. Clin Nutr. 2020;40(5):3082–93.
71. Liu F, Pan X, Zhao S, Ren R, Chang G, Mao Y. Effect of home enteral nutritional support compared with normal oral diet in postoperative subjects with upper gastrointestinal cancer resection: a meta-analysis. Front Surg. 2022;9:844475.
72. Komatsu S, Konishi T, Matsubara D, Soga K, Shimomura K, Ikeda J, Taniguchi F, Iwase H, Kubota T, Shioaki Y, Otsuji E. Night home enteral nutrition as a novel enforced and physiologically effective nutrition therapy following total gastrectomy for gastric cancer. Sci Rep. 2022;12(1):14922.
73. Miyazaki Y, Omori T, Fujitani K, Fujita J, Kawabata R, Imamura H, Okada K, Moon JH, Hirao M, Matsuyama J, Saito T, Takahashi T, Kurokawa Y, Yamasaki M, Takiguchi S, Mori M, Doki Y, Osaka University Clinical Research Group for Gastroenterological Study. Oral nutritional supplements versus a regular diet alone for body weight loss after gastrectomy: a phase 3, multicenter, open-label randomized controlled trial. Gastric Cancer. 2021;24(5):1150–9.
74. Nose Y, Yamashita K, Takeoka T, Momose K, Saito T, Tanaka K, Yamamoto K, Makino T, Takahashi T, Kurokawa Y, Yamasaki M, Shiraishi O, Miyata H, Yasuda T, Yano M, Eguchi H, Doki Y. Perioperative ghrelin administration attenuates postoperative skeletal muscle loss in

patients undergoing esophagectomy for esophageal cancer: secondary analysis of a randomized controlled trial. Ann Surg Oncol. 2022;29(6):3604–12.
75. Ford KL, Prado CM, Weimann A, Schuetz P, Lobo DN. Unresolved issues in perioperative nutrition: a narrative review. Clin Nutr. 2022;41:1578–90.

Part III
Surgical Specialties

Chapter 10
Risk Reduction in Diabetic Patients Undergoing Orthopaedic Surgery

Michael S. Pinzur

Introduction

Most experts herald the 1999 publication from the Institute of Medicine, "*To Err is Human*", as the beginning of the "*Patient Safety Movement*" [1]. This seminal report estimated that up to 98,000 deaths occurred yearly in the United States due to preventable errors occurring during the delivery of health care. Avoiding error became the focus during the early phase of this paradigm shift. Early adopters borrowed on the concepts of entropy that we learned in high school physics, appreciating that a system left to its own devices, would revert to disorder. It was felt that this systemic disorder was responsible for the errors that led to patient harm. Patient care pathways and clinical algorithms evolved as the methodology to standardize clinical care and counteract these error-producing forces. They borrowed the principles of decision support from the business world to develop clinical systems that were designed to lessen the risk for deviation and error.

The by-product of this thinking was likely a strong motivating force that led to the development of Hospitalist-Orthopaedic co-management programs. Introducing internal medicine principles led to the development of clinical algorithms designed to not only decrease the risk for error, but also decrease the risks of co-morbidity disease-impact on clinical care. The final step leading to the most forward thinking delivery of health care was the asking the question when performing elective surgery … If we make sick patients less sick, will their clinical outcomes be improved? This evolution in thinking allowed the Patient Safety Movement to evolve from the simple avoidance of treatment errors, to the current approach that medically

M. S. Pinzur (✉)
Department of Orthopaedic Surgery and Rehabilitation, Loyola University Medical Center, Maywood, IL, USA
e-mail: mpinzu1@lumc.edu

© The Author(s), under exclusive license to Springer Nature Switzerland AG 2024

J. Faintuch, S. Faintuch (eds.), *Recent Strategies in High Risk Surgery*,
https://doi.org/10.1007/978-3-031-56270-9_10

optimizes patients' co-morbidities, thus allowing *sick* patients to take advantage of modern clinical innovations at a reasonable risk tolerance.

The United States Centers for Disease Control currently estimates that there are over 30 million diabetes in the United States, a number approaching 10% of our population, with an estimated over 80 million additional individuals over 18 years of age being pre-diabetic [2]. This objective of this chapter to provide physicians the clinical tools to employ the modern methods of medical optimization for complex diabetic patients undergoing emergent, urgent and elective Orthopaedic Surgery [3].

Diabetic Organ System Disease

The primary initiator of diabetic organ system disease is the presence of elevated blood sugar over time. Elevated blood sugar binds with hemoglobin within red blood cells to form glycosylated hemoglobin, which is clinically measured as hemoglobin A1C. This glycosylated hemoglobin leads to a release of free radicals, which damages the basement membrane of all vessels in the arterial tree, leading to a similar level of disease expression in all key organ systems [4, 5]. We have long viewed the presence of peripheral neuropathy, as measured by insensitivity to the Semmes-Weinstein 5.07 monofilament, as an important risk factor in diabetics (Fig. 10.1). Instead of viewing insensitivity to the monofilament as a risk

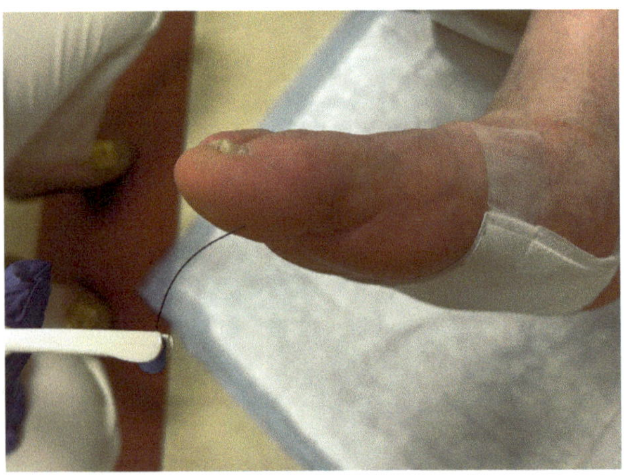

Fig. 10.1 Semmes-Weinstein 5.07 monofilament. This monofilament imparts 10 g of pressure to the tuft of the hallux. When patients cannot, perceive this amount of pressure, they exhibit a level of sensory peripheral neuropathy that is associated with other diabetic organ system disease. Long thought of as a *risk factor* for associated organ system disease, this level of peripheral neuropathy should be considered as a disease marker, as patients with peripheral neuropathy also have a level of cardiac, pulmonary, renal disease and osteoporosis

factor, we should view the presence of peripheral neuropathy as a measure of disease expression.

When caring for patients, we view the serum level of hemoglobin A1C, as a measure of estimated serum glucose levels over the past 3 months. We use the measurement of serum glucose as a temporal measure of real-time blood sugar. It is this measurement that allows the poorly controlled diabetic to develop both the acute and chronic consequences of life-threatening ketoacidosis. Management of serum glucose will be expanded when we discuss the *hard stops* of care for diabetic patients.

Hospitalist Co-management

The increasing complexities associated with the delivery of complex medical care led to the development of the Hospitalist, as a medical specialty. First described by Wachter in 1996, the care of hospitalized medical patients has been assumed by physicians who could focus on inpatient medical care, without the associated stresses of an outpatient medical practice [6, 7]. Early adopters to the Hospitalist patient care model expanded this concept to develop co-management partnerships with Orthopaedic and other surgical colleagues. Patients could then have the added advantage of medical expertise when clinical care could be managed as a team effort. While these programs were not initially able to improve the metrics of health care, experience has led to improved clinical outcomes, decreased rates of complications and hospital re-admissions, and substantial cost savings [8–11].

Most musculoskeletal care is currently provided in the ambulatory setting. Total hip and knee arthroplasty is increasingly being performed on healthy individuals without hospital admission. Therefore, virtually all patients undergoing inpatient urgent or elective Orthopaedic surgery have sufficient medical co-morbidities to warrant the routine utilization of a Hospitalist-Orthopaedic co-management patient care model [12].

The *Hard Stops*

There are four medical co-morbidities that have clearly been associated with increased rates of death, poor clinical outcomes, surgical site infections, perioperative complications, hospital re-admission and impaired metrics of health care [3, 13]. Glucose management in both diabetics and non-diabetics, cardio-pulmonary function, anemia and hypertension, are the critical medical co-morbidities that must be addressed, regardless of the nature of surgery. We call these four medical co-morbidities *hard stops*, as they must be addressed when both performing emergent or urgent surgery, and have the potential to be optimized prior to elective surgery.

Blood Sugar/Hemoglobin A1C

Management of blood glucose is the first objective when discussing either longitudinal medical management or surgical intervention in diabetic individuals. The level of glycosylated hemoglobin, that is, Hemoglobin A1C provides the treating physician an estimation of daily blood glucose levels over the past 90 days. The United States Centers for Disease Control define levels under 5.7% as normal. Levels in patients between 5.7–6.4% designate the patient as being *pre-diabetic*, with values over 6.5% designating the patient as having clinical diabetes [14]. There is growing literature that the target for optimal glucose management is 6.5%, and that elective surgery should be delayed if levels are above 8% [15–18].

Morbid Obesity

The current accepted cutoff for performing elective Orthopaedic surgery is a BMI of 40. While this value is controversial, the current recommendation for performing elective Orthopaedic surgery in morbidly obese patients is to develop and institutional methodology to address these patients. Best practice organizations have these individuals evaluated by a local hyperbaric program. Many of these patients can achieve significant weight loss with structured diet. Some will benefit from so-called *weight loss* surgery. There should be a screening process to determine which patients have made a substantial effort to decrease their BMI, and thus, decrease their risk for perioperative morbidity. This programming makes the BMI value of 40 as a soft target, allowing for surgery in patients that lower their BMI, albeit even if they do get attain the *hard stop* value of 40 [3, 19].

Anemia

Anemia, as defined by a hemoglobin level below 12 g/dL, has been demonstrated to be associated with less than favorable clinical outcomes, and an increased risk for perioperative complications in elective Orthopaedic surgery [3, 19, 20]. A local program can be developed to use oral iron supplementation, targeted medication and dietary modification to address this co-morbidity.

Hypertension/Elevated Diastolic Blood Pressure

The final of the four hard stops is a diastolic blood pressure greater than 110 mmHg, which has been associated with increased perioperative complications [3, 19]. This value should be addressed before safely proceeding with elective surgery.

A *best practice* initiative advises the development of checklists to be utilized during all phases of care. The checklist can be even utilized in preparing patients for emergent or urgent surgery, so that all participating physicians have a clear understanding of the level of co-morbid disease. The checklist can be expanded for patients undergoing elective surgery to additionally include the so-called *soft stops* [3, 13].

The *Soft* Stops

SOFT stops are medical co-morbidities that can be improved prior to proceeding with elective Orthopaedic surgery. The degree that one addresses these conditions will vary with the delay tolerance prior to performing the elective surgery. These medical co-morbid conditions include smoking cessation, nutrition, and sleep apnea. When addressing the geriatric population, many patients being evaluated for treatment have some element of malnutrition. Several investigations have demonstrated that patients with metrics associated with malnutrition are more likely to develop delayed wound healing and postoperative infection [3, 13, 21–24]. Each individual health system needs to address how much medical optimization should be undertaken prior to proceeding with elective reconstructive Orthopaedic surgery.

The Perioperative Period

The modern patient safety movement has demonstrated that organizations that develop standardization of health care delivery are more likely to delivery improved metrics of care, lower rates of perioperative complication, and a decreased rate of hospital re-admission. The application of standardized care is accomplished when physicians within an organization agree to use *in common* perioperative checklists and electronic medical record order sets [3, 13].

Perioperative Glucose Management

Glucose monitoring and control are crucial during the perioperative management of diabetics. The accepted range should be between 140 and 200 mg/dL during the perioperative period. Blood sugar should be measured and monitored in all Orthopaedic patients, as up to 25% of patients undergoing Orthopaedic surgery will experience severe hyperglycemia during the perioperative period, regardless of whether they carry a pre-operative diagnosis of diabetes [18, 25]. This is likely due to the high incidence of patients who are pre-diabetic, and only exhibit symptoms associated with the stress of surgery [5]. Performing surgery on diabetics early in the day takes advantage of diurnal glucose levels [2, 6]. Careful postoperative glucose monitoring is essential, one of the earliest signs of impending surgical site infection is worsening glycemic control [26].

Known diabetic patients are advised to hold their medications on the day of surgery, with exception of metformin. Patients taking metformin are instructed to stop taking the medication the evening prior to surgery to decease the development of lactic acidosis [22]. Oral medications can be re-introduced when blood sugars are stable within the accepted range.

Perioperative Hypertension

Cardio-vascular disease and hypertension are frequently associated with diabetes due to the deleterious effects at the basement membrane level [4, 5]. When stressed during the perioperative period, hypertension can be complicated with heart attack and stroke [17]. Careful monitoring and perioperative management are associated with improved patient outcomes [27]. The use of regional anesthesia as opposed to general anesthesia should be considered when feasible and when regional methods prove adequate.

Antibiotic Prophylaxis

Surgical site infection is the leading cause of perioperative complication, increased length of stay and hospital re-admission in diabetics undergoing Orthopaedic surgery [28–30]. Prophylactic appropriate perioperative antibiotics initiated less than 1 h prior to surgical incision and continued for no more than 24 following surgery have been demonstrated to decrease the risk of surgical site infection [3, 13].

Venous Thromboembolism (VTE) Prophylaxis

Diabetic individuals are likely at a higher risk for developing perioperative venous thromboembolism, likely secondary to both biochemical and biomechanical considerations [19, 31–33]. Prophylaxis should combine early ambulation, mechanical methods (venous compression devices) and some element of chemical prophylaxis. Building local checklists and electronic medical record *order sets* allow both standardization of care and the individualization necessary to address the unique needs of the individual patient [3, 13].

Medical Optimization of Patients Undergoing Urgent or Emergent Orthopaedic Surgery

Very few musculoskeletal conditions require emergent surgery. This section will focus on patients with life or limb-threatening conditions. The most-common condition in this category is the patient with abscess or infection that requires acute decompression of the abscess, removal of sepsis-producing infected tissue or amputation. Since the natural history of these conditions lead to death or limb-loss, time to surgery is of the essence.

A thoughtful collaboration between the Internal Medicine Hospitalist, Infectious Disease Specialist, Anesthesiologist, and Surgeon should be undertaken to address the *Hard Stops* discussed earlier. There should be an attempt to address cardiac function, and control blood pressure and blood sugar levels as close to the safe range as possible. Due to the essence of time, medical optimization of co-morbidities needs to be delayed until the need for surgery has been addressed.

Medical Optimization of Patients Undergoing Urgent Orthopaedic Surgery

The prototype musculoskeletal conditions that require urgent surgical treatment are geriatric hip and femur fractures. It is now well accepted that those patients who have surgery within the first 24 h post injury, have the most favorable clinical outcomes. The mortality rate and incidence of perioperative complications is greatly increased when surgery is performed greater than 24 h post injury [34]. It appears that the most favorable clinical outcomes are achieved with the development of Hospitalist-Orthopaedic co-management practice patterns [12, 34].

Geriatric patients that can be safely prepared for surgery the morning after sustaining a hip or femur fracture, should be admitted to the hospital to a co-management service that appreciates the urgency of having the patient medically prepared for surgery the next morning. Those patients with unstable medical co-morbidities that preclude readiness for surgery the next morning should be admitted to a traditional medical service, where their unstable medical co-morbidities can be optimized prior to temporally stabilized prior to undergoing surgery.

The primary co-morbidity that delays the surgical treatment of unstable fractures is an acute myocardial infarction associated with the fracture or an unstable cardiac arrhythmia. The goal is to stabilize these conditions as soon as possible, to allow performing the life-saving surgery.

Blood glucose levels need to be brought down to the previously described *safe* range. This often requires consultation among Internal Medicine Hospitalist, Endocrinologist, and Anesthesiologist. Interdisciplinary co-ordination is often required to address time constraints.

The next most common impediment to surgical readiness is observed in patients being treated with anticoagulant medications. Patients managed longitudinally with warfarin are generally monitored with protime (PT), partial thromboplastin time (PTT), or a laboratory derived ration, and/or the so-called international normalized ratio (INR). The effects of the warfarin can be reversed with vitamin K. Depending on the number of hours before the planned surgery, this reversal can be accomplished by intravenous, intramuscular, or oral vitamin K. A locally agreed upon algorithm for normalizing coagulation metrics is associated with timely care that avoids the complications associated with anticoagulation. Many of the modern anticoagulation medications do not have to be stopped prior to safely performing surgery.

Medical Optimization of Patients Undergoing Elective Orthopaedic Surgery

Modern reconstructive Orthopaedic Surgery often uses techniques that expose patients to prolonged surgical anesthesia, extensive surgical approach, and levels of blood loss far greater than seen in a previous era. Modern shared risk-benefit decision-making is necessary when exposing patients to such risks. Unlike the constraints imposed by emergent or urgent Orthopaedic surgery, time can be taken to medically optimize patients before exposing them to the risks associated with surgery. Multidisciplinary medical optimization programs have been demonstrated to decrease the rate of perioperative complication, reduce hospital length of stay (LOS), reduce postoperative emergency department (ED) visits, reduce the rate of hospital re-admission and increase the rate of discharge to home following surgery [3, 13, 35].

Patients undergoing elective surgery have the time to effectively address the *Hard Stops* associated with surgery. We avoid the term *medical clearance,* as this term seems to imply some sort of *guarantee*. Instead, we attempt to risk stratify, improving medical conditions when feasible. Patients with cardiac co-morbidities can be evaluated by a Cardiology consultant, who often has the capacity to initiate medical therapy or perform a procedure that improves cardiac status, thus decreasing the risk for perioperative cardiac complication. The judicious use of consultant allows a similar medical optimization with other medical co-morbidities, such as hypertension, renal failure, or chronic pulmonary disease.

Each organization should develop a local set of guidelines to address elective musculoskeletal surgery in morbidly obese patients. While a target BMI less than 40 is the accepted standard, many investigations have demonstrated reasonable clinical outcomes in patients with a BMI greater than 40. That said, it should be understood that clinical outcomes are improved as we approach the target BMI of 40. A *Best Practice* initiative would allow each individual patient to be evaluated by a team, that includes a physician member of a bariatric program. Patients should be evaluated by this team and demonstrate some effort to improve their risk stratification. Once the team feels that the patient has made a reasonable effort, risk stratification and surgical planning can be initiated.

The subtle, but more difficult medical co-morbidities that require addressing are the *Soft Stops* that we have discussed earlier. The most difficult of these co-morbidities are smoking and malnutrition. A local strategy should address these co-morbidities, so that the decision-making is consistent.

References

1. Kohn LT, Corrigan JM, Donaldson MS, editors. To Err is Human. Institute of Medicine; 2000.
2. Goldin A, Beckman JA, Schmidt AM, Creager MA. Advanced glycation end products. Sparking the development of diabetic vascular injury. Circulation. 2006;114:597–605.
3. https://www.aaos.org/quality/quality-programs/quality-toolkits/?embed_path=modexm%253DEmbedStart%2526toolkit%253DSurgical%252520Risk%252520Reduction%252520Toolkit. Accessed 22 Feb 2023.

4. Rogers LC, Frykberg RG, Armstrong DG, Boulton AJM, Edmonds M, Ha Van G, Hartemann A, Game F, Jeffcoate W, Jirkovska A, Jude E, Morbach S, Morrison W, Pinzur M, Pitocco D, Sanders L, Wukich DK, Uccioli L. The diabetic Charcot foot syndrome: a report of the joint task force on the Charcot foot by the American Diabetes Association and the American podiatric medical association. Diabetes Care. 2011;34:2123–9.
5. https://www.facs.org/quality-programs/strong-for-surgery/. Accessed 28 Feb 2023.
6. Wichita R, Goldman L. The emerging role of "hospitalists" in the American health care system. N Engl J Med. 1996;335:514–7. https://doi.org/10.1056/NEJM199608153350713.
7. https://www.hospitalmedicine.org/about/history-mission/. Accessed 24 Feb 2023.
8. Auerbach AD, Wachter RM, Cheng HQ, et al. Comanagement of surgical patients between neurosurgeons and hospitalists. Arch Intern Med. 2010;170(22):2004–10. https://doi.org/10.1001/archinternmed.2010.432.
9. Huddleston JM, Long KH, Naessens JM, et al. Medical and surgical comanagement after elective hip and knee arthroplasty: a randomized, controlled trial. Ann Intern Med. 2004;141(1):28–38. https://doi.org/10.7326/0003-4819-141-1-200407060-00012.
10. Lyons M, McGregor P, Pinzur MS, Adams W, Wilkos-Prostran L. Risk reduction and perioperative complications in diabetics with multiple medical comorbidities undergoing Charcot foot reconstruction. Foot Ankle Int. 2021;42(7):902–9.
11. Pinzur MS, Gurza E, Kristopaitis T, et al. Hospitalist-orthopedic co-management of high-risk patients undergoing lower extremity reconstruction surgery. Orthopedics. 2009;32(7):495. https://doi.org/10.3928/01477447-20090527-14.
12. http://tools.hospitalmedicine.org/Implementation/Co-ManagementWhitePaper-final_5-10-10.pdf. Accessed 22 Feb 2023.
13. https://www.facs.org/quality-programs/strong-for-surgery/. Accessed 25 Feb 2023.
14. https://www.niddk.nih.gov/health-information/diabetes. Accessed 25 Feb 2023.
15. Chrastil J, et al. Is hemoglobin A1c or perioperative hyperglycemia predictive of periprosthetic joint infection or death following primary total joint arthroplasty? J Arthroplasty. 2015;30(7):1197–202.
16. Leung V, Ragbir-Toolsie K. Perioperative management of patients with diabetes. Health Serv Insights. 2017;10:1178632917735075Published 2017 Nov 15. https://doi.org/10.1177/1178632917735075.
17. Lizano-Díez I, Poteet S, Burniol-Garcia A, Cerezales M. The burden of perioperative hypertension/hypotension: a systematic review. PLoS One. 2022;17(2):e0263737. https://doi.org/10.1371/journal.pone.0263737.
18. Stryker LS. Modifying risk factors: strategies that work diabetes mellitus. J Arthroplast. 2016;31(8):1625–7. https://doi.org/10.1016/j.arth.2016.02.084.
19. Piazza G, Goldhaber SZ, Kroll A, Goldberg RJ, Emery C, Spencer FA. Venous thromboembolism in patients with diabetes mellitus. Am J Med. 2012;125(7):709–16. https://doi.org/10.1016/j.amjmed.2011.12.004.
20. Greenky M, Gandhi K, Pulido L, Restrepo C, Parvisi J. Pre-operative anemia in total joint arthroplasty: is it associated with periprosthetic joint injection. Clin Orthop Relat Res. 2012;470:2695–701.
21. Blevins K, Aalirezaie A, Shohat N, Parvizi J. Malnutrition and the development of periprosthetic joint infection in patients undergoing primary elective total joint arthroplasty. J Arthroplast. 2018;33(9):2971–5. https://doi.org/10.1016/j.arth.2018.04.027. Epub 2018 Apr 23.
22. Deren ME, Huleatt J, Winkler MF, Rubin LE, Salzler MJ, Behrens SB. Assessment and treatment of malnutrition in orthopaedic surgery. JBJS Rev. 2014;2(9):e1. https://doi.org/10.2106/JBJS.RVW.M.00125.
23. Emara K, Hirose CB, Rogero R. What preoperative optimization should be implemented to reduce the risk of surgical site infection/periprosthetic joint infection (SSI/PJI) in patients undergoing total ankle arthroplasty. Foot Ankle Int. 2019;40(1_suppl):6S–8S.
24. Golladay GJ, Satpathy J, Jiranek WA. Patient optimization-strategies that work: malnutrition. J Arthroplast. 2016;31(8):1631–4. https://doi.org/10.1016/j.arth.2016.03.027. Epub 2016 Mar 24.

25. Althoff A, Cancienne JM, Cooper MT, Werner BC. Patient-related risk factors for periprosthetic ankle joint infection: an analysis of 6977 total ankle arthroplasties. J Foot Ankle Surg. 2018;57(2):269–72. https://doi.org/10.1053/j.jfas.2017.09.006.
26. Sanz París A, García JM, Gómez-Candela C, et al. Malnutrition prevalence in hospitalized elderly diabetic patients. Nutr Hosp. 2013;28:592–9.
27. DiNardo M, Donihi AC, Forte P, Gieraltowski L, Korytkowski M. Standardized glycemic management and perioperative glycemic outcomes in patients with diabetes mellitus who undergo same-day surgery. Endocr Pract. 2011;17(3):404–11. https://doi.org/10.4158/EP10316.OR.
28. Martin ET, Kaye KS, Knott C, et al. Diabetes and risk of surgical site infection: a systematic review and meta-analysis. Infect Control Hosp Epidemiol. 2016;37(1):88–99. https://doi.org/10.1017/ice.2015.249.
29. Thomas R, Chou L. Diabetic foot disease. In: Orthopaedic knowledge update 5, foot and ankle. Rosemont: American Academy of Orthopaedic Surgeons; 2014. p. 67–83.
30. Wukich DK, Lowery NJ, McMillen RL, Frykberg RG. Postoperative infection rates in foot and ankle surgery: a comparison of patients with and without diabetes mellitus. J Bone Jt Surg Am. 2010;92(2):287–95. https://doi.org/10.2106/JBJS.I.00080.
31. Chang W, Wang B, Li Q, Zhang Y, Xie W. Study on the risk factors of preoperative deep vein thrombosis (DVT) in patients with lower extremity fracture. Clin Appl Thromb Hemost. 2021;27:10760296211002900. https://doi.org/10.1177/10760296211002900. PMID: 33754840; PMCID: PMC7995307.
32. Chung WS, Lin CL, Kao CH. Diabetes increases the risk of deep-vein thrombosis and pulmonary embolism. A population-based cohort study. Thromb Haemost. 2015;114(4):812–8.
33. Petrauskiene V, Falk M, Waernbaum I, Norberg M, Eriksson JW. The risk of venous thromboembolism is markedly elevated in patients with diabetes. Diabetologia. 2005;48(5):1017–21.
34. https://www.aaos.org/quality/quality-programs/lower-extremity-programs/hip-fractures-in-the-elderly/. Accessed 22 Feb 2023.
35. Dlott CC, Moore A, Nelson C, et al. Preoperative risk factor optimization lowers hospital length of stay and postoperative emergency department visits in primary total hip and knee arthroplasty patients. J Arthroplast. 2020;35(6):1508–1515.e2.

Chapter 11
Advanced Trauma Life Support

Christopher R. Parrino, Ryan B. Fransman, Andrew J. Varone, and Samuel M. Galvagno Jr.

Initial Assessment

Implementing a systematic approach to the initial assessment of a trauma patient is critical. By following a methodical system, the trauma team may rapidly identify and address immediate life-threatening injuries. If done well, it can also serve to provide a degree of organization to a frequently chaotic environment. A successful initial assessment starts before the patient arrives. The team leaders must identify themselves and begin the room setup and team task allocation. This includes identifying personnel available to assist, establishing roles and expectations for each role, and ensuring the availability of appropriate equipment for procedures. Involved personnel often include clinicians to help secure the airway; respiratory therapy personnel; X-ray technologists; and nurses to establish rapid intravenous (IV) access, obtain vital signs, administer medications, and document critical events. Additional staff may be useful to assist with cardiopulmonary resuscitation (CPR) or other procedures, if indicated. It is also important to ensure the room is quiet and that closed loop communication is employed. Procedural supplies should include difficult airway kits, chest tubes with appropriate drainage systems, large bore central venous access kits, intra-arterial blood pressure monitoring systems, rapid IV infusers, and blood product availability.

C. R. Parrino · S. M. Galvagno Jr. (✉)
Department of Anesthesiology, University of Maryland School of Medicine, Baltimore, MD, USA
e-mail: Christopher.Parrino@som.umaryland.edu; Sgalvagno@som.umaryland.edu

R. B. Fransman
Department of Surgery, Grady Memorial Hospital, Atlanta, GA, USA

A. J. Varone
Program in Trauma, University of Maryland School of Medicine, Baltimore, MD, USA
e-mail: andrew_varone@brown.edu

© The Author(s), under exclusive license to Springer Nature Switzerland AG 2024

J. Faintuch, S. Faintuch (eds.), *Recent Strategies in High Risk Surgery*,
https://doi.org/10.1007/978-3-031-56270-9_11

A, B, C, D, E

The most widely used trauma initial assessment includes a primary and secondary survey. The primary survey is encapsulated by the mnemonic "ABCDE" (Airway, Breathing, Circulation, Disability, Exposure); however, massive exsanguination should be controlled immediately when identified. Particularly for those who do not routinely perform trauma assessments, it is important to address each step sequentially rather than in parallel to ensure nothing is missed. An axiom during the primary survey is "resuscitate first." For instance, in a severely hypotensive patient who requires definitive airway management, blood transfusions should occur before and during airway management. The primary survey can and should be repeated whenever deemed necessary, given any clinical change or deterioration. Once the primary survey is complete, the team can perform a secondary survey which includes a thorough history and head-to-toe physical examination, complemented by appropriate imaging modalities.

Primary Survey

It is important to note that while basic life support (BLS), advanced cardiovascular life support (ACLS), and some military trauma programs now prioritize circulation and massive exsanguination over airway and breathing, current algorithms for advanced trauma life support (ATLS®) still maintain the traditional "ABCDE" pathway [1].

Airway management is addressed in a subsequent section of this chapter. Once the airway has been secured, evaluation of breathing demands assessment of the patient's ability to ventilate. Assessment includes the visual inspection of breathing, respiratory rate and effort, and auscultation of bilateral breath sounds. If hemodynamically unstable patients are found to have diminished or absent breath sounds in the appropriate setting, this should prompt concern for tension pneumothorax and may indicate the need for rapid decompression. Chest decompression should involve placement of a needle, finger, or tube thoracostomy in the fourth or fifth intercostal space in the anterior axillary line. Several studies have demonstrated higher success of needle decompression with the anterior axillary position compared to the previously accepted second intercostal space in the midclavicular line [2–4].

Shock Prevention

The priority is establishing the patient's vital signs and rapidly identifying potential shock states. If found to be in shock, hemorrhagic shock should be considered and resuscitation with blood products should commence as soon as possible. Up to 1 L of crystalloid in 500 mL increments is still an acceptable starting point, particularly if non-hemorrhagic causes of shock are still being considered; however, these fluids have often already been administered in the field. If a patient remains hypotensive after initial crystalloid resuscitation, blood product transfusion should be considered. If available, whole blood may be superior to traditional low-ratio 1:1:1 (1 unit of packed red blood cells [PRBCs] to 1 unit of fresh frozen plasma [FFP] to 1 unit of platelets) resuscitation and should also be considered for patients in hemorrhagic shock.

Large bore IV access should be rapidly obtained. If unable to obtain peripheral IV access efficiently, central access should not be delayed. Any external hemorrhage must also be identified and controlled. Peripheral pulses should be evaluated in each extremity and discrepancies between the extremities noted and appropriately evaluated during the secondary survey.

Glasgow Score

Disability refers to prompt evaluation of the patient's neurologic status, to identify time-sensitive traumatic brain or spinal cord injuries. A Glasgow Coma Scale (GCS) score should be obtained on presentation. If possible, it is preferred to obtain a full GCS prior to administration of paralytics and sedation to identify a baseline and any need for urgent osmotic therapy or time sensitive imaging.

Exposure involves removal of the patient's clothing and a full body inspection. This is particularly important in penetrating trauma patients who may have hidden wounds in their skin folds, axilla, or perineum that could drastically alter subsequent management. The patient should be rolled and their back as well as cervical spine examined for posterior injuries.

Imaging Procedures

In critically ill or hemodynamically unstable patients, it may be important to obtain adjunct testing immediately after completion of the primary survey, to help identify the potential source of their current clinical status. These tests are often essential to help guide surgical planning and exploration (i.e., which body cavity to enter), particularly in the setting of blunt trauma with an unknown source of hemorrhage. These adjuncts include chest X-ray; Focused Assessment with Sonography for Trauma (FAST) examination or Extended-FAST (e-FAST), which includes a pleural assessment; and pelvic X-ray. In addition to allowing rapid identification of life-threatening pneumothorax or hemothorax and position of invasive lines or tubes, chest X-rays also provide insight into the mediastinum and aortic knob and sometimes may indicate aortic injury and associated mediastinal hematoma.

The FAST exam can be done quickly at the bedside to assess the dependent portions of the abdomen for free fluid as well as examine the pericardium in the subxiphoid location to evaluate for tamponade. However, sensitivity and specificity of this examination remains operator dependent. E-FAST adds the evaluation of lung sliding on the anterior chest, which if done properly may be more sensitive for smaller pneumothoraces than chest X-ray. Chest radiographs and FAST examinations can and should be repeated if a relevant change in clinical status is noted.

Pelvic radiographs can be done quickly to identify unstable pelvic fractures which are often accompanied by vascular injuries. Identification of an unstable pelvic fracture should prompt application of a pelvic binder and early discussion with specialists from interventional radiology, vascular surgery, and orthopedic surgery, depending on the patient's clinical status.

Secondary Inspection

A secondary survey, including a full history and head-to-toe physical examination should be completed after the primary survey is conducted. Neurologic and vascular examinations of each extremity should be performed and documented. Medications, particularly anticoagulants and cardiac medications, should be noted as these agents may have significant impacts on the patient's trauma physiology and the trauma team's approach to interventions.

Once the primary and secondary surveys and adjunct testing are complete, further laboratory and radiographic testing should be undertaken based on the patient's clinical status and signs and symptoms, as appropriate.

Airway and Ventilation Management

Many severely injured patients will require definitive airway management. A definitive airway is defined as a cuffed tube, placed in the trachea, which enables the provision of positive pressure ventilation. Endotracheal intubation is the most employed technique; only about 0.3% of trauma patients will require a surgical airway, either in the form of cricothyrotomy or tracheostomy [5]. Intubation may be required in situations of trauma-associated cardiac arrest, agitation, inability to protect the airway (e.g., blood pooling, emesis, altered mental status, GCS $\leq$8), or impending risk of airway obstruction (e.g., neck hematoma, inflammatory changes associated with noxious chemical inhalation).

Intubation may also be used when high opioid use is required for pain control. The technique with the highest likelihood of success based on clinical acumen should be employed. Multiple studies have compared video laryngoscopy to direct laryngoscopy with varying results. Video laryngoscopy is likely superior to direct laryngoscopy for patients with predicted difficult airways and has a higher first pass success rate [6].

Aspiration of Gastric Contents

Injured patients who present to the hospital should be presumed to have a full stomach and identified as high risk for pulmonary aspiration. Therefore, rapid sequence induction and intubation (RSII) should be performed. The key principles behind RSII are avoidance of mask ventilation, and pre-oxygenation should be performed via passive methods (e.g., nasal cannula, non-rebreather mask). Patients with spontaneous respiratory effort who do not achieve adequate ventilation due to soft tissue obstruction in the oropharynx may benefit from placement of a nasopharyngeal or oropharyngeal airway. Mixed data supports the avoidance of nasopharyngeal tubes in patients believed to have unstable midface and base of skull fractures.

The "Sellick maneuver" (i.e., cricoid pressure) is no longer recommended in traumatic airway management due to its potential to worsen optimal intubation views, and because of the lack of training for potential assistants to apply effective cricoid pressure. The clinician responsible for airway management should be prepared to complete laryngoscopy with a cervical collar in place. Yet, with well-trained personnel and clear communication, manual in-line stabilization with removal of the anterior segment of the cervical collar will be of benefit to hasten laryngoscopic placement and assist in optimal mouth opening. Care should be taken to avoid neck hyperextension and maintenance of a sniffing position.

Anesthetics and Vasoactive Interactions

Patient hemodynamics and mechanism of injury will assist in determining which induction agents will be appropriate. In patients with profound hypotension, propofol is typically avoided due to its systemic vasodilatory properties. More hemodynamically neutral induction agents such as etomidate and ketamine are better tolerated in hypotensive patients. Small doses of benzodiazepines (e.g., midazolam) or opioids (e.g., fentanyl) may be used as adjuncts to decrease the dose of other sedative-hypnotics required for unconsciousness.

For paralysis, succinylcholine may be used if rapid reversibility is desired, but its administration should be avoided in patients with identified motor neuron disease, prior history of paralysis, muscular dystrophies, crush injury, and high injury severity scale poly-trauma, and severe burns more than 24 h after onset.

In children receiving succinylcholine, an anticholinergic agent such as atropine or glycopyrrolate should be co-administered due to risk for succinylcholine-induced bradycardia. Rocuronium, a non-depolarizing neuromuscular blocking agent, may be used at a higher dose (1.2 mg/kg) for RSII to achieve quicker onset and similar intubating conditions to succinylcholine [7]. Patients arriving to the trauma resuscitation bay in cardiac arrest may be intubated without medications, and sedation later initiated if return of spontaneous circulation is achieved.

Intubation and Ventilation

Endotracheal tubes (ETTs) are sized according to their internal diameter in millimeters. An 8.0 mm ETT is usually appropriate for most adult males, and a 7.0 mm is usually appropriate for most adult females. New recommendations include the use of cuffed ETTs for pediatric patients according to the following formula: Cuffed ETT Size = (Age ÷ 4) + 3.5. Uncuffed ETTs should be used only in infants. If intubation and mask ventilation both prove impossible, a supraglottic airway should be inserted, according to the American Society of Anesthesiologists difficult airway algorithm [8]. Care should be taken to limit peak airway pressures when a supraglottic airway is in place, to avoid insufflating the stomach. If insertion of a supraglottic airway proves unsuccessful, then placement of a surgical airway should be undertaken.

Moderate Ventilation Peaks

Lung-protective ventilation with tidal volumes of 6–8 mL/kg of ideal body weight should be employed after a secure airway is established. Peak and plateau pressures should be monitored closely due to the potential for positive pressure ventilation to worsen hemodynamic instability and any pre-existing airway or pulmonary pathology. If hemodynamic collapse occurs after initiation of positive pressure ventilation, hypovolemia and tension pneumothorax should be assumed and bilateral needle/finger/tube thoracostomies performed expeditiously, while infusing IV fluids or blood products. As discussed later in this chapter, a lower $PaCO_2$ of 30–35 mmHg should be targeted for patients with suspected impending intracerebral herniation from an associated traumatic brain injury.

Shock

Shock is defined as a state of relative end organ hypoperfusion and may progress to multisystem organ failure if allowed to proceed unchecked. Resuscitation in trauma should be aimed at maintaining and reassessing adequate oxygen delivery. If intravenous access is not immediately obtained in the unstable trauma patient, intraosseous access should be obtained. The proximal or distal tibia and the proximal humerus are the preferred sites, and commercially available devices/kits should be employed for safety and efficacy. Most patients following trauma will benefit as well from the placement of arterial catheters for closer hemodynamic monitoring, as much as for large bore central venous catheters.

Though the most common etiology of shock in trauma is hemorrhagic shock, other etiologies such as cardiogenic, obstructive, distributive, and neurogenic should be considered. The FAST examination is employed to rapidly exclude common life-threatening injuries such as pericardial tamponade, abdominal organ injury, and with the e-FAST, pneumothorax.

Fluid Replenishment

Hemorrhage is classified by the American College of Surgeons into a four-tiered system (Table 11.1) [1]. Recent updates to ATLS® include the addition of pulse pressure and base excess, as both have been shown to correlate with the degree of hypovolemia due to hemorrhage [9, 10]. Limited crystalloid may be appropriate for resuscitation from Class I or Class II hemorrhage; When blood products are available, blood should be the mainstay of volume resuscitation until hemorrhage has been controlled. When hemorrhage is ongoing, damage control resuscitation is undertaken, allowing permissive hypotension with systolic blood pressure (SBP) ≥90 mmHg and a mean arterial pressure (MAP) of 50–65 mmHg. Once hemorrhage is controlled, a MAP of ≥65 is ideal for sufficient end organ perfusion.

Patients with hemorrhagic shock following trauma should receive blood products and possibly tranexamic acid (TXA; ideally with the first dose administered within 1 h of injury). Crystalloid administration should be limited because it causes hemodilution and decreases clot formation and strength. In emergent situations where blood typing has not yet occurred, type O blood should be given. Rh-negative

Table 11.1 Classification of hemorrhage

	Class I	Class II	Class III	Class IV
Blood loss (% of blood volume)	<15%	15–30%	31–40%	>40%
Heart rate	↔	↔/↑	↑	↑/↑↑
Blood pressure	↔	↔	↔/↓	↓
Pulse pressure	↔	↓	↓	↓
Respiratory rate	↔	↔	↔/↑	↑
Urine output	↔	↔	↓	↓↓
Glasgow Coma Scale	↔	↔	↓	↓
Base excess	0 to −2 mEq/L	−2 to −6 mEq/L	−6 to −10 mEq/L	−10 mEq/L or less
Resuscitation required?	No	Crystalloid or blood	Blood	Massive transfusion
Responsive to fluid bolus?	Responsive	Transiently responsive, then worsening	Transiently responsive, then worsening	Non-responsive
Need for surgical intervention?	Possibly	Likely	More likely	Most likely

Adapted from American College of Surgeons Committee on Trauma. Advanced Trauma Life Support (ATLS®) Student Course Manual, 10th, 2018 [1]

blood should be given to women of childbearing age to avoid alloimmunization that may complicate future pregnancies; for those pregnant, Rho(D) immune globulin should be administered.

A widely adopted protocol for blood and blood products recommends a ratio of 1 unit of PRBCs to 1 unit of FFP to 1 unit of platelets. Whole blood may be superior to this component therapy, but actual benefit has yet to be determined in larger randomized controlled trials. Ionized calcium levels decrease with massive transfusion and should be monitored closely and repleted empirically (i.e., 1 g calcium chloride for every 4–6 units of blood transfused).

Tissue Perfusion and Coagulation

Adequacy of resuscitation may be assessed in many ways, including the monitoring of serial blood lactate levels, base excess, urine output, mental status, and central venous oxygen saturation. Patients who have sustained traumatic injuries frequently present to the hospital with coagulopathy. Hypothermia and acidosis present on admission can negatively impact coagulopathy and mortality, so resuscitation fluids should be warmed before administration. Point of care coagulation testing, namely thromboelastography [TEG] or rotational thromboelastometry [ROTEM] can provide valuable information about the patient's coagulation status. Administration of TXA was shown to improve all-cause mortality in the CRASH-2 trial [11], but its use continues to be debated.

Neurogenic Circulatory Shock

Neurogenic shock should be suspected in patients with spinal cord injuries with concomitant bradycardia and hypotension. In patients with neurogenic shock without hemorrhagic shock, norepinephrine, epinephrine, selective alpha-1 agonists, and volume resuscitation with crystalloid should be used to maintain adequate perfusion of the spinal cord and end organs to avoid secondary insults.

Thoracic Trauma

Thoracic injuries occur in 10–30% of all trauma patients [12, 13]. Most injuries to the chest can be managed non-operatively with less than 10% of blunt chest injuries and between 15–30% of penetrating chest injuries requiring an operation [1]. Occult pneumothoraces and hemothoraces (i.e., seen on CT scan but not on chest X-ray) in an otherwise stable patient may even be observed with repeat imaging—without tube thoracostomy—pending the patient's clinical course. If tube thoracostomy is indicated for pneumothorax or hemothorax, minor bleeding and most air leaks will cease on their own with pleural apposition, if a well-positioned chest tube is placed.

Rib Fractures

They are associated with a poor prognosis and increased mortality in the elderly population, and pain is treated aggressively to avoid respiratory splinting which may lead to atelectasis and pneumonia. In severe cases, epidural analgesia may be offered. Studies have demonstrated a mortality and pneumonia risk of approximately 20–30% in those older than 65, with a 19% increase in mortality per additional rib fracture [14]. Although most thoracic trauma is non-operative, prompt recognition of critical thoracic injuries is essential. Immediate life-threatening chest injuries requiring urgent intervention include tension pneumothorax/hemothorax, massive hemothorax, cardiac tamponade, and thoracic aortic injury.

Tension Pneumothorax

Tension pneumothorax should be diagnosed based on physiology, history, and physical exam alone. A trauma patient with decreased breath sounds, tachycardia, and hypotension should be considered to have a tension pneumothorax with impending cardiovascular collapse and a decompressive procedure (i.e., needle, finger, or tube thoracostomy) should be performed to prevent cardiac arrest.

Physiologically this occurs in the setting of a "one way valve" leading to ongoing air accumulation in the pleural space and increased intrathoracic pressure. Ultimately, this increase in pressure begins to compromise venous return with subsequent cardiovascular collapse. Physical exam findings include tracheal deviation away from the side of injury; jugular venous distention; and hyper-resonance to percussion on the affected side. Jugular venous distention may not be appreciated in massive hemothorax if the patient is intravascularly depleted.

Tension pneumothorax may be addressed either by tube thoracostomy or in prehospital situations, needle decompression. ATLS® has now adopted the anterior axillary approach in the fifth intercostal space as the preferred location for needle decompression of a pneumothorax [1–4].

Major Hemothorax

Massive hemothorax is defined as a hemothorax with more than 1500 mL blood evacuated with initial chest tube placement or more than 200 mL/h. over 4 h. This degree of ongoing bleeding suggests that the source of hemorrhage is significant and unlikely to resolve with simple chest tube placement and pleural apposition. Surgical exploration is indicated to identify the underlying source of bleeding and stop the hemorrhage. On physical examination, massive hemothorax is associated with dullness to percussion and collapsed neck veins due to intravascular volume depletion from massive hemorrhage. For the treatment of any hemothorax, ATLS® previously recommended placement of a large bore tube thoracostomy. Recent studies have demonstrated that the diameter (size) of the tube does not affect the ability to evacuate a fresh traumatic hemothorax. Therefore, ATLS® now recommends placement of a smaller 28–32 Fr chest tube for any acute hemothorax that is visible on chest radiograph [15].

Aortic Damage

Blunt thoracic aortic injury may be life threatening. If no contraindication exists, ATLS® now recommends impulse control with a short-acting beta-1 blocker (i.e., esmolol) to decrease the heart rate to <80 beats per minute and a target mean arterial pressure of 60–70 mmHg with the goal of reducing wall stress and thus the risk for rupture or worsening of an existing injury. Early computed tomography angiography (CTA) should be considered as well as consultation with a vascular or cardiothoracic surgeon. Endovascular repair of aortic injuries has largely replaced open repair as the preferred technique. Large commercial stents suitable for the proximal aorta can now be introduced and positioned through the femoral artery. In exceptional conditions when the damage encompasses the origin of large branches (carotid, subclavian artery), customized stents can be ordered, although these are extremely costly and take some time to be manufactured.

Cardiac Damage and Pericardial Tamponade

Significant cardiac injury is relatively uncommon in both blunt and penetrating trauma but can be highly lethal due to gradual accumulation of blood in the pericardial sac causing tamponade. Hypotensive patients with chest trauma should have prompt investigation of the pericardium with cardiac ultrasonography. This is most often performed during the initial FAST exam or later by a formal echocardiogram. A concomitant left-sided hemothorax may obscure the traditional ultrasound windows, contributing to false positive or false negative results. If tamponade is identified, the patient will likely require a sternotomy for exploration of the heart and definitive repair. Sternal fractures may also be noted in patients with blunt cardiac injury.

The most common presenting rhythm in blunt cardiac injury is sinus tachycardia, although other arrhythmias such as atrial fibrillation are possible. Elevations in cardiac troponin are common with blunt cardiac injury, and levels should be trended. The Eastern Association for the Surgery of Trauma (EAST) guidelines allow the trauma team to rule out a blunt cardiac injury in those with a normal electrocardiogram (ECG) and negative troponins, thus obviating the need for further cardiac monitoring. Continuous telemetry monitoring should be undertaken in those with new onset arrhythmias. The role of echocardiography is in those with a persistent new arrhythmia or in those with hypotension without an evident source of hemorrhage.

Penetrating Abdominal Trauma (Gunshot or Stab Wound), Unstable

Patients with penetrating truncal trauma who are hemodynamically unstable, have peritonitis on physical examination, or have evisceration warrant surgical exploration in the form of a laparotomy after primary survey. Adjuncts in the form of a chest X-ray and foreign body X-ray series in gunshot victims may serve to provide additional clues regarding trajectory and retained projectiles, however should not delay operative intervention.

Penetrating Abdominal Trauma, Gunshot, Stable

Patients who present after gunshot to the abdomen almost universally require abdominal exploration if peritoneal violation is suspected. Many institutions advocate for proceeding to the operating room emergently for exploratory laparotomy after primary survey, chest X-ray, and foreign body series X-rays. A FAST examination may be helpful, though it is not mandatory as a negative FAST does not rule out peritoneal violation, hollow viscus injury, and retroperitoneal organ pathology. Computed tomography (CT) scan often does not change management and simply prolongs time to surgical incision, although some high-volume centers routinely perform pre-operative CT scan to help guide operative planning with trajectory assessment, if it can be done efficiently.

If there is suspicion of a tangential gunshot wound (i.e., does not enter the peritoneum), a CT scan may be helpful and can often indicate in favor of non-operative management. There are some high-volume trauma centers that manage isolated, stable right upper quadrant hepatic gunshot wounds with CT imaging and observation, with or without angioembolization, though this approach is still debated [16].

Penetrating Abdominal Trauma, Stab Wound, Stable

If there is evidence of peritonitis or evisceration on arrival, the patient should proceed for operative intervention. If there is no peritonitis or evident evisceration, EAST guidelines recommend obtaining CT imaging with contrast to help stratify patients [16]. CT imaging with IV contrast, encompassing rectal contrast for penetrating flank wounds, remains widely utilized however continues to be a topic of debate. Diagnostic laparoscopy has been proposed as a method of screening to determine peritoneal violation in these patients. If positive for peritoneal violation, the procedure in most cases is converted to a laparotomy for formal exploration. Diagnostic laparoscopy has also been used for thoracoabdominal stab wounds in the evaluation of diaphragmatic injuries.

As advancements in minimally invasive surgery continue, some institutions are performing laparoscopic exploration and repair of simple injuries, though this remains highly dependent on surgeon experience and skill. If non-operative management is pursued for an equivocal diagnosis, serial abdominal exams are performed for 24 h unless there is clear evidence that the peritoneum was not violated. Less commonly used methods include diagnostic peritoneal lavage and local wound exploration to determine peritoneal violation. Both have been found to result in higher rates of non-therapeutic laparotomy.

Penetrating Flank/Back Trauma, Stab Wound, Stable

Without violation of the peritoneum, patients may not develop peritonitis until late in their clinical course. They should undergo augmented CT imaging with double or triple contrast (oral, rectal, IV, or both IV and enteral) to evaluate retroperitoneal structures for violation; the specific protocol is institution dependent. Oral contrast should opacify the entire duodenum and rectal contrast should reach the ileocecal valve for the study to be adequate.

Penetrating Pelvic Trauma

Penetrating pelvic trauma can result in highly devastating injuries which are difficult to diagnose and treat. Major vascular injuries are possible as are bladder, ureteral, and rectal injuries. Trans-pelvic injuries may also enter the abdomen and cause intraperitoneal damage. Ideally, a CT scan with rectal and IV contrast should be obtained, although variability in rectal tube placement may result in false negative studies due to incomplete visualization of the distal rectum. If higher concern for rectal injury exists, direct visualization with proctoscopy can be performed. Delayed phase images and CT cystography may help identify genitourinary and bladder injuries.

Blunt Abdominal Trauma, Unstable

In general, blunt abdominal trauma patients with hemodynamic instability or peritonitis should proceed to the operating room for formal exploration without CT imaging after initial evaluation. These patients frequently present with significant abdominal tenderness, guarding, and rigidity, although concomitant traumatic brain or spinal cord injuries may cloud a thorough abdominal examination.

Blunt Abdominal Trauma, Stable

Most blunt trauma patients will have sustained some trauma to the chest, abdomen, or pelvis. If hemodynamically stable, these patients will typically undergo a CT scan with IV contrast. CT is a useful tool for evaluating solid organ, vascular, and genitourinary injuries, but it can miss hollow viscus injuries. A small amount of free fluid in the abdomen or thickening of a loop of bowel or mesentery should prompt concern for a bowel injury, thus indicating the need for observation, repeat imaging, or exploration.

Blunt Pelvic Trauma

Blunt trauma resulting in significant pelvic fractures can result in life-threatening hemorrhage. This can be due either to direct injury of major vasculature or to disruption of the sacral venous plexus. Patients may present with an open book or unstable pelvic fracture on physical examination, which should prompt quick application of a pelvic binder and closed reduction of the pelvis to help reduce this potential space. Expeditious consultation with an orthopedic surgeon should occur, and if ongoing bleeding is suspected, resuscitation with blood products should continue. Options for intervention include surgical preperitoneal packing, angioembolization, or placement of a zone three resuscitative endovascular balloon occlusion of the aorta (REBOA) device [17].

Head Trauma

Any patient with altered mental status following trauma should be considered to have acute neurologic injury. GCS is the most used method of evaluating the severity of any head injury (Table 11.2). Eye opening, verbal response, and motor response are evaluated as part of the GCS with a minimum of 1 and a maximum of 4, 5, and 6 points awarded in each category, respectively. When part of the evaluation is unable to be completed (e.g., when a patient is intubated), that category is designated as "non-testable" or "NT." Severe head trauma is suspected when the presenting GCS is ≤ 8. Comorbid cervical spine injuries may also be seen in this patient population, as discussed elsewhere in this chapter.

Management of patients with traumatic brain injury is focused on maintaining cerebral perfusion pressure (CPP) and avoiding increased intracranial pressure

Table 11.2 Glasgow Coma Scale

Parameter	Score
Eye opening	
Spontaneous	4
To sound	3
To pressure	2
None	1
Non-testable	NT
Verbal response	
Oriented	5
Confused	4
Words	3
Sounds	2
None	1
Non-testable	NT
Motor response	
Obeys commands	6
Localizes	5
Normal flexion	4
Abnormal flexion	3
Extension	2
None	1
Non-testable	NT

Adapted from American College of Surgeons Committee on Trauma. Advanced Trauma Life Support (ATLS®) Student Course Manual, 10th, 2018 [1]

(ICP). The equation for cerebral perfusion pressure is as follows: **CPP = MAP – ICP**. The Brain Trauma Foundation recommends targeting a CPP of between 60–70 mmHg and ICP ≤22 mmHg. These targets are derived from a number of international trauma centers that require invasive intracerebral monitoring. Duration of systemic hypotension is inversely correlated with outcomes, likely due to secondary brain injury and ischemia [18]. Hyperventilation is a rescue maneuver that can be employed temporarily to decrease ICP by targeting a $PaCO_2$ of 30–35 mmHg. Administration of prophylactic anti-epileptics is recommended to prevent post-traumatic seizures in the instance of an intraparenchymal, subdural, or epidural hemorrhage.

Spine and Spinal Cord Trauma

Up to 8% of patients with a head injury will also have a cervical spine injury [19]. ATLS® guidelines have recently de-emphasized the use of "spinal immobilization" and instead favor "restriction of spinal motion." Backboard use should be limited and backboards removed promptly after arrival of the patient to the trauma bay, due to the potential for pressure injuries from the hard surface. The Canadian C-Spine Rule [20] and National Emergency X-Radiography Utilization Study (NEXUS)

Table 11.3 Summary of Canadian and NEXUS cervical spine rules for ruling out injury to the cervical spine [20, 21]

Canadian	NEXUS
Radiography **NOT** necessary if: Simple rear-end motor vehicle crash Sitting position in emergency department Ambulatory (at any time since injury) Delayed onset of neck pain No midline cervical spine tenderness Can rotate neck actively 45° to the right and left	Radiography **NOT** necessary if: No posterior midline cervical spine tenderness No evidence of intoxication Normal level of alertness No focal neurologic deficits No painful distracting injuries
Radiography **NECESSARY** before removal of cervical collar: Age >65 years Paresthesias in extremities Dangerous mechanism (fall from >3 feet [1 m] or 5 stairs, axial load to head, motor vehicle crash with high speed/ejection/rollover, motorized recreational vehicle or bike collision)	

criteria [21] have utility in excluding patients at low risk for cervical spine injury who may benefit from early removal of a cervical collar (Table 11.3).

Primary Neurogenic Shock

Patients with spinal cord injury may manifest with spinal shock or neurogenic shock with neurologic deficits. Brady-arrhythmias and loss of sympathetic tone may be seen within 30 min of injury and may persist for up to 6 weeks. Avoidance of hypotension in these patients is critical to prevent secondary ischemic insults to the spinal cord, that may worsen any preexisting neurologic deficits.

Musculoskeletal Trauma

While the majority of musculoskeletal trauma is not considered life threatening and the management of orthopedic injuries is beyond the scope of this chapter, trauma teams should have fundamental knowledge of some orthopedic emergencies. Femur fractures may be life threatening secondary to massive blood loss in the thigh from the bone vascular complexes, surrounding musculature, and major vasculature near the fracture. Early discussion with an orthopedic surgeon is imperative to ensure early stabilization and operative repair.

As with all fractures, if reduction or manipulation is attempted, it is necessary to obtain a distal neurovascular exam before and after intervention. If an urgent or emergent reduction is necessary due to concern for concomitant vascular pathology with absent distal pulses or altered neurologic examination, repeated examinations should be undertaken and the findings closely monitored. Arterial indices should be monitored in any major peripheral vascular injury associated with long bone fractures. Angiography may be performed if there is concern for vascular compromise.

Open fractures necessitate administration of prophylactic antibiotics. Most often cefazolin is sufficient, though more extensive injuries or those with overt contamination may require alternative regimens [22]. Tetanus immunization status should be assessed and the vaccine administered if vaccination status is unknown.

Thermal Injuries

Patients with severe burns are best cared for at designated burn treatment centers. Treatment depends on the severity and extent of the body burned. Total body surface area (TBSA) burned is measured in percentage points according to the Lund–Browder chart (the "Rule of Nines"). Only second- and third-degree burns are included in the TBSA calculation. Children and the elderly, due to their more friable skin, are at increased risk of severe burn injuries.

Patients with burns ≥20% TBSA require early and aggressive fluid replacement. Either 2 mL (modified Brooke formula) or 4 mL (Parkland formula) per kilogram of body weight per % burned TBSA of isotonic crystalloid (e.g., lactated Ringer's solution) should be administered in the first 24 h, with the first half of the volume administered in the first 8 h since injury and the second half administered in the following 16 h. Recent ATLS® guidelines recommend closely monitoring urine output and adjusting the infusion rate to achieve a urine output of 0.5–1.0 mL/kg/h [1]. Care should be taken to avoid excessive fluid and blood administration, as fluid overload can cause right heart failure, pulmonary edema, pleural effusions and multiple compartment syndrome (i.e., compartment syndromes of the abdomen or extremities). Small children and infants should receive dextrose in their resuscitation fluids because their risk for hypoglycemia is high.

Burn Shock

Blood loss is also common in patients with massive burns. Serial hemoglobin and hematocrit levels should be obtained and blood transfused accordingly to a hemoglobin goal of 7.0 g/dL unless prior coronary artery disease or active acute coronary syndrome are present, in which case a hemoglobin goal of 8.0 g/dL may be indicated.

Though burns are often the only external manifestation of thermal injury, care should be taken to evaluate the airway early. Smoke inhalation and caustic material ingestion often accompany burns, and may predispose the patient to progressive airway swelling and impending respiratory distress. Singed nasal hairs and oropharyngeal deposits of soot are predictors that deeper penetration of smoke may have occurred. Tachypnea, stridor, and altered mental status are later signs of airway compromise that may necessitate endotracheal intubation. Early assessment with laryngoscopy, pharyngoscopy, bronchoscopy, and esophagoscopy may be required for baseline anatomical assessment and evaluation.

Succinylcholine curarization more than 24 h after burn injury can cause fatal hyperkalemia, so other curarizing agents should be preferred, if necessary. Carboxyhemoglobinemia may occur in patients who have inhaled smoke and may cause falsely elevated readings from the pulse oximeter. Oxygenation should therefore be evaluated with arterial blood gases or co-oximetry. Hyperbaric oxygen therapy is an effective therapy for clinically significant carboxyhemoglobinemia.

Early transport to tertiary burn centers has demonstrated a mortality benefit in this population. It is imperative to continue active reassessment of these patients during the initial 72 h of resuscitation to identify the need for early debridement and escharotomies.

Electrical Injuries

Electrical shocks and lightning strikes may induce cardiac arrhythmias. Ventricular fibrillation is a life-threatening arrhythmia that may be encountered by emergency medical services in the prehospital environment. Arrhythmias should be treated in accordance with Advanced Cardiac Life Support guidelines (acls.net/aclsalg). Patients should have an ECG performed on admission and should receive continuous cardiac monitoring in case delayed arrhythmias develop. Electrical damage may induce cardiomyocyte damage, so any patients with any chest pain should have troponin levels evaluated.

Pediatric Trauma

Trauma is the leading cause of death and disability for children in the United States. As of 2020, firearm-related injury surpassed motor vehicle accidents as the principal cause of death in children, according to the Centers for Disease Control [23]. Other causes of death in decreasing order include drug overdose/poisoning, suffocation, drowning, and burns. In Europe, the leading cause of death remains motor vehicle accidents [24]. The majority of homicides in infants (children <1 year of age) is accounted for by non-accidental trauma (battered child syndrome). Signs include multiple subdural hemorrhages, metaphyseal long bone fracture, posterior rib fractures, and bilateral retinal hemorrhages. Even treatable, reversible cases may require formal legal reporting, depending on institutional rules and local legislation.

Ventilatory Assistance and Shock

The care of infants and children following trauma demands a multidisciplinary team approach to address both the medical and psychological sequelae of trauma and to offer the child the best chances for a quick recovery. The most common reason for unsuccessful resuscitation of the pediatric patient includes failure to secure the airway and manage ventilation, as well as failure to recognize and treat intracranial and intra-abdominal hemorrhage. When evaluating a young child, the use of a Broselow tape or ribbon (a length-based, color-coded resuscitation aid) is endorsed by the Pediatric Advanced Life Support, even though controversies emerge, particularly concerning overweight and obese children. Criticisms notwithstanding, it contributes to standardize initial care, minimize medication errors, and assist with properly sized equipment selection.

If intravenous access is not obtained in an emergent situation, intraosseous access is indicated, with the anteromedial proximal tibia and distal femur as the preferred sites.

Central Nervous System Trauma

The relatively large size of a child's head compared with the rest of their body increases angular momentum and predisposes them to trauma of the head and cervical spine. Bones in pediatric patients are not yet fully calcified, meaning that bony manifestations of trauma may not be apparent, even when severe blunt trauma may have occurred. Care should be taken to perform a thorough evaluation of intracranial, intrathoracic, and intra-abdominal structures when the mechanism of injury indicates possible lesions, even if there is no associated overlying bony deformity. However exposure of the child to radiation (e.g., for a CT scan) should be limited wherever possible according to the As Low As Reasonably Achievable (ALARA) guidelines [25].

The spleen is the most commonly injured organ following blunt abdominal trauma, followed by the liver. Small bowel perforations at the ligament of Treitz are more common in children, as are bladder rupture injuries (due to the shallow depth of the pediatric pelvis).

Endotracheal Intubation

Decreased pulmonary functional residual capacity is seen in children, predisposing them to rapid desaturation when apnea is induced. Thus, adequate pre-oxygenation should be undertaken prior to endotracheal intubation whenever possible. A long, floppy epiglottis is present in young children, and a straight (e.g., Miller) blade may be preferred over a curved (e.g., Macintosh) blade for direct laryngoscopy. Surgical cricothyroidotomy is rarely indicated in children <12 years of age, due to inability to palpate the cricothyroid membrane. If tension pneumothorax is suspected, needle decompression should be accomplished at the second intercostal space in the mid-clavicular line.

Challenges in Diagnosis of Shock

Children have increased physiologic reserve, and hypotension may not manifest until 30% or more of the total blood volume has been lost. Progression from tachycardia to bradycardia often accompanies hypotension in children. The lower limit of normal Systolic Blood Pressure in children may be obtained with the following formula: Lowest acceptable SBP = (2 * age in years) + 70 mmHg. In the hypotensive child, fluid resuscitation with 20 mL/kg of isotonic crystalloid is indicated prior to initiation of transfusion of 10–20 mL/kg of balanced ratios of PRBCs, FFP, and platelets.

Transfer to a designated pediatric trauma center is critical after initial stabilization. Awaiting transfer, consultation with pediatric subspecialists will aid resuscitative efforts. It is important to recognize that infants and children have unique physiology that requires an in-depth understanding, and may inform a different approach to trauma care.

Geriatric Trauma

Though the mechanisms of injury are similar across age groups, the mortality of these injuries in geriatric patients is higher. This may be due to improper triage, senescence of organ systems, and a higher incidence of pre-existing medical conditions at the time of injury [26]. The most common mechanisms of trauma in the geriatric population include falls, motor vehicle accidents, burns, and penetrating injuries [27]. Those with hepatic cirrhosis, coagulopathy, chronic obstructive pulmonary disease, ischemic heart disease, or diabetes mellitus are more likely to die. Traumatic injuries due to another medical condition (i.e., motor vehicle accident after myocardial infarction or seizure) should be considered during initial presentation and workup.

Brain Trauma

Geriatric patients are at increased risk for traumatic brain injury and its associated morbidity and mortality due to their pre-existing conditions (e.g., cognitive deficits) and prescription drugs (sleep medication, anticoagulants, and/or antiplatelet agents). Furthermore, it may be difficult to distinguish between pre-existing dementia and a new-onset neurologic deficit; presence of family members at the bedside may assist clinicians in determining changes in mental status.

Reversal of Anticoagulants

This is a novel and quickly evolving field and is indicated in the instance of life-threatening bleeding. Warfarin may be reversed with administration of fresh frozen plasma, vitamin K, prothrombin complex concentrate (Kcentra, CSL Behring), or recombinant Factor VIIa. The Factor Xa inhibitors apixaban (Eliquis, Bristol Myers Squibb), rivaroxaban (Xarelto, Bayer), and edoxaban (Lixiana, Savaysa, Daiichi Sankyo) may be reversed with andexanet alfa (AndexXa, Astra Zeneca) or with a four-factor prothrombin complex concentrate. The direct thrombin inhibitor dabigatran (Pradaxa, Boehringer Ingelheim) may be reversed with idarucizumab (Praxbind, Boehringer Ingelheim). Low molecular weight heparin (enoxaparin, Lovenox, Winthrop) and unfractionated heparin can be reversed with well-known protamine sulfate.

Bones and Joints

Arthritic changes may complicate airway management due to restricted motion of the cervical spine. Rib fractures are more common due to age-related osteopenia and may be associated with splinting on respiration, leading to increased risk for pneumonia, atelectasis, and mortality. The risk of pneumonia and mortality increases for each additional rib fractured [1]. Pelvic fractures in the elderly are associated with a four-fold increase in mortality compared to similar injuries in younger patients.

Mandatory Legal Reporting

As may be noted in other vulnerable populations such as pregnant patients and children, maltreatment of aged persons should be considered. When history and clinical findings are suggestive of abuse or neglect, an expeditious social work consultation should be undertaken and the authorities contacted.

Ideal patient-centered care may be accomplished by having early goals of care discussions with both the patient and their family. Because age is such an important risk factor for morbidity and mortality following trauma, these conversations provide a useful framework for structuring future discussions regarding aggressive en of life care, should a patient's clinical condition worsen. A preliminary exchange regarding social, familial, cultural, and religious beliefs and priorities should convert potentially painful questions into less challenging ones.

Trauma in Pregnancy

Approximately 6–8% of pregnant patients will experience a traumatic injury, most commonly from motor vehicle incidents [28]. It is important to recognize that up to 8% of pregnant patients presenting with blunt trauma may be victims of domestic violence instead [29]. The obstetric team is ideally present for admission of any pregnant patient to the trauma bay to monitor both the parturient and fetus and to perform an expedient delivery if emergently indicated. Fetal heart tones should be continuously monitored after 20–24 weeks of gestation. It is important to note that pregnancy causes relevant anatomic and physiologic changes that can inform care (Table 11.4).

IV access should be obtained above the diaphragm in case of caval compression by the gravid uterus, and patients placed in a modified left lateral decubitus position to offload the vena cava and optimize venous return. The risk of gastroesophageal reflux and aspiration is increased in pregnant patients in the second and third trimesters, so each patient should be assumed to have a full stomach and the airway managed with RSII as described earlier in this chapter. Fluid retention during pregnancy may distend the oropharyngeal tissues and displace airway structures from their normal location, complicating endotracheal intubation. Video laryngoscopy is the preferred method for airway management.

Pregnant patients presenting in cardiac arrest should have perimortem cesarean delivery performed within 5–10 min, which may improve both maternal and fetal

Table 11.4 Selected anatomic, physiologic, and laboratory changes of pregnancy [28–31]

Anatomic and physiologic changes of pregnancy
Increased
Heart rate and cardiac output
Mucosal engorgement of nasal and oral cavities
Minute ventilation (mostly from increased from tidal volume)
Oxygen consumption
Plasma volume
Uterine size (fundal height reaches umbilicus at 20 weeks gestation)
Decreased
Functional residual capacity
Lower esophageal sphincter pressure
Rate of gastric emptying (principally during labor)
Systemic vascular resistance and blood pressure (starting in second trimester)

Normal laboratory values (**non-pregnant**)	Parameter	Normal laboratory values (**pregnant**)
22–26	Bicarbonate (mmol/L)	20
0.6–1.2	Creatinine (mg/dL)	0.4–0.7
12–16	Hemoglobin (g/dL)	11
40	$PaCO_2$ (mmHg)	30
7.40	pH	7.44

survival [30, 31]. Perimortem cesarean delivery should be performed at the site of the arrest, because transport to an operating room comes at the cost of time and high-quality resuscitative efforts. There is no evidence that any medication used during ACLS is teratogenic or harmful to the fetus. Therefore, especially in traumatic arrest, the ATLS® approach to resuscitation in conjunction with ACLS should not be altered.

Amniotic fluid embolism is a life-threatening complication that involves the entry of amniotic fluid into the maternal vascular space and is associated with disseminated intravascular coagulation.

Immunoglobulin therapy (Rho[D] immune globulin, several manufacturers) should be given to all Rh-negative parturients (intramuscular or intravenous route, depending on product) unless the injury site is remote from the abdomen and isolated. As mentioned above, many parturients fall victim to physical abuse, so this should be considered in the right clinical context.

Transferring to Definitive Care

Trauma patients benefit from receiving care at trauma centers for a variety of reasons. If transfer to a designated trauma center is being considered, early consultation with the receiving trauma center should be initiated to help guide further management, imaging, and transfer priorities. It should also be noted that tertiary referral centers are frequently at maximum capacity, which may also delay transport. Studies demonstrate that a significant portion of trauma patients undergo CT imaging prior to transport, which has been shown to lead to lengthy delays in definitive care [32]. There occurs a high rate of repeat CT scans at receiving facilities, which is associated with increased healthcare costs and radiation exposure for patients [33, 34].

All available records, laboratory data, and imaging obtained at the initial hospital should be transmitted to the receiving institution for review. Ideally, this occurs electronically during the initial transfer request phone call. When giving handoff to another team, a systematic approach or framework such as the SBAR protocol (situation, background, assessment, and recommendation) may be helpful in maintaining brevity in communication, yet ensuring that vital information has been relayed to formulate an effective care plan.

References

1. American College of Surgeons Committee on Trauma. Advanced Trauma Life Support (ATLS) Student Course Manual, 10th. web4.facs.org/ebusiness/ProductCatalog/ProductCategory.aspx?ID=26. Accessed 30 June 2023.
2. Laan DV, Vu TDN, Thiels CA, et al. Chest wall thickness and decompression failure: a systematic review and meta-analysis comparing anatomic locations in needle thoracostomy. Injury. 2016;47(4):797–804.
3. Leatherman ML, Held JM, Fluke LM, et al. Relative device stability of anterior versus axillary needle decompression for tension pneumothorax during casualty movement: preliminary analysis of a human cadaver model. J Trauma Acute Care Surg. 2017;83(1 Suppl 1):S136–41.

4. Powers WF, Clancy TV, Adams A, West TC, Kotwall CA, Hope WW. Proper catheter selection for needle thoracostomy: a height and weight-based criteria. Injury. 2014;45(1):107–11.
5. Stephens CT, Kahntroff S, Dutton RP. The success of emergency endotracheal intubation in trauma patients: a 10-year experience at a major adult trauma referral center. Anesth Analg. 2009;109(3):866–72.
6. Jungbauer A, Schumann M, Brunkhorst V, Börgers A, Groeben H. Expected difficult tracheal intubation: a prospective comparison of direct laryngoscopy and video laryngoscopy in 200 patients. Br J Anaesth. 2009;102(4):546–50.
7. Tran DTT, Newton EK, Mount VAH, Lee JS, Wells GA, Perry JJ. Rocuronium versus succinylcholine for rapid sequence induction intubation. Cochrane Database Syst Rev. 2015;10:CD002788.
8. Apfelbaum JL, Hagberg CA, Connis RT, et al. 2022 American Society of Anesthesiologists practice guidelines for management of the difficult airway. Anesthesiology. 2022;136(1):31–81.
9. Mutschler M, Nienaber U, Brockamp T, et al. Renaissance of base deficit for the initial assessment of trauma patients: a base deficit-based classification for hypovolemic shock developed on data from 16,305 patients derived from the TraumaRegister DGU®. Crit Care. 2013;17(2):R42.
10. Mutschler M, Nienaber U, Brockamp T, et al. A critical reappraisal of the ATLS classification of hypovolaemic shock: does it really reflect clinical reality? Resuscitation. 2013;84(3):309–13.
11. CRASH-2 Trial Collaborators, Shakur H, Roberts I, et al. Effects of tranexamic acid on death, vascular occlusive events, and blood transfusion in trauma patients with significant haemorrhage (CRASH-2): a randomised, placebo-controlled trial. Lancet. 2010;376(9734):23–32.
12. Battle CE, Hutchings H, Evans PA. Risk factors that predict mortality in patients with blunt chest wall trauma: a systematic review and meta-analysis. Injury. 2012;43(1):8–17.
13. LoCicero J, Mattox KL. Epidemiology of chest trauma. Surg Clin N Am. 1989;69(1):15–9.
14. Bulger EM, Arneson MA, Mock CN, Jurkovich GJ. Rib fractures in the elderly. J Trauma. 2000;48(6):1040–6.
15. Inaba K, Lustenberger T, Recinos G, et al. Does size matter? A prospective analysis of 28–32 versus 36–40 French chest tube size in trauma. J Trauma Acute Care Surg. 2012;72(2):422–7.
16. Como JJ, Bokhari F, Chiu WC, et al. Practice management guidelines for selective nonoperative management of penetrating abdominal trauma. J Trauma. 2010;68(3):721–33.
17. Cullinane DC, Schiller HJ, Zielinski MD, et al. Eastern Association for the Surgery of Trauma practice management guidelines for hemorrhage in pelvic fracture—update and systematic review. J Trauma. 2011;71(6):1850–68.
18. Pietropaoli JA, Rogers FB, Shackford SR, Wald SL, Schmoker JD, Zhuang J. The deleterious effects of intraoperative hypotension on outcome in patients with severe head injuries. J Trauma. 1992;33(3):403–7.
19. Demetriades D, Charalambides K, Chahwan S, et al. Nonskeletal cervical spine injuries: epidemiology and diagnostic pitfalls. J Trauma. 2000;48(4):724–7.
20. Stiell IG, Wells GA, Vandemheen KL, et al. The Canadian C-spine rule for radiography in alert and stable trauma patients. JAMA. 2001;286(15):1841–8.
21. Hoffman JR, Mower WR, Wolfson AB, Todd KH, Zucker MI. Validity of a set of clinical criteria to rule out injury to the cervical spine in patients with blunt trauma. National Emergency X-radiography utilization study group. N Engl J Med. 2000;343(2):94–9.
22. Hoff WS, Bonadies JA, Cachecho R, Dorlac WC. East practice management guidelines work group: update to practice management guidelines for prophylactic antibiotic use in open fractures. J Trauma. 2011;70(3):751–4.
23. Goldstick JE, Cunningham RM, Carter PM. Current causes of death in children and adolescents in the United States. N Engl J Med. 2022;386(20):1955–6.
24. Kyu HH, Stein CE, Boschi Pinto C, et al. Causes of death among children aged 5–14 years in the WHO European region: a systematic analysis for the global burden of disease study 2016. Lancet Child Adolesc Health. 2018;2(5):321–37.
25. Strauss KJ, Kaste SC. ALARA in pediatric interventional and fluoroscopic imaging: striving to keep radiation doses as low as possible during fluoroscopy of pediatric patients—a white paper executive summary. J Am Coll Radiol. 2006;3(9):686–8.

26. Brooks SE, Peetz AB. Evidence-based care of geriatric trauma patients. Surg Clin N Am. 2017;97(5):1157–74.
27. Hruska K, Ruge T. The tragically hip: trauma in elderly patients. Emerg Med Clin N Am. 2018;36(1):219–35.
28. Huls CK, Detlefs C. Trauma in pregnancy. Semin Perinatol. 2018;42(1):13–20.
29. Krywko DM, Toy FK, Mahan ME, Kiel J. Pregnancy trauma. StatPearls; 2022. ncbi.nlm.nih.gov/books/NBK430926/.
30. Einav S, Kaufman N, Sela HY. Maternal cardiac arrest and perimortem caesarean delivery: evidence or expert-based? Resuscitation. 2012;83(10):1191–200.
31. Katz VL, Dotters DJ, Droegemueller W. Perimortem cesarean delivery. Obstet Gynecol. 1986;68(4):571–6.
32. Onzuka J, Worster A, McCreadie B. Is computerized tomography of trauma patients associated with a transfer delay to a regional trauma centre? CJEM. 2008;10(3):205–8.
33. Quick JA, Bartels AN, Coughenour JP, Barnes SL. Trauma transfers and definitive imaging: patient benefit but at what cost? Am Surg. 2013;79(3):301–4.
34. Jones AC, Woldemikael D, Fisher T, Hobbs GR, Prud'homme BJ, Bal GK. Repeated computed tomographic scans in transferred trauma patients: indications, costs, and radiation exposure. J Trauma Acute Care Surg. 2012;73(6):1564–9.

Chapter 12
Severe Traumatic Brain Injury: A Review for the General and Trauma Surgeon

Corrado P. Marini, John McNelis, and Patrizio Petrone

Introduction

According to the Glasgow Coma Score (GCS), mild, moderate, and severe traumatic brain injury (TBI) correspond to decreasing GCS scores in the corresponding ranges of 15–13, 12–9, and 8–3 [1, 2]. Another assessment method is shown in Table 12.1. A more comprehensive definition of severe TBI (sTBI) includes a depressed GCS (<8), loss of consciousness >24 h, and/or amnesia >7 days [3]. The 30-day mortality of patients with sTBI ranges from 35 to 45%. Those who survive incur neurological sequelae for 6–12 months or even longer, as revealed by Glasgow Outcome Scale (GOS) or extended GOS (GOSE) [4]. Scores <4 are consistent with poor functional results for both of them.

It is recommended that the initial GCS should be re-evaluated after completion of the resuscitation and stabilization phases, in order to predict more accurately the 14-day and 6-months outcomes (CrasH or IMPACT [5, 6]).

C. P. Marini
New York Medical College, Jacobi Medical Center, Bronx, NY, USA
e-mail: corradom@nychhc.org

J. McNelis
Department of Surgery, Albert Einstein College of Medicine, Jacobi Medical Center, Bronx, NY, USA
e-mail: John.McNelis@nychhc.org

P. Petrone (✉)
Department of Surgery, NYU Grossman Long Island School of Medicine, NYU Langone Hospital—Long Island, Mineola, NY, USA
e-mail: patrizio.petrone@nyulangone.org

© The Author(s), under exclusive license to Springer Nature Switzerland AG 2024

J. Faintuch, S. Faintuch (eds.), *Recent Strategies in High Risk Surgery*,
https://doi.org/10.1007/978-3-031-56270-9_12

Table 12.1 Alternate classification

Severity	GCS	Loss of consciousness	Structural imaging
Mild	13–15	<20 min to 1 h	Normal
Moderate	9–12	1–24 h	Normal/abnormal
Severe	3–8	>24 h	Abnormal

GCS Glasgow Coma Scale

Available and Innovative Variables

Intracranial pressure (ICP), bi-frontal near infrared spectroscopy regional oxygen saturation (rSO_2), brain tissue oxygen ($PbtO_2$), external ventricular drainage (EVD), cerebral blood flow (CBF), and cerebral microdialysis (CMD) are among the most mentioned multimodality measures within this context. Other predictive tools such as Marshall, Rotterdam, CrasH, and IMPACT, along with existing clinical and patho-anatomic classifications targeting injury subtypes, should not be overlooked either [6–8].

Their utilization should obviously be examined in the light of invasiveness, safety, convenience, and cost but also of potential advantages concerning both mortality and long-term recovery. In other words, the most favorable effectivity, risk/benefit, and cost/benefit ratios should be sought.

Primary Lesions

Most centers classify sTBI in accordance with computerized tomography findings (CT scan) as follows: (1) epidural hematoma; (2) hemorrhagic contusion/hematoma; (3) diffuse axonal injury; (4) subdural hematoma; (5) subarachnoid/intraventricular hemorrhage; and (6) diffuse swelling, as a result of the trauma itself. Secondary injury is frequent as a result of uncorrected hypoxemia, hypotension, and intracranial fluid dynamics. Instead of occurring in the initial seconds, it tends to appear within hours or even many days, depending on restoration of brain perfusion and physiology. Diffuse axonal injury or swelling, hemorrhagic contusions, and intraventricular or parenchymal traumatic hemorrhage represent the most unpredictable lesions, as corrective interventions are often unavailable or ineffective, allowing for ongoing neuronal damage.

Intracranial Pressure Dynamics

The Monro–Kellie hypothesis (1783) states that the sum of the three components contained within the rigid skull, namely blood (arterial and venous blood, 10%), cerebrospinal fluid (CSF, 10%), and brain parenchyma (80%), is constant. An increase in one requires a reciprocal decrease in one or the other two. The intracranial pressure (ICP) represents the pressure within the brain parenchyma and CSF. ICP increases with corresponding reductions in cerebral blood flow (CBF) can be caused by elevated cerebral blood volume (arterial or venous), increased CSF volume or enlarged brain parenchyma (edema), and also abnormal brain expansion (mass lesion).

While most surgeons are familiar with the numeric value of ICP and of its implication on brain integrity, few can interpret the waveform of the ICP tracing and understand the associated information that can be gathered from it. The three characteristic peaks, namely, P1, P2, and P3, have different physiologic meanings and should be individually analyzed (Figs. 12.1 and 12.2).

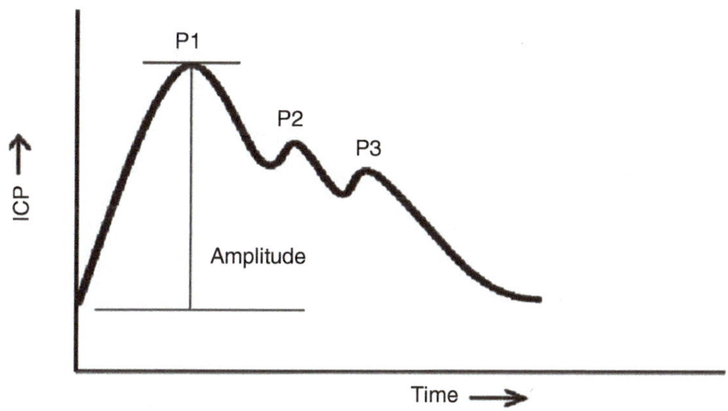

Fig. 12.1 *ICP* intracranial pressure, *P1* P1 wave, *P2* P2 wave, *P3* P3 wave

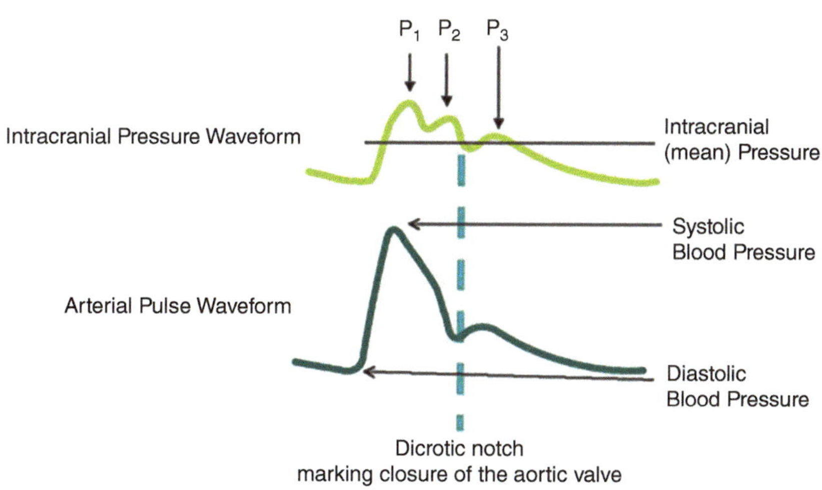

Fig. 12.2 *P1* P1 wave, *P2* P2 wave, *P3* P3 wave

Intracranial Hypertension (IH)

IH affects the characteristics of the waveform. An increase in amplitude of the three peaks indicates a mean increase in ICP. A reduced amplitude of P1 suggests decreased cerebral perfusion pressure (CPP), and an increase in the P2 peak above P1 is indicative of decreased cerebral compliance (CC). A P2/P1 ratio >1 correlates with increased ICP and a loss of CC, with an r of 0.94 [9] (Fig. 12.3). The mean P2/P1 ratio has a sensitivity of 100%, specificity of 45.4%, a positive predictive value (PPV) of 36.8%, and negative predictive value (NPV) of 100% to predict IH with a cutoff value of 1.06. Of note, P2/P1 >1 precedes the increase in the absolute mean value of the ICP. This supports the hypothesis that morphological changes of the brain volume-pressure curve precede IH.

Cerebral Blood Flow (CBF)

Normal range of CBF is 50–65 mL/100 g/min, accompanied by low venous pressure (2–5 mmHg) [10]. Brain vessels increase or reduce perfusion depending on oxygen requirements, as a phenomenon of cerebral autoregulation (CA) [11]. CBF <10–15 mL/100 g/min (tissue oxygen tension/$PbtO_2$ <15 mmHg) is usually incompatible with neuronal survival. Reversible damages are triggered by CBF 15–20 mL/100 g/min and electroencephalographic aberrations around 25 mL/100 g/min.

Cerebral perfusion pressure (CPP) = mean arterial pressure (MAP) − ICP (Fig. 12.4) [12]. Constant CBF is linked to cerebral vessel resistance in the settings of increased or decreased CPP, respectively. Above and below the lower and upper limits of 50 and 160 mmHg, CA is lost and CBF becomes dependent on mean CPP in a linear fashion.

Impaired Cerebral Autoregulation

Some degree of loss is observed in 49–87% of affected cases soon after sTBI [13–15], and it contributes markedly to secondary brain injury. Continuous transcranial Doppler ultrasonography (TCD) of the middle cerebral artery flow and calculation

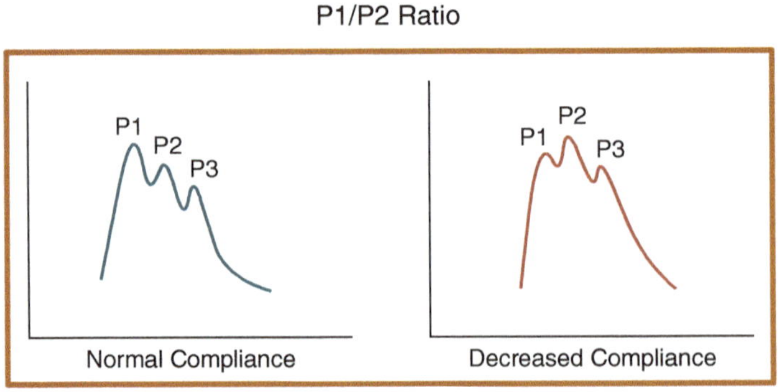

Fig. 12.3 P1/P2 ratio. *P1* P1 wave, *P2* P2 wave, *P3* P3 wave

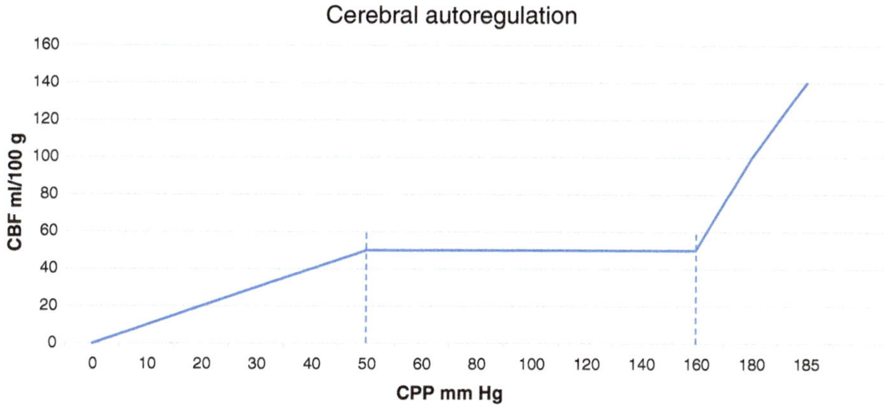

Fig. 12.4 Cerebral autoregulation. *CBF* cerebral blood flow, *CPP* cerebral perfusion pressure

of the pressure reactivity index (PRx), related to the slow waves in ICP and MAP, are well known tools to follow CA.

MAP Norepinephrine Challenge

This is another option to test CA integrity, even though less reliable than PRx calculation. MAP is raised during 10–20 min by norepinephrine infusion, and MAP, CPP, ICP, and $PbtO_2$ are repeatedly documented. ICP will diminish (2–5 mmHg within 3–5 min) if CA is present, whereas no change or elevation will be observed if CA was lost [16].

Open Versus Closed TBI

In both circumstances, GCS is widely used, more recently complemented by the Neurological Outcome Scale for Traumatic Brain Injury (NOS-TBI) [17]. Both modalities of trauma are similarly followed by various degrees of vasospasm, which may not alleviate before 5–7 days, thus aggravating low tissue perfusion (Table 12.2) [18, 19].

Subsequent Brain Damage

After sTBI, several cellular and metabolic shifts can be detected, encompassing calcium influx into neuronal cells and increased tissue levels of glutamate, aspartate, and free radicals. All of these contribute toward cerebral edema, intracranial hypertension, impaired CA, and decreased CBF, further damaging the affected brain [20–22]. Systemic hypotension should be prevented, including after hospital admission, when

Table 12.2 Glasgow Coma Scale

Behavior	Response	Score
Eye opening response	Spontaneously	4
	To speech	3
	To pain	2
	No response	1
Best verbal response	Oriented to time, space, and person	5
	Confused	4
	Inappropriate words	3
	Incomprehensible sounds	2
	No response	1
Best motor response	Obeys commands	6
	Moves to localized pain	5
	Flexion withdrawal from pain	4
	Abnormal flexion (decorticate)	3
	Abnormal extension (decerebrate)	2
	No response	1
Total score	Best response	15
	Comatose	≤8
	Unresponsive	3

Available at glasgowcomascale.org/

the patient is transferred to the intensive care unit (ICU), as it is a strong driver of mortality (55–150% elevation) [23, 24]. Marked brain edema is another well-described ominous development, as brain herniation could precipitate abrupt demise.

CT Predictive Models

The Marshall model is more than 30 years old; however, it is still useful, notably for early outcome, in the first 4 weeks. The Rotterdam guideline is deemed more trustworthy for long-term course, being recommended for 6-month prediction (Tables 12.3 and 12.4) [7, 25–27]. The International Mission for Prognosis and Analysis of Clinical Trials (IMPACT) is also a recommended score and has the advantage of online calculation (Table 12.5) (tbi-impact.org/?p=impact/calc) [28].

Immediate Management

Upon arrival at the emergency unit, all patients with sTBI should be intubated and ventilated to a PCO_2 range of 35–45. In case of IH, the level is set at 32–35 mmHg, and an intermittent bolus of mannitol 0.25–1.0 g/kg is prescribed. Normal saline <2000 mL is preferred over Lactated Ringers based on the results of the

Table 12.3 Marshall CT classification

Category	Definition
Diffuse injury I	No intracranial pathology
Diffuse injury II	Cisterns present with midline shift <5 mm and/or lesion densities present. No high or mixed density lesion >25 cm^3
Diffuse injury III	Cisterns compressed or absent with midline shift 0–5 mm
Diffuse injury IV	Midline shift >5 mm, no high or mixed density >25 cm^3
Evacuated mass lesion	Any lesion evacuated surgically
Non-evacuated mass lesion	High or mixed density lesion >25 cm^3, not evacuated surgically

Available at radiopaedia.org/articles/marshall-classification-of-traumatic-brain-injury

Table 12.4 Rotterdam CT classification

CT finding	Score
Basal cisterns	0
Normal	1
Compressed absent	2
Midline shift	
≤5 mm	0
>5 mm	1
Epidural mass lesion	
Present	0
Absent	1
Intraventricular or subarachnoid hemorrhage	
Absent	0
Present	1
Sum score	+1

Available at radiopaedia.org/articles/rotterdam-ct-score-of-traumatic-brain-injury

1 point is added as a sum score to make the grade numerically total 6 points consistent with the motor score of the GHCS and the Marshall Classification. (Maas AI, et al. Neurosurgery 2005;57(6):1173–82)

PROMMTT study that showed the superiority of saline for prehospital fluid replenishment [29, 30]. Lactated Ringer's solution seems superior when the patient is hypothermic.

CT scan of the head is required in all patients suspected of having suffered for sTBI. A group of patients with sTBI requires immediate craniotomy or primary decompressive craniectomy. Those who do not require an immediate procedure should undergo multimodality monitoring and goal-directed therapy, as soon as they are resuscitated and transported to the ICU. The exceptions are those with unsurvivable brain injuries, who could become organ donors depending on systemic conditions and family ethical consent. These are basically cases with GCS 3 along with fixed or unreactive pupils, severe damage to the brain or brainstem, or absence of cerebral blood flow with imaging methods.

Table 12.5 IMPACT (International Mission for Prognosis and Analysis of Clinical Trials in TBI)

Admission characteristics	Value
Core	
Age (14–99)	
Motor score	1–6
Pupils	Both reactive, one, none
Core + CT	
Hypoxia	Yes or no
Hypotension	Yes or no
CT classification	Marshall I–IV, evacuated mass lesion, non-evacuated mass lesion
tSAH on CT	Yes or no
Epidural mass on CT	Yes or no
Core + CT + lab	
Glucose (3–20 mmol/L)	
Hb (6–17 g/dL)	

Available at tbi-impact.org/?p=impact/calc
Prediction models for 6-month outcome after TBI
ISAH intraventricular or subarachnoid hemorrhage, *Hb* hemoglobin concentration

Advanced Monitoring—ICP

Parenchymal or intraventricular ICP monitoring is a widely recognized technique to prevent secondary brain injury from IH (ICP >20 mmHg). In the USA, 90% of level I and II trauma centers adopt it; however, not more than 37% in Europe [31]. Indeed, there is some controversy in the literature about its usefulness [32, 33]. Nevertheless most specialists admit that in conjunction with a three-tier algorithm, it can improve clinical results [34, 35]. An external ventricular drain (EVD) encompassing a pressure transducer provides reliable ICP monitoring and CSF drainage, in circumstances of marked pressure elevations. ICP-guided therapy requires data on cerebral tissue oxygenation ($PbtO_2$) for optimal benefits.

Near Infrared Spectroscopy (NIRS)–Regional Cerebral Oxygen Saturation (rSO_2)

Oxygen demand-supply aberrations in the territory of the anterior and middle cerebral arteries (rSO_2 <55%) can be followed with this technique. Usually, a low rSO_2 is compatible with elevated oxygen extraction due to decreased CBF.

Brain Tissue Oxygen Tension ($PbtO_2$)

Current Guidelines for the Management of Severe Traumatic Brain Injury, fourth ed., do not advise $PbtO_2$ monitors for direct brain tissue oxygenation measurement; however, a consensus of experts supports the use treatment protocols based on both $PbtO_2$ and ICP [36, 37]. The results of the BOOST II trial and of other studies provide further evidence of the usefulness of such an apporach [38, 39].

Raising Brain Tissue Oxygen Tension

When $PbtO_2$ is <20 mmHg, if ICP is >20 mmHg, an oxygen challenge (5 min 100% FiO_2) could be attempted. If positive, the percentage is reduced to <60% as persistent normobaric hyperoxia is dangerous. If ICP is <20 mmHg, the norepinephrine challenge (with intact CA) will benefit CPP and $PbtO_2$, however, not ICP. Brain oxygen consumption can also be diminished, if CA is lost or does not respond to elevation of CPP, with an infusion of fentanyl, midazolam, and propofol (burst suppression), as detected on continuous EEG.

Normothermia Versus Hypothermia

Fever above 38.3 °C is frequent in the first week after sTBI [40] and is deleterious regarding brain edema [41–43]. Normothermic control seems safer, as therapeutic hypothermia could increase mortality and long-term functional impairment [44]. Prophylactic hypothermia is not endowed with clear benefits either [36, 45, 46]. Several temperature control devices are available in the market (Artic Sun, Medivance, Inc.; Louisville, CO, USA, and others), and for patient comfort, anti-shivering therapy should be added [47–49].

Enteral Feeding

Basal calorie expenditure replenishment should be achieved in 5–7 days [36]. Given the impact of multiple prescribed drugs and possible associated injuries and complications, the calculation of calories requirements using conventional predictive equations such as the Harris-Benedict, Penn State University, or Mifflin St Jeor or ASPEN equations can lead to significant variability; therefore, indirect calorimetry is recommended [50, 51]. Selected patients may suffer from severe hypermetabolism (up to 160% elevation) and massive nitrogen loss (up to 16 g/day) [52]. We believe that the amount of nutritional support proposed by the Brain Trauma Foundation, to provide more than 50% of resting energy expenditure (REE) for 2 weeks, is too conservative. It is not uncommon to observe 25% or more of increase in measured resting energy expenditure (mREE), confirming substantial energy loss. According to some studies, not only length of stay in the hospital and immune function can be negatively influenced by insufficient alimentation, but also mortality [53, 54].

We prefer jejunal tubes along with a peptide formula, for easier absorption. Gastric feeding with a nasogastric tube using conventional diets is an alternative; however, metoclopramide 10 mg IV qid eventually complemented by erythromycin 250 mg IV qid should be considered in circumstances of intolerance. The CORTRAK 2 Enteral Access System (EAS), endowed with an electromagnetic sensing device, can be convenient for optimal tube positioning in comatose patients, especially in the jejunum.

Multimodality Monitoring and Goal-Directed Therapy Protocol (MM&GDTP)

The pillars of our proposal are normothermia (37° ± 0.2 ° C) along with ICP, $PbtO_2$, CPP, and rSO_2 control. Hourly cerebral microdialysis (CMD) data (lactate, glucose, pyruvate, glutamate, and derived lactate/pyruvate ratio [LPR]) supplies metabolic information, and continuous EEG with BS should be considered as well. These measures are started 2–4 h after admission, or promptly after immediate craniotomy/craniectomy, if that was necessary, and maintained for 3–5 days.

Despite lack of consensus in the literature and increased hospital expenditures, gathering such physiologic data is justified by the ability to predict outcomes better than intermittent data [52, 55]. They should be added to early and effective nutritional therapy for more favorable survival and long-term functional end points [56]. As MM&GDTP has not been tested yet in controlled trials, it should still be classified as investigational. The suggested therapeutic algorithm is outlined in Table 12.6.

Rehabilitation

Given the immediate, intermediate, and late functional repercussions of sTBI, this population demands rehabilitation protocols starting in the trauma unit, proceeding to the subsequent hospitalization phase, and continuing after discharge. Experienced trauma and neuroplasticity teams are adept at dealing with coma and arousal states, weaning off mechanical ventilation, and early mobilization. Although late rehabilitation is an option for enhancing functional recovery, the earlier it is started the best [57, 58].

Table 12.6 Treatment algorithm

Type A
ICP ≤20 mmHg; CPP ≥70 mmHg; NIRS >55%; $PbtO_2$ ≥20 mmHg; CMD L/P <40
No further therapy needed
Type B
Sustained ICP >20 mmHg; CPP ≥70 mmHg; NIRS >55%; $PbtO_2$ ≥20 mmHg, CMD L/P <40
Therapy aimed at decreasing ICP
Tier 1
Elevated head of bed to 30°
Maintain normothermia (37 °C)
Drain CSF
Adjust sedation with midazolam/propofol
3% Normal saline to serum Na 155–160 mEq/L
Mannitol 0.25–0.50 g/kg IV bolus to serum osmolality 320 mOsm/kg/H_2O or Osm gap <20
Tier 2: ICP >20 mmHg for >15 min for 1 h during first 72 h despite tier 1 therapy
Increase respiratory rate to keep PCO_2 32–35 mmHg
High dose mannitol 1.0–1.5 g/kg IV bolus if Osm <320 mOSm/L
BS (2–4 burst/min on cEEG) with midazolam to 10–15 mg/h and propofol to 75–100 μg/kg/min
Repeat CT scan head to assess mass lesion progression
If ICP refractory, and there is increased mass effect, decompressive craniectomy
Type C
ICP <20 mmHg; CPP ≥70 mmHg; NIRS <55%; $PbtO_2$ <20 mmHg; CMD L/P >40 with glucose <0.8 mmol/L and pyruvate <120 μmol/L
Therapy aimed at increasing $PbtO_2$ and decreasing LPR
Tier 1
Increase CPP up to 100 mmHg in increments of 10 mmHg with infusion NE, if ICP decreases ≥3 mmHg with increasing CPP. Do not proceed if ICP does not decrease or rises with increasing CPP
Optimize sedation
Increase FiO_2 100 then keep at 60%
Increase PEEP to 10 cm H_2O
Do not increase PaO_2 >150 mmHg for sustained periods of time
Tier 2
Increase midazolam to 10–15 mg/h and propofol to 75–100 μg/kg/min
Setup cEEG to BS 2–4 bursts/minute
Drain CSF <15 mmHg
If Hg <7 g/dL transfuse 3 units PRBCs less than 7 days old

ICP intracranial pressure, *CPP* cerebral perfusion pressure, *NIRS* near infrared spectroscopy, *$PbtO_2$* brain tissue oximetry, *CMD L/P* cerebral microdialysis lactate/pyruvate ratio, *CSF* cerebrospinal fluid, *PCO_2* partial pressure of CO_2, *BS* burst suppression, *NE* norepinephrine, *PEEP* positive end expiratory pressure

References

1. Taylor CA. Traumatic brain injury-related emergency department visits, hospitalizations, and deaths—United States, 2007 and 2013. MMWR Surveill Summ. 2017;66:1.
2. Teasdale G, Jennett B. Assessment of coma and impaired consciousness. A practical scale. Lancet. 1974;2(7872):81–4.
3. Blyth BJ, Bazarian JJ. Traumatic alterations in consciousness: traumatic brain injury. Emerg Med Clin N Am. 2010;28(3):571–94.
4. Wilson JT, Pettigrew LE, Teasdale GM. Structured interviews for the Glasgow outcome scale and the extended Glasgow outcome scale: guidelines for their use. J Neurotrauma. 1998;15(8):573–85.
5. Collaborators MCT. Predicting outcome after traumatic brain injury: practical prognostic models based on large cohort of international patients. BMJ. 2008;336(7641):425–9.
6. Roozenbeek B, Lingsma HF, Lecky FE, et al. Prediction of outcome after moderate and severe traumatic brain injury: external validation of the international mission on prognosis and analysis of clinical trials (IMPACT) and corticoid randomisation after significant head injury (CRASH) prognostic models. Crit Care Med. 2012;40(5):1609–17.
7. Maas AIR, Hukkelhoven CWPM, Marshall LF, Steyerberg EW. Prediction of outcome in traumatic brain injury with computed tomographic characteristics: a comparison between the computed tomographic classification and combinations of computed tomographic predictors. Neurosurgery. 2005;57(6):1173–82.
8. Charry JD, Falla JD, Ochoa JD, et al. External validation of the Rotterdam computed tomography score in the prediction of mortality in severe traumatic brain injury. J Neurosci Rural Pract. 2017;8(Suppl 1):S23–6.
9. de Moraes FM, Rocha E, Duarte Barros FC, et al. Wave morphology as a surrogate for ICP monitoring: a comparison between an invasive and a noninvasive method. Neurocrit Care. 2022;37:219–27.
10. Rafols JA. Control of the brain microcirculation following traumatic brain injury and stroke. Brain Circ. 2015;1:146–58.
11. Aaslid R, Lindegaard KF, Sorteberg SW, Nornes H. Cerebral autoregulation dynamics in humans. Stroke. 1989;20:45–52.
12. Lasses LA. Cerebral blood flow and oxygen consumption in man. Physiol Rev. 1959;39:183–238.
13. Bouma GJ, Muizelaar JP, Bandoh K, Marmarou A. Blood pressure and intracranial pressure-volume dynamics in severe head injury: relationship with cerebral blood flow. J Neurosurg. 1992;77(1):15–9.
14. Alali AS, Fowler RA, Mainprize TG, et al. Intracranial pressure monitoring in severe traumatic brain injury: results from the American College of Surgeons trauma quality improvement program. J Neurotrauma. 2013;30(20):1737–46.
15. Bouma GJ, Muizelaar JP, Stringer WA, Choi SC, Fatouros P, Young HF. Ultra-early evaluation of regional cerebral blood flow in severely head-injured patients using xenon-enhanced computerized tomography. J Neurosurg. 1992;77(3):360–8.
16. Johnson U, Lewén A, Ronne-Engström E, Howells T, Enblad P. Should the neurointensive care management of traumatic brain injury patients be individualized according to autoregulation status and injury subtype? Neurocrit Care. 2014;21(2):259–65.
17. Wilde EA, McCauley SR, Kelly TM, et al. Feasibility of the neurological outcome scale for traumatic brain injury (NOS-TBI) in adults. J Neurotrauma. 2010;27(6):975–81.
18. Oertel M, Boscardin WJ, Obrist WD, Glenn TC, McArthur DL, Gravori T, Lee JH, Martin NA. Posttraumatic vasospasm: the epidemiology, severity, and time course of an under-estimated phenomenon: a prospective study performed in 299 patients. J Neurosurg. 2005;103(5):812–24.
19. Bouma GJ, Muizelaar JP. Cerebral blood flow, cerebral blood volume, and cerebrovascular reactivity after severe head injury. J Neurotrauma. 1992;9(Suppl 1):S333–48.

20. Marmarou A, Signoretti S, Fatouros PP, Portella G, Aygok GA, Bullock MR. Predominance of cellular edema in traumatic brain swelling in patients with severe head injuries. J Neurosurg. 2006;104(5):720–30.
21. DeWitt DS, Prough DS. Traumatic cerebral vascular injury: the effects of concussive brain injury on the cerebral vasculature. J Neurotrauma. 2003;20(9):795–825.
22. Stiefel MF, Tomita Y, Marmarou A. Secondary ischemia impairing the restoration of ion homeostasis following traumatic brain injury. J Neurosurg. 2005;103(4):707–14.
23. Chesnut RM, Marshall LF, Klauber MR, et al. The role of secondary brain injury in determining outcome from severe head injury. J Trauma. 1993;34(2):216–22.
24. Chesnut RM, Marshall SB, Piek J, Blunt BA, Klauber MR, Marshall LF. Early and late systemic hypotension as a frequent and fundamental source of cerebral ischemia following severe brain injury in the Traumatic Coma Data Bank. Acta Neurochir Suppl (Wien). 1993;59:121–5.
25. Marshall LF, Marshall SB, Klauber MR, et al. A new classification of head injury based on computerized tomography. J Neurosurg. 1991;75(Suppl):S14–20.
26. Jacobs B, Beems T, van der Vliet TM, et al. Outcome prediction in moderate and severe traumatic brain injury: a focus on computed tomography variables. Neurocrit Care. 2013;19(1):79–89.
27. Mata-Mbemba D, Mugikura S, Nakagawa A, et al. Early CT findings to predict early death in patients with traumatic brain injury. Acad Radiol. 2014;21(5):605–11.
28. Marmarou A, Lu J, Butcher I, et al. IMPACT database of traumatic brain injury: design and description. J Neurotrauma. 2007;24(2):239–50.
29. Holcomb JB, del Junco DJ, Fox EE, et al. The prospective, observational, multicenter, major trauma transfusion (PROMMTT) study: comparative effectiveness of a time-varying treatment with competing risks. JAMA Surg. 2013;148(2):127–36.
30. Rowell SE, Fair KA, Barbosa RR, et al. The impact of pre-hospital Administration of Lactated Ringer's solution versus normal saline in patients with traumatic brain injury. J Neurotrauma. 2016;33(11):1054–9.
31. Stocchetti N, Penny KI, Dearden M, et al. Intensive care management of head-injured patients in Europe: a survey from the European brain injury consortium. Intensive Care Med. 2001;27(2):400–6.
32. Chesnut RM, Temkin N, Carney N, et al. A trial of intracranial-pressure monitoring in traumatic brain injury. N Engl J Med. 2012;367(26):2471–81.
33. Kramer AH, Couillard PL, Zygun DA, Aries MJ, Gallagher CN. Continuous assessment of "optimal" cerebral perfusion pressure in traumatic brain injury: a cohort study of feasibility, reliability, and relation to outcome. Neurocrit Care. 2019;30(1):51–61.
34. Hawryluk GWJ, Aguilera S, Buki A, et al. A management algorithm for patients with intracranial pressure monitoring: the Seattle International Severe Traumatic Brain Injury Consensus Conference (SIBICC). Intensive Care Med. 2019;45(12):1783–94.
35. Asgari S, Vespa P, Bergsneider M, Hu X. Lack of consistent intracranial pressure pulse morphological changes during episodes of microdialysis lactate/pyruvate ratio increase. Physiol Meas. 2011;32(10):1639–51.
36. Carney N, Totten AM, O'Reilly C, et al. Guidelines for the management of severe traumatic brain injury. Neurosurgery. 2017;80(1):6–15.
37. Chesnut R, Aguilera S, Buki A, et al. A management algorithm for adult patients with both brain oxygen and intracranial pressure monitoring: the Seattle International Severe Traumatic Brain Injury Consensus Conference (SIBICC). Intensive Care Med. 2020;46(5):919–29.
38. Stiefel MF, Gracias VH, Bloom S. Conventional neurocritical care and cerebral oxygenation after traumatic brain injury. J Neurosurg. 2006;105:8.
39. Okonkwo DO, Shutter LA, Moore C, et al. Brain tissue oxygen monitoring and Management in Severe Traumatic Brain Injury (BOOST-II): a phase II randomized trial. Crit Care Med. 2017;45(11):1907–14.
40. Stocchetti N, Rossi S, Zanier E, et al. Pyrexia in head-injured patients admitted to intensive care. Intensive Care Med. 2002;28:1555–62.

41. Suehiro E, Fujisawa H, Ito H, Ishikawa T, Maekawa T. Brain temperature modifies glutamate neurotoxicity in vivo. J Neurotrauma. 1999;16(4):285–97.
42. Chatzipanteli K, Alonso OF, Kraydieh S, Dietrich WD. Importance of posttraumatic hypothermia and hyperthermia on the inflammatory response after fluid percussion brain injury: biochemical and immunocytochemical studies. J Cereb Blood Flow Metab. 2000;20(3):531–42.
43. Bayir H, Adelson PD, Wisniewski SR, et al. Therapeutic hypothermia preserves antioxidant defenses after severe traumatic brain injury in infants and children. Crit Care Med. 2009;37(2):689–95.
44. Andrews PJD, Sinclair HL, Rodriguez A, et al. Hypothermia for intracranial hypertension after traumatic brain injury. N Engl J Med. 2015;373(25):2403–12.
45. Cooper DJ, Nichol AD, Bailey M, et al. Effect of early sustained prophylactic hypothermia on neurologic outcomes among patients with severe traumatic brain injury: the POLAR randomized clinical trial. JAMA. 2018;320(21):2211.
46. Olson DM, Grissom JL, Williamson RA, Bennett SN, Bellows ST, James ML. Interrater reliability of the bedside shivering assessment scale. Am J Crit Care. 2013;22(1):70–4.
47. Sadaka F, Krause K, Tow M, Wilcox M, O'Brien J. Induced normothermia after severe traumatic brain injury: a prospective observational pilot safety and feasibility study. J Neurol Res. 2015;4(5–6):127–31.
48. Kilpatrick MM, Lowry DW, Firlik AD, Yonas H, Marion DW. Hyperthermia in the neurosurgical intensive care unit. Neurosurgery. 2000;47(4):850–6.
49. Yokobori S, Yokota H. Targeted temperature management in traumatic brain injury. J Intensive Care. 2016;4(1):28.
50. Frankenfield DC, Ashcraft CM. Estimating energy needs in nutrition support patients. J Parenter Enter Nutr. 2011;35(5):563–70.
51. Pavlidou E, Petridis D, Tolia M, et al. Estimating the agreement between the metabolic rate calculated from prediction equations and from a portable indirect calorimetry device: an effort to develop a new equation for predicting resting metabolic rate. Nutr Metab. 2018;15:41.
52. Krakau K, Omne-Pontén M, Karlsson T, Borg J. Metabolism and nutrition in patients with moderate and severe traumatic brain injury: a systematic review. Brain Inj. 2006;20(4):345–67.
53. Härtl R, Gerber LM, Ni Q, Ghajar J. Effect of early nutrition on deaths due to severe traumatic brain injury. J Neurosurg. 2008;109(1):50–6.
54. Maxwell J, Gwardschaladse C, Lombardo G, et al. The impact of measurement of respiratory quotient by indirect calorimetry on the achievement of nitrogen balance in patients with severe traumatic brain injury. Eur J Trauma Emerg Surg. 2017;43(6):775–82.
55. Roh D, Park S. Brain multimodality monitoring: updated perspectives. Curr Neurol Neurosci Rep. 2016;16(6):56.
56. Marini CP, Petrone P, McNelis J, et al. Treatment of patients with severe traumatic brain injury: a 7-year single institution experience. J Neurocrit Care. 2021;14(1):36–45.
57. Turner-Stokes L. Evidence for the effectiveness of multi-disciplinary rehabilitation following acquired brain injury: a synthesis of two systematic approaches. J Rehabil Med. 2008;40(9):691–701.
58. Johnston MV. Plasticity in the developing brain: implications for rehabilitation. Dev Disabil Res Rev. 2009;15(2):94–101.

Chapter 13
Current Management of Post-operative Mesenteric Ischemia

Rohan N. Kulkarni and Mohammad H. Eslami

Acute Mesenteric Ischemia

Acute mesenteric ischemia (AMI) is a sudden, severe decrease in blood flow to the intestines due to thrombosis or embolism and is considered a medical emergency requiring urgent intervention. If left untreated, acute mesenteric ischemia can progress to bowel infarction, perforation, and sepsis. Globally, the incidence of AMI is rare, estimated to be 0.1–0.2% of all hospital admissions; however, certain surgical procedures especially with prolonged hypotension are precipitating mechanisms, of the non-occlusive modality however encompassing thrombosis as well. Mortality rate depends on many factors, ranging from 10 to 50% [1–6]. Classic acute mesenteric ischemia can result from various causes including thrombosis of the mesenteric arteries due to atherosclerosis, embolism of cardiac or aortic origin, and arterial dissection. Vasospasm can be a contributing phenomenon. The most common cause of AMI is embolic occlusion usually from cardiac sources such as atrial fibrillation, myocardial infarction, or endocarditis [7, 8]. Thrombotic occlusion of the mesenteric arteries can also cause AMI, usually in patients with underlying atherosclerosis or hypercoagulable states [9].

The clinical presentation of acute mesenteric ischemia is often abrupt, with patients experiencing some or all of the following: severe abdominal pain, nausea, vomiting, diarrhea, and bloody stools. The pain is usually out of proportion to the physical exam and is often described as cramping, colicky, or diffuse with associated abdominal tenderness, rebound tenderness, and/or absent bowel sounds [10, 11]. Patients with acute mesenteric ischemia may also have signs of systemic inflammation such as fever, leukocytosis, and metabolic acidosis [12]. Imaging

R. N. Kulkarni (✉) · M. H. Eslami
Division of Vascular Surgery, Department of Surgery, UPMC Heart and Vascular Institute, UPMC Presbyterian Hospital, Pittsburgh, PA, USA
e-mail: kulkarnirn@upmc.edu; mohammad.eslami@vandaliahealth.org

© The Author(s), under exclusive license to Springer Nature Switzerland AG 2024

J. Faintuch, S. Faintuch (eds.), *Recent Strategies in High Risk Surgery*,
https://doi.org/10.1007/978-3-031-56270-9_13

studies such as computed tomography angiography (CTA), magnetic resonance angiography (MRA), or duplex ultrasonography may confirm the diagnosis of AMI.

The management of acute mesenteric ischemia starts with infusion of fluids, anticoagulants, and antibiotics. It involves as well emergent revascularization to restore blood flow to the affected mesenteric arteries. Options for revascularization include surgical intervention such as thromboembolectomy, bypass grafting, or endarterectomy, or endovascular intervention such as catheter-directed thrombolysis or angioplasty with stenting. Typically, open or laparoscopic surgical exploration is required alongside revascularization to assess the viability of the bowel and may involve bowel resection. Old age, chronic renal disease, patient dependency, arrhythmias, cardiac failure, hypotension, large bowel involvement, acidosis (lactate), delay to surgery and inotropes are all ominous markers as concerns mortality. Bowel wall thickening and notably timely anticoagulation and revascularization seem to improve survival [1].

Chronic Mesenteric Ischemia

Chronic mesenteric ischemia (CMI) is a gradual, progressive decrease in blood flow to the intestines due to atherosclerotic narrowing of the mesenteric arteries [8]. CMI is a rare condition that accounts for less than 5% of all cases of mesenteric ischemia, typically affects patients over the age of 60 with a history of atherosclerotic disease, and can be associated with other systemic manifestations of atherosclerosis [13]. Other causes of CMI include vasculitis, fibromuscular dysplasia, and radiation-induced vasculopathy.

The clinical presentation of chronic mesenteric ischemia is often insidious and may include post-prandial abdominal pain, weight loss, food fear, and diarrhea [14]. The pain is usually located in the epigastric or periumbilical region and may be relieved by fasting or lying down. Patients with chronic mesenteric ischemia may also have signs of malnutrition, such as hypoalbuminemia, anemia, or vitamin deficiencies [15].

The management of chronic mesenteric ischemia involves revascularization to restore blood flow to the affected mesenteric arteries [8]. The choice of treatment depends on the severity and location of the arterial stenosis or occlusion. Endovascular interventions, such as percutaneous transluminal angioplasty (PTA) and stenting, are considered first-line treatment for chronic mesenteric ischemia [16]. In patients with extensive atherosclerosis or multiple arterial stenoses, open surgical revascularization such as mesenteric artery bypass or endarterectomy may be preferred over endovascular intervention or may be necessary in cases where endovascular interventions have failed [17, 18].

Non-occlusive Mesenteric Ischemia (NOMI)

NOMI is also known as mesenteric vasoconstriction syndrome. NOMI is a type of mesenteric ischemia that occurs when blood flow to the intestines is reduced due to high doses or prolonged use of vasopressors in critically ill patients, notably with refractory shock. These patients typically have underlying medical conditions such as heart failure, liver cirrhosis, or sepsis [19, 20]. This then leads to vasoconstriction in the mesenteric circulation resulting in reduced blood flow and oxygen delivery to the intestines [21]. The pathophysiology of vasopressor-induced NOMI is complex and not fully understood. It is thought to involve multiple factors, including the direct effects of vasoconstrictive medications on the mesenteric vessels, impaired autoregulation of mesenteric blood flow, and the effects of systemic hypoperfusion and hypoxia in critically ill patients [22].

The diagnosis of NOMI can be challenging as imaging studies may not show a clear obstruction in the mesenteric vessels [23]. Diagnosis is typically based on a high index of clinical suspicion, along with imaging findings such as thickened bowel walls, decreased contrast enhancement, or pneumatosis intestinalis on CT scans [24].

Management of vasopressor-induced NOMI involves maintaining hemodynamic support despite sharp reduction or discontinuation of vasopressors and providing adequate oxygenation and fluid resuscitation. This is not an easy challenge for hypotensive patients with severe derangements of the macro and micro circulation. Additional treatments may include pharmacologic vasodilators, such as direct prostaglandin infusion in the superior mesenteric artery (Alprostadil/prostaglandin E1, UCB Pharma, Monheim, Germany) or endovascular interventions such as angioplasty or stenting [3, 25]. With irreversible ischemia, surgery will be necessary to remove damaged or necrotic bowel.

Mesenteric Venous Ischemia

Mesenteric venous ischemia is a condition in which a blood clot forms in one of the primary veins draining the intestines resulting in massive congestion within the mesenteric circulation. The superior mesenteric vein (SMV) is the most commonly affected vein in mesenteric venous thrombosis (MVT), accounting for approximately two-thirds of cases; however, the portal vein is also commonly involved, either alone or in combination with the SMV [26]. The exact cause of MVT is often not clear, but risk factors can include hypercoagulable states, abdominal surgeries, inflammatory bowel disease, pregnancy and the post-partum period, liver disease, pancreatitis, and certain medications [26–28].

Venous mesenteric ischemia can either present suddenly with severe diffuse abdominal pain or insidiously over the course of days to weeks [29]. Diagnosis requires a high index of suspicion given the patients history and physical exam, and typically requires a CTA with a dedicated venous phase, although a duplex ultrasound scan can be performed in those that cannot undergo CTA [30].

The treatment of venous mesenteric ischemia involves anticoagulation therapy, initially with heparin or low-molecular-weight heparin to prevent the progression of thrombosis, followed by bowel rest, and supportive care for complications such as sepsis, dehydration, and electrolyte imbalance [31, 32]. This is followed by long-term anticoagulation with warfarin or direct oral anticoagulants (DOACs) to prevent recurrence.

Depending on the severity of bowel ischemia, surgery may be indicated. Surgical treatment includes both open and endovascular options with or without bowel resection. In the most severe cases, an intestinal transplant may be necessary.

Initial Post-operative Assessment and Monitoring

After surgery, patients with mesenteric ischemia require close monitoring to assess their condition and ensure that they are recovering properly. Post-operative monitoring is critical to ensure adequate blood flow to the intestines and prevent further complications, as many of the described syndromes can be progressive or with delayed repercussions. Close observation and prompt recognition of any signs of complications are necessary to facilitate early reintervention and minimize morbidity and mortality.

Vascular Procedures

After revascularization with or without bowel resection, patients are typically monitored in the intensive care unit (ICU) to ensure stable hemodynamics and adequate organ perfusion.

Secondary Embolism, Thrombosis, Non-occlusive Ischemia

For patients experiencing AMI secondary to an embolic source, the pre- and post-op exams should be identical to rule out any new emboli. Patients with CMI may also have peripheral vascular disease in multiple distributions and are at risk of non-occlusive mesenteric ischemia in the event of post-operative hypotension or vasopressor support [33, 34]. In either case an early thorough vascular exam can help significantly in identifying post-operative complications and determining the nature of its cause.

Blood pressure monitoring is essential in the post-operative period to assess the patient's hemodynamic stability [34]. Multi-lumen central lines are maintained for resuscitation and medication administration along with invasive monitoring via arterial lines to provide accurate and continuous blood pressure readings. Persistent post-operative hypotension should raise concerns for hypovolemia, bleeding, cardiac dysfunction, or sepsis and should be monitored in conjunction with serial physical exams, urine output, and laboratory values.

Ongoing/Recurrent Abdominal Pain

Patients who experience new or worsening abdominal pain and distension or signs of bleeding may require additional imaging studies to monitor the patency of the revascularized arteries and evaluate intestinal perfusion. Post-operative imaging modalities may include computed tomography angiography (CTA), magnetic resonance angiography (MRA), or duplex ultrasound [35–37]. CTA is typically preferred for imaging mesenteric vessels as compared to MRA as it provides faster imaging and higher spatial resolution for the detection and localization of vascular stenoses, is more widely available, allows better visualization of calcification, and is more resistant to patient motion [38–40]. Additionally, when ordered along with a venous phase, CTA allows for interrogation of bowel ischemia. These studies can be performed within the first 24–48 h after revascularization and may be repeated as needed.

Laboratory Work Up

1. Coagulation studies: Coagulation studies such as prothrombin time (PT), activated partial thromboplastin time (aPTT), and international normalized ratio (INR) help in monitoring coagulation status and can be used in conjunction with the CBC. A thromboelastogram (TEG) may also be utilized to identify any specific deficiencies in the patient's ability to form clot. Disseminated intravascular coagulation (DIC) is not a common finding, with an incidence between 5 and 20% for acute mesenteric ischemia and less than 5% for chronic; however, the development of DIC in mesenteric ischemia is associated with worse outcomes, including higher mortality rates [6, 41–44].
2. Serial post-operative serum lactate levels are often utilized to monitor bowel perfusion recovery and aid in detecting any signs of continued hypoxia or hypoperfusion. Persistently elevated serum lactate levels after revascularization should prompt concerns for continued tissue ischemia and is associated with worse patient outcomes [45].

Medical Management

Medical management of mesenteric ischemia may involve several measures to support the patient's hemodynamic status and address underlying comorbidities. These measures include fluids and electrolytes, antibiotics, pain medication, and parenteral/enteral feeding, depending on gastrointestinal tolerance [46–48].

Anticoagulation therapy: Heparin, low-molecular-weight heparin, or direct oral anticoagulants (DOACs) may be used. Many patients experience acute mesenteric ischemia secondary to atrial fibrillation–related embolic events after discontinuation of anticoagulation for other reasons [49]. In this setting it is important to communicate with the surgical team the timing for restarting therapeutic anticoagulation as continuing to hold it can put them at further embolic risk [50].

Second-Look Operations

In the past, second-look procedures were common, and in certain circumstances even an open-abdomen option was adopted, despite catastrophic complications [51–56]. Intestinal perfusion was typically documented when it was already too late, and gangrenous bowel carried an ominous mortality. Today, efficient hemodynamic and oxygenation markers provide a useful picture of the post-operative course, even though regional perfusion deficits or imbalances are harder to detect and, in most circumstances, anticipate potential or imminent troubles. Metabolic acidosis, hypoxia, intramural pneumatosis, and signs of sepsis continue to carry prognostic relevance. If a high level of suspicion for ongoing bowel ischemia remains, imaging methods should be repeated, and further interventions planned.

Nutritional Support

Tolerance of the oral diet may be markedly delayed or insufficient even after successful revascularization; notably, if enteral resection was required, thus enteral nutrition could be delivered via a nasogastric or nasoenteric tube. Exceptionally a percutaneous gastrostomy or jejunostomy tube may be placed to facilitate enteral feeding. Short bowel syndrome is a possibility after total small bowel ischemia, and intestinal transplantation should be considered depending on the circumstances [57–62].

Treatment Options: Arterial

The choice of treatment option depends on various factors such as patient age, comorbidities, and the severity of the disease and influences post-operative care algorithms. Endovascular interventions have been increasingly utilized over the last decade, and they have been shown to be a safe and effective alternative to open surgery [3, 63].

Endovascular Interventions

Percutaneous transluminal angioplasty (PTA): PTA involves the use of a balloon catheter to dilate the stenotic or occluded segment of the mesenteric artery to improve blood flow and relieve ischemia. Angioplasty is typically utilized in conjunction with stenting in patients with chronic mesenteric ischemia.

Stenting: Stenting involves the placement of a bare metal (uncovered) or covered stent graft within the mesenteric artery, usually the SMA, to maintain patency and improve blood flow. Stenting may be used in conjunction with PTA or performed primarily. Often times after stenting, a patient will need to be placed on antiplatelet medications to prevent stent thrombosis. The most commonly used antiplatelet agents after vascular stenting are aspirin and P2Y12 receptor inhibitors (such as clopidogrel, ticagrelor, or prasugrel) [64]. P2Y12 receptor inhibitors are often prescribed in addition to aspirin and are usually continued for a period of 1–12 months, depending on the type of stent [65]. When patients are newly placed on a P2Y12 inhibitor, they should be monitored closely for signs or symptoms of bleeding.

Common access sites include the brachial or common femoral arteries. They should be closely monitored in the immediate post-operative period for any bleeding, hematoma formation, or pseudoaneurysm development. It is extremely important to have a full pulse/signal exam performed and documented at the end of any endovascular case.

Retrograde open mesenteric stenting (ROMS): When percutaneous stenting has no indication or has failed, an alternative is to access the affected artery through an exploratory laparotomy incision via direct percutaneous access into the distal SMA [46]. Aspirin and/or P2Y12 inhibitors will need to be administered in the post-operative setting.

Open Surgical Interventions

Thrombectomy and bowel resection, with eventual bypass grafting of the mesenteric artery, were used during decades. In the era of endovascular first approach, open arterial proposals deserve much less interest. By the same token, mesenteric venous thrombosis is most often handled with systemic anticoagulation without surgical revascularization. Catheter-directed thrombectomy and thrombolysis could be attempted depending on angiographic findings [66–68]. Non-occlusive mesenteric ischemia, as alluded to, is primarily a non-surgical condition, except in circumstances of late diagnosis, when bowel gangrene already occurred and demands resection.

Post-operative Management: Mesenteric Venous Thrombosis (MVT)

Unlike arterial mesenteric ischemia which is typically considered a surgical emergency, symptoms of mesenteric venous thrombosis are often less severe and may develop gradually over time. Treatment is often via anticoagulation alone, although surgical intervention may be necessary in extreme cases. Diagnosis is made by CT scan in 90% of patients, and management depends on the presence or absence of bowel necrosis [67, 68]. Long-term management should be directed toward treatment of the underlying cause, and regular follow-up after MVT is essential in evaluating the response to treatment. Up to 25% of patients will experience recurrent thromboses of the mesenteric circulation within the first 30 days. This rate is lowered to 3% if maintained on therapeutic oral anticoagulation [32, 68].

References

1. Sumbal R, Ali Baig MM, Sumbal A. Predictors of mortality in acute mesenteric ischemia: a systematic review and meta-analysis. J Surg Res. 2022;275:72–86.
2. Acosta S, Björck M. Acute thrombo-embolic occlusion of the superior mesenteric artery: a prospective study in a well defined population. Eur J Vasc Endovasc Surg. 2003;26(2):179–83.
3. Acosta S. Mesenteric ischemia. Curr Opin Crit Care. 2015;21(2):171–8.
4. Stoney RJ, Cunningham CG. Acute mesenteric ischemia. Surgery. 1993;114(3):489–90.
5. Schoots I, Koffeman G, Legemate D, Levi M, Van Gulik T. Systematic review of survival after acute mesenteric ischaemia according to disease aetiology. J Br Surg. 2004;91(1):17–27.
6. Oldenburg WA, Lau LL, Rodenberg TJ, Edmonds HJ, Burger CD. Acute mesenteric ischemia: a clinical review. Arch Intern Med. 2004;164(10):1054–62.
7. Björnsson S, Resch T, Acosta S. Symptomatic mesenteric atherosclerotic disease—lessons learned from the diagnostic workup. J Gastrointest Surg. 2013;17:973–80.
8. Clair DG, Beach JM. Mesenteric ischemia. NEJM. 2016;374(10):959–68.
9. Acosta S, Ögren M, Sternby N-H, Bergqvist D, Björck M. Clinical implications for the management of acute thromboembolic occlusion of the superior mesenteric artery: autopsy findings in 213 patients. Ann Surg. 2005;241(3):516.
10. Carver TW, Vora RS, Taneja A. Mesenteric ischemia. Crit Care Clin. 2016;32(2):155–71.
11. Park WM, Gloviczki P, Cherry KJ Jr, Hallett JW Jr, Bower TC, Panneton JM, et al. Contemporary management of acute mesenteric ischemia: factors associated with survival. J Vasc Surg. 2002;35(3):445–52.
12. Kougias P, Lau D, El Sayed HF, Zhou W, Huynh TT, Lin PH. Determinants of mortality and treatment outcome following surgical interventions for acute mesenteric ischemia. J Vasc Surg. 2007;46(3):467–74.
13. Roobottom C, Dubbins P. Significant disease of the celiac and superior mesenteric arteries in asymptomatic patients: predictive value of Doppler sonography. AJR Am J Roentgenol. 1993;161(5):985–8.
14. Bjorck M, Koelemay M, Acosta S, Bastos Goncalves F, Kolbel T, Kolkman J, et al. Editor's Choice-Management of the diseases of mesenteric arteries and veins: clinical practice guidelines of the European Society of Vascular Surgery (ESVS). Eur J Vasc Endovasc Surg. 2017;53(4):460.
15. van Dijk LJ, van Noord D, de Vries AC, Kolkman JJ, Geelkerken RH, Verhagen HJ, et al. Clinical management of chronic mesenteric ischemia. Eur Gastroenterol J. 2019;7(2):179–88.
16. Schermerhorn ML, Giles KA, Hamdan AD, Wyers MC, Pomposelli FB. Mesenteric revascularization: management and outcomes in the United States, 1988–2006. J Vasc Surg. 2009;50(2):341–8.e1.
17. Atkins MD, Kwolek CJ, LaMuraglia GM, Brewster DC, Chung TK, Cambria RP. Surgical revascularization versus endovascular therapy for chronic mesenteric ischemia: a comparative experience. J Vasc Surg. 2007;45(6):1162–71.
18. Kruger AJ, Walker PJ, Foster WJ, Jenkins JS, Boyne NS, Jenkins J. Open surgery for atherosclerotic chronic mesenteric ischemia. J Vasc Surg. 2007;46(5):941–5.
19. Acosta S. Epidemiology of mesenteric vascular disease: clinical implications. Semin Vasc Surg. 2010;23(1):4–8.
20. Benjamin E, Oropello JM. Acute mesenteric ischemia: pathophysiology, diagnosis, and treatment. Dis Mon. 1993;39(3):134–210.

21. Al-Diery H, Phillips A, Evennett N, Pandanaboyana S, Gilham M, Windsor JA. The pathogenesis of nonocclusive mesenteric ischemia: implications for research and clinical practice. J Int Care Med. 2019;34(10):771–81.
22. Bailey RW, Bulkley GB, Hamilton SR, Morris JB, Haglund UH. Protection of the small intestine from nonocclusive mesenteric ischemic injury due to cardiogenic shock. Am J Surg. 1987;153(1):108–16.
23. Trompeter M, Brazda T, Remy CT, Vestring T, Reimer P. Non-occlusive mesenteric ischemia: etiology, diagnosis, and interventional therapy. Eur Radiol. 2002;12:1179–87.
24. Howard TJ, Plaskon LA, Wiebke EA, Wilcox MG, Madura JA. Nonocclusive mesenteric ischemia remains a diagnostic dilemma. Am J Surg. 1996;171(4):405–8.
25. Boley SJ, Sprayregan S, Siegelman SS, Veith FJ. Initial results from an aggressive roentgenological and surgical approach to acute mesenteric ischemia. Surgery. 1977;82(6):848–55.
26. Kumar S, Kamath PS. Acute superior mesenteric venous thrombosis: one disease or two? Am J Gastroenterol. 2003;98(6):1299–304.
27. Kumar S, Sarr MG, Kamath PS. Mesenteric venous thrombosis. NEJM. 2001;345(23):1683–8.
28. Harnik IG, Brandt LJ. Mesenteric venous thrombosis. Vasc Med. 2010;15(5):407–18.
29. North J, Wollenman O Jr. Venous mesenteric occlusion in the course of migrating thrombophlebitis. Surg Gynecol Obstet. 1952;95(6):665–71.
30. Zhang J, Duan Z, Song Q, Luo Y, Xin S, Zhang Q. Acute mesenteric venous thrombosis: a better outcome achieved through improved imaging techniques and a changed policy of clinical management. Eur J Vasc Endovasc Surg. 2004;28(3):329–34.
31. Abdu RA, Zakhour B, Dallis D. Mesenteric venous thrombosis—1911–1984. Surgery. 1987;101(4):383–8.
32. Amitrano L, Guardascione MA, Scaglione M, Pezzullo L, Sangiuliano N, Armellino MF, et al. Prognostic factors in noncirrhotic patients with splanchnic vein thromboses. Am J Gastroenterol. 2007;102(11):2464–70.
33. Mythen M, Webb A. The role of gut mucosal hypoperfusion in the pathogenesis of post-operative organ dysfunction. Int Care Med. 1994;20:203–9.
34. Chang JB, Stein TA. Mesenteric ischemia: acute and chronic. Ann Vasc Surg. 2003;17(3):323–8.
35. Perko MJ, Just S, Schroeder TV. Importance of diastolic velocities in the detection of celiac and mesenteric artery disease by Duplex ultrasound. J Vasc Surg. 1997;26(2):288–93.
36. Zwolak RM. Can duplex ultrasound replace arteriography in screening for mesenteric ischemia? Semin Vasc Surg. 1999;12(4):252–60.
37. Meaney J. Non-invasive evaluation of the visceral arteries with magnetic resonance angiography. Eur Radiol. 1999;9:1267–76.
38. Kolkman JJ, Geelkerken RH. Diagnosis and treatment of chronic mesenteric ischemia: an update. Best Pract Res Clin Gastroenterol. 2017;31(1):49–57.
39. Fleischmann D. Multiple detector-row CT angiography of the renal and mesenteric vessels. Eur J Radiol. 2003;45:S79–87.
40. Horton KM, Fishman EK. Multidetector CT angiography in the diagnosis of mesenteric ischemia. Radiol Clin N Am. 2007;45(2):275–88.
41. Kurland B, Brandt LJ, Delany HM. Diagnostic tests for intestinal ischemia. Surg Clin N Am. 1992;72(1):85–105.
42. Wiesner W, Khurana B, Ji H, Ros PR. CT of acute bowel ischemia. Radiology. 2003;226(3):635–50.
43. Yağmurdur MC, Ozdemir A, Topaloğlu S, Kilinç K, Ozenç A. Effects of alpha tocopherol and verapamil on liver and small bowel following mesenteric ischemia-reperfusion. Turk J Gastroenterol. 2002;13(1):40–6.
44. Akyıldız HY, Sözüer E, Uzer H, Baykan M, Oz B. The length of necrosis and renal insufficiency predict the outcome of acute mesenteric ischemia. Asian J Surg. 2015;38(1):28–32.
45. Acosta S, Nilsson T. Current status on plasma biomarkers for acute mesenteric ischemia. J Thromb Thrombol. 2012;33:355–61.
46. Wyers MC. Acute mesenteric ischemia: diagnostic approach and surgical treatment. Semin Vasc Surg. 2010;23(1):9–20.

47. Safioleas, Moulakakis, Papavassiliou, Kontzoglou, Kostakis. Acute mesenteric ischaemia, a highly lethal disease with a devastating outcome. Vasa. 2006;35(2):106–11.
48. Kozuch P, Brandt L. Diagnosis and management of mesenteric ischaemia with an emphasis on pharmacotherapy. Aliment Pharmacol Ther. 2005;21(3):201–15.
49. Endean ED, Barnes SL, Kwolek CJ, Minion DJ, Schwarcz TH, Mentzer RM Jr. Surgical management of thrombotic acute intestinal ischemia. Ann Surg. 2001;233(6):801.
50. Lange H, Jäckel R. Usefulness of plasma lactate concentration in the diagnosis of acute abdominal disease. Eur J Surg. 1994;160(6–7):381–4.
51. Meng X, Liu L, Jiang H. Indications and procedures for second-look surgery in acute mesenteric ischemia. Surg Today. 2010;40:700–5.
52. Boley S, Feinstein F, Sammartano R, Brandt L, Sprayregen S. New concepts in the management of emboli of the superior mesenteric artery. Surg Gynecol Obstet. 1981;153(4):561–9.
53. Lindblad B, Håkansson H. The rationale for "second-look operation" in mesenteric vessel occlusion with uncertain intestinal viability at primary surgery. Acta Chir Scand. 1987;153(9):531–3.
54. Shaw R. The "second look" after superior mesenterial embolectomy or reconstruction for mesenteric infarction. Curr Surg Manag. 1965;509.
55. Tola M, Portoghese A, Maniga A. Laparoscopic second-look in acute intestinal ischemia. Minerva Chir. 1997;52(5):527–30.
56. Kaminsky O, Yampolski I, Aranovich D, Gnessin E, Greif F. Does a second-look operation improve survival in patients with peritonitis due to acute mesenteric ischemia? A 5-year retrospective experience. World J Surg. 2005;29:645–8.
57. Cheatham ML, Safcsak K, Brzezinski SJ, Lube MW. Nitrogen balance, protein loss, and the open abdomen. Crit Care Med. 2007;35(1):127–31.
58. Friese RS. The open abdomen: definitions, management principles, and nutrition support considerations. Nutr Clin Pract. 2012;27(4):492–8.
59. Ivatury R, Kolkman K, Johansson K. Management of open abdomen. Acta Clin Belg. 2007;62(sup1):206–9.
60. Lewis SJ, Andersen HK, Thomas S. Early enteral nutrition within 24 h of intestinal surgery versus later commencement of feeding: a systematic review and meta-analysis. J Gastrointest Surg. 2009;13:569–75.
61. Schroeder D, Gillanders L, Mahr K, Hill GL. Effects of immediate postoperative enteral nutrition on body composition, muscle function, and wound healing. JPEN J Parent Enter Nutr. 1991;15(4):376–83.
62. Sagar S, Harland P, Shields R. Early postoperative feeding with elemental diet. Br Med J. 1979;1(6159):293–5.
63. Block TA, Acosta S, Björck M. Endovascular and open surgery for acute occlusion of the superior mesenteric artery. J Vasc Surg. 2010;52(4):959–66.
64. Giustino G, Baber U, Sartori S, Mehran R, Mastoris I, Kini AS, et al. Duration of dual antiplatelet therapy after drug-eluting stent implantation: a systematic review and meta-analysis of randomized controlled trials. J Am Coll Cardiol. 2015;65(13):1298–310.
65. Wyers MC, Powell RJ, Nolan BW, Cronenwett JL. Retrograde mesenteric stenting during laparotomy for acute occlusive mesenteric ischemia. J Vasc Surg. 2007;45(2):269–75.
66. Singal AK, Kamath PS, Tefferi A. Mesenteric venous thrombosis. Mayo Clin Proc. 2013;88(3):285–94.
67. Dentali F, Ageno W, Witt D, Malato A, Clark N, Garcia D, et al. Natural history of mesenteric venous thrombosis in patients treated with vitamin K antagonists. Thromb Haemost. 2009;102(09):501–4.
68. Hollingshead M, Burke CT, Mauro MA, Weeks SM, Dixon RG, Jaques PF. Transcatheter thrombolytic therapy for acute mesenteric and portal vein thrombosis. J Vasc Interv Radiol. 2005;16(5):651–61.

Chapter 14
Safety and Success in Modern Liver Transplantation

Madelynn Zhang, Navdeep Singh, William K. Washburn, and Austin D. Schenk

Abbreviations

ARDS	Acute respiratory distress syndrome
BD	Brain dead
CIT	Cold ischemic time
CMV	Cytomegalovirus
CRRT	Continuous renal replacement therapy
DAA	Direct-acting antiretroviral
DCD	Deceased from cardiac death
DILI	Drug-induced liver injury
EAD	Early allograft dysfunction
EBV	Epstein-Barr virus
ESLD	End-stage liver disease
HAT	Hepatic arterial thrombosis
HCC	Hepatocellular carcinoma
HCV	Hepatitis C virus
HIV	Human immunodeficiency virus
HPS	Hepatopulmonary syndrome
HSV	Herpes simplex virus
IC	Ischemic cholangiopathy
LDLT	Living donor liver transplant
MARS	Molecular adsorbent recirculation system
MELD	Model for end-stage liver disease

M. Zhang
The Ohio State University College of Medicine, Columbus, OH, USA
e-mail: madelynn.zhang@osumc.edu

N. Singh · W. K. Washburn · A. D. Schenk (✉)
Department of Surgery, Division of Transplantation, The Ohio State University Wexner Medical Center, Columbus, OH, USA
e-mail: navdeep.singh@osumc.edu; ken.washburn@osumc.edu; austin.schenk@osumc.edu

© The Author(s), under exclusive license to Springer Nature Switzerland AG 2024

J. Faintuch, S. Faintuch (eds.), *Recent Strategies in High Risk Surgery*,
https://doi.org/10.1007/978-3-031-56270-9_14

NASH	Non-alcoholic steatohepatitis
PBC	Primary biliary cirrhosis
PNF	Primary non-function
POPH	Portopulmonary hypertension
PSC	Primary sclerosing cholangitis
SIRS	Systemic inflammatory response syndrome
SMV	Superior mesenteric vein
SRTR	Scientific Registry of Transplant Recipients
TPA	Tissue plasminogen activator

Introduction

In the six decades since Dr. Thomas Starzl performed the world's first successful liver transplant [1], significant improvements in surgical technique, anesthetic practice, and critical care have allowed liver transplantation to become standard-of-care treatment for patients with end-stage liver disease (ESLD). Without doubt, liver transplantation remains one of the most complex and high-risk abdominal surgical procedures performed. This chapter is intended to provide a practical overview of adult liver transplantation with emphasis on modern strategies employed to mitigate risk and achieve ideal recipient outcomes.

Indications for Liver Transplantation

The Scientific Registry of Transplant Recipients (SRTR) groups the indications for liver transplantation into the 10 categories shown in Table 14.1 [2]. As of 2021, 33.9% of patients awaiting liver transplantation carried the diagnosis of alcoholic liver disease [3]. Non-alcoholic steatohepatitis (NASH) is the second most common indication for liver transplantation comprising 19.2% of the waiting list, and notably

Table 14.1 Potential indications for liver transplantation

Non-alcoholic steatohepatitis (NASH)
Alcoholic liver disease
Hepatitis B or C
Cholestatic liver disease
Autoimmune liver disease
Metabolic liver disease
Malignant liver disease
Liver graft failure
Acute liver failure
Other modalities of acute or chronic liver failure

this number has increased by 250% over the last 10 years. Hepatitis C (HCV) was historically a leading indication for liver transplantation, and a common cause of early graft failure sometimes necessitating re-transplantation [4]. The advent of direct-acting antiretroviral (DAA) medications has greatly reduced the prevalence of HCV, need for HCV-related liver transplantation, and has even allowed for expansion of the donor pool wherein HCV-positive donor livers can be transplanted followed by recipient treatment with DAAs, allowing for excellent long-term outcomes [5, 6].

The category of cholestatic liver diseases includes primary biliary cirrhosis (PBC), primary sclerosing cholangitis (PSC), IgG4-related sclerosing cholangitis, and genetic diseases such as Caroli's disease that lead to progressive cholestasis. Not infrequently there are mixed disorders in which autoimmune and cholestatic etiologies intersect. Liver transplantation for metabolic diseases is far more common in the pediatric population; however, patients with alpha-1-antitrypsin deficiency, hemochromatosis, and Wilson's disease are often transplanted in adulthood. Hepatocellular carcinoma (HCC) is by far the most common malignancy treated with liver transplantation; however, the field of transplant oncology is rapidly evolving [7] to include intrahepatic and hilar cholangiocarcinoma, colon cancer with unresectable liver metastases, and neuroendocrine tumors [8]. Common causes of acute liver failure include acetaminophen overdose and other forms of drug-induced liver injury (DILI), acute alcoholic hepatitis, viral etiologies, and acute Budd-Chiari syndrome.

Preoperative Evaluation for Liver Transplantation

Liver transplantation provides full cure for appropriately chosen recipients, but also it has potential to shorten overall length of life when offered to unsuitable candidates [9, 10].

Evaluation typically begins with an electrocardiogram, echocardiogram, stress test, and assessment of cardiac risk factors. Risk factors for coronary artery disease including tobacco use, peripheral vascular disease, diabetes, hypertension, hyperlipidemia, and obesity are considered, and left heart catheterization is generally pursued in patients with multiple risk factors. Right heart catheterization is warranted in any candidate with elevated right ventricular systolic pressures or other suggestions of possible right heart dysfunction, and the combination of echocardiography and right heart catheterization are generally used to identify and distinguish between hepatopulmonary syndrome (HPS) and portopulmonary hypertension (POPH). Arterial blood gases should be obtained in all candidates, and formal pulmonary function testing should be pursued in patients with abnormal blood gases, a baseline oxygen requirement, significant exercise-induced desaturation, and smoking history or radiographic evidence of obstructive pulmonary disease.

Two-dimensional liver imaging (CT or MRI) is recommended for all potential candidates and serves dual purposes. Because cirrhosis increases risk for hepatocellular carcinoma, preoperative imaging is used to identify, stage, and plan bridging therapies for candidates with HCC. From a surgical perspective, preoperative imaging allows the transplant surgeon to verify portal vein patency or select alternative inflow, decipher hepatic arterial anatomy, and measure the dimensions of the right upper quadrant in order to select an appropriately sized donor. In cases of acute or decompensated cirrhosis where candidates are unstable for transport to radiology, a bedside Doppler ultrasound can substitute.

Oncology Screening

Upper endoscopy is generally performed to treat esophageal varices prior to wait-listing. Searching for occult malignancies is warranted as these lesions will blossom with the initiation of immunosuppression, and thus colonoscopy should also be performed for all candidates over the age of 50 or with increased risk factors for colon cancer. Likewise guidelines for other age-related cancer screenings are followed including mammograms in all female candidates over the age of 40, Papanicolaou (PAP) smear testing in women without hysterectomy, and prostate specific antigen (PSA) testing in men. Alfa fetoprotein levels are also checked in all candidates as an additional screen for HCC.

Several additional components round out the pretransplant work-up. Dental screening is recommended, and critical dental issues should be addressed pretransplant. Formal or informal clinical frailty assessment is absolutely essential to identify candidates who can complete the rigorous recovery that follows liver transplantation [11]. Psychiatric and neurocognitive testing can be useful to assess readiness for transplant in cases of addictive disease (e.g. alcohol or drug-related HCV) and to ensure medication adherence and baseline stability in cases of comorbid psychiatric disease (e.g. schizophrenia, bipolar disease).

Transplant centers generally verify the willingness of at-home support resources for transplant candidates, particularly in cases where physical or mental barriers decrease recipient independence and necessitate intensive care-giving. Financial and insurance assessments help verify transplant center reimbursement and also ensure that transplant-related costs will not be bankrupting for the recipient. Lastly, preoperative bloodwork is used to calculate model for end-stage liver disease (MELD) score, assess renal function, measure cytomegalovirus (CMV), Epstein-Barr virus (EBV), and herpes simplex virus (HSV) serostatus, and exclude syphilis, active hepatitis, human immunodeficiency virus (HIV) and tuberculosis. Most programs also include drug and alcohol screening in candidate bloodwork (Table 14.2).

Table 14.2 Essential evaluation for liver transplantation

Cardiovascular screening
Electrocardiogram
Echocardiogram
Stress test
Right and left heart catheterization (if indicated)
Pulmonary testing
Chest X-ray
Arterial blood gas
Pulmonary function tests
Liver imaging (CT, MRI, or Doppler US)
Frailty assessment
Upper gastrointestinal endoscopy
Age and gender appropriate cancer screening
Dental screening
Psychiatric and neurocognitive assessment
Verification of at-home support
Financial and insurance assessment
Bloodwork

CT Computed tomography, *MRI* Magnetic resonance imaging, *US* Ultrasonography

Absolute Contraindications to Liver Transplantation

Flow-limiting coronary artery disease not amenable to percutaneous or open surgical intervention is a rare but absolute contraindication to liver transplantation. Likewise, non-correctable severe valvular disease and conditions causing significant non-reversible depression of the ejection fraction prohibit transplantation. Due to the proximity and "in-series" relationship of the liver and right ventricle, dynamic right heart function is essential for safe liver transplantation. Regardless of etiology, non-correctable conditions causing a mean pulmonary artery pressure >40 mmHg are generally considered an absolute contraindication [12]. Extra-hepatic malignancy is almost always a contraindication to liver transplantation, as are uncontrolled psychiatric illness, lack of adequate social support, and inability to pay for post-transplant medications.

Relative Contraindications to Liver Transplantation

There is no recommended maximum age for liver transplant recipients, and certainly transplant recipients in their seventies and even eighties can experience excellent outcomes [13, 14]. Rather, age must be considered in the context of functional

Table 14.3 Contraindications to Liver Transplantation

Absolute	
	Flow-limiting coronary artery disease
	Severe valvular disease
	Reduced left ventricular ejection fraction
	Severe right heart dysfunction
	Mean pulmonary artery pressure > 40 mmHg
	Extra-hepatic malignancy
	Uncontrolled psychiatric illness
	Absence of social support
	Inability to pay for post-transplant medications
Relative	
	Advanced age with significant co-morbid conditions
	Advanced frailty
	Severe obesity
	Non-treatable infections or SIRS, sepsis, ARDS
	Absence of surgical options for portal inflow
	Untreated drug/alcohol addiction

SIRS Systemic inflammatory response syndrome, *ARDS* Acute respiratory distress syndrome

status and comorbid conditions. Without doubt, older recipients have a more difficult time recovering from liver transplantation. Accordingly, they should have fewer comorbidities and a better functional status than otherwise similar younger candidates (Table 14.3).

Frailty

Although age and frailty do not strictly correlate, it is often true that frailty increases with increasing age. Preoperative assessment of frailty is important in any potential candidate for liver transplantation [15, 16]. Grip strength or number of transitions between sitting and standing in a fixed time period are combined with nutritional assessment and sometimes quantification of muscle mass. Although there is not, as yet, a universally agreed upon frailty index for liver transplantation, most transplant providers utilize a personal gestalt in judging physical readiness for transplant. Unless the candidate has been recently hospitalized and has had a precipitous decline, persistent non-ambulatory status is highly concerning.

Obesity

Akin to age, there is no recommended maximum body mass index for transplant candidates [17, 18]. Despite this, all transplant surgeons will acknowledge that operative difficulty increases with increasing recipient BMI, notably in the presence of ascites and a high degree of intra-abdominal (visceral) adiposity.

Hepatocellular Carcinoma (HCC)

The Milan criteria [19] proposed that favorable transplant outcomes could be achieved for single tumors <5 cm in size and for up to 2–3 tumors, provided each is less than 3 cm in size. More recently UCSF [20] (a single tumor ≤6.5 cm or ≤3 tumor each less than ≤4.5 cm in size with a cumulative diameter of ≤8 cm.) and Toronto criteria [21, 22] (no limit on tumor size or number, provided there is no extra-hepatic extension and tissue biopsy is free of vascular invasion or poorly differentiated cell morphology) have been adopted.

Infection

Infection is sometimes, but not always, a contraindication to liver transplantation [23–25]. Common recipient infections include spontaneous bacterial peritonitis, pneumonia, bacteremias, *C. Difficile* infection, and active lower extremity cellulitis. Localized infections that are actively being treated are usually not a barrier to successful transplantation. Infections not amenable to rapid clearance (e.g. endocarditis) and systemic infections causing systemic inflammatory response syndrome (SIRS), sepsis or acute respiratory distress syndrome (ARDS) are contraindications to liver transplant.

Recipient Anatomy

Anatomic considerations rarely preclude liver transplantation. Nevertheless technical success requires robust portal and arterial inflow to the liver, unobstructed venous outflow, and ability to reconstruct the biliary tract. Hepatic venous outflow into the inferior vena cava is rarely an issue except in certain patients with

Budd-Chiari syndrome, or tumor margins close to the vena cava. Problems with the recipient hepatic artery do not preclude liver transplantation because arterial conduits built with donor iliac vessels can be anastomosed to the supraceliac or infrarenal aorta; however, severe atherosclerosis of the recipient celiac tree *and* abdominal aorta is problematic. Portal vein thrombosis or absence (cavernous transformation of the portal vein) pose unique technical challenges but do not preclude liver transplantation unless all other sources of alternative portal inflow are unsuitable. Biliary reconstruction can be difficult but is always achievable using a duct-to-duct anastomosis, Roux-en-Y hepaticojejunostomy, or even choledochoduodenostomy.

Active Substance Abuse

Active substance abuse is not uncommon in liver transplant candidates [26, 27]. Center polices on marijuana use are variable and national guidelines do not exist [28]. Active use of "hard" drugs (cocaine, heroine, amphetamine, ecstasy) is generally considered a contraindication to transplant. Alcohol use is controversial. Many centers have protocols for selection and transplantation of patients with acute alcoholic hepatitis, often with excellent results [29, 30]. In cases of established alcoholism where patients have previously been advised by a physician to stop drinking, a period of complete sobriety and participation in substance abuse counseling are generally required. The necessity of counseling and the length of sobriety required are complex issues because alcohol-related recidivism has been notoriously difficult to predict in liver transplant recipients [31, 32].

Acute/Fulminant Liver Failure

Transplant professionals must carefully weigh the magnitude of critical illness against the ability to rapidly and completely correct the proximal causes of illness [33, 34]. Most transplant centers will consider intubated candidates so long as the fraction of inspired oxygen (FiO_2) and degree of ventilatory support are not excessively high. Likewise most centers will proceed with candidates on low doses of one or two vasopressors but not candidates on near-maximal support. Renal failure can be managed both intraoperatively and postoperatively and need not be a contraindication. Neurologic evaluation is essential, and CT-imaging is generally used to monitor for cerebral edema. High-dose continuous renal replacement therapy (CRRT) [35, 36] and/or adjunctive therapies such as the molecular absorbent recirculation system (MARS) [37, 38] should be used to clear ammonia and other toxins from the circulation. Hypernatremia is an ominous sign [39].

Living Versus Deceased Donor Liver Transplant

All transplant candidates should be considered for both living and deceased liver transplantation. Currently, liver allocation in the United States is guided by "sickest-first" prioritization wherein the MELD score [40, 41] is used to quantify the degree of illness and rank-order candidates. The median MELD score at transplant in the United States is approximately 29 [42], with a range from 6–40 (the higher the score, the worse the prognosis), and the median waiting time from listing to transplant is 13.5 months [43]. MELD-based allocation strongly favors acutely ill candidates. There are many candidates with significant symptoms and a poor quality of life who face long waiting times to transplant because of low-medium MELD scores that do not rise rapidly [44]. For these candidates, living donor liver transplantation (LDLT) can offer the fastest route to transplantation and cure.

Living Versus Deceased Donor

Most studies suggest that long-term graft and patient survival are slightly superior for living donor recipients [45, 46]. These findings must be tempered by knowledge that living donor recipients are carefully selected. Nonetheless, because living donors are exceedingly healthy and the transplanted liver mass is typically pristine, superior graft survival is expected. This advantage of living donor liver transplantation is counterbalanced by increased rates of biliary complications and hepatic arterial thrombosis (HAT) [47]. The re-intervention rate following living donation, including percutaneous, endoscopic, and operative procedures, is generally much higher than that seen following transplantation with a deceased donor allograft. The increased re-intervention rate is easily explained by the technical challenges of the smaller sized vessels present on the donor hemi-liver.

Due to the increased technical complexity of living donor liver transplant, not every candidate is appropriate for this operation. Candidates with prior upper abdominal surgery, extensive portal vein thrombosis, or need for caval replacement require careful preoperative consideration if living donation is to be used. Additionally, selected recipients should have a baseline level of stamina and fitness that will allow them to endure the re-interventions that are common following LDLT. Recipient selection for LDLT depends heavily on center expertise and the program maturity of the LDLT center.

Brain Dead (BD) Versus Cardiac Death (DCD) Donors

BD donors are generally considered favorable because these organs are never subjected to a period of asystole during which tissues are warm, non-oxygenated, and prone to microvascular clot formation. Recognized complications of DCD liver transplantation include ischemic cholangiopathy (IC) and early allograft dysfunction (EAD) [48–50]. Historically, DCD liver transplantation was associated with both decreased patient and graft survival; however, recent reports suggest that equivalent outcomes can be achieved by experienced centers with rigorous DCD protocols [51]. Just as in LDLT, recipient selection is critical to success in DCD liver transplantation. Short cold ischemic times are required to mitigate the risk of IC and therefore, an expeditious hepatectomy is required. For this reason, candidates with complex prior surgical histories or extensive portal vein thrombosis are sometimes avoided in DCD transplantation. Interestingly, recent advances in normothermic oxygenated perfusion pumps [52, 53] and normothermic regional perfusion [54, 55] offer opportunity to offer DCD liver transplantation to a far wider pool of potential recipients.

Overall, donor and recipient pairing is an exercise in risk management. Critically ill recipients and frail recipients have the least capacity to withstand complications and benefit from high-quality donor allografts with low risk for primary non-function (PNF), EAD, or IC. As recipient acuity drops donor selection can be liberalized. The risk of waitlist mortality should always be compared against the risk of perioperative mortality when non-ideal donor allografts are used [56].

Timing and Team Coordination

Logistics and timing are crucial to success in liver transplantation. Numerous studies highlight the importance of minimizing allograft cold ischemic time (CIT) [57, 58]. CITs of 12 h are considered maximally acceptable and are only appropriate for the healthiest donor organs. With meticulous planning and coordinated teamwork, CITs of 4–8 h are routinely achievable. Most donor operations occur at some distance from the transplant center, and the donor and recipient teams must remain in close communication. To prioritize recipient safety, the recipient operation is typically not started until the donor allograft has been visualized, cross-clamped, flushed, and carefully examined on the back-table at the donor hospital. Some centers begin the recipient hepatectomy while the donor organ is in transit to the transplant center, and others wait until the organ has arrived. In either case it is imperative to have prompt transport of the recipient to the operating room and efficient preparation for surgery.

The Donor Operation

Although operative details of the donor hepatectomy are beyond the scope of this chapter, several critical aspects of the donor operation deserve emphasis. First, visual and tactile assessment of the donor liver are critically important components of donor selection. Experienced donor surgeons can detect early fibrosis, steatosis, and other anatomic concerns (e.g. calcified vessels in the porta hepatis) that might necessitate non-transplantation of the liver. When donor quality is uncertain, liver biopsies can be obtained. Identification and preservation of accessory or variant hepatic arterial anatomy is important. Thorough flushing of the donor liver with preservation solution is imperative, and rapid external cooling of the liver with ice is recommended. Once the donor liver has been flushed, safe but rapid explant is necessary followed by a careful inspection for iatrogenic surgical damage on the donor-hospital back-table, and rapid transportation to the transplant center. In DCD procurements these critical steps happen on a very accelerated timescale and require an experienced surgeon.

Operative Set-Up and Recipient Preparation

Larger operating suites are preferred for liver transplantation to accommodate the equipment and personnel required. Electrocautery and argon plasma coagulation are generally considered essential. A variety of other surgical energy devices are variably utilized including bipolar, ultrasonic, and radiofrequency vessel sealing devices. Intraoperative blood salvage devices are frequently utilized. Anesthetic equipment must include a fluid warmer and rapid infusion device. Historically, liver transplantation was performed using veno-veno bypass; however, this invasive approach is now used less commonly [59].

Recipients are positioned supine with arms extended. Following intubation naso- or orogastric decompression is recommended and a Foley urinary catheter is placed. Arterial and central venous access are obtained. Use of a multi-lumen access catheter is preferred as the introducer portion allows for pulmonary artery catheter insertion and the infusion ports allow for rapid large-volume resuscitation. Additional large-bore intravenous access is highly recommended. Most liver transplant anesthesiologists employ either pulmonary artery catheter monitoring or continuous transesophageal echocardiographic monitoring, for minute-to-minute feedback on volume status and resuscitation needs. Preoperative antibiotics should include broad-spectrum Gram-positive and Gram-negative coverage. Antifungals are recommended in large-volume transfusions cases and are sometimes used in special circumstances (e.g. normothermic machine perfusion of the donor liver). Preoperative doses of steroid and calcineurin inhibitor are generally given. True inductive immunosuppression with lymphocyte depleting agents or other agents are not necessary. Coordination with the hospital blood bank is critical.

Intraoperative Anesthetic Care

Hemodynamics are typically labile during liver transplantation with large fluctuations in intravascular volume and significant acid-base shifts. Anesthetic care must be responsive and dynamic. Constant assessment of left ventricular filling and left ventricular function are keys to a safe operative course. Acute kidney injury and even renal failure requiring dialysis are common complications following liver transplantation, and these are best avoided with constant attention to volume status and effective communication between the surgical and anesthesia teams. Intraoperative CRRT is sometimes required to manage volume status in renal failure patients or acidosis in acute liver failure patients. Neuroprotection is equally important and requires monitoring of serum sodium and osmolarity, particularly in non-compensated recipients with acute liver failure. Active preparation for the hypotension, hyperkalemia, acidosis, and blood loss that can accompany allograft reperfusion are needed. Right heart dysfunction and intracardiac thrombosis are also risks.

Recipient Hepatectomy

A bilateral subcostal incision, with or without upward midline extension to the xiphoid, is commonly used for liver transplantation. A variety of other incisions including midline incisions, "hockey stick" incisions (right subcostal with midline extension), and "inverted T" incisions (bilateral subcostal with caudad midline extension) can be used in recipients with an accommodating body habitus. The falciform ligament is commonly recanalized and is usually divided with ties or a vascular stapler. The liver is fully mobilized taking down the right and left triangular ligaments. The anterior surface of the right and left-middle hepatic veins is exposed, and the right adrenal gland is released to allow visualization of the vena cava beneath the right hepatic lobe. The *pars flaccida* is opened. Excellent retraction is critical for success in liver transplantation and can be achieved with a variety of fixed retraction systems.

Once the liver is fully mobilized, the *porta hepatis* is dissected. Goals are to identify and carefully divide the hepatic artery and bile duct and to fully skeletonize the portal vein. It is important to preserve sufficient length on the hepatic artery and bile duct to allow for tension-free anastomoses to the donor equivalents. In deceased donor transplantation, dissection at the level of the mid-porta is usually sufficient. In LDLT, dissection takes place as close to the hilar plate as possible to preserve maximal length on all structures. In deceased donor transplantation, the proper hepatic artery may be used for anastomosis if it is of sufficient caliber, or dissection can proceed proximal to the gastroduodenal artery or even to the take-off of the splenic artery from the celiac trunk (Fig. 14.1). In LDLT, the gallbladder is retracted and the right hepatic artery is dissected all the way onto the cystic plate in an effort to attain maximal length and a caliber that will size-match well with the donor artery. The portal vein should be divided at its bifurcation in deceased donor transplantation and the right and left branches are usually taken individually in LDLT. The choice of when to divide the portal vein is situation-specific. Early division allows for greater mobility of the liver and can facilitate caval dissection, but prolonged

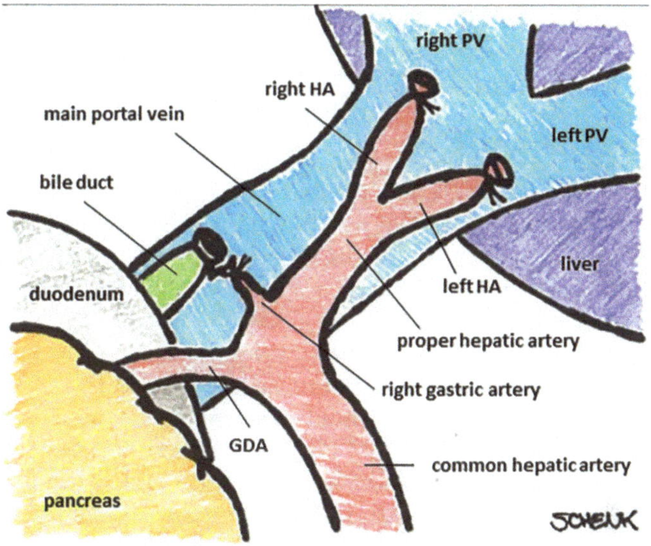

Fig. 14.1 Ideal dissection of the recipient hepatic artery during hepatectomy. With this exposure the proper hepatic artery can be clamped and the arterial anastomosis created where the right and left hepatic arteries bifurcate. Alternatively, the common hepatic artery can be clamped proximal to the gastroduodenal artery/GDA, the GDA can be divided, and the arterial anastomosis can be created using the common hepatic artery at the level of the GDA take-off

portal clamping times in patients without collateralization can lead to bowel edema and loss of domain.

The recipient hepatectomy is then typically completed in one of two ways. If caval interposition is planned, clamps are placed circumferentially about the suprahepatic vena cava and distal vena cava between the right adrenal vein and right renal vein. The liver is then cut out sharply preserving cuffs of tissue on the proximal and distal cavae to allow for subsequent anastomoses to the donor vena cava. If "piggyback" technique is employed, the short hepatic veins are ligated with clips and ties. The liver is "peeled off" of the cava until the right hepatic vein and left-middle hepatic veins can be divided and the liver fully explanted.

There are several keys to a successful recipient hepatectomy. Speed and efficiency are important to minimize cold ischemic time and reduce blood loss. Blood loss is sometimes vigorous, and two-way communication with the anesthesia team is important. Interval clamping the portal vein prior to its division can reduce blood loss from the liver itself, reduce liver volume to allow for better visibility, and portal venous congestion can be relieved by removing the portal vein clamp prior to final division of the portal vein. Prior to implantation, it is absolutely essential to verify that the portal vein and hepatic artery will provide the necessary vascular inflow and that the vena cava is clamped in a manner that will allow creation of unobstructed venous outflow. All potential inflow and outflow issues should be addressed before the donor liver is brought to the field for implantation.

Unique Vascular Considerations

Portal Vein Complications

Preoperatively the recipient surgeon should review CT or MR imaging and identify major porto-systemic collaterals. If portal flow is sluggish, ligation of collaterals can restore normal hepatopetal flow. Left renal vein ligation is a convenient strategy for closing splenorenal shunts [60, 61]. If portal vein thrombosis is encountered, eversion thromboendovenectomy [62] is the preferred approach. If the clot cannot be removed, donor iliac vein is generally attached to the superior mesenteric vein (SMV), and this "SMV jump graft" is tunneled to the porta in retrocolic fashion. If the SMV is unsuitable or inaccessible, alternative inflow options include large upper abdominal varices and the left renal vein [63, 64]. In emergent situations, portacaval transposition [65] or arterialization of the portal vein [66] can be considered. In LDTL, portal inflow can sometimes be too robust for the smaller living donor graft. Attenuation of portal flow is best achieved through splenic artery ligation or splenectomy [67].

Hepatic Artery Handling

If the recipient hepatic artery dissects or is otherwise unusable, donor iliac artery is used to create an aortic conduit. Preoperatively, it is useful to review recipient imaging and know the atherosclerotic burden in various sections of the aorta in case an aortic conduit is needed. If the conduit is created during the anhepatic phase, the supraceliac aorta is usually accessible. If the recipient hepatic artery dissects or thromboses during or after implantation, it is sometimes difficult to expose the supraceliac aorta, and in these cases, an infrarenal aortic conduit can be created. The ligament of Treitz is taken down to expose the infrarenal aorta and the conduit is tunneled to the porta in retrogastric retrocolic fashion. If the entire aorta is atherosclerotic, donor iliac arteries can be joined end-to-end, and a long conduit can be brought to the porta from the common or external iliac artery. Regardless of technique, robust arterial and portal inflow are essential to the success and longevity of any transplant (Table 14.4).

Table 14.4 Surgical options for portal vein problems

Ligation of porto-systemic collaterals to augment hepatopetal flow
Eversion thromboendovenectomy
Superior mesenteric vein jump grafting
Varicoportal anastomosis
Renoportal bypass
Portacaval transposition
Arterialization of the portal vein

Implantation

Implantation begins with the caval anastomosis. If caval interposition is used end-to-end, anastomoses are created between the donor and recipient suprahepatic and lower cavae (Fig. 14.2). In piggyback technique, several variants are possible. One option is to preserve length on the hepatic veins during hepatectomy. The hepatic veins can then be clamped at their junction with the cava. The donor suprahepatic cava is then sewn to either the left-middle hepatic vein orifice (while the right is oversewn) or to a large common orifice created by joining the left-middle and right

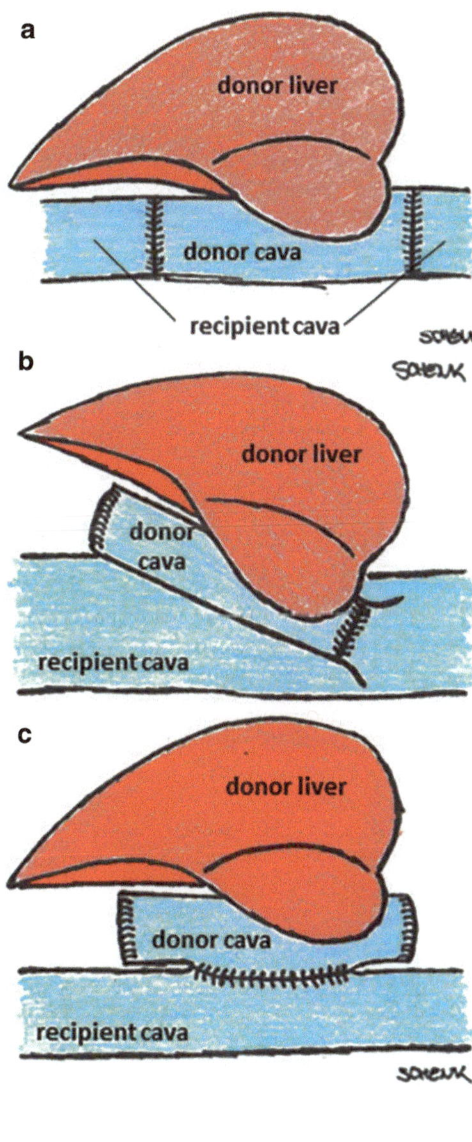

Fig. 14.2 Techniques for venous anastomosis during implantation. (**a**) Caval interposition technique, (**b**) piggyback technique using the recipient native hepatic vein orifices, (**c**) piggyback technique using a side-to-side anastomosis of the donor and recipient vena cava

hepatic veins. The lower cava is closed and never connected. Alternatively, a partially occluding clamp can be placed longitudinally along the recipient vena cava and a long longitudinal cavotomy is made (Fig. 14.3).

The suprahepatic and lower vena cavae on the donor are closed and a matching cavotomy is made along the undersurface of the donor cava. The liver is positioned in the right abdomen, and the donor and recipient cavae are joined in side-to-side

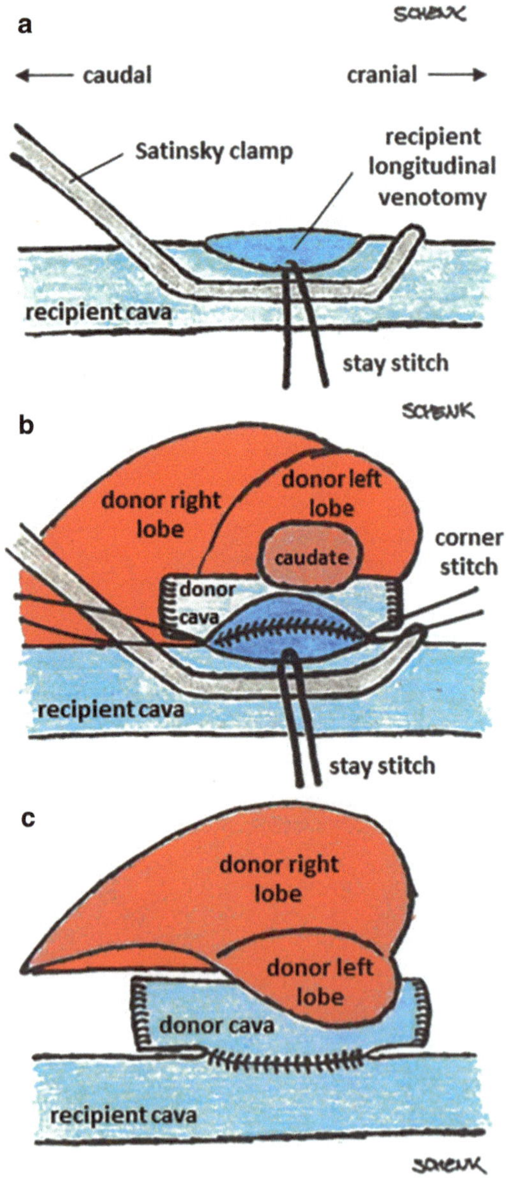

Fig. 14.3 Technique for side-to-side cavocavostomy. (**a**) A Satinsky clamp is placed longitudinally along the recipient vena cava such that it only partially occludes flow. A longitudinal venotomy is made. A stay stitch can be used to open the venotomy. (**b**) The donor liver is placed in the right upper quadrant such that the donor and recipient cavae lie adjacent. The back wall of the cavocavostomy is completed from the inside and the front wall is completed from the outside. (**c**) Final configuration following side-to-side cavocavostomy

fashion. Irrespective of technique, unobstructed outflow is essential. Venous outflow obstruction can cause venous congestion, hepatic dysfunction, ascites, and even thrombosis and allograft failure. In LDLT, the hepatic vein or veins are generally sewn to large cavotomies on the right-lateral side of the recipient cava so that the small hemi-liver can lie in the right abdomen, without twisting the recipient cava and obstructing hepatic venous outflow (Fig. 14.4).

Following the caval anastomosis, the donor and recipient portal veins are joined in end-to-end fashion taking care to shorten the donor vein as much as possible to avoid redundant bowing that can cause thrombosis. The arterial anastomosis can be completed before or after reperfusion of the allograft. A "parachuting" technique can facilitate rapid anastomosis when the arterial sewing angles are challenging. In DCD liver transplantation time to arterial reperfusion should be minimized to avoid ischemic cholangiopathy, and many centers infuse tissue plasminogen activator (TPA) via the hepatic artery prior to anastomosis to eliminate thrombi in the biliary microvasculature [68, 69].

Liver allograft reperfusion poses unique challenges [70]. Potassium and lactate loads, as well as cold preservation solution released from the donor liver, can cause substantial cardiac dysfunction as well as systemic vasoplegia. These are best avoided by thoroughly flushing and warming the liver. This can be achieved by opening the portal vein while the caval clamps remain in position. Blood fills the donor liver and can be drained through an open lower vena cava (in piggyback technique) or through a venting hole in an untied caval anastomosis (in caval interposition or LDLT). Once the liver is sufficiently "blood flushed" the caval anastomosis can be tied or the lower vena cava can be rapidly closed with a vascular stapler. The

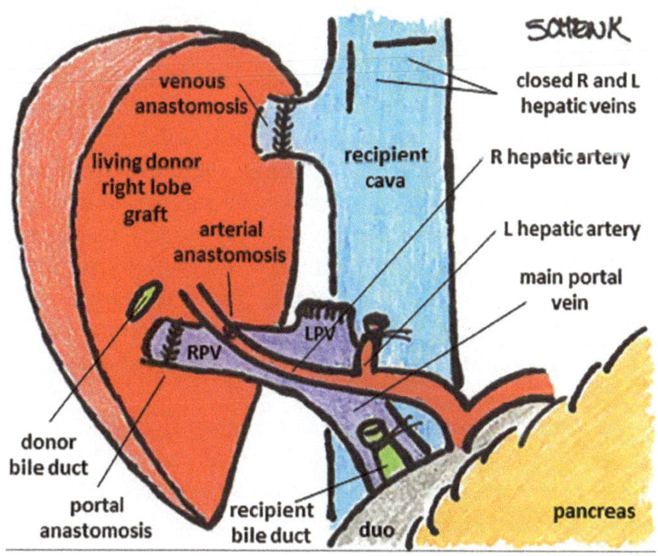

Fig. 14.4 Anatomic configuration of a living donor right lobe graft following venous, portal, and arterial anastomoses but prior to biliary reconstruction

caval clamps are then removed and the donor liver is then in full continuity with the recipient circulation. This technique markedly reduces the incidence of post-reperfusion arrest.

Biliary Reconstruction

Whenever possible, end-to-end anastomosis of the donor and recipient bile duct is preferred. Care is taken to make sure the anastomosis is well vascularized, tension-free, and non-redundant in length. Duct-to-duct anastomoses enable relatively easy post-transplant biliary interventions via endoscopic retrograde cholangio-pancreatography, which can be particularly useful in cases of biliary leak or stricture. Certain disease states (e.g. primary sclerosing cholangitis) or technical complications (e.g. dense scarring of the recipient duct in a re-operative scenario) prohibit use of the recipient duct. In these cases, biliary continuity is best restored with a Roux-en-Y hepaticojejunostomy. Choledochoduodenostomy has also been described and can be useful if the bowels are "frozen" from prior surgical procedures [71].

Hemostasis

Reoperation for post-operative bleeding occurs commonly in liver transplantation. Causative factors include raw surface area within the abdominal cavity, delayed production of clotting factors by the freshly transplanted liver, acidosis, hypothermia, and sometimes massive-transfusion coagulopathy. Meticulous attention to hemostasis during the hepatectomy and after implantation is necessary. Aside from balanced resuscitation with red cells, fresh frozen plasma, platelets and cryoprecipitate, adjunctive agents including aminocaproic acid, tranexamic acid, and prothrombin complex concentrate are sometimes used [72]. Intraoperative use of thromboelastography is particularly useful to guide balanced resuscitation [73]. It is crucial to understand that clotting factor replacement is extremely dynamic in the operating room and early post-operative period. A perfectly resuscitated patient may again suffer from coagulopathy due to ongoing factor consumption and submaximal production by the recovering allograft.

Both lab values and drain output character and quantity should be used to guide post-operative resuscitation in the intensive care unit, and administered products should be given promptly and should be warmed if possible. Abdominal packing and use of a temporary abdominal closure can be considered in cases where surgical or medical hemostasis is particularly challenging.

Complications

Current national one-year survival following adult liver transplantation in the US is estimated at 92% [3]. Causes of morbidity and mortality are varied but can be divided into intraoperative, perioperative, and remote events. Intraoperative catastrophes including fatal hemorrhage, air embolism, intraoperative myocardial infarction, post-reperfusion arrest, pulmonary embolism, and new right heart failure are all described. Fortunately, despite these possibilities, chances for on-table death during liver transplantation are exceedingly low in the modern era.

Primary Non-function (PNF)

This Primary non-function is a rare but ominous occurrence estimated to occur in ~2% of liver transplants [74]. Patients are urgently re-listed for liver transplantation. Occasionally the failing allograft acts similar to an abscess and patients can actually be stabilized by explanting the failed allograft, creating a portacaval shunt, and supporting the anhepatic patient in the intensive care unit prior to re-transplantation. More commonly, recipients experience early allograft dysfunction (EAD) [50] with elevated aminotranferases, bilirubin, or INR which reflect delayed or submaximal functioning of the allograft. The exact relationship between EAD and long-term allograft survival is controversial, but EAD certainly leads to increased length of stay and vulnerability to other in-hospital complications.

Hepatic artery thrombosis (HAT) and bile leak are uncommon but serious perioperative complications. HAT can, but does not always, manifest with deranged aminotransferases. Some centers perform routine post-transplant ultrasonography to surveil for HAT. If caught early, HAT can sometimes be salvaged with arterial thrombectomy, revision or the creation of a new arterial conduit. If undetected, HAT leads to progressive cholangiopathy, development of intrahepatic abscesses, and need for re-transplantation [75]. Bile leaks are estimated to occur following ~5–20% of liver transplants [76] and are typically detected via drain output, imaging, or a downturn in clinical trajectory. When a standard duct-to-duct biliary anastomosis was used, ERCP and stenting offer opportunity to control the leak. Reoperation for washout and wide drainage is sometimes necessary depending on the volume of bile spilled and the efficacy of the post-operative drains previously placed. Operative revision of the biliary anastomosis itself can be undertaken but is usually technically challenging in an inflamed or infected field with compromised tissue quality. Conversion to Roux-en-Y hepaticojejunostomy is often a preferred option when surgical revision is necessary. Percutaneous transhepatic cholangiocatheters are very useful for bile diversion in complex leaks.

Biliary stricture and ischemic cholangiopathy (IC) are often considered the Achilles' heels of liver transplantation. Biliary strictures are estimated to occur in 15–30% of deceased donor liver transplant recipients and 30–60% of LDLT recipients [77, 78]. Stenting and balloon dilation are the mainstays of management. IC can occur following any type of liver transplant but is typically associated with DCD donors. Historically, 8–12% rates of IC have been reported in DCD liver transplantation; however, rates as low as 1–2% have been reported in modern series [51]. IC can be of varying severity and can be categorized by location within the biliary tree [48]. Some forms of IC are amenable to endoscopic intervention and others require re-transplantation.

Late Complications

In the months and years following liver transplantation, recipients are monitored for rejection, common complications of immunosuppression, and recurrent liver disease. Rare but devastating conditions such as post-transplant lymphoproliferative disorder (PTLD) and graft-versus-host-disease (GVHD) do occur. Infections typically associated with lifelong immunosuppressive use include cytomegalovirus (CMV), Epstein-Barr virus, and *Pneumocystis carini* pneumonia (PCP). Leading causes of late mortality in liver transplant recipients include de novo malignancies, cardiovascular complications, and infection (Table 14.5).

Table 14.5 Complications of liver transplantation

Intra-operative
Hemorrhage
Air embolism
Intraoperative myocardial infarction
Post-reperfusion arrest
Pulmonary embolism
New right heart failure
Perioperative
Primary non-function (PNF)
Early allograft dysfunction (EAD)
Hepatic arterial thrombosis (HAT)
Bile leak
Early and late post-operative
Biliary stricture
Ischemic cholangiopathy (IC)
Rejection
Renal failure
Recurrent liver disease
Post-transplant lymphoproliferative disease (PTLD)
Graft-versus host disease (GVHD)
CMV, EBV, HSV, PCP infections
de novo malignancy
Cardiovascular complications

CMV Cytomegalovirus, *EBV* Epstein-Barr virus, *HSV* Herpes simplex virus, *PCP* Pneumocystis carini

Post-Operative Care

The average hospital length of stay following liver transplantation is 10 days. Many recipients require additional nursing care or physical therapy following hospital discharge which can involve a rehabilitation facility or at-home services. Most common immunosuppression regimens include a calcineurin inhibitor, mycophenolate mofetil, and a corticosteroid taper [79]. Bloodwork is usually checked twice weekly initially and with reduced frequency as time passes. Particular attention must be paid to calcineurin inhibitor levels. High levels are nephrotoxic and cause a wide range of side effects, and low levels may precipitate rejection. Proactive long-term care of liver transplant recipients includes regular dermatology follow-up, timely cancer screening, attention to modifiable cardiovascular risk factors, monitoring of bone density and renal function, and the provision of appropriate immunizations.

Measuring Success

One-year patient and graft survival, though valuable, fail to address the overall efficacy of the transplant center in serving a population of patients with ESLD and also fail to capture patient experience and satisfaction [80]. There is increasing interest in composite metrics, such as "textbook outcome," that capture transplant center performance in multiple domains and offer more holistic definitions of quality and success [81]. Regulatory monitoring is evolving as well. Transplant centers are now accountable for risk-adjusted waitlist mortality and organ offer acceptance rates, in addition to patient and graft survival [82]. Lastly, numerous disparities in access to liver transplantation have been identified. Organ allocation policy has been substantially revised in an effort to promote equity [83].

Future Perspectives

Despite harrowing origins in which liver transplantation was described by some as unethical, liver transplantation is now widely recognized as safe standard-of-care therapy for patients with otherwise incurable liver disease. The future of liver transplantation is bright. Indications for liver transplantation, particularly within the emerging domain of transplant oncology, are expanding. Growing world-wide experience with LDLT has increased the safety profile of this operation. Broader donor utilization is now possible because of advances in organ preservation and maturation of the techniques required for safe utilization of DCD donors. Long-term patient and graft survival continue to improve. Better immunosuppressive drugs are in development and transplant immunobiologists are moving closer to the goal of immunologic tolerance. Moving forward, the field is challenged to identify all potential beneficiaries and ensure broad, rapid, and equal access to liver transplantation for all patients in need.

References

1. Cazes B. 1st world attempt at homotransplantation of the liver in man (Denver, Colorado, USA). Presse Med. 1963;71:1695–6.
2. Scientific Registry of Transplant Recipients STAR File Data Dictionary. srtr.org/requesting-srtr-data/saf-data-dictionary. Accessed 31 July 2023.
3. OPTN/SRTR 2021 Annual Data Report. HHS/HRSA; 2023. srtr.transplant.hrsa.gov/annual_reports/Default.aspx. Accessed 31 July 2023.
4. Jimenez-Perez M, Gonzalez-Grande R, Rando-Munoz FJ. Management of recurrent hepatitis C virus after liver transplantation. World J Gastroenterol. 2014;20(44):16409–17.
5. Sobotka LA, Mumtaz K, Wellner MR, et al. Outcomes of hepatitis C virus seropositive donors to hepatitis C virus seronegative liver recipients: a large single center analysis. Ann Hepatol. 2021;24:100318.
6. Kapila N, Menon KVN, Al-Khalloufi K, et al. Hepatitis C virus NAT-positive solid organ allografts transplanted into hepatitis C virus-negative recipients: a real-world experience. Hepatology. 2020;72(1):32–41.
7. Quaresima S, Melandro F, Giovanardi F, et al. New insights in the setting of transplant oncology. Medicina. 2023;59(3)
8. Shannon AH, Ruff SM, Schenk AD, Washburn K, Pawlik TM. Updates and expert opinions on liver transplantation for gastrointestinal malignancies. Medicina. 2023;59(7)
9. Martin P, DiMartini A, Feng S, Brown R Jr, Fallon M. Evaluation for liver transplantation in adults: 2013 practice guideline by the American Association for the Study of Liver Diseases and the American Society of Transplantation. Hepatology. 2014;59(3):1144–65.
10. Kriss M, Biggins SW. Evaluation and selection of the liver transplant candidate: updates on a dynamic and evolving process. Curr Opin Organ Transplant. 2021;26(1):52–61.
11. Lai JC, Sonnenday CJ, Tapper EB, et al. Frailty in liver transplantation: an expert opinion statement from the American Society of Transplantation Liver and Intestinal Community of Practice. Am J Transplant. 2019;19(7):1896–906.
12. Krowka MJ, Plevak DJ, Findlay JY, Rosen CB, Wiesner RH, Krom RA. Pulmonary hemodynamics and perioperative cardiopulmonary-related mortality in patients with portopulmonary hypertension undergoing liver transplantation. Liver Transpl. 2000;6(4):443–50.
13. Mousa OY, Nguyen JH, Ma Y, et al. Evolving role of liver transplantation in elderly recipients. Liver Transpl. 2019;25(9):1363–74.
14. Mohan BP, Iriana S, Khan SR, Yarra P, Ponnada S, Gallegos-Orozco JF. Outcomes of liver transplantation in patients 70 years or older: a systematic review and meta-analysis. Ann Hepatol. 2022;27(6):100741.
15. Lai JC, Shui AM, Duarte-Rojo A, et al. Association of frailty with health-related quality of life in liver transplant recipients. JAMA Surg. 2023;158(2):130–8.
16. Lai JC, Shui AM, Duarte-Rojo A, et al. Frailty, mortality, and health care utilization after liver transplantation: From the Multicenter Functional Assessment in Liver Transplantation (FrAILT) Study. Hepatology. 2022;75(6):1471–9.
17. Kaur N, Emamaullee J, Lian T, et al. Impact of morbid obesity on liver transplant candidacy and outcomes: national and regional trends. Transplantation. 2021;105(5):1052–60.
18. Dick AA, Spitzer AL, Seifert CF, et al. Liver transplantation at the extremes of the body mass index. Liver Transpl. 2009;15(8):968–77.
19. Mazzaferro V, Regalia E, Doci R, et al. Liver transplantation for the treatment of small hepatocellular carcinomas in patients with cirrhosis. NEJM. 1996;334(11):693–9.
20. Yao FY, Ferrell L, Bass NM, et al. Liver transplantation for hepatocellular carcinoma: expansion of the tumor size limits does not adversely impact survival. Hepatology. 2001;33(6):1394–403.
21. DuBay D, Sandroussi C, Sandhu L, et al. Liver transplantation for advanced hepatocellular carcinoma using poor tumor differentiation on biopsy as an exclusion criterion. Ann Surg. 2011;253(1):166–72.

22. Sapisochin G, Goldaracena N, Laurence JM, et al. The extended Toronto criteria for liver transplantation in patients with hepatocellular carcinoma: a prospective validation study. Hepatology. 2016;64(6):2077–88.
23. Verna EC, Pereira MR. Transplanting patients with active bacterial infection. Clin Liver Dis. 2017;9(4):81–5.
24. McDonald DP, Leithead JA, Gunson BK, Ferguson JW. Subclinical spontaneous bacterial peritonitis at the time of liver transplantation does not impact on outcomes. Eur J Gastroenterol Hepatol. 2016;28(1):101–6.
25. Bert F, Larroque B, Paugam-Burtz C, et al. Microbial epidemiology and outcome of bloodstream infections in liver transplant recipients: an analysis of 259 episodes. Liver Transpl. 2010;16(3):393–401.
26. Marroni CA, Fleck AM Jr, Fernandes SA, et al. Liver transplantation and alcoholic liver disease: history, controversies, and considerations. World J Gastroenterol. 2018;24(26):2785–805.
27. Webzell I, Ball D, Bell J, et al. Substance use by liver transplant candidates: an anonymous urinalysis study. Liver Transpl. 2011;17(10):1200–4.
28. Kotwani P, Saxena V, Dodge JL, Roberts J, Yao F, Hameed B. History of marijuana use does not affect outcomes on the liver transplant waitlist. Transplantation. 2018;102(5):794–802.
29. Herrick-Reynolds KM, Punchhi G, Greenberg RS, et al. Evaluation of early vs standard liver transplant for alcohol-associated liver disease. JAMA Surg. 2021;156(11):1026–34.
30. Weeks SR, Sun Z, McCaul ME, et al. Liver transplantation for severe alcoholic hepatitis, updated lessons from the world's largest series. J Am Coll Surg. 2018;226(4):549–57.
31. Choudhary NS, Saraf N, Mehrotra S, Saigal S, Soin AS. Recidivism in liver transplant recipients for alcohol-related liver disease. J Clin Exp Hepatol. 2021;11(3):387–96.
32. Chuncharunee L, Yamashiki N, Thakkinstian A, Sobhonslidsuk A. Alcohol relapse and its predictors after liver transplantation for alcoholic liver disease: a systematic review and meta-analysis. BMC Gastroenterol. 2019;19(1):150.
33. Queck A, Weiler N, Trebicka J. Transplantation in acute-on-chronic liver failure: feasibility and futility. Clin Liver Dis. 2022;19(5):191–3.
34. Engelmann C, Thomsen KL, Zakeri N, et al. Validation of CLIF-C ACLF score to define a threshold for futility of intensive care support for patients with acute-on-chronic liver failure. Crit Care. 2018;22(1):254.
35. Cardoso FS, Gottfried M, Tujios S, Olson JC, Karvellas CJ, Group USALFS. Continuous renal replacement therapy is associated with reduced serum ammonia levels and mortality in acute liver failure. Hepatology. 2018;67(2):711–20.
36. Slack AJ, Auzinger G, Willars C, et al. Ammonia clearance with haemofiltration in adults with liver disease. Liver Int. 2014;34(1):42–8.
37. Garcia Martinez JJ, Bendjelid K. Artificial liver support systems: what is new over the last decade? Ann Intensive Care. 2018;8(1):109.
38. Mitzner SR. Extracorporeal liver support-albumin dialysis with the Molecular Adsorbent Recirculating System (MARS). Ann Hepatol. 2011;10(Suppl 1):S21–8.
39. Bernardi M, Zaccherini G. Approach and management of dysnatremias in cirrhosis. Hepatol Int. 2018;12(6):487–99.
40. Malinchoc M, Kamath PS, Gordon FD, Peine CJ, Rank J, ter Borg PC. A model to predict poor survival in patients undergoing transjugular intrahepatic portosystemic shunts. Hepatology. 2000;31(4):864–71.
41. Sacleux SC, Samuel D. A critical review of MELD as a reliable tool for transplant prioritization. Semin Liver Dis. 2019;39(4):403–13.
42. Median MELD at transplant by 250 nautical mile circles around liver transplant programs and median PELD at transplant within the nation. https://www.optn.transplant.hrsa.gov/media/ko5n33do/mts_distribution_document_2022mar8.pdf. Accessed 31 July 2023.
43. Office of the Inspector General; Fostering Equity in Patient Access to Transplantation: Differences in Waiting times for Livers. https://www.oig.hhs.gov/oei/reports/oei-01-99-00210.pdf. Accessed 31 July 2023.

44. Saab S, Ibrahim AB, Shpaner A, et al. MELD fails to measure quality of life in liver transplant candidates. Liver Transpl. 2005;11(2):218–23.
45. Roberts JP, Hulbert-Shearon TE, Merion RM, Wolfe RA, Port FK. Influence of graft type on outcomes after pediatric liver transplantation. Am J Transplant. 2004;4(3):373–7.
46. Cotter TG, Minhem M, Wang J, et al. Living donor liver transplantation in the United States: evolution of frequency, outcomes, center volumes, and factors associated with outcomes. Liver Transpl. 2021;27(7):1019–31.
47. Abu-Gazala S, Olthoff KM. Current status of living donor liver transplantation in the United States. Annu Rev Med. 2019;70:225–38.
48. Croome KP, Mathur AK, Aqel B, et al. Classification of distinct patterns of ischemic cholangiopathy following DCD liver transplantation: distinct clinical courses and long-term outcomes from a multicenter cohort. Transplantation. 2022;106(6):1206–14.
49. Mourad MM, Algarni A, Liossis C, Bramhall SR. Aetiology and risk factors of ischaemic cholangiopathy after liver transplantation. World J Gastroenterol. 2014;20(20):6159–69.
50. Olthoff KM, Kulik L, Samstein B, et al. Validation of a current definition of early allograft dysfunction in liver transplant recipients and analysis of risk factors. Liver Transpl. 2010;16(8):943–9.
51. Limkemann AJ, Singh N, Helfrich K, et al. Safely expanding the liver donor pool by utilization of organs from donation after circulatory death with comparable results to donation after brain death, a large single-center experience. J Gastrointest Surg. 2022;26(7):1453–61.
52. Duran M, Calleja R, Hann A, et al. Machine perfusion and the prevention of ischemic type biliary lesions following liver transplant: what is the evidence? World J Gastroenterol. 2023;29(20):3066–83.
53. Sousa Da Silva RX, Weber A, Dutkowski P, Clavien PA. Machine perfusion in liver transplantation. Hepatology. 2022;76(5):1531–49.
54. Schiff T, Koziatek C, Pomerantz E, et al. Extracorporeal cardiopulmonary resuscitation dissemination and integration with organ preservation in the USA: ethical and logistical considerations. Crit Care. 2023;27(1):144.
55. Pasrija C, Tipograf Y, Shah AS, Trahanas JM. Normothermic regional perfusion for donation after circulatory death donors. Curr Opin Organ Transplant. 2023;28(2):71–5.
56. Merion RM, Schaubel DE, Dykstra DM, Freeman RB, Port FK, Wolfe RA. The survival benefit of liver transplantation. Am J Transplant. 2005;5(2):307–13.
57. Feng S, Goodrich NP, Bragg-Gresham JL, et al. Characteristics associated with liver graft failure: the concept of a donor risk index. Am J Transplant. 2006;6(4):783–90.
58. Park JB, Kwon CH, Choi GS, et al. Prolonged cold ischemic time is a risk factor for biliary strictures in duct-to-duct biliary reconstruction in living donor liver transplantation. Transplantation. 2008;86(11):1536–42.
59. Lapisatepun W, Lapisatepun W, Agopian V, Xia VW. Venovenous bypass during liver transplantation: a new look at an old technique. Transplant Proc. 2020;52(3):905–9.
60. Singh N, Washburn K, Black S, Schenk A. Techniques for management of portal vein thrombosis during liver transplantation. Case Rep Transplant. 2020;2020:8875196.
61. Slater RR, Jabbour N, Abbass AA, et al. Left renal vein ligation: a technique to mitigate low portal flow from splenic vein siphon during liver transplantation. Am J Transplant. 2011;11(8):1743–7.
62. Robles R, Fernandez JA, Hernandez Q, et al. Eversion thromboendovenectomy in organized portal vein thrombosis during liver transplantation. Clin Transpl. 2004;18(1):79–84.
63. Alexopoulos SP, Thomas E, Berry E, Whang G, Matsuoka L. The portal vein-variceal anastomosis: an important technique for establishing portal vein inflow. Clin Transpl. 2014;28(1):52–7.
64. Quintini C, Spaggiari M, Hashimoto K, et al. Safety and effectiveness of renoportal bypass in patients with complete portal vein thrombosis: an analysis of 10 patients. Liver Transpl. 2015;21(3):344–52.
65. Ceulemans B, Aerts R, Monbaliu D, et al. Liver transplantation using cavoportal transposition: an effective treatment in patients with complete splanchnic venous thrombosis. Transplant Proc. 2005;37(2):1112–4.

66. Paloyo S, Nishida S, Fan J, et al. Portal vein arterialization using an accessory right hepatic artery in liver transplantation. Liver Transpl. 2013;19(7):773–5.
67. Yoshizumi T, Mori M. Portal flow modulation in living donor liver transplantation: review with a focus on splenectomy. Surg Today. 2020;50(1):21–9.
68. Jayant K, Reccia I, Virdis F, Shapiro AMJ. Systematic review and meta-analysis on the impact of thrombolytic therapy in liver transplantation following donation after circulatory death. J Clin Med. 2018;7(11)
69. Hashimoto K, Eghtesad B, Gunasekaran G, et al. Use of tissue plasminogen activator in liver transplantation from donation after cardiac death donors. Am J Transplant. 2010;10(12):2665–72.
70. Gurusamy KS, Naik P, Abu-Amara M, Fuller B, Davidson BR. Techniques of flushing and reperfusion for liver transplantation. Cochrane Database Syst Rev. 2012;14(3):CD007512.
71. Truong R, Moore HB, Sauaia A, et al. Choledochoduodenostomy continues to be a safe alternative for biliary reconstruction in deceased-donor liver transplantation. Am J Surg. 2022;224(6):1398–402.
72. Yoon U, Bartoszko J, Bezinover D, et al. Intraoperative transfusion management, antifibrinolytic therapy, coagulation monitoring and the impact on short-term outcomes after liver transplantation-a systematic review of the literature and expert panel recommendations. Clin Transpl. 2022;36(10):e14637.
73. Roullet S, Freyburger G, Cruc M, et al. Management of bleeding and transfusion during liver transplantation before and after the introduction of a rotational thromboelastometry-based algorithm. Liver Transpl. 2015;21(2):169–79.
74. Hartog H, Hann A, Perera M. Primary nonfunction of the liver allograft. Transplantation. 2022;106(1):117–28.
75. Mourad MM, Liossis C, Gunson BK, et al. Etiology and management of hepatic artery thrombosis after adult liver transplantation. Liver Transpl. 2014;20(6):713–23.
76. Kochhar G, Parungao JM, Hanouneh IA, Parsi MA. Biliary complications following liver transplantation. World J Gastroenterol. 2013;19(19):2841–6.
77. Fasullo M, Patel M, Khanna L, Shah T. Post-transplant biliary complications: advances in pathophysiology, diagnosis, and treatment. BMJ Open Gastroenterol. 2022;9(1):e000778.
78. Rao HB, Prakash A, Sudhindran S, Venu RP. Biliary strictures complicating living donor liver transplantation: problems, novel insights and solutions. World J Gastroenterol. 2018;24(19):2061–72.
79. Montano-Loza AJ, Rodriguez-Peralvarez ML, Pageaux GP, Sanchez-Fueyo A, Feng S. Liver transplantation immunology: immunosuppression, rejection, and immunomodulation. J Hepatol. 2023;78(6):1199–215.
80. Mathur AK, Talwalkar J. Quality measurement and improvement in liver transplantation. J Hepatol. 2018;68(6):1300–10.
81. Schenk AD, Han JL, Logan AJ, et al. Textbook outcome as a quality metric in liver transplantation. Transplant Direct. 2022;8(5):e1322.
82. OPTN Enhanced Transplant Program Performance Metrics. optn.transplant.hrsa.gov/media/r5lmmgcl/mpsc_performancemetrics_3242022b.pdf. Accessed 4 Aug 2023.
83. Chan E, Logan AJ, Sneddon JM, et al. Dynamic impact of liver allocation policy change on donor utilization. Am J Transplant. 2022;22(7):1901–8.

Part IV
Protocols of Special Relevance

Chapter 15
Immunization Routines for Surgical Splenectomy

Michelle Lippincott and Vic Velanovich

Splenic Anatomy and Function

The spleen is the largest secondary lymphoid organ in the body and is unique in structure and function. It is the only portion of the lymphatic system with a direct blood supply. This feature allows it to filter non-functional or damaged blood cells and opsonized particulates. Furthermore, by facilitating otherwise low-probability interactions between antigen-presenting cells (APCs) and cognate lymphocytes, it serves as a bridge between the adaptive and innate immune response [1].

The splenic parenchyma consists of three distinct functional "zones." These are termed the white pulp, red pulp, and marginal zone (also the perifollicular zone). The red pulp makes up the majority of the splenic parenchyma. It consists of a system of cords that lack endothelium and allow for direct interaction of red pulp macrophages with the contents of the blood [2]. These macrophages serve to remove damaged or opsonized cells or pathogens [1, 3]. The white pulp is the primary site of adaptive immune response in the spleen. It is analogous to lymph nodes containing distinct T and B cell zones. The white pulp's adaptive response results from interactions between antigen-presenting cells and B or T lymphocytes [2–4]. This interaction produces highly specific antibodies against encountered pathogens for adaptive immunity [3]. The marginal zone abuts the white pulp and contains marginal zone B cells. These act as the primary response against bloodborne pathogens. These B cells form IgM antibodies that promote T-cell responses [3]. Marginal zone location of memory B cells that produce IgM, which is critical for the opsonization of encapsulated bacteria [4].

M. Lippincott · V. Velanovich (✉)
Department of Surgery, Morsani College of Medicine, The University of South Florida, Tampa, FL, USA
e-mail: mlippincott@usf.edu; vvelanov@usf.edu

© The Author(s), under exclusive license to Springer Nature Switzerland AG 2024

J. Faintuch, S. Faintuch (eds.), *Recent Strategies in High Risk Surgery*,
https://doi.org/10.1007/978-3-031-56270-9_15

Overwhelming Post-splenectomy Infection

Increased risk of infection is a well-known complication of splenectomy [5–7]. Overwhelming post-splenectomy infection (OPSI) describes fulminant sepsis unique to asplenic patients. Without opsonization, infection with encapsulated organisms can quickly progress to life-threatening sepsis. Notably, *Streptococcus pneumoniae* causes 50–90% [6, 8] of these infections, followed by *Haemophilus influenzae* and *Neisseria meningitidis* [4, 5]. Other implicated organisms with higher disease risk in asplenic patients include *Plasmodium falciparum*, *Babesia microti*, and *Capnocytophaga canimorsus* [8]. Asplenic patients also have an increased risk of infection from non-encapsulated organisms [5].

The incidence of invasive infection in patients undergoing splenectomy for all indications is 3.2% [5]. Although the incidence is low, the mortality rate is 50–70% [7], with death resulting from septic shock, multisystem organ failure, disseminated intravascular coagulation, and adrenal hemorrhage.

The concern about OPSI leads to various techniques for splenic salvage in hopes of preserving splenic function. It is not the purpose of this chapter to review such techniques, but these include operative splenic salvage, partial splenectomy, and selective splenic artery branch embolization [9]. Nevertheless, despite these efforts, splenectomy for trauma and disease may be unavoidable.

One of the potential consequences of splenic trauma, with or without splenectomy, is splenosis. Splenosis occurs with fragments of the injured implant onto various surfaces of the peritoneal cavity, with the most likely location being the omentum [10]. Although splenosis at one time was thought to provide some immune function, this function is not sufficient to provide a reliable method to prevent OPSI [10]. Therefore, the presence of splenosis, or accessory spleens for that matter, should not be the reason to avoid post-splenectomy immunizations.

The data regarding OPSI is limited by the wide variety of indications for splenectomy and the need for subgroup analysis. We know that the incidence of post-splenectomy sepsis is similar in adults and children, though the mortality is higher in children [5]. Adult patients who undergo splenectomy for non-traumatic causes carry a higher risk of infection than their traumatic counterparts; this includes infections with non-encapsulated organisms [11]. In both adults and children, infection rates are highest in patients undergoing splenectomy for thalassemia major and sickle cell anemia [5]. The timing of OPSI after splenectomy is not well agreed upon though the quoted overall mean time to the onset of infection was 22.6 months for all causes of splenectomy [5].

The mainstay of treatment of post-splenectomy sepsis involves early identification and treatment with empiric broad-spectrum antibiotics. Early identification and treatment may reduce mortality by 10% [12].

Lastly, although OPSI is the most feared of post-splenectomy complications, other infectious adverse outcomes also occur. These include intra-abdominal abscesses, pneumonia, surgical site infections, as well as others [13]. These infections tend to occur in the peri-operative period, whereas OPSI tends to occur months or years after splenectomy.

Immunization Recommendation for Asplenic or Hyposplenic Patients

Indications and Timing

Post-splenectomy vaccines are mandated in all patients undergoing splenectomy for any indication. Immunizations are not recommended in patients who have undergone angioembolization as these patients have preserved splenic immune function [14]. For the purpose of this book, guidelines for vaccinations are limited to adults.

In cases of elective splenectomy, the initial dose of vaccines should be given at least 14 days before surgery, and in some cases, are recommended 4–6 weeks preoperatively [15]. In cases of unplanned splenectomy, they should be given immediately post-operatively once the patient's condition is stable [16].

Pneumococcal Pneumoniae

The United States Centers for Disease Control (CDC) recommendations for vaccination of anatomically or functional asplenic adults are as follows [16]:

- PCV13 vaccine either pre-operatively or immediately post-op
- PPSV23 8 weeks after PCV 13
- PPSV23 5 years following the first dose of PPSV23

Neisseria Meningitidis

CDC recommendations for Neisseria meningitidis vaccination in asplenic patients consist of recommendations for ACWY serotypes and B serotypes as listed below [16]:

Meningococcal Serotypes—ACWY:

- 2 dose series of either MenAWCY vaccine 8 weeks apart [MenACWY-CRM (Menevo) OR MenACWY-D (Menactra)]
- Repeat in 5 years if last dose was at age >7, 3 years if last dose at age <7
- Of note, MenACWY-D should not be given concomitantly with PCV13 but instead 4 weeks afterward as this can attenuate antibody response to PCV13. MenAVWY-CRM can be given concomitantly with PCV13.

Meningococcal B:

- Two-dose series of MenB-4C (Bexsero), 1 month apart OR
- Three-dose series of MenB-FHbp (Trumenba) with dose 2 at 1–2 months and dose 3 at 6 months
- Either can be given concomitantly with Men-ACWY
- There are no recommendations for boosters for MenB

Hemophaelous Influenzae

- One-time dose of *Haemophilus influenzae* type B conjugate vaccine [16].

Influenza

- Administer seasonal influenza vaccine to asplenic patients to mitigate the risk of secondary pneumonia [15].
- Asplenic patients should not receive live attenuated vaccines.

Challenges with Immunizations

As one can see by the schedule provided above, obtaining the appropriate vaccinations can be a daunting task and requires 7–9 vaccinations within the first 12 months post-splenectomy. The studied booster compliance rate is poor [17–19]. Suggested interventions to improve compliance include patient education and surgeon ownership of the vaccine schedule [15].

Prophylactic Antibiotics

In addition to immunizations, the asplenic patient, as well as their family members, need to be appraised of the early signs and symptoms of OPSI. This is vital as OPSI is a rapidly progressing disease, and the time period from first symptoms to death can be short, measured in hours to a few days. Therefore, the American Society of Hematology recommends prophylactic antibiotics, depending on age, time since splenectomy, degree of immunocompromise, or prior episodes of sepsis for adults of penicillin VK 250 mg orally twice a day (or cephalexin 250 mg orally twice a day for patients with penicillin allergies). For patients with early signs of sepsis (e.g., fever), emergency antibiotic administration prior to arrival to an emergency department of amoxicillin-clavulanate 875/125 mg orally twice a day [20]. Therefore, asplenic patients should have such antibiotics on hand for immediate use if symptoms of infections occur.

Conclusions

Vaccinations in splenectomized patients are of the utmost importance in preventing life-threatening infections. Although well defined, the current guidelines for vaccination can be confusing for patients and providers. Furthermore, the logistical challenge of providing these vaccines can lead to poor compliance and suboptimal benefit regarding infection prevention. This challenge highlights the importance of surgeon involvement in maintaining up-to-date knowledge of these vaccine schedules and identifying barriers to obtaining such immunizations.

References

1. Lewis SM, Williams A, Eisenbarth SC. Structure and function of the immune system in the spleen. Sci Immunol. 2019;4 https://doi.org/10.1126/sciimmunol.aau6085.
2. Mebius RE, Kraal G. Structure and function of the spleen. Nat Rev Immunol. 2005;5:606–16. https://doi.org/10.1038/nri1669.
3. Kuchar E, Miśkiewicz K, Karlikowska M. A review of guidance on immunization in persons with defective or deficient splenic function. Brit J Haematol. 2015;171:683–94. https://doi.org/10.1111/bjh.13660.
4. Sabatino AD, Carsetti R, Corazza GR. Post-splenectomy and hyposplenic states. Lancet. 2011;378:86–97. https://doi.org/10.1016/s0140-6736(10)61493-6.
5. Bisharat N, Omari H, Lavi I, Raz R. Risk of infection and death among post-splenectomy patients. J Infection. 2001;43:182–6. https://doi.org/10.1053/jinf.2001.0904.
6. Spelman D, Buttery J, Daley A, et al. Guidelines for the prevention of sepsis in asplenic and hyposplenic patients. Intern Med J. 2008;38:349–56. https://doi.org/10.1111/j.1445-5994.2007.01579.x.
7. Holdsworth RJ, Cuschieri A, Irving AD. Postsplenectomy sepsis and its mortality rate: actual versus perceived risks. Br J Surg. 1991;78:1031–8. https://doi.org/10.1002/bjs.1800780904.
8. Sinwar PD. Overwhelming post splenectomy infection syndrome—review study. Int J Surg. 2014;12:1314–6. https://doi.org/10.1016/j.ijsu.2014.11.005.
9. Coccolini F, Montori G, Catena F, et al. Splenic trauma: WSES classification and guidelines for adult and pediatric patients. World J Emerg Surg. 2017;12:40. https://doi.org/10.1186/s13017-017-0151-4.
10. Connell NT, Brunner AM, Kerr CA, Schiffman FJ. Splenosis and sepsis: the born-again spleen provides poor protection. Virulence. 2011;2:4–11. https://doi.org/10.4161/viru.2.1.14611.
11. Camejo L, Nandeesha N, Phan K, et al. Infectious outcomes after splenectomy for trauma, splenectomy for disease and splenectomy with distal pancreatectomy. Langenbecks Arch Surg. 2022;407:1685–91. https://doi.org/10.1007/s00423-022-02446-3.
12. Brigden M, Pattullo AL. Prevention and management of overwhelming postsplenectomy infection—an update. Crit Care Med. 1999;27:836–42.
13. Vagholkar DK. Complications of splenectomy. Int J Surg Sci. 2020;4:218–22. https://doi.org/10.33545/surgery.2020.v4.i2d.420.
14. Freeman JJ, Yorkgitis BK, Haines K, et al. Vaccination after spleen embolization: a practice management guideline from the Eastern Association for the Surgery of Trauma. Injury. 2022;53:3569–74. https://doi.org/10.1016/j.injury.2022.08.006.
15. Casciani F, Trudeau MT, Vollmer CM. Perioperative immunization for splenectomy and the surgeon's responsibility. JAMA Surg. 2020;155:1068–77. https://doi.org/10.1001/jamasurg.2020.1463.
16. Kroger A, Bahta L, Long S, Sanchez P. Advisory Committee on Immunization Practices (ACIP) general best guidance for immunization; 2023. https://www.cdc.gov/vaccines/hcp/acip-recs/general-recs/downloads/general-recs.pdf. Accessed 29 March 2023.
17. Gonzalez RA, Robbins JM, Garwe T, et al. Effect of post-splenectomy booster vaccine program on vaccination compliance in trauma patients. Am Surg. 2021;87:796–804. https://doi.org/10.1177/0003134820956274.

18. Alvarado AR, Udobi K, Berry S, et al. An opportunity for improvement in trauma care: 8-week booster vaccination adherence among patients after trauma splenectomy. Surgery. 2018;163:415–8. https://doi.org/10.1016/j.surg.2017.09.037.
19. Bianchi FP, Stefanizzi P, Spinelli G, et al. Immunization coverage among asplenic patients and strategies to increase vaccination compliance: a systematic review and meta-analysis. Expert Rev Vaccines. 2021;20:297–308. https://doi.org/10.1080/14760584.2021.1886085.
20. Lee GM. Preventing infections in children and adults with asplenia. Hematology. 2020;2020:328–35. https://doi.org/10.1182/hematology.2020000117.

Chapter 16
Management of the Difficulty Airway in the Perioperative Period (A Surgical Perspective)

R. H. Kelley, D. C. Sullivan, and J. A. Scott

Introduction

Complications associated with airway management are the leading cause of death or permanent brain damage in otherwise healthy patients who undergo anesthesia for elective procedures [1]. A one-year review of major airway complications at National Health Services Hospitals, UK (NAP4) found 46 events per million general anesthetics, with an associated mortality of 5.6 per million. Difficult or delayed intubation, failed intubation and a catastrophic scenario now referred to as "can't intubate can't oxygenate" accounted for an estimated 39% of events [2].

There is evidence that repeated conventional tracheal intubation attempts contributes to patient morbidity. A practice analysis of emergent intubations showed that beyond two intubation attempts there is an increase in hypoxemia, esophageal intubation, regurgitation, aspiration, bradycardia, airway trauma and cardiac arrest [3].

Airway complications can result in adverse outcomes including brain injury, cardiopulmonary arrest, airway trauma, need for emergency surgical airway access and unanticipated ICU stay [3–5]. Data from the United States published in 2009 shows mortality rate of 1.1 per million for patients undergoing anesthesia, with 2.3% of deaths attributed to failed or difficult intubation [6]. Respiratory complications that occur during emergency airway management are estimated to account for one third of all anesthetic deaths [3].

R. H. Kelley
Department of Anesthesiology & Perioperative Medicine, UMass Chan Medical School, Worcester, MA, USA
e-mail: Rosemary.Kelley@umassmed.edu

D. C. Sullivan · J. A. Scott (✉)
Division of Critical Care, Department of Anesthesiology & Perioperative Medicine, UMass Chan Medical School, Worcester, MA, USA
e-mail: Daniel.Sullivan@umassmemorial.org; aaron.scott@umassmemorial.org

© The Author(s), under exclusive license to Springer Nature Switzerland AG 2024

J. Faintuch, S. Faintuch (eds.), *Recent Strategies in High Risk Surgery*,
https://doi.org/10.1007/978-3-031-56270-9_16

In otherwise healthy patients, difficulty with airway management leading to a severe outcome occurs with a frequency of 11.6 per million [1]. According to 2019 claims analysis, in recent years difficult tracheal intubations tended to occur in sicker patients, with 76% of difficult intubations between 2000 and 2012 involving ASA III-V categories [5].

Difficult Airway

It corresponds to anticipated or unanticipated barriers or failure by a trained anesthesia provider in any of the following areas: face mask ventilation, laryngoscopy, ventilation with supraglottic airway, tracheal intubation, extubation or invasive airway [4].

While the overall incidence of difficult airways is estimated to be low (1.4–5.0% [7, 8]), there is significant mortality. Impossible face mask ventilation occurs at an estimated rate of 0.07–0.16% [9]. Difficult intubation occurs at a rate of 1.6 per 1000 with the incidence of failed intubation being 1.3 per 10,000 [1]. Any of these scenarios can lead to a "cannot intubate, cannot oxygenate" scenario, which occurs in less than 1 out every 5000 elective cases. This requires a surgical airway rescue in less than 1 out of every 50,000 cases, nevertheless accounts for 25% of anesthesia-related deaths [10]. Delays in surgical airway initiation during these emergencies remains an issue.

Increased Serious Complications

A 2019 claims analysis revealed that despite similar incidence of difficult intubations, incidence of brain damage or death at induction of anesthesia was 5.5 times higher between 2000 and 2012 when compared to 1993–1990 [5]. Two-thirds of difficult intubations occur at induction in the operating room, 13–14% occur during the procedure, 14–16% at extubation and 4–7% occur during recovery in the post-anesthesia care unit [5]. Failure to predict and plan for a patient with a difficult airway remains the most important factor contributing to catastrophic events [2, 4, 5, 10].

Airway Assessment

Risk assessment for predicting challenging airways has been a significant topic of research in anesthesiology. Despite this, anticipation of difficult airways remains incredibly difficult. A 2015 cohort study involving 188,064 patients had 3391 difficult tracheal intubations and 857 cases of difficult mask ventilation [11]. Notably 93% of the difficult tracheal intubations were unanticipated. Difficult mask ventilation was unanticipated in 94% of cases. According to a 2018 Cochrane Review with 844,206 participants, there is no current bedside screening test alone or in combination, that is entirely reliable in detecting an unanticipated difficult airway [12].

History

A thorough history and physical examination is vital emphasizing prior diseases and episodes of difficult intubation, neck surgery or injury, snoring or related medical conditions including obstructive sleep apnea (OSA). A history of difficult intubations is the most predictive risk factor [10].

Facial Features and Anatomical Measures

The "3-3-2 Rule" can be applied for mouth and neck anatomical evaluation (see Table 16.1). Additional criteria include head and neck mobility, neck circumference, presence of a beard (indicator of difficult face mask ventilation), and ability to prognath (the upper lip bite test).

The upper lip bite test is the best pre-operative indicator of difficult airway. The inability to project forward the lower jaw, and thus bite any part of the upper lip with the lower incisors, has 60% sensitivity for detection of difficulty in tracheal intubation [10]. Conversely, the ability to extend teeth above the lower border of the upper lip is predictive of a reduced risk intubation. These tests are less predictive in cases with edentulism.

Indices for difficult airway evaluation include neck circumference to thyromental distance, height to thyromental distance, and thyromental to hyomental distance ratios.

Table 16.1 Visual representation of the important features distinguishing possible easy versus difficult airway with the 3-3-2 Rule for Difficult Airway Evaluation. Created by Dr. Sullivan

The "3–3-2 Rule" for Difficult Airway Evaluation		
	Easy	Difficult
Interincisor distance (mouth opening)	≥3 fingerbreadths	<3 fingerbreadths
Hyoid-mental distance	≥3 fingerbreadths	<3 fingerbreadths
Hyoid-thyroid cartilage distance	≥2 fingerbreadths	<2 fingerbreadths

Table 16.2 Graphical representation of the important anatomic features differentiating a Class 1 to Class 4 airway in the Modified Mallampati Scoring system. Created by Dr. Sullivan

Modified Mallampati Scoring				
	Visible			
	Soft palate	Fauces	Uvula	Tonsillar pillars
Class 1	Yes	Yes	Full	Yes
Class 2	Yes	Yes	Partial	No
Class 3	Yes	No	Base	No
Class 4	No	No	No	No

Mallampati Scoring

Despite being more than 40 years old, it is still widely used. Modified Mallampati scoring [13, 14] allows for quick evaluation of the anatomy of the mouth and oropharynx. The patient is instructed to extend their neck and protrude their tongue to their maximum ability. The anatomy is then classified into class 1–4 based on visible structures (Table 16.2).

Ultrasound

Several upper airway ultrasound (UA-US) index tests have been cited in the literature including the following: DSE, distance from skin to epiglottis; DSHB, distance from skin to hyoid bone; DSVC, distance from skin to vocal cords; E-VC, distance from the epiglottis to the midpoint of distance between the vocal cords.

Distance from skin to epiglottis (DSE) seems accurate to predict difficult laryngoscopy based on 10 studies considering 1812 patients [15]. DSE is assessed using a linear probe placed in a transverse plane and measuring the thickness of the pre-epiglottic space at the midline, with higher values of DSE having a significant association with difficult intubation. The positive predictive value ranged from 30.26% to 49.4% while the negative predictive value ranged from 94.61% to 97.53%. Due to the low prevalence of patients with difficult airway in the target population, a negative test represents a probability of an easy laryngoscopy being about 95%–97%.

It may help to rule out the probability of a true difficult laryngoscopy in a selected population with uncertain difficult airways based on clinical assessment. However, further studies needed with better standardization of US assessment to limit heterogeneity.

Physiologic Difficult Airway

In addition to the anatomic features described above, there are physiologic features which may contribute to difficult airway management. Physiologic derangements include hypoxemia, hypotension, severe metabolic acidosis, and right ventricular failure, which increase the risk of cardiovascular collapse from airway management due to transition to positive pressure ventilation, and/or difficulty with optimizing gas exchange [16]. Additional physiologic considerations include the presence of a full stomach, increasing education and aspiration risk.

Obesity

Obesity is a significant predictor of airway difficulty due a combination of anatomic and physiologic factors listed above. In addition to the anatomic factors listed above, physiologically, patients with obesity have reduced functional capacity, resulting in a decrease in the duration of apnea before desaturation [16]. Patients with obesity twice as likely to have severe airway complications as those who are not obese [2]. Patients with body mass index great above 40 are four times more likely to have a severe complication.

Airway Management

According to the 2022 Difficult Airway Algorithm, prior to attempting intubation, the clinician managing the airway should choose either an awake or post-induction airway strategy. Any one factor alone, including assessed difficulty with intubation, ventilation, or aspiration or desaturation risk, may be clinically important enough to warrant an awake intubation. Patients with a suspected difficult laryngoscopy and at least one additional risk factor including suspected difficult face mask/supraglottic airway, increased risk of aspiration or increased risk of rapid desaturation should undergo awake intubation [4]. Throughout the algorithm there is repeated emphasis on limiting attempts alternating and optimizing techniques and avoiding task fixation and maintaining an awareness of the passage of time, this is likely due to known human factors which contribute to failed airways as discussed below.

Pre-Oxygenation

ASA guidelines emphasize optimization of oxygenation prior to and in between intubation attempts through low- or high-flow nasal cannula and elevated head position throughout procedure [4]. Pre-oxygenation followed by apneic oxygenation is an effective maneuver for prolonging safe apnea time. Apnea time is the time before oxygen desaturation. Apneic oxygenation traditionally is provided using low-flow nasal oxygen at flow rates up to 15 L/min while the patient is apneic [17, 18]. It is effective in prolonging apnea time before desaturation prior to intubation. Pre-oxygenation is recommended to be performed in all patients undergoing anesthesia although there is special emphasis on pre-oxygenation if there is an anticipated interruption of O_2 delivery such as before and during awake fiberoptic intubation [17].

In patients with morbid obesity, it has been shown that high-flow nasal oxygenation compared to conventional oxygenation provides longer safe apnea time by 40% (76 s) and higher minimum SpO_2 during anesthesia induction [19, 20].

In critically ill patients with acute hypoxic respiratory failure, pre-oxygenation with non-invasive or high-flow oxygen therapy did not change the risk of severe hypoxemia [21].

Face Mask Ventilation

Face mask ventilation is a maneuver associated with airway management that is often overlooked. In an unanticipated difficult airway scenario, face mask ventilation can be used as a rescue maneuver between tracheal intubation attempts or while pursuing surgical options. Additionally difficulty with face mask ventilation can be an important indicator as 25% of patients who are difficult face mask ventilation are difficult to intubate [9]. Effective face mask ventilation can be confirmed by the following: rise in chest, capnographic tracing and increase in oxygen saturation. There are four classifications of face mask ventilation [20], described in Table 16.3.

Troubleshooting aids in face mask ventilation include oropharyngeal or nasopharyngeal airway, modified two-handed ventilation with exaggerated jaw life. Jaw-thrust and chin life maneuvers are performed to keep the airway open [22].

Direct Laryngoscopy

When difficulty is encountered during a direct laryngoscopy, a changing the operator or changing to video laryngoscopy for a second or third attempt should always

Table 16.3 Graphical representation of qualities differentiating Grade 1 to Grade 4 face mask ventilation. Created by Dr. Sullivan

Face mask ventilation	
Grade	Description
1	Easy one-provider ventilation achieved
2	Possible with oral airway or other adjuvant
3	Difficult; inadequate, unstable, or requiring additional providers
4	Impossible

be considered [23].

Video Laryngoscopy

Video laryngoscopy overcomes the requirement to align the anatomic axes by using a camera attached near the tip of the laryngoscope blade to capture a live image that is projected on a portable monitor [24]. There are now numerous devices that can be utilized for video laryngoscopy. The first attempt and overall success rate for tracheal intubation via video laryngoscopy is often higher compared to direct layrngoscopy [25]. Success rate of tracheal intubation with video laryngoscope is 97.1%–99.6% overall and 95.8%–100% when a difficult airway is suspected [26, 27]. A 2016 Cochrane review comparing video laryngoscopy with direct laryngoscopy concluded that video laryngoscopy may reduce the number of failed tracheal intubations, particularly among patients with a difficult airway [28]. However, there was insufficient evidence that the use of a video laryngoscope reduces the number of tracheal intubation attempts or the incidence of hypoxia or respiratory complications. This may be due to a lack of evidence that the use of a video laryngoscope affects the time required for tracheal intubation.

The presence of blood in the airway, airway edema, cervical immobility and obesity are associated with increased odds of first attempt failure with video laryngoscopy in an ICU [24].

Awake Intubation

Awake intubation techniques include tracheal intubation with the aid of a flexible bronchoscope, video laryngoscopy, direct laryngoscopy, combined techniques and retrograde wire-aided intubation [4]. Awake tracheal intubation has a high success rate and a favorable safety profile; however, it is often considered underutilized in anticipated difficult airway management [29].

Tracheal intubation while the patient is awake involves applying topical airway anesthesia and securing the airway, with or without the use of sedation [29]. Ideally, the patient is sufficiently conscious and breathing spontaneously. Otherwise, a patient's responsiveness to stimuli, airway reflexes, and ability to maintain spontaneous ventilation is impaired by deep sedation [30]. Unfortunately both excessive sedation and inadequate sedation can increase the difficulty of bronchoscopic intubation [31]. Poorly managed sedation during "awake" intubation was a contributing factor noted in the NAP4 study [2].

Awake fiberoptic intubation is highly reliable with a low number of complications and a success rate ranging from 88% to 100% depending on operator experience [32]. There have been a wide variety of medications described in the literature for use during "awake" fiberoptic intubation including benzodiazepines, opioids (fentanyl, remifentanil), propofol, dexmedetomidine, and ketamine [32–34].

Surgical Airway

In a patient with either an anticipated or an unanticipated difficult airway, the situation may arise where a surgical airway may become the only option to secure the airway. Available options include open, percutaneous or needle cricothyroidotomy or open tracheostomy. The time available to the proceduralist may guide decision making.

The "Three-Step Emergency Cricothyroidotomy," as described by the military, is where a scalpel is used to incise the skin vertically superficial to the cricothyroid membrane, the non-dominant finger is used to palpate the membrane, quickly following with a horizontal incision through the cricothyroid membrane. An elastic bougie is then inserted into the trachea, allowing for placement of an endotracheal tube over the bougie and into the airway before removal of the bougie and inflation of the endotracheal tube cuff [35]. This method is now frequently referred to as the "scalpel, finger, bougie" technique.

Percutaneous cricothyroidotomy involves palpation of the cricothyroid membrane, followed by insertion of a needle through the cricothyroid membrane and into the trachea. Using the Seldinger technique, a wire is then advanced through the needle that then allows for the placement of an emergency airway tube through the cricothyroid membrane [36].

Needle cricothyroidotomy allows for emergency oxygenation by placing a large bore IV cannula (typically 14 g) through the cricothyroid membrane. Once in place, oxygen can be administered via a three-way stop cock or jet ventilation to allow for oxygenation. Needle cricothyroidotomy generally does not allow for adequate carbon dioxide management and a more definitive airway should be pursued to ensure proper ventilation [36].

In some situations, the decision may be made to perform a surgical tracheotomy, rather than a cricothyroidotomy. This can be performed asleep or awake based on the situation. The procedural description is beyond the scope of this chapter. The entire team should be in communication to ensure the best decision is made given the circumstances.

In 2019, DeVore et al. published a systematic review that found that, overall, the rate of complications for both cricothyrotomy and tracheotomy was comparable. The most frequent early complications were failure to obtain an airway (1.6%) and hemorrhage (5.6%). Airway stenosis was the most common long-term complication (0.22%–7.0%). They concluded that both approaches present similar risks and management should depend on clinician experience and patient characteristics [37].

Extubation of Difficult Airway

An overlooked aspect of airway management, the post-operative course and extubation period is critical when considering the overall picture of managing the difficult airway. Joffe et al. point out that "only one article regarding extubation is published for every 36 regarding tracheal intubation [5]." A number of factors play into the decision of when, where, and how to extubate the patient with a known (or unknown) difficult airway; these include factors associated with the surgical procedure itself, as well as the patient's own anatomy and physiology.

Mechanical ventilation carries time-dependent risks, with complications like ventilator-associated pneumonia, barotrauma, non-pulmonary complications like hypotension, acute kidney injury, and gastric stress ulcers, as well as overall mortality increasing as time on the ventilator increases [38]. Timely and efficient strategies toward extubation remains the best preventative measure in preventing these complications [39].

General Extubation Criteria

Anesthesiologists employ a number of criteria when deciding whether or not a patient is ready to extubate in the operating room. These criteria can be applied broadly to every patient undergoing mechanical ventilation, whether immediately postoperatively in the operating room, in the post-anesthesia care unit (PACU), or in the intensive care setting. Safely dictating the timing of extubation in difficult airway patients is a critical aspect of ensuring successful liberation from the ventilator [39].

When considering extubation, several broad criteria must first be applied to assess the patient's level of readiness for liberation from mechanical ventilatory support. These criteria can be best summed up by the acronym "MOVE": mental status, oxygenation, ventilation, and expectoration [40]. These criteria are summarized in Table 16.4.

Mental status is traditionally assessed by asking the patient to perform simple commands, such as hand squeeze, sustained head lift, and deep inspiratory effort. The Glasgow Coma Scale has been shown to be a reliable scoring system for prediction of extubation success, with higher scores indicating a higher likelihood of success [41–43]; studies have shown, however, that patients with GCS <8 can safely be extubated if the clinical picture allows [44]. Required support of oxygenation and ventilation should be minimized prior to attempted extubation; while these factors can be optimized via the use of non-invasive measures such as high-flow nasal

Table 16.4 Graphical representation of the MOVE criteria used to support potential for successful extubation. Created by Dr. Sullivan

"MOVE" criteria for extubation	
Criteria	Indicator of successful extubation
Mental status	Glascow coma scale ≥ 8[a]
Oxygenation	$FiO_2 \leq 50\%$, PEEP ≤ 8; PaO_2/FiO_2 ratio >150
Ventilation	Rapid shallow breathing index (RSBI) >105
Expectoration	Subjective; thin/scant secretions, strong cough/gag reflex

[a]Patients with GCS <8 should be considered for extubation depending on the rest of the clinical picture

cannula and non-invasive positive pressure ventilation, patients with PaO_2/FiO_2 ratios less than 150, as well as those requiring FiO_2 greater than 0.50 and PEEP greater than 8 cmH_2O to maintain adequate oxygenation, are poor candidates for extubation [39]. Rapid shallow breathing index (RSBI) greater than 105 breaths/min/L has shown high sensitivity (97%) for predicting patients who will pass spontaneous breathing trial, but only moderate specificity (65%), conferring no benefit to survival and no reduction in extubation failure or tracheostomy while prolonging the weaning process [45]. Assessment of airway secretions (qualitative and quantitative) and the patient's ability to clear them remains subjective but should be taken into consideration on a case-by-case basis [43].

Additional criteria to consider when deciding whether a patient is ready for spontaneous breathing trial and extubation are numerous and vary widely based on the clinical picture. Patients who are likely to return to the operating room for additional procedures under general anesthesia within 24 h should not be extubated, as repeated airway instrumentation for intubation increases the risk of airway trauma and edema. Cardiovascular instability requiring escalating measures of support is generally accepted to be a relative contraindication for extubation, though extubation can be considered if support is minimal and there are no other contraindications to removal of mechanical ventilatory support [40].

In patients who have had a prolonged course on the ventilator, or those who have undergone repeated instrumentation of the airway (prior failed extubation, repeated intubation for surgical procedures, head/neck surgery, etc.), additional assessment of the airway may be necessary prior to extubation. The cuff-leak test can be performed using qualitative and quantitative means to assess the airway for laryngeal edema that could cause post-extubation stridor. Qualitatively, the test is performed by listening for a leak with a stethoscope over the upper trachea when the balloon is deflated. To assess for a cuff-leak quantitatively, the patient should be placed on volume-control ventilation, and the balloon deflated. The difference between inspired and expired tidal volume is then measured ($V_{Tinsp} - V_{Texp} = \Delta V_T$). Quantitative cutoff points are subject to some debate; ΔV_T of 10% [46], 12% [45], and 15.5% [44] of the V_{Tinsp} have been suggested as a positive cuff leak. In patients with no cuff-leak on assessment prior to planned extubation, a four-dose course of corticosteroids prior to extubation has been supported by recent meta-analyses and societal guidelines [46, 47].

Timing of Extubation

In addition to the criteria listed above, consideration must be given to both the timing and the setting of withdrawal of mechanical ventilatory support. The operating room is a highly controlled environment, with ample support staff and equipment available in the event of a catastrophic failure. The intensive care unit has the potential to be a far less-supported setting, requiring logistical preparation when considering the extubation of a difficult airway. Multiple factors specific to the postoperative patient make this period a high-risk stage in the patient's care; pharmacologically, use and timing of neuromuscular blockers and opioids play an important role in extubation-readiness. Surgical factors including fluid balance, patient positioning (i.e., prolonged steep head-down positioning), and location of surgical site (head/neck surgery) also increase the likelihood of difficulty with liberation from mechanical ventilatory support.

When considering extubation of the difficult airway in the intensive care setting, preparation is critical to ensure the highest chance of success. It is our opinion that a team-based approach including physicians from all necessary teams (critical care, anesthesiology, surgery, and ENT as indicated), nursing, respiratory therapy, and pharmacy ensures the best likelihood of a positive outcome. Equipment should be made available to progress down the difficult airway algorithm (outlined above) should failure be imminent. This includes video laryngoscope, fiberoptic bronchoscope, laryngeal mask airway, bougie introducers, as well as equipment for cardiopulmonary resuscitation [46]. It may also be advisable to have tracheostomy or cricothyrotomy kits (as well as personnel trained in their usage) available at bedside in case of surgical airway emergency.

The use of post-extubation ventilatory support should be discussed and prepared ahead of time whenever possible. Evidence has shown that non-invasive positive pressure ventilation has utility in preventing re-intubation in select high-risk patient groups, including those with COPD and other causes of hypercapnia [48, 49]. High-flow oxygen has also shown benefit in this regard in subsets of patients with hypoxemic respiratory failure [49, 50].

Human Factors and Team Approach to Difficult Airway Management

Human Factors Associated with Difficult Airways

Significant advances have been made in airway management over recent years. A 2018 study of greater than 400,000 anesthetics found that rates of difficult and failed tracheal intubation decreased fourfold between 2002 and 2015 [51]. Despite this improvement, outcomes associated with difficult tracheal intubation remain poor [5]. There is considerable evidence that a lack of adequate planning for intubation difficulty or failure contributes to patient harm [2, 4, 5]. In the NAP4 study, 40% of serious airway complications were attributed to human factors such as poor situational awareness. In the 2019 claims analysis a judgment error described as perseveration was noted in 25% of claims. Perseveration is defined as consistent application of airway management technique or tool in three or more attempts without deviation or change, or the return to a technique or tool that was previously unsuccessful [5].

Team Approach

Literature around team-based approaches to difficult airway management started with the Difficult Airway Response Team (DART) at Hopkins [52] has expanded to numerous hospital systems since. In their decade review of their DART program, Mark et al. reported responding to over 1000 events in a 10-year time period with no resultant adult airway related adverse events or morbidity [53]. This approach is now frequently included in literature describing of airway management in critical illness [54]. While typically used for emergency airway management in the emergency room, inpatient floor and intensive care unit, some hospitals mobilize their airway response teams for intraoperative activations as well. Knowing the resources available at your institution is a vital part of perioperative difficult airway management.

Summary

Care for the patient in the perioperative period involves both surgical and sedation/anesthetic risk assessment. Any patient receiving moderate sedation or anesthesia care must have their airway evaluated to assess the potential for difficult airway management. A focused history and physical examination, looking for visible characteristics that predict difficult airway, is vital. Preparation to optimize physiologic reserve, including pre-oxygenation, pairs with basic and advanced airway skills, such as face mask ventilation and Direct/Video Laryngoscopy, to manage the airway in normal circumstances. In the event of an anticipated difficult airway, a fiberoptic intubation may be pre-determined; however, an unanticipated difficult airway may put the surgical team in a position to proceed with surgical airway management. Extubation is a frequently overlooked aspect of airway management in the perioperative period but is nonetheless an important consideration. Communication is key between members of the perioperative team in any potential scenario to provide the safest care possible to the patient.

References

1. Schiff JH, Welker A, Fohr B, et al. Major incidents and complications in otherwise healthy patients undergoing elective procedures: results based on 1.37 million anaesthetic procedures. Br J Anaesth. 2014;113(1):109–21. https://doi.org/10.1093/bja/aeu094.
2. Cook TM, Woodall N, Frerk C, et al. Major complications of airway management in the UK: results of the Fourth National Audit Project of the Royal College of Anaesthetists and the Difficult Airway Society. Part 1: anaesthesia. Br J Anaesth. 2011;106(5):617–31. https://doi.org/10.1093/bja/aer058.
3. Mort TC. Emergency tracheal intubation: complications associated with repeated laryngoscopic attempts. Anesth Analg. 2004;99(2):607–13, table of contents.

4. Apfelbaum JL, Hagberg CA, Connis RT, et al. 2022 American Society of Anesthesiologists Practice Guidelines for management of the difficult airway. Anesthesiology. 2022;136(1):31–81. https://doi.org/10.1097/ALN.0000000000004002.
5. Joffe AM, Aziz MF, Posner KL, et al. Management of difficult tracheal intubation: a closed claims analysis. Anesthesiology. 2019;131(4):818–29. https://doi.org/10.1097/ALN.0000000000002815.
6. Li G, Warner M, Lang BH, et al. Epidemiology of anesthesia-related mortality in the United States, 1999-2005. Anesthesiology. 2009;110(4):759–65. https://doi.org/10.1097/aln.0b013e31819b5bdc.
7. Kheterpal S, Han R, Tremper KK, et al. Incidence and predictors of difficult and impossible mask ventilation. Anesthesiology. 2006;105(5):885–91. https://doi.org/10.1097/00000542-200611000-00007.
8. Langeron O, Masso E, Huraux C, et al. Prediction of difficult mask ventilation. Anesthesiology. 2000;92(5):1229–36. https://doi.org/10.1097/00000542-200005000-00009.
9. Kheterpal S, Martin L, Shanks AM, et al. Prediction and outcomes of impossible mask ventilation: a review of 50,000 anesthetics. Anesthesiology. 2009;110(4):891–7. https://doi.org/10.1097/ALN.0b013e31819b5b87.
10. Detsky ME, Jivraj N, Adhikari NK, et al. Will this patient be difficult to intubate?: the rational clinical examination systematic review. JAMA. 2019;321(5):493–503. https://doi.org/10.1001/jama.2018.21413.
11. Nørskov AK, Rosenstock CV, Wetterslev J, et al. Diagnostic accuracy of anaesthesiologists' prediction of difficult airway management in daily clinical practice: a cohort study of 188 064 patients registered in the Danish Anaesthesia Database. Anaesthesia. 2015;70(3):272–81. https://doi.org/10.1111/anae.12955.
12. Roth D, Pace NL, Lee A, et al. Airway physical examination tests for detection of difficult airway management in apparently normal adult patients. Cochrane Database Syst Rev. 2018;5(5):CD008874. https://doi.org/10.1002/14651858.CD008874.pub2.
13. Mallampati SR, Gatt SP, Gugino LD, et al. A clinical sign to predict difficult tracheal intubation: a prospective study. Can Anaesth Soc J. 1985;32(4):429–34.
14. Samsoon GL, Young JR. Difficult tracheal intubation: a retrospective study. Anaesthesia. 1987;42(5):487–90. https://doi.org/10.1111/j.1365-2044.1987.tb04039.x.
15. Carsetti A, Sorbello M, Adrario E, et al. Airway ultrasound as predictor of difficult direct laryngoscopy: a systematic review and meta-analysis. Anesth Analg. 2022;134(4):740–50. https://doi.org/10.1213/ANE.0000000000005839.
16. Mosier JM, Joshi R, Hypes C, et al. The physiologically difficult airway. West J Emerg Med. 2015;16(7):1109–17. https://doi.org/10.5811/westjem.2015.8.27467.
17. Nimmagadda U, Salem MR, Crystal GJ. Preoxygenation: physiologic basis, benefits, and potential risks. Anesth Analg. 2017;124(2):507–17. https://doi.org/10.1213/ANE.0000000000001589.
18. Ramachandran SK, Cosnowski A, Shanks A, et al. Apneic oxygenation during prolonged laryngoscopy in obese patients: a randomized, controlled trial of nasal oxygen administration. J Clin Anesth. 2010;22(3):164–8. https://doi.org/10.1016/j.jclinane.2009.05.006.
19. Wong DT, Dallaire A, Singh KP, et al. High-flow nasal oxygen improves safe apnea time in morbidly obese patients undergoing general anesthesia: a randomized controlled trial. Anesth Analg. 2019;129(4):1130–6. https://doi.org/10.1213/ANE.0000000000003966.
20. Moon TS, Tai K, Kim A, et al. Apneic oxygenation during prolonged laryngoscopy in obese patients: a randomized, double-blinded, controlled trial of nasal cannula oxygen administration. Obes Surg. 2019;29(12):3992–9. https://doi.org/10.1007/s11695-019-04077-y.
21. Frat JP, Ricard JD, Quenot JP, et al. Non-invasive ventilation versus high-flow nasal cannula oxygen therapy with apnoeic oxygenation for preoxygenation before intubation of patients with acute hypoxaemic respiratory failure: a randomised, multicentre, open-label trial. Lancet Respir Med. 2019;7(4):303–12. https://doi.org/10.1016/S2213-2600(19)30048-7.

22. Fei M, Blair JL, Rice MJ, et al. Comparison of effectiveness of two commonly used two-handed mask ventilation techniques on unconscious apnoeic obese adults. Br J Anaesth. 2017;118(4):618–24. https://doi.org/10.1093/bja/aex035.
23. Aziz MF, Brambrink AM, Healy DW, et al. Success of intubation rescue techniques after failed direct laryngoscopy in adults: a retrospective comparative analysis from the Multicenter Perioperative Outcomes Group. Anesthesiology. 2016;125(4):656–66. https://doi.org/10.1097/ALN.0000000000001267.
24. Joshi R, Hypes CD, Greenberg J, et al. Difficult airway characteristics associated with first-attempt failure at intubation using video laryngoscopy in the intensive care unit. Ann Am Thorac Soc. 2017;14(3):368–75. https://doi.org/10.1513/AnnalsATS.201606-472OC.
25. Aziz MF, Dillman D, Fu R, et al. Comparative effectiveness of the C-MAC video laryngoscope versus direct laryngoscopy in the setting of the predicted difficult airway. Anesthesiology. 2012;116(3):629–36. https://doi.org/10.1097/ALN.0b013e318246ea34.
26. Aziz MF, Healy D, Kheterpal S, et al. Routine clinical practice effectiveness of the Glidescope in difficult airway management: an analysis of 2,004 Glidescope intubations, complications, and failures from two institutions. Anesthesiology. 2011;114(1):34–41. https://doi.org/10.1097/ALN.0b013e3182023eb7.
27. Aziz MF, Abrons RO, Cattano D, et al. First-attempt intubation success of video laryngoscopy in patients with anticipated difficult direct laryngoscopy: a multicenter randomized controlled trial comparing the C-MAC D-blade versus the GlideScope in a mixed provider and diverse patient population. Anesth Analg. 2016;122(3):740–50. https://doi.org/10.1213/ANE.0000000000001084.
28. Lewis SR, Butler AR, Parker J, et al. Videolaryngoscopy versus direct laryngoscopy for adult patients requiring tracheal intubation. Cochrane Database Syst Rev. 2016;11(11):CD011136. https://doi.org/10.1002/14651858.CD011136.pub2.
29. Ahmad I, El-Boghdadly K, Bhagrath R, et al. Difficult Airway Society guidelines for awake tracheal intubation (ATI) in adults. Anaesthesia. 2020;75(4):509–28. https://doi.org/10.1111/anae.14904.
30. Lodenius Å, Maddison KJ, Lawther BK, et al. Upper airway collapsibility during dexmedetomidine and propofol sedation in healthy volunteers: a nonblinded randomized crossover study. Anesthesiology. 2019;131(5):962–73. https://doi.org/10.1097/ALN.0000000000002883.
31. Heidegger T, Schnider TW. "Awake" or "Sedated": safe flexible bronchoscopic intubation of the difficult airway. Anesth Analg. 2017;124(3):996–7. https://doi.org/10.1213/ANE.0000000000001748.
32. Cabrini L, Baiardo Redaelli M, Ball L, et al. Awake fiberoptic intubation protocols in the operating room for anticipated difficult airway: a systematic review and meta-analysis of randomized controlled trials. Anesth Analg. 2019;128(5):971–80. https://doi.org/10.1213/ANE.0000000000004087.
33. Joseph TT, Gal JS, DeMaria S, et al. A retrospective study of success, failure, and time needed to perform awake intubation. Anesthesiology. 2016;125(1):105–14. https://doi.org/10.1097/ALN.0000000000001140.
34. Johnston KD, Rai MR. Conscious sedation for awake fibreoptic intubation: a review of the literature. Can J Anaesth. 2013;60(6):584–99. https://doi.org/10.1007/s12630-013-9915-9.
35. MacIntyre A, Markarian MK, Carrison D, et al. Three-step emergency cricothyroidotomy. Mil Med. 2007;172(12):1228–30. https://doi.org/10.7205/milmed.172.12.1228.
36. Bribriesco A. Cricothyroid approach for emergency access to the airway. Thorac Surg Clin. 2018;28:435.
37. DeVore EK, Redmann A, Howell R, et al. Best practices for emergency surgical airway: a systematic review. Laryngoscope Investig Otolaryngol. 2019;4(6):602–8. https://doi.org/10.1002/lio2.314.
38. Esteban A, Anzueto A, Frutos F, et al. Characteristics and outcomes in adult patients receiving mechanical ventilation: a 28-day international study. JAMA. 2002;287(3):345–55.
39. Boles JM, Bion J, Connors A, et al. Weaning from mechanical ventilation. Eur Respir J. 2007;29(5):1033–56. https://doi.org/10.1183/09031936.00010206.

40. Saeed F, Lasrado S. Extubation. [Updated 2023 Feb 9]. In: StatPearls [Internet]. Treasure Island (FL): StatPearls Publishing; 2024 Jan-. Available from: https://www.ncbi.nlm.nih.gov/books/NBK539804/.
41. Igarashi Y, Ogawa K, Nishimura K, et al. Machine learning for predicting successful extubation in patients receiving mechanical ventilation. Front Med (Lausanne). 2022;9:961252. https://doi.org/10.3389/fmed.2022.961252.
42. Mogase LG, Koto MZ. Failed extubation in a tertiary-level hospital intensive care unit, Pretoria, South Africa. South Afr J Crit Care. 2021;37(3) https://doi.org/10.7196/SAJCC.2021.v37i3.446.
43. Torrini F, Gendreau S, Morel J, et al. Prediction of extubation outcome in critically ill patients: a systematic review and meta-analysis. Crit Care. 2021;25(1):391. https://doi.org/10.1186/s13054-021-03802-3.
44. Coplin WM, Pierson DJ, Cooley KD, et al. Implications of extubation delay in brain-injured patients meeting standard weaning criteria. Am J Respir Crit Care Med. 2000;161(5):1530–6. https://doi.org/10.1164/ajrccm.161.5.9905102.
45. Tanios MA, Nevins ML, Hendra KP, et al. A randomized, controlled trial of the role of weaning predictors in clinical decision making. Crit Care Med. 2006;34(10):2530–5. https://doi.org/10.1097/01.CCM.0000236546.98861.25.
46. Girard TD, Alhazzani W, Kress JP, et al. An Official American Thoracic Society/American College of Chest Physicians Clinical Practice Guideline: liberation from mechanical ventilation in critically ill adults. Rehabilitation protocols, ventilator liberation protocols, and cuff leak tests. Am J Respir Crit Care Med. 2017;195(1):120–33. https://doi.org/10.1164/rccm.201610-2075ST.
47. Kuriyama A, Umakoshi N, Sun R. Prophylactic corticosteroids for prevention of postextubation stridor and reintubation in adults: a systematic review and meta-analysis. Chest. 2017;151(5):1002–10. https://doi.org/10.1016/j.chest.2017.02.017.
48. Agarwal R, Aggarwal AN, Gupta D, et al. Role of noninvasive positive-pressure ventilation in postextubation respiratory failure: a meta-analysis. Respir Care. 2007;52(11):1472–9.
49. Fernando SM, Tran A, Sadeghirad B, et al. Noninvasive respiratory support following extubation in critically ill adults: a systematic review and network meta-analysis. Intensive Care Med. 2022;48(2):137–47. https://doi.org/10.1007/s00134-021-06581-1.
50. Xu Z, Li Y, Zhou J, et al. High-flow nasal cannula in adults with acute respiratory failure and after extubation: a systematic review and meta-analysis. Respir Res. 2018;19(1):202. https://doi.org/10.1186/s12931-018-0908-7.
51. Schroeder RA, Pollard R, Dhakal I, et al. Temporal trends in difficult and failed tracheal intubation in a regional community anesthetic practice. Anesthesiology. 2018;128(3):502–10. https://doi.org/10.1097/ALN.0000000000001974.
52. Mark LJ, Herzer KR, Cover R, et al. Difficult airway response team: a novel quality improvement program for managing hospital-wide airway emergencies. Anesth Analg. 2015;121(1):127–39. https://doi.org/10.1213/ANE.0000000000000691.
53. Mark L, Lester L, Cover R, et al. A decade of difficult airway response team: lessons learned from a hospital-wide difficult airway response team program. Crit Care Clin. 2018;34(2):239–51. https://doi.org/10.1016/j.ccc.2017.12.008.
54. Scott JA, Heard SO, Zayaruzny M, et al. Airway management in critical illness: an update. Chest. 2020;157(4):877–87. https://doi.org/10.1016/j.chest.2019.10.026.

Part V
Fluids, Electrolytes and Shock

Chapter 17
Damage Control Resuscitation: Massive Transfusion Protocols and Pharmacologic Adjuncts

David Ray Velez

Abbreviations

EAST	Eastern Association for the Surgery of Trauma
FAST	Focused Assessment with Sonography in Trauma
MTP	Massive transfusion protocol
pRBC	Packed red blood cells
TEG	Thrombelastography
TXA	Tranexamic acid

Introduction

In the United States, hemorrhagic shock is responsible for 1.5 million deaths annually [1]. In this disproportionately young population, it results in nearly 75 million years of life lost. Over the last 400 years, management has significantly evolved. Caring for injured gladiators, Galen (129–210) was closely familiar with hemorrhage and accepted the Hippocratic theory of the four bodily humors. From this theory he advocated bloodletting in the management of hemorrhage and the first 1600 years of the modern era were heavily influenced by his work [1]. With the discovery of blood circulation in the 1600s, the first transfusions were seen—first from dog-to-dog, then lamb-to-human, and eventually human-to-human in 1795 [1].

Through the 1800s, there were multiple attempts at intravenous fluid administration using various products. These including formulations such as water with ascetic acid, alkali-containing fluids, and even milk. Saline was first pioneered during the

D. R. Velez (✉)
Department of Surgery, University of Nevada, Las Vegas, Las Vegas, NV, USA
e-mail: david.velez@unlv.edu

© The Author(s), under exclusive license to Springer Nature Switzerland AG 2024

J. Faintuch, S. Faintuch (eds.), *Recent Strategies in High Risk Surgery*,
https://doi.org/10.1007/978-3-031-56270-9_17

cholera epidemic and became more widely available during World War I [1]. The introduction of crystalloid resuscitation resulted in improved outcomes and decreased mortality although later was found to cause damage at the cellular level by inciting a systemic inflammatory response with reperfusion injury [2, 3]. Transition to resuscitation with blood and blood products is now emphasized while limiting this crystalloid infusion. More recently, a significant coagulopathy has been noted, especially by the military during Operation Iraqi Freedom and Operation Enduring Freedom [4, 5]. An acute traumatic coagulopathy (ATC) was present in 24.4% of the patients and was associated with high mortality [4, 5]. ATC has also been referred to as trauma-induced coagulopathy (TIC).

The term "damage control" was first used in 1993 to describe abbreviated surgical procedures that were aborted early after control of life-threatening injuries and contamination to allow for physiologic resuscitation prior to definitive managements. The term was based on a United States Navy principle to describe the emergency management of sinking watercraft. "Damage Control Resuscitation" was a concept codified as a United States Department of Defense clinical practice guideline in 2004, during the military conflicts in the Middle East [6, 7].

Today there are numerous approaches in the management of hemorrhagic shock and multiple adjuncts have been proposed. The surrounding literature is extensive and complex. This review seeks to condense and summarize the plethora of concepts to make it more accessible to the practicing surgeon. It will explain modern damage control resuscitation, the various approaches to massive transfusion, and the numerous pharmacologic adjuncts.

Pathophysiology of Hemorrhagic Shock

The word "shock" stems from the French "choc", meaning a violent act, such as the impact of jousting lance. Today, hemorrhagic shock is generally described as inadequate tissue prefusion due to blood loss. However, despite the significant advancements in its understanding, the exact definition still remains murky. In fact, the more poetic definitions of the past may be better at capturing the true sense of "shock" than are phrases that deconstruct ideas of tissue perfusion [8].

Hemorrhage results in many physiologic and compensatory changes that are directly related to the degree of blood loss [9]. These changes are described by the classes of shock and are summarized in Table 17.1. Class I hemorrhagic shock occurs with loss of less than 15% total blood volume and shows minimal change in vital signs. Class II occurs when 15–30% of total blood volume is lost and we begin to see low-level tachycardia and decreased pulse pressure although blood pressure remains normal. Class III occurs once over 30% of total blood volume is lost and it is at this point that hypotension, tachypnea, and oliguria are seen. Class IV shock occurs when over 40% of total blood volume is lost and the patient will show marked tachycardia, significant hypotension, negligible urine output, and lethargy.

During hemorrhagic shock oxygen delivery is unable to meet oxygen demand at the cellular level. Aerobic metabolism is converted to anaerobic metabolism with

Table 17.1 Classification of hemorrhagic shock

Class	Blood loss (percentage total blood volume)	Heart rate (*beats/min*)	Blood pressure	Pulse pressure	Respiratory rate (*breaths/min*)	Urine output	Mental status
I	<750 cc (<15%)	<100	Normal	Normal	14–20	Normal	Slightly anxious
II	750–1500 cc (15–30%)	100–120	Normal	Narrow	20–30	Normal	Mildly anxious
III	1500–2000 cc (30–40%)	120–140	Decreased	Narrow	30–40	Decreased	Confused, anxious
IV	>2000 cc (>40%)	>140	Decreased	Narrow	> 40	Negligible	Confused, lethargic

the resultant oxygen debt [10]. This results in a buildup of oxygen free radicals [10]. Additionally, lactic acid and inorganic phosphates accumulate [10]. A systemic inflammatory response is ignited by the release of damage-associated molecular patterns (DAMPs) [11]. Hypovolemia additionally causes vasoconstriction, causing end-organ hypoperfusion and damage. Major blood flow impairment to the heart and brain can be immediately followed by serious arrhythmias and cerebral anoxia [12].

It has been shown that hemorrhagic shock results in a diffuse coagulopathy due to multiple complex mechanisms [13]. Activated protein C (APC) inactivates factors Va and VIIIa, thereby inhibiting coagulation. Increased activity of activated protein C has been noted after trauma, which is believed to be due to increased activity of thrombomodulin [14, 15]. Thrombomodulin promotes activated protein C activation and is activated in the setting of hypoperfusion. The endothelial glycocalyx layer has anticoagulant components such as chondroitin sulfate and heparan sulfate [13]. The endothelial glycocalyx layer can "shed" after injury due to yet undetermined mechanisms [13]. Although the clotting cascade is activated locally to physiologically stop the bleed, distant sites see an increase in fibrinolytic activity, likely to prevent microvascular thrombosis [13, 16]. In addition, platelet numbers are depleted, migration is decreased, and their function is impaired [10]. With hemorrhagic shock the lethal triad of hypothermia, acidosis, and coagulopathy results in significant morbidity and devastating outcomes [17].

Damage Control Resuscitation

Damage control resuscitation encompasses stopping the bleeding, reducing excessive crystalloid replenishment, prompt however carefully managed blood transfusion, permissive hypotension, and attention to coagulopathy, acidosis, and hypothermia.

As with any trauma, resuscitation begins with an efficient primary and secondary survey following Advanced Trauma Life Support (ATLS) algorithms. Physiologic compensation occurs early in hemorrhagic shock and it often takes a loss of 30% total blood volume before hypotension is seen. Some of the earliest signs to beware include tachycardia and cutaneous vasoconstriction. A cold-pale patient with tachycardia should be presumed to be in shock until proven otherwise. Hemorrhagic shock in injured patients is most common although any form of shock can be present and once identified, the cause should be sought. Diagnosis, however, should not delay appropriate resuscitation.

Prompt actions to stop the bleed are critical. Temporary control of extremity wounds should be obtained with direct pressure, suture closure, hemostatic dressings, or proximal tourniquet. Thoracic and abdominal bleeding, however, are non-compressible. Patients in hemorrhagic shock do not afford the luxury of CT evaluation and require immediate intervention. Surgeons may consider resuscitative endovascular balloon occlusion of the aorta (REBOA) for patients in hemorrhagic shock due to abdominopelvic hemorrhage although there are strict contraindications and to date there is no high-grade evidence demonstrating improved survival or outcomes.

Initial fluid therapy starts with 1–2 L of a warmed lactated Ringer's solution. In the pediatric patient, bolus should be limited to 20 cc/kg if weight is under 40 kg. Balanced crystalloids such as lactated Ringer are preferred over normal-saline as it has been shown to cause hyperchloremic metabolic acidosis with increased risk for renal dysfunction and increased mortality [18, 19]. There was previously a concern with giving lactated Ringer in the setting of blood transfusion due to an increased risk of clot formation and tubing dysfunction. However, at the high transfusion rates used in standard trauma resuscitation this is not an issue [20].

Further management is then based on the patient's response to this initial bolus which is indictive of shock class. "Rapid responders" likely have class I hemorrhagic shock. "Transient responders" will initially respond but then begin to show signs of deterioration, indicating class II–III hemorrhagic shock. Patients with minimal-no response are highly concerning for exsanguination with class IV hemorrhagic shock. Rapid responders require no further immediate fluid boluses. Both transient responders and non-responders should be further resuscitated with blood or blood products. For hypotensive patients with immediate concern for class III–IV hemorrhagic shock this initial crystalloid bolus should be bypassed and transfusion with blood and blood products should begin immediately. When significant volumes of blood transfusion are anticipated massive transfusion protocols should be activated and consideration for pharmacologic adjuncts should be given.

Maintaining a "normal" blood pressure was historically highlighted by the early resuscitation strategies [21]. Rapid resuscitation in a bleeding patient, however, is now thought to worsen bleeding. This rapid fluid resuscitation decreases the viscosity of blood, disrupts fragile new clots, and worsens elements of the lethal triad. Although originally proposed by Walter Cannon during World War I, the 1990s–2000s saw a reinvigorated interest in the idea of "hypotensive resuscitation" [22]. This was also referred to as "permissive hypotension" or "controlled resuscitation". A lower blood pressure goal, often a systolic blood pressure of ≥70 mmHg, is initially targeted until the physician is able to achieve definitive hemostasis, [23].

aiming to lower blood loss, use of blood products, and higher survival [23]. A significant contraindication would be the suspicion of traumatic brain injury (TBI) in which maintenance of cerebral perfusion pressure is essential to limit secondary brain injury. In the presence of traumatic brain injury initial goal systolic blood pressures should be ≥110 mmHg for ages 15–49, ≥100 mmHg for ages 50–69 or ≥110 mmHg for ages ≥70 [24]. However, fluid resuscitation will allow recovery only once the bleeding has been stopped. The ultimate goal for all patients must be definitive hemorrhage control.

Massive Transfusion Protocol (MTP)

Only in the 1960s we began to separate blood into its components: red cells, platelets, and plasma [25]. Over the next 10–20 years, this "component therapy" began to replace the traditional use of whole blood [26]. Trauma only represents a small proportion of blood transfusions (10–15%) and individualized therapies with specific components are frequently preferred [26, 27]. "Component therapy", as opposed to whole blood, lengthened storage times and reduced blood product waste [26], becoming the preferred transfusion approach to trauma by the 1990s.

With the recognition of acute traumatic coagulopathy, the understanding has evolved that severely injured patients require not just pRBC transfusions but also plasma and platelets. Massive transfusion protocol (MTP) is typically defined as ≥10 units pRBC in 24 h or ≥4 units pRBC in 1 h. MTP activation has historically proceeded with hemostatic resuscitation although the use of thrombelastography and whole blood are evolving.

MTP Activation Indications

MTP improves patient survival, decreases the use of blood products, and decreases costs [28]. MTP should be activated as soon as large-volume transfusions are anticipated although the exact determination is debated. Over a dozen scoring systems have been developed to predict the need for MTP activation. They differ in their criteria and the significance applied to each value. Some of the most common criteria include a positive Focused Assessment with Sonography in Trauma (FAST) exam, hypotension with systolic blood pressure ≤90 mmHg, tachycardia with heart rate ≥120 beats/min, unstable pelvic fracture, and decreased hemoglobin.

A recent systematic review compared 15 of the most commonly described scores [29]. They found that when using a combination of clinical assessment, laboratory values, and FAST the Trauma-Associated Severe Hemorrhage (TASH) score was the most well validated. When laboratory results are unavailable the Assessment of Blood Consumption (ABC) score "balances accuracy with ease of use". When FAST is not available the Vandromme score is most accurate but the Schreiber score is most sensitive. If all that is available to the surgeon is clinical assessment, the Shock Index has fair performance. Ultimately, a universal set of indications is doubtful. Scoring systems should be individualized and each hospital system should implement what is feasible based on their own available resources.

Hemostatic Resuscitation

"Damage Control Resuscitation" was an approach codified by the United States Department of Defense (DOD) as a clinic practice guideline during the military operations in the Middle East in 2004 [6, 7]. The most critically ill trauma patients were transfused at a ratio of 1:1 pRBC and plasma [6, 30]. With the addition of platelets this converted into the "1:1:1" ratio [31].

In the large PROPPR trial death due to exsanguination diminished at 24 hours, however not all-cause mortality [31]. In another analysis hemostatic resuscitation did benefit outcomes and mortality [28], and many have adopted it as the historical "Gold Standard" during blood transfusion in trauma.

Thrombelastography (TEG)

TEG measures the viscoelastic properties of clot formation in real-time to guide transfusion efforts. TEG was created in 1940s Germany although the first clinical use was during the Vietnam War (1955–1975) [32, 33]. In the late twentieth century it was adopted by cardiac and liver surgeons although with newer more reliable and rapid machines it has seen renewed interest in trauma [33]. Conventional coagulation testing performed in the laboratory takes longer than the point-of-care TEG. In trauma, conventional results are often inaccurate by the time they result due to transfusion and rapid physiologic changes. From time of admission in the resuscitation bay until results are available RapidTEG takes 30.8 min, standard TEG takes 41.5 min, and conventional tests take 64.9 min [34]. This is further amplified when considering that TEG can be viewed in real-time with some useful data available much sooner.

There has been one past randomized control trial evaluating the use of TEG in trauma [35]. It evaluated 111 trauma patients after MTP activation. Patients were given an initial 4 U pRBC and then further transfusion was guided by either TEG or conventional coagulation assays. The study found decreased 28-day mortality with the largest impact in the first 6 h after injury. There were however potential weaknesses to the study as physicians could request unblinding if the felt TEG was either indicated or contraindicated, eight of which did so. They were not truly evaluating a 1:1:1 resuscitation as the median transfusion at 6 h for the conventional coagulation assay group had only 8 U pRBC, 5 U plasma, and 1 U platelets. There is also consideration that the results may be too good as patients treated by TEG had nearly one-quarter the mortality at 6 h and one-half at 28 days, questioning risk of other bias.

To date studies have mostly been retrospective and observational. TEG has allowed for a more rapid goal-directed resuscitation although definitive high-grade evidence that it decreases transfusion requirements or improves mortality is lacking [36, 37]. The use of TEG does involve some complexity requiring understanding of the results and how to respond although simple algorithms can be followed. Increased R-Time indicates insufficient factors and should be treated with FFP. Increased K-time or decreased alpha-angle indicates insufficient fibrinogen and requires cryoprecipitate. Decreased maximum amplitude (MA) indicates insufficient or inhibited platelets and should be treated with either platelet transfusion or DDAVP depending on the situation. An elevated lysis at 30 min (LY-30) indicates rapid clot breakdown and should be treated with TXA.

Whole Blood

Military conflicts in Iraq and Afghanistan have renewed interest in the use of whole blood transfusion, partially due to the need in austere far-forward environments where access to conventional blood bank supplies are limited [38, 39]. Although it has primarily been used in the military setting with "fresh" whole blood from an available "walking blood bank" of prescreened soldiers, it is now being utilized in some civilian trauma centers [40]. Multiple factors have limited its use such as the misconceptions that whole blood must be type ABO specific, whole blood cannot be leukoreduced, whole blood cannot maintain platelets, or that cold storage of whole blood causes loss of platelet function. These, however, have all been overcome [41].

After storage and dilution, blood products being given during a balanced resuscitation with a 1:1:1 ratio have a hematocrit 29%, coagulation factor concentration 65% of normal, and platelet count 88,000 [42, 43]. In the immediate post-transfusion period 5–10% of red blood cells are lost and only two-thirds of the administered platelets will be viable [44, 45]. Effective concentration of transfusion in a 1:1:1 ratio is therefore only hematocrit 26%, coagulation factor concentration 65% of normal, and platelet count 59,000. At these levels, transfusion with blood products alone barely keep levels above traditional transfusion indications. Adding more of one component further dilutes the other two and the addition of fluids will dilute all three. Whole blood however has a hematocrit 35–38%, coagulation factor concentration 85% of normal, and platelet count 150,000–200,000 [43].

Studies evaluating the use of whole blood compared to component therapy are mostly observational or retrospective with significant heterogeneity. The only randomized control trial to date was a single center pilot feasibility trial with insufficient power to detect mortality differences. A 2020 systematic review found an overall poor quality of evidence [46]. There have been some retrospective studies to suggest decreased transfusion requirements and mortality although sufficient high-quality evidence is currently lacking with no major randomized control trial [40,

47]. Despite this, many advocate whole blood as the best resuscitation product. Although availability is currently limited, it is being used with increasing frequency and rapidly spreading among major trauma centers.

Pharmacologic Adjuncts

Recombinant Activated Factor VIIa (rVIIa)

Recombinant activated factor VIIa (rVIIa) binds to the surface of activated platelets and promotes the activation of factor X with thrombin generation. It was first used in 1999 for the management of uncontrolled hemorrhage but today trauma remains an off-label use in the United States [48]. Dosing has varied although both past randomized control trials have used 200 μg/kg initially followed by 100 μg/kg at 1 and 3 h [49, 50]. Although early retrospective analysis was promising, further studies have failed to consistently show benefit. Both past randomized control trials, including the CONTROL trial, indicated reduced blood product use, significantly so after blunt trauma, however no difference in mortality was seen [49, 50].

Although there was initially great hope with its introduction and some retrospective cohort studies saw reduced mortality, when taken together current literature has failed to show any high-grade evidence of decreased transfusion requirements or improved mortality [28]. To date no change in the rate of venous thromboembolism formation has been seen [28]. 2017 Eastern Association for the Surgery of Trauma (EAST) guidelines were unable to recommend for or against its use [28]. At this time, with no clear benefit, the use of recombinant activated factor VIIa has mostly fallen out of favor.

Tranexamic Acid (TXA)

TXA inhibits plasminogen conversion to the active protease plasmin, thereby inhibiting fibrinolysis and clot breakdown. Similar to recombinant activated factor VIIa, its use in trauma remains off-label in the United States. TXA is typically given as a 1 g bolus followed by a second 1 g infused over 8 h.

CRASH-2, the largest study to date, was an international randomized control trial throughout 40 countries with over 20,000 patients [51]. It saw significantly decreased risk of death due to bleeding and decreased risk of all-cause mortality [51]. Subgroup analysis saw significantly decreased risk of mortality if given within 3 h of injury but increased risk if given after 3 h [52]. CRASH-2 was an excellent trial however there were potential weaknesses that should be recognized. There was selection bias as physicians could exclude patients if the felt TXA was either indicated or contraindicated and there was no report in how many were excluded in this way. There is also a significant question of external validity due to wide variation in trauma systems with the majority of patients being treated in countries that do not routinely provide rapid access to blood products, damage control surgery, or advanced critical care [53].

Other retrospective observational studies such as the military MATTERs and MATTERs II have also evaluated TXA use [51, 54–56]. Although some studies have shown improved mortality, when results are combined there is no clear mortality benefit or difference in transfusion requirements [28]. Risk for venous thromboembolism is unknown at this time due to lack of standardization in its reporting [28]. Based largely on the CRASH-2 findings, 2017 EAST guidelines did give a conditional recommendation for its use [28]. TXA is recommended in the early management of significant traumatic hemorrhage but only if given within 3 h of injury and potential limitations should be noted.

Cryoprecipitate (Cryo)

Fibrinogen is the first coagulation factor to reach critically low concentrations in major blood loss and low levels in the trauma patient have been associated with worse outcomes [57, 58]. Cryoprecipitate serves as the standard source for fibrinogen administration. High-grade research has been limited. CRYOSTAT-1 was a United Kingdom feasibility randomized control trial evaluating the use of early cryoprecipitate in trauma by giving two early pools of cryoprecipitate within a goal of less than 90 min [59]. Results suggested reduced mortality, although the difference was not significant ($P = 0.14$) [59]. CRYOSTAT-2 will follow up with a larger multicenter randomized control trial throughout the United Kingdom. By retrospective observation in the United States, MATTERs II found a mortality benefit of cryoprecipitate similar to TXA and proposed that cryoprecipitate may independently add to the survival benefit of TXA if given together [56]. MATTERs II however is limited due to the potential bias in the retrospective observational nature and venous thromboembolism rates were not reported. Current evidence to guide the use of cryoprecipitate is insufficient with no clear guidelines and further evaluation is needed.

Vasopressors

Vasopressors have previously been considered heresy in the treatment of hemorrhagic shock. Research has demonstrated increased mortality with most vasopressors and their use had mostly been abandoned [60]. However, the potential is again being questioned. A recent systematic review evaluating vasopressor use found that the only randomized control trial was "too imprecise to yield meaningful results" and that although all the observational studies found increased short-term mortalities, with relative risk 2.31–7.39, there was high risk of bias as patients receiving vasopressors were significantly more ill [61]. The review concluded that the existing data were of low quality [61]. When Sperry et al. evaluated the use of early vasopressors they found significantly increased mortality, however on logistic regression arginine vasopressin (AVP) was the only vasopressor not associated with significantly increased mortality [60]. Collier et al. then found increased risk of mortality with the use of arginine vasopressin, however 84% received it in combination with other vasopressors making it difficult to draw strong conclusions [62].

Arginine vasopressin, specifically, has recently been reevaluated. In hemorrhagic shock, the baroreceptor-mediated secretion of this pituitary hormone is impaired and the circulating levels are rapidly depleted [63]. The AVERT-Shock trial evaluated the use of low-dose arginine vasopressin on the early resuscitation of adult trauma patients who received at least 6 units of blood product within 12 h of injury [64]. It was randomized, double-blind, and placebo-controlled. Patients were given a 4-unit bolus of arginine vasopressin, started on a 0.04-unit/min infusion, and then titrated following definitive hemorrhage control. They saw decreased transfusion requirements but no change in mortality [64]. There was no increased risk of complications however, unexpectedly, venous thromboembolism risk was significantly reduced by the use of arginine vasopressin [64]. At this time, with no improvement in mortality seen the definitive use of arginine vasopressin in trauma remains questioned.

Conclusion

The understanding of damage control resuscitation is essential to the management of the critically injured patient. It generally begins with 1–2 L of a warmed lactated Ringer's fluid bolus. For patients that fail to mount an appropriate response rapidly, additional crystalloid infusion should be forgone, and the patient should be transitioned to blood and blood products. Hemodynamically unstable patients in class III–IV hemorrhagic shock should immediately be transfused with blood products and the initial crystalloid bolus should be bypassed. Massive Transfusion Protocols should be activated in more critical conditions, encompassing a 1:1:1 approach although the use of whole blood is reemerging and considered by many to be superior, if available. TEG-guided resuscitation should be considered as a potentially valuable resource.

Among the various pharmacologic adjuncts available, TXA can be administered within 3 h of injury if large volumes are likely to be required. Cryoprecipitate or arginine vasopressin are other options, used it at the surgeon's discretion. Recombinant factor VIIa, although once showed significant promise, has now mostly fallen out of favor. "Permissive hypotension" is contraindicated in the presence of traumatic brain damage or previous hypertension. Definitive control of bleeding must be the ultimate goal.

References

1. Velez DR. The history of hemorrhagic shock and damage control resuscitation. Am Surg. 2022;88(11):2656–9.
2. Mattox KL. The ebb and flow of fluid (as in resuscitation). Eur J Trauma Emerg Surg. 2015;41(2):119–27.
3. Pope A, French G, Longnecker DE. Fluid resuscitation: state of the science for treating combat casualties and civilian injuries. Washington, DC: National Academic Press; 1999.
4. MacLeod JB, Lynn M, McKenney MG, et al. Early coagulopathy predicts mortality in trauma. J Trauma. 2003;55:39–44.
5. Brohi K, Singh J, Heron M, Coats T. Acute traumatic coagulopathy. J Trauma. 2003;54:1127–30.
6. Hess JR, Holcomb JB, Hoyt DB. Damage control resuscitation: the need for specific blood products to treat the coagulopathy of trauma. Transfusion. 2006;46(5):685–6.
7. Holcomb JB, Jenkins D, Rhee P, et al. Damage control resuscitation: directly addressing the early coagulopathy of trauma. J Trauma. 2007;62(2):307–10.
8. Milham FH. A brief history of shock. Surgery. 2010;148(5):1026–37.
9. Advanced Trauma Life Support (ATLS) student course manual, 10th ed. Am Coll Surg; 2018.
10. Cannon JW. Hemorrhagic shock. N Engl J Med. 2018;378(4):370–9.
11. Zhang Q, Raoof M, Chen Y, Sumi Y, Sursal T, Junger W, Brohi K, Itagaki K, Hauser CJ. Circulating mitochondrial DAMPs cause inflammatory responses to injury. Nature. 2010;464(7285):104–7.
12. Tisherman SA, Alam HB, Rhee PM, Scalea TM, Drabek T, Forsythe RM, Kochanek PM. Development of the emergency preservation and resuscitation for cardiac arrest from trauma clinical trial. J Trauma Acute Care Surg. 2017;83(5):803–9.
13. Chang R, Cardenas JC, Wade CE, Holcomb JB. Advances in the understanding of trauma-induced coagulopathy. Blood. 2016;128(8):1043–9.
14. Holcomb JB, del Junco DJ, Fox EE, Wade CE, Cohen MJ, Schreiber MA, Alarcon LH, Bai Y, Brasel KJ, Bulger EM, et al. The Prospective, Observational, Multicenter, Major Trauma Transfusion (PROMMTT) Study: comparative effectiveness of a time-varying treatment with competing risks. JAMA Surg. 2013;148(2):127–36.
15. Cohen MJ, Kutcher M, Redick B, Nelson M, Call M, Knudson MM, Schreiber MA, Bulger EM, Muskat P, Alarcon LH, et al. Clinical and mechanistic drivers of acute traumatic coagulopathy. J Trauma Acute Care Surg. 2013;75(1 Suppl 1):S40–7.
16. Hoffman M, Cichon LJH. Practical coagulation for the blood banker. Transfusion. 2013;53(7):1594–602.
17. Cosgriff N, Moore EE, Sauaia A, Kenny-Moynihan M, Burch JM, Galloway B. Predicting life-threatening coagulopathy in the massively transfused trauma patient: hypothermia and acidosis revisited. J Trauma. 1997;42(5):857–61.
18. Hoorn EJ. Intravenous fluids: balancing solutions. J Nephrol. 2017;30(4):485–92.
19. Semier MW, Self WH, Wanderer JP, et al. Balanced crystalloids versus saline in critically ill adults. N Engl J Med. 2018;378(9):829–39.
20. Lorenzo M, Davis JW, Negin S, et al. Can Ringer's lactate be safely used with blood transfusions? Am J Surg. 1998;175(4):308–10.
21. Cannon WB, Fraser J, Cowell EM. The prevention of wound shock. JAMA. 1918;70:618–21.
22. Dutton RP, Mackenzie CF, Scalea TM. Hypotensive resuscitation during active hemorrhage: impact on in-hospital mortality. J Trauma. 2002;52(6):1141–6.
23. Tran A, Yates J, Lau A, et al. Permissive hypotension versus conventional resuscitation strategies in adult trauma patients with hemorrhagic shock: a systematic review and meta-analysis of randomized controlled trials. J Trauma Acute Care Surg. 2018;84(5):802–8.
24. Carney N, Totten AM, O'Reilly C, et al. Guidelines for the management of severe traumatic brain injury, fourth edition. Neurosurgery. 2017;80(1):6–15.
25. Das PC, Smit Sibinga CT, Halie MR. Supportive therapy in haematology. Boston, MA: Martinus Nijhoff Publishing; 1985.

26. Hall S, Murphy MF. Limitations of component therapy for massive haemorrhage: is whole blood the whole solution? Anesthesia. 2015;70(5):511–4.
27. Como JJ, Dutton RP, Scalea TM, et al. Blood transfusion rates in the care of acute trauma. Transfusion. 2004;44(6):809–13.
28. Cannon JW, Khan MA, Raja AS, Cohen MJ, Como JJ, Cotton BA, Dubose JJ, Fox EE, Inaba K, Rodriguez CJ, et al. Damage control resuscitation in patients with severe traumatic hemorrhage: a practice management guideline from the eastern Association for the Surgery of Trauma. J Trauma Acute Care Surg. 2017;82(3):605–17.
29. Shih AW, Khan SA, Wang AY, Dawe P, Young PY, Greene A, Hudoba M, Vu E. Systematic reviews of scores and predictors to trigger activation of massive transfusion protocols. J Trauma Acute Care Surg. 2019;87(3):717–29.
30. Borgman MA, Spinella PC, Perkins JG, et al. The ratio of blood products transfused affects mortality in patients receiving massive transfusions at a combat support hospital. J Trauma. 2007;63(4):805–13.
31. Holcomb JB, Tilley BC, Baraniuk S, et al. Transfusion of plasma, platelets and red blood cells in a 1:1:1 vs a 1:1:2 ratio and mortality in patients with severe trauma: the PROPPR randomized clinical trial. JAMA. 2015;313(5):471–82.
32. Hartert H. Blutgerinnungsstudien Mit Der Thrombelastographie; Einem Neuen Untersuchungs Verfahren. Klin Wochenschr. 1948;26(37–38):577–83.
33. Walsh M, Fritz S, Hake D, et al. Targeted thromboelastographic (TEG) blood component and pharmacologic hemostatic therapy in traumatic and acquired coagulopathy. Curr Drug Targets. 2016;17(8):954–70.
34. Jeger V, Zimmerman H, Exadaktylos AE. Can RapidTEG accelerate the search for coagulopathies in the patient with multiple injuries? J Trauma. 2009;66(4):1253–7.
35. Gonzalez E, Moore EE, Moore HB, et al. Goal-directed hemostatic resuscitation of trauma-induced coagulopathy: a pragmatic randomized clinical trial comparing a viscoelastic assay to conventional coagulation assays. Ann Surg. 2016;263(6):1051–9.
36. Unruh M, Reyes J, Helmer SD, Haan JM. An evaluation of blood product utilization rates with massive transfusion protocol: before and after thromboelastography (TEG) use in trauma. Am J Surg. 2019;218(6):1175–80.
37. Mohamed M, Majeske K, Sachwani GR, et al. The impact of early thromboelastography directed therapy in trauma resuscitation. Scand J Trauma Resusc Emerg Med. 2017;15(1):99.
38. Repine TB, Perkins JG, Kauvar DS, Blackborne L. The use of fresh whole blood in massive transfusion. J Trauma. 2006;60(6 Suppl):S59–69.
39. Vanderspurt CK, Spinella PC, Cap AP, et al. The use of whole blood in US military operations in Iraq, Syria, and Afghanistan since the introduction of low-titer type O whole blood: feasibility, acceptability, challenges.
40. Pivalizza EG, Stephens CT, Sridhar S, et al. Whole blood for resuscitation in adult civilian trauma in 2017: a narrative review. Anesth Analg. 2018;127(1):157–62.
41. Spinela PC, Pidcoke HF, Strandenes G, et al. Whole blood for hemostatic resuscitation of major bleeding. Transfusion. 2016;56(2):S190–202.
42. Mays JA, Hess JR. Modelling the effects of blood component storage lesions on the quality of hemostatic resuscitation in massive transfusion for trauma. Blood Transfus. 2017;15(2):153–7.
43. Cap AP, Beckett A, Benov A, et al. Whole blood transfusion. Mil Med. 2018;183(Suppl 2):44–51.
44. Bosman GJ. Survival of red blood cells after transfusion: process and consequences. Front Physiol. 2013;4:376.
45. Armand R, Hess JR. Treating coagulopathy in trauma patients. Transfus Med Rev. 2003;17(3):223–31.
46. Avery P, Morton S, Tucker H, et al. Whole blood transfusion versus component therapy in adult trauma patients with acute major haemorrhage. Emerg Med J. 2020;37(6):370–8.
47. Spinella PC, Perkins JG, Grathwohl KW, et al. Warm fresh whole blood is independently associated with improved survival for patients with combat-related traumatic injuries. J Trauma. 2009;66(4 Suppl):S69–76.

48. Boffard KD, Riou B, Warren B, et al. Recombinant factor VIIa as adjunctive therapy for bleeding control in severely injured trauma patients: two parallel randomized, placebo-controlled, double-blind clinical trials. J Trauma. 2005;59(1):8–15.
49. Hauser CJ, Boffard K, Dutton R, et al. Results of the CONTROL trial: efficacy and safety of recombinant activated factor VII in the management of refractory traumatic hemorrhage. J Trauma. 2010;69(3):489–500.
50. Spinella PC, Perkins JG, McLaughlin DF, et al. The effect of recombinant activated factor VII on mortality in combat-related casualties with severe trauma and massive transfusion. J Trauma. 2008;64(2):286–94.
51. CRASH-2 Trial Collaborators, Shakur H, Roberts I, et al. Effects of tranexamic acid on death, vascular occlusive events, and blood transfusion in trauma patients with significant Haemorrhage (CRASH-2): a randomised, placebo-controlled trial. Lancet. 2010;376(9734):23–32.
52. CRASH-2 Trial Collaborators, Roberts I, Shakur H, et al. The importance of early treatment with tranexamic acid in bleeding trauma patients: an exploratory analysis of the CRASH-2 randomized control trial. Lancer. 2011;377(9771):1096–101.
53. Gruen RL, Jacobs IG, Reade MC, PATCH-Trauma Study. Trauma and tranexamic acid. Med J Aust. 2013;199(5):310–1.
54. Cole E, Davenport R, Willett K, Brohi K. Tranexamic acid use in severely injured civilian patients and the effects on outcomes: a prospective cohort study. Ann Surg. 2015;261(2):390–4.
55. Morrison JJ, Dubose JJ, Rasmussen TE, Midwinter MJ. Military application of tranexamic acid in trauma emergency resuscitation (MATTERs) study. Arch Surg. 2012;147(2):113–9.
56. Morrison JJ, Ross JD, Dubose JJ, et al. Association of cryoprecipitate and tranexamic acid with improved survival following wartime injury: findings from the MATTERs II study. JAMA Surg. 2013;148(3):218–25.
57. Hiippala ST, Myllyla GJ, Vahtera EM. Hemostatic factors and replacement of major blood loss with plasma-poor red cell concentrates. Anesth Analg. 1995;81(2):360–5.
58. Rourke C, Curry N, Khan S, et al. Fibrinogen levels during trauma hemorrhage, response to replacement therapy, and association with patient outcomes. J Thromb Haemost. 2012;10(7):1342–51.
59. Curry N, Rourke C, Davenport R, et al. Early cryoprecipitate for major Haemorrhage in trauma: a randomized controlled feasibility trial. Br J Anaesth. 2015;115(1):76–83.
60. Sperry JL, Minei JP, Frankel HL, et al. Early use of vasopressors after injury: caution before constriction. J Trauma. 2008;64(1):9–14.
61. Hylands M, Toma A, Beaudoin N, et al. Early vasopressor use following traumatic injury: a systematic review. BMJ Open. 2017;7(11):e017559.
62. Collier B, Dossett L, Mann M, et al. Vasopressin use is associated with death in acute trauma patients with shock. J Crit Care. 2010;25(1):173.e9–14.
63. Sims CA, Guan Y, Bergey M, et al. Arginine vasopressin, copeptin, and the development of relative AVP deficiency in hemorrhagic shock. Am J Surg. 2017;214(4):589–95.
64. Sims CA, Holena D, Kim P, et al. Effects of low-dose supplementation of arginine vasopressin on need for blood product transfusion in patients with trauma and hemorrhagic shock. JAMA Surg. 2019;154(11):994–1003.

Chapter 18
Perioperative Fluid Management and Volume Assessment

Raksha Bangalore, Kathryn Jan, Jennifer Elia, and Kunal Karamchandani

Introduction

While optimal fluid therapy serves to ensure adequate end-organ perfusion by maintaining cardiac preload and stroke volume, both insufficient and excessive fluid administration have serious implications during the perioperative period [1–5]. Hypovolemia leads to a decrease in organ perfusion which may result in myocardial demand ischemia, acute kidney injury, multiorgan failure, and even death. Alternatively, hypervolemia can lead to pulmonary congestion, postoperative ileus, nausea/vomiting, dilutional coagulopathy, and death in predisposed patients.

Fluid Physiology During the Perioperative Period

In a homeostatic adult, approximately 60% of the total body weight is composed of water. In the elderly population it is progressively reduced to 50% [6, 7]. At the cellular level, a third of the total body water content is extracellular while the remainder is intracellular. Within the extracellular volume, a quarter is represented by blood plasma and the remainder is interstitial [2, 3, 8]. Fluid may shift between these compartments based on the hydrostatic, oncotic, and osmotic pressure

R. Bangalore · K. Jan · K. Karamchandani (✉)
Department of Anesthesiology and Pain Management, University of Texas Southwestern Medical Center, Dallas, TX, USA
e-mail: Raksha.bangalore@utsouthwestern.edu; Kathryn.Jan@UTSouthwestern.edu; kunal.karamchandani@utsouthwestern.edu

J. Elia
Department of Anesthesiology & Perioperative Care, University of California, Irvine, CA, USA

© The Author(s), under exclusive license to Springer Nature Switzerland AG 2024

J. Faintuch, S. Faintuch (eds.), *Recent Strategies in High Risk Surgery*,
https://doi.org/10.1007/978-3-031-56270-9_18

gradients, considering that the vascular endothelium separating the plasma and interstitial tissue as well as cellular membranes are permeable to water.

Frank-Starling Curve

Intravascular fluid serves as preload to the heart which then ejects it as stroke volume to perfuse vital organs. This is called the Frank-Starling relationship and is based on the relationship between the length of myocardial fibers and the force generated by their contraction. It is depicted by the Frank-Starling curve which relates preload or the left ventricular end-diastolic pressure to cardiac performance, measured as ventricular stroke volume (SV), or as cardiac output (CO) which corresponds to SV X heart rate (Fig. 18.1). When the myocardial performance is normal, myocardial contractility increases with more massive preload. However, the contractility reaches a maximum point limited by the cardiac muscle fibers, after which any further increase in preload does not benefit CO.

During states of increased left ventricular contractility, for example due to infusion of inotropic drugs, there is a greater cardiac performance for a given preload, represented graphically as an upward shift of the normal curve. Conversely, during states of decreased left ventricular contractility, such as systolic heart failure, the opposite occurs representing a downward shift of the normal curve. This relationship can be used to identify patients that are fluid responsive during the perioperative period (Fig. 18.1).

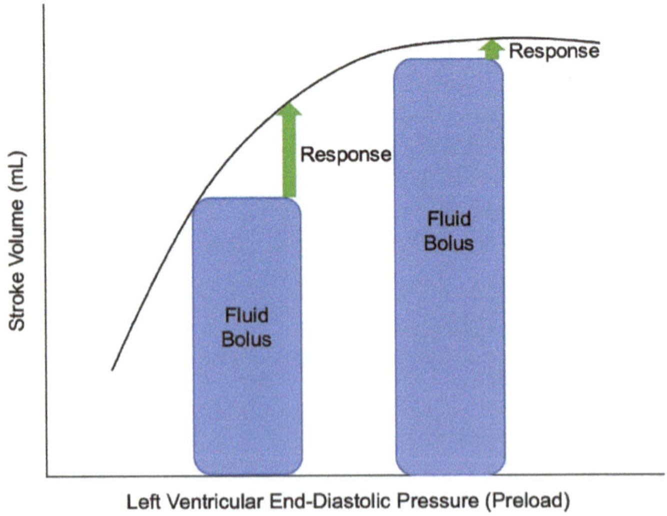

Fig. 18.1 Frank-starling curve

Fluid Responsiveness (FL)

An augmentation in SV or CO by 10–15% with moderate volume administration is defined as FL [9]. Likewise, when SV or CO is unchanged with a fluid bolus, the patient is considered volume non-responsive.

Factors Impacting Fluid Status During the Perioperative Period

Preoperative Fasting

Dehydration before elective surgery is common and is compounded by longer preoperative fasting times [10]. Historically, the increased risk of aspiration, as described by Mendelson, led to recommendations of 'nil by mouth after midnight' prior to surgery requiring general anesthesia [11, 12]. Currently both European and American guidelines promote the intake of clear fluids up to 2 h before elective surgery [13, 14]. Additionally, the advent of enhanced recovery after surgery (ERAS) protocols, has led to promoting the intake of carbohydrate-containing clear liquids up to 2 h prior to surgery to improve patient comfort (thirst, hunger) and glycemic control, usually without increasing the risk of aspiration [15–20].

However, especially for patients with lower health literacy, nil by mouth after midnight is still commonly instructed instead of established guidelines [20]. Mechanical bowel preparation can also be a mechanism of fluid loss [7]. Pediatric patients are instructed to drink clear fluids up until an hour before induction of anesthesia, and there is a renewed interest in adopting the same guideline for all age groups [21, 22]. Similarly, mechanical bowel preparation before colorectal surgery is less practiced in recent years [21].

Intraoperative Fluid Losses

Insensible losses (breathing, evaporation, sweating) are related to induction of anesthesia and surgical exposure and should be added to measured or estimated blood and other bodily fluid losses, all of which lead to a decrease in effective circulatory blood volume [23, 24]. Larger wounds with more exposed viscera tend to have higher fluid losses; these are less in laparoscopic surgery as compared to open procedures. However, evaporative losses still exist due to insufflation. Minor wounds with slightly exposed viscera lose approximately 2 mL/h of fluid, whereas for major wounds with a completely exposed abdomen up to 32 mL/h should be expected [24]. Insensible losses due to anesthesia-induced vasodilation potentially contribute to hypovolemia. Intraoperative insensible losses from a patient's skin and airway alone are estimated to be 0.3 mL/kg/h [23, 24].

Postoperative Factors

Although hypovolemia may persist postoperatively through continued bleeding as well as drainage from the surgical site or high ostomy output, other factors lead to generalized fluid retention, with possible edema as well as hypervolemia. Antidiuretic hormone, aldosterone, cortisol, and atrial natriuretic peptide are secreted after surgical interventions and lead to increased sodium and water retention as well as decreased diuresis [4].

Surgical stress and trauma can additionally promote capillary permeability via release of cytokines such as interleukin-6, tumor necrosis factor, substance-P, and bradykinin. Due to such inflammatory mediators, patients frequently become intravascularly depleted while showing signs of extravascular fluid overload, edema occurring mostly in the lungs, gut, and subcutaneous tissues. This combination of systemic and regional phenomena contributes to classic "third-spacing" in directly manipulated or damaged tissues (anastomoses, dissected peritoneal surfaces, zones of accidental or surgical trauma). When significant amounts of fluid remain in the local interstitial tissue (third space) rather than the cardiocirculatory system, such will lead to intravascular volume contraction [2, 5].

Perioperative Volume Assessment and Fluid Responsiveness

Physical exam signs such as skin turgor, capillary refill, and neck vein assessments can preliminarily suggest overall volume status, however monitoring of static and dynamic parameters as well as of fluid responsiveness are essential for improvement in clinical outcomes.

Static Parameters

They include blood pressure, heart rate, central venous pressure (CVP), pulmonary artery occlusion pressure (PAOP), inferior vena cava (IVC) diameter, and left ventricular end-diastolic volume, which provide a single time point evaluation of the patient's volume status. Historically, CVP and PAOP have also been used to determine fluid responsiveness, but they are unreliable predictors of improvement in cardiac output due to volume administration [25, 26]. This is likely due to a combination of the inability to accurately measure preload by these variables, the complex relationship between SV and ventricular preload, and the critical effect of ventricular contractility on cardiac output [25, 27].

Dynamic Parameters

Classically in mechanically ventilated patients, during inspiration positive intrathoracic pressure decreases venous return to the heart, leading to a reduction in right ventricular SV, resulting in reduced left ventricular preload and SV. During expiration, the opposite is observed where both right ventricular and left ventricular SV increase. These cyclic changes may be accentuated in patients who are hypovolemic, and contribute to evaluate volume responsiveness [28]. More modern investigations focus on pulse pressure variation (PPV), systolic pressure variability (SPV), stroke volume variation (SVV), and pulse oximetry plethysmography variability index (PVI), and their ability to predict fluid responsiveness [29].

Pulse Pressure Variation

PPV is calculated using the following equation:

$$\mathrm{PPV}(\%) = \left(\frac{\mathrm{PPmax} - \mathrm{PPmin}}{\left(\frac{\mathrm{PPmax} + \mathrm{PPmin}}{2} \right)} \right) \times 100$$

PPV along with SVV have been documented in several small series, and their value for detecting fluid responsiveness is promising [30]. PPV can be less reliable during spontaneous ventilation, low tidal volumes in mechanically ventilated patients, high-frequency ventilation such as jet ventilation, presence of pulmonary hypertension, limited lung compliance, altered chest compliance such as open chest conditions, aberrant cardiac rhythms, and elevated intraabdominal pressure [9].

Systolic Pressure Variability

SPV is the difference between the maximal and minimal systolic blood pressure (SBP) following a positive pressure breath and can be calculated using measurements from an arterial waveform. In patients receiving positive pressure ventilation, systolic pressure variability has utility in assessing volume responsiveness. SPV can be calculated using this equation:

$$\mathrm{SPV}(\mathrm{mmHg}) = \left(\frac{\mathrm{SBPmax} - \mathrm{SBPmin}}{\left(\frac{\mathrm{SBPmax} + \mathrm{SBPmin}}{2} \right)} \right)$$

In intravascularly depleted patients, a significant SPV can be expected, and an SPV >10 mmHg is consistent with fluid responsiveness [31, 32].

Stroke Volume Variation

SVV is given by the following equation:

$$\mathrm{SVV}(\%) = \left(\frac{\mathrm{SVmax} - \mathrm{SVmin}}{\mathrm{SVmean}} \right) \times 100$$

SV can be estimated using invasive or non-invasive hemodynamic monitoring devices including echocardiography. Some devices that provide direct or indirect SVV measurements during the perioperative period include, LiDCO LXi™, Masimo Corporation, Irvine, CA, USA), FloTrac/Vigileo® and ClearSight™ (Edwards Lifesciences, Irvine, CA, USA), PiCCO (Pulse Index Contour Cardiac Output, Getinge, Wayne, NJ, USA), Argos® (Retia Medical, White Plains, NY, USA).

These devices tend to provide a much less invasive method compared to pulmonary artery (PAC) or Swan Ganz catheter derived measurements of CO, and have been shown to measure similar mean CO values, albeit with inconsistencies in measuring the dynamic trends among various techniques [33].

The FLoTrac® needs a specific transducer whereas the Argos® monitor does not require a special transducer as it analyzes information from the regular arterial transducer and incorporates its proprietary Multi-Beat Analysis (MBA™) to calculate the cardiac output and other hemodynamic variables. The ClearSight™ depends on a noninvasive finger cuff. As with some other measurements, complex computation is essential to calculate SVV, potentially introducing errors in the estimate [34].

Like PPV, an SVV > 13% can predict volume responsiveness [29, 31]. Although, in mechanically ventilated patients with tidal volume <6 mL/kg, SVV may have limited ability in recognizing a fluid responder [36]. By increasing the tidal volume from 6 to 8 mL/kg and causing a greater impact to preload, volume responsiveness can be identified using the absolute change in SVV. The threshold for ΔSVV is 2.5% with a sensitivity of 81% and specificity of 80% [35, 36]. The presence of normal sinus rhythm, absence of valvular heart disease, relatively normal lung and chest compliance, and normal intraabdominal pressure are generally required for SVV to accurately predict fluid responsiveness.

Plethysmographic Variability Index (PVI) and Perfusion Index (PI).

Perfusion index (PI) is the ratio of pulsatile blood flow to the non-pulsatile blood in peripheral tissues, and most pulse oximetry devices can display PI continuously. With PI values, PVI can be obtained using this equation:

$$\text{PVI}(\%) = \left(\frac{\text{PImax} - \text{PImin}}{\text{PImax}}\right) \times 100$$

PVI is a dynamic index between 0 and 100 with higher values indicating increased variability, signaling a higher likelihood that a patient may be fluid responsive [37–39].

Nevertheless PPV and SVV are more widely employed. One meta-analysis focusing these two indexes indicated reduced mortality (odds ratio 0.55, 95% CI 0.30–1.03) and ICU-related costs (−1619, 95% CI −2174 to −1063 USD) for critically ill patients [40, 41].

Clinical Tests for Fluid Responsiveness

Passive Leg Raising

The passive leg raising (PLR) test allows a clinician to directly observe the response to augmented cardiac output with an increase in preload. To accurately test for fluid responsiveness, the patient is positioned in a semi-recumbent position with the head of the bed at a 45° angle as shown in Fig. 18.2 with legs extended, and a baseline CO is obtained. The bed is then positioned to elevate the legs, and CO is measured again within a minute. This positional shift mobilizes approximately 300 cc of fluid from the legs to the central venous system, thereby increasing the preload to the right heart, which would increasing the CO by 10% in volume-responsive patients [9]. CO measurement is superior to arterial blood pressure in predicting hemodynamics that will improve with volume expansion [40, 41].

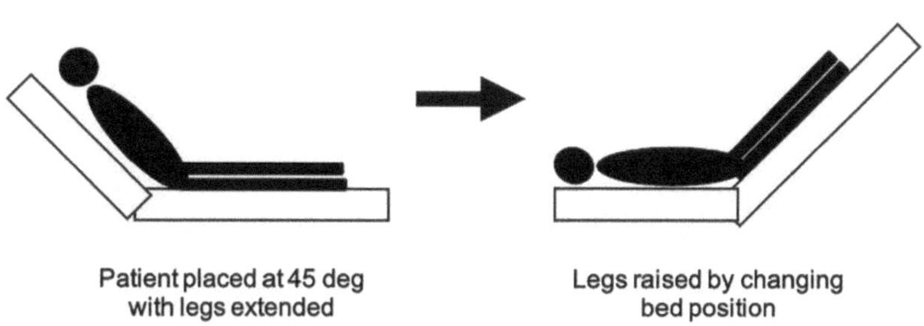

Fig. 18.2 Passive leg raising test. The patient is positioned with head of the bed raised to 45° elevating the torso while the legs remain flat. The position is shifted to elevate the legs 45° above the heart to augment preload. The cardiac output is measured at baseline (on the left) which is compared to the cardiac output with change in position (on the right)

End-Expiratory Occlusion Test

In situations where PLR cannot be performed, the end-expiratory occlusion (EEO) test is an alternative for volume assessment during passive ventilation. At the end of expiration, ventilation is paused for 15–30 s while evaluating for any changes in cardiac output. With a ventilatory pause, there is a physiologic increase in venous return to the right side leading to increased preload and, in turn, an augmented CO. If the measured CO is greater than 5% from baseline, it is indicative of fluid responsiveness [42, 43]. EEO may be able to detect volume responsiveness during the intraoperative and postoperative periods independent of ventilatory settings and the duration of the expiratory hold [43]. Nevertheless it is not a standard procedure in most services yet.

Echocardiography

Both transesophageal (TEE) and transthoracic (TTE) echocardiography have been around for decades, yet they are not recommended by guidelines nor are they routinely employed in the perioperative period, except for specific interventions notably concerning cardiac surgery. Both suffer from quality limitations, compared to CT and magnetic resonance imaging, and TEE utilization can be followed by upper gastrointestinal injuries. Imaging shortcomings have been substantially improved by more modern three-dimensional echocardiography (3D-TEE).

Echocardiographic measurement of left ventricular end-diastolic volume can be used as a surrogate for preload, and the subaortic velocity time integral (VTI) measured at the left ventricular outflow tract (LVOT) can reflect SV and thus help assess volume responsiveness. Additionally, ultrasonographic examination of the IVC can also help evaluate fluid status and gauge fluid responsiveness.

LVOT and VTI

In the parasternal long-axis view, the LVOT diameter can be measured at 0.5 cm into the ventricle from the aortic cusp insertion (Fig. 18.3). In the apical five-chamber view, a doppler signal placed across the LVOT and tracing along the ejection signal is calculated to be the VTI representing the blood flow during the cardiac cycle (Fig. 18.4). Similar to SV, variation in VTI is observed during the cardiac cycle and is calculated using the following equation.

$$\text{VTI variation}(\%) = \left(\frac{\text{VTImax} - \text{VTImin}}{\left(\frac{\text{VTImax} + \text{VTImin}}{2} \right)} \right) \times 100$$

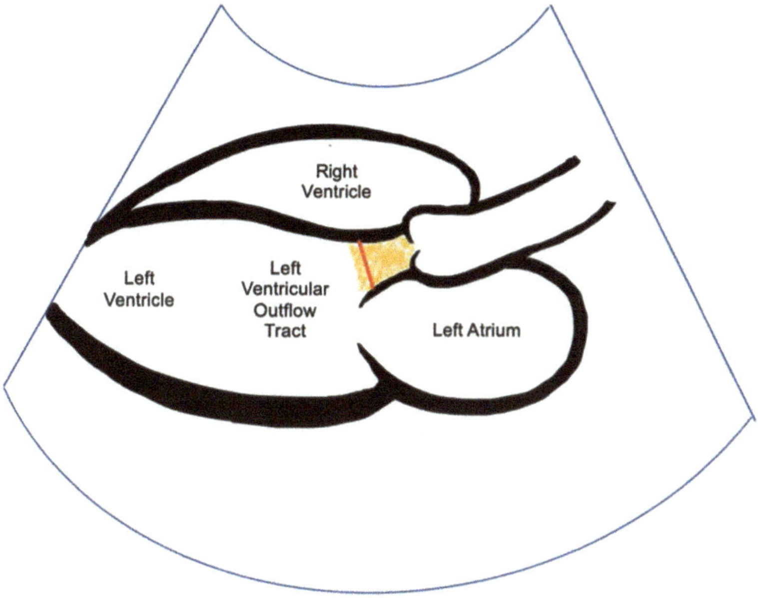

Fig. 18.3 Parasternal long-axis view. The diameter of the left ventricular outflow tract is measured as shown in red

VTImax represents the highest value while VTImin represents the lowest value measured during 10 cardiac cycles.

In septic mechanically ventilated patients, a VTI variation of 15.9% can detect volume responsiveness with a sensitivity of 87.5% and specificity of 95% [44]. LVOT VTI can also be used with the PLR test, and an increase in VTI >12% is indicative of volume responsiveness [45]. Additionally, a series of calculations using the LVOT diameter and VTI can be used to estimate the CO (Fig. 18.4).

$$\text{Cardiac Output} = \text{Stroke Volume} \times \text{Heart Rate}$$

$$\text{Stroke Volume} = \text{LVOT area} \times \text{LVOT VTI}$$

$$\text{LVOT area} = \pi\left(\frac{\text{LVOT diameter}}{2}\right)$$

IVC Diameter

From the subxiphoid view, the IVC diameter can be visualized (Fig. 18.5). It is a static parameter that approximates the CVP or right atrial pressure. An IVC diameter of <2.1 cm is consistent with right atrial pressures between 0 and 5 mmHg and a diameter >2.1 cm is indicative of pressure between 10 and 20 mmHg. However,

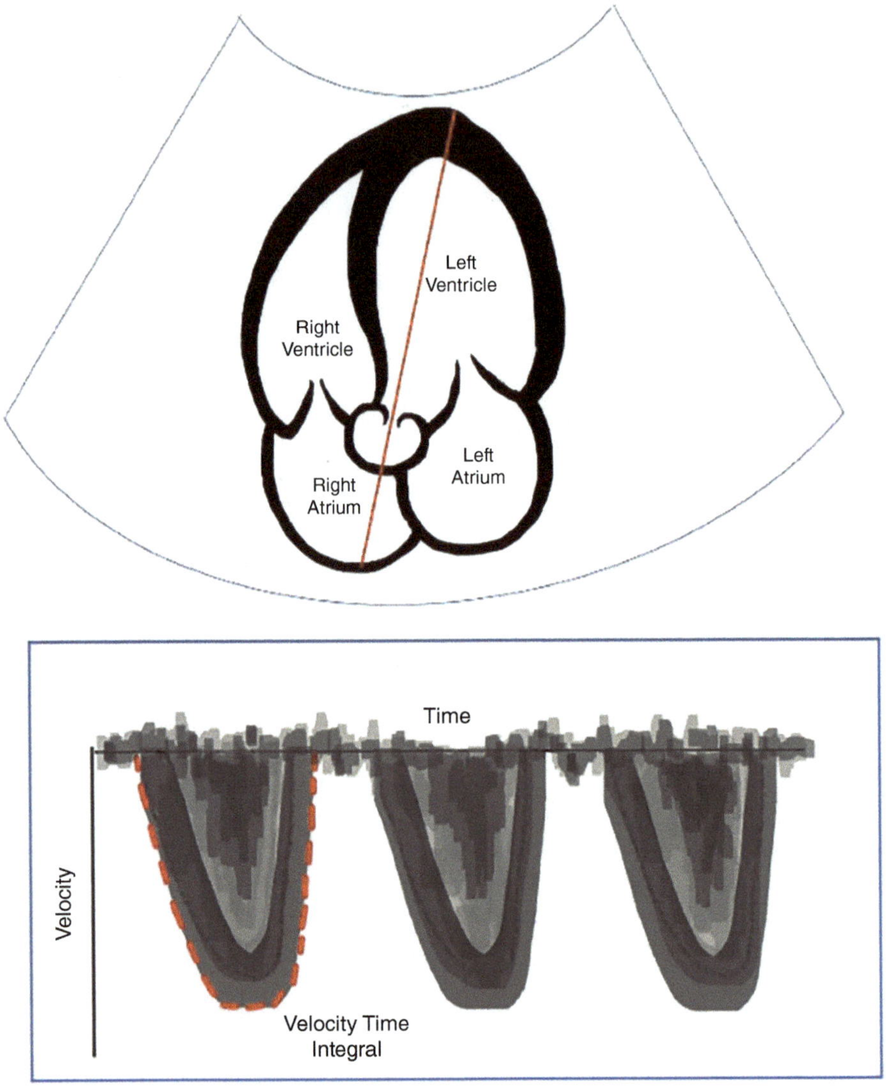

Fig. 18.4 Apical five-chamber view with doppler across left ventricular outflow tract (Top). Doppler placed as shown in red to obtain velocity time integral by tracing around the curve (Bottom)

like CVP and PAOP, the diameter of IVC, when used alone, is a poor marker for volume responsiveness [21]. On the contrary, the variance of the inferior vena cava throughout the respiratory cycle, as a dynamic marker, can be used to evaluate volume responsiveness [46]. The collapsibility of the IVC can be calculated using the equation:

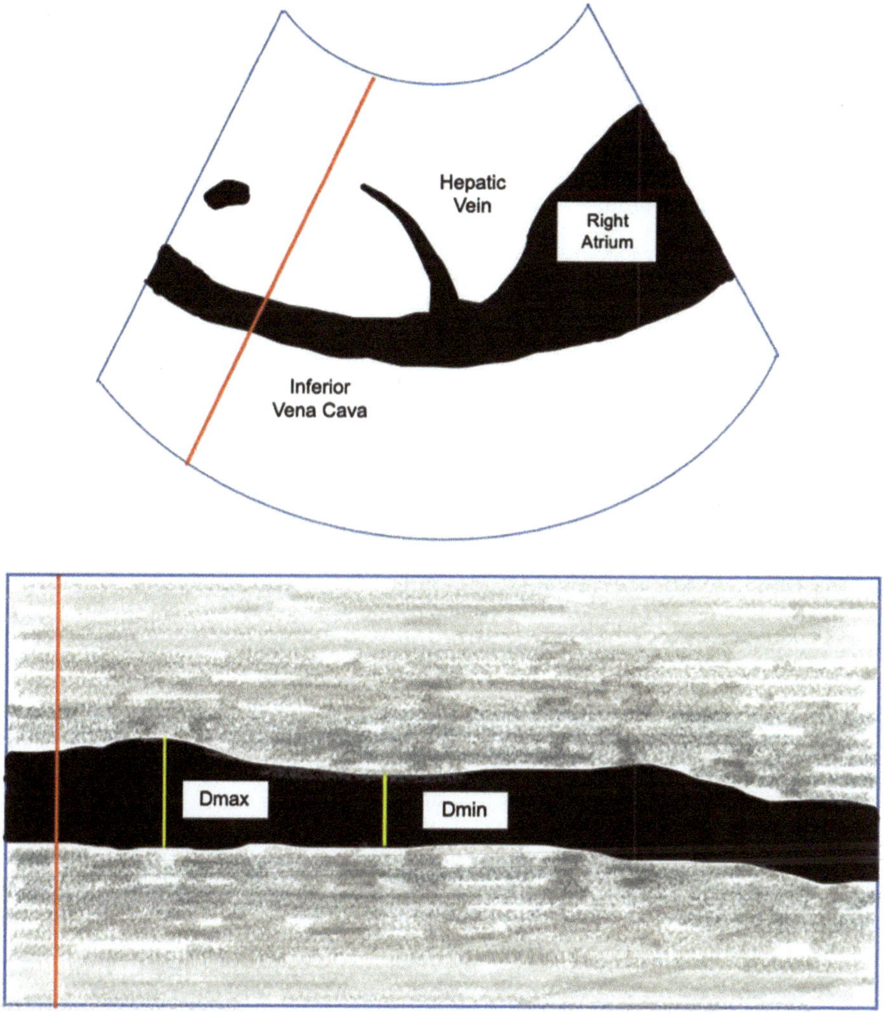

Fig. 18.5 Inferior Vena Cava in the subcostal view with doppler. (Top) M-Mode view of inferior vena cava with maximum and minimal diameter. (Bottom) *D*max Maximum diameter, *D*min Minimum diameter

$$\text{IVC Collapsibility} = \left(\frac{D\max - D\min}{\left(\frac{D\max + D\min}{2} \right)} \right) \times 100$$

where *D*max is the maximal diameter and *D*min is the minimal diameter of the IVC during the respiratory cycle.

IVC diameter and collapsibility have been shown to accurately estimate CVP and right atrial pressure, particularly in spontaneously breathing patients [47]. The diagnostic accuracy is less consistent in mechanically ventilated patients, making this assessment less useful for patients under general anesthesia. The collapsibility index of >12% is indicative of volume responsiveness in a spontaneously breathing patient. In mechanically ventilated patients, the distensibility of the IVC can be measured and volume responsiveness is likely if the distensibility index >18% [21].

$$\text{IVC Distensiblity} = \left(\frac{D\max - D\min}{(D\min)} \right) \times 100$$

Perioperative Fluid Management

The commonly used 0.9% normal saline (NS) is an unbalanced isotonic crystalloid as it has a non-physiologic chloride concentration [48, 49]. More balanced alternatives are shown in Table 18.1.

In spite of controversial reports, the SMART (Isotonic Solutions and Major Adverse Renal Events) protocol demonstrated less renal complications and less mortality with balanced preparations [50–55].

Table 18.1 Composition of commonly used crystalloid solutions

	3% Saline	0.9% Saline	Plasma-lyte	Lactated ringers	D5 ½ NS	½ NS
Sodium (mmol/L)	513	154	140	130	77	77
Chloride (mmol/L)	513	154	98	109	77	77
Potassium (mmol/L)	0	0	5	4	0	0
Magnesium (mmol/L)	0	0	3	0	0	0
Calcium (mmol/L)	0	0	0	3	0	0
Acetate (mmol/L)	0	0	27	0	0	0
Gluconate (mmol/L)	0	0	23	0	0	0
Lactate (mmol/L)	0	0	0	28	0	0
Dextrose (mEq/L)	0	0	0	0	25	0
Osmolarity (mOsm/L)	1026	308	294	273	280	154
pH	5	5	7.4	6.5	4.5	5.6

D5 5% Dextrose, *NS* Normal saline, *D5 ½ NS* 5% Dextrose combined with diluted normal saline, *½ NS* Normal saline diluted in water 1:1

Colloids

They have been widely prescribed in the past, as a means of minimizing capillary leakage, replacing expensive and not always available blood transfusions [56]. However, morbidity and mortality increased and their use has been discontinued.

At this moment only human serum albumin (5% and 25% formulations) is an option, for selected cases of decompensated cirrhosis, ascites as well as other rare conditions, not for routine administration. Synthetic colloids still exist in the market; however, most countries discourage their use [57].

Crystalloids Versus Colloids

After traumatic brain injury (TBI), mortality rate was higher and neurologic outcomes poorer when albumin was administered [58, 59]. In contrast, a post-hoc analysis showed a decreased risk of mortality in patients with septic shock when receiving albumin to correct hypoalbuminemia [60]. The Surviving Sepsis Guidelines recommend considering albumin in patients who have received large-volume crystalloid resuscitation [61–63].

Liberal Versus Restrictive Fluid Management

In a 2003 study, patients in the liberal group gained 4 kg compared to 1 kg in the restrictive group by the first postoperative day [64]. There has been much variability in the practice of perioperative fluid administration over the past two decades, as outcomes research has prompted changes in practice [64–67]. Current existing evidence comparing liberal and restrictive fluid replacement strategies is rather inconclusive. In earlier studies, liberal fluid management strategy was associated with increased perioperative morbidity, hospital costs, and length of stay [68]. After colorectal surgery, fluid overload is still incriminated for postoperative ileus [66], and surgical complications such as pneumonia and anastomotic leakage, seem more frequent in the same circumstances of excessive fluid utilization after esophagectomy [67].

In a large randomized controlled trial focusing major abdominal surgery, no difference in overall 1-year survival was observed; however, patients in the restrictive group had a higher incidence of acute kidney injury [69]. A subsequent meta-analysis found no difference in early or late postoperative mortality [70].

Enhanced Recovery After Surgery (ERAS)

Despite not uncommon criticisms, the increasingly popular ERAS programs advocate for a "zero-balance" fluid goal [17, 71]. For high-risk surgical patients, ERAS guidelines endorse goal-directed fluid therapy techniques, which are discussed below [16, 19].

Goal-Directed Therapy

Goal-directed therapy (GDT) is a strategy that aims to provide clear objectives for fluid administration during the perioperative period. This approach involves real-time assessments of hemodynamic and cardiac output parameters to guide fluid therapy. A predefined algorithm, as illustrated in Fig. 18.6, is selected depending on the operation, setting, and experience of the team, to determine when a fluid bolus is necessary. For example, if SVV remains above 13% for 5–10 min, and the patient is also hypotensive, this may indicate that the patient could benefit from additional fluid administration.

The evidence supporting GDT is not entirely conclusive, much like the fluid strategies described earlier [72–75].

A large meta-analysis found moderate evidence of benefit only concerning infectious postoperative complications and anastomotic leakage [76]. One should

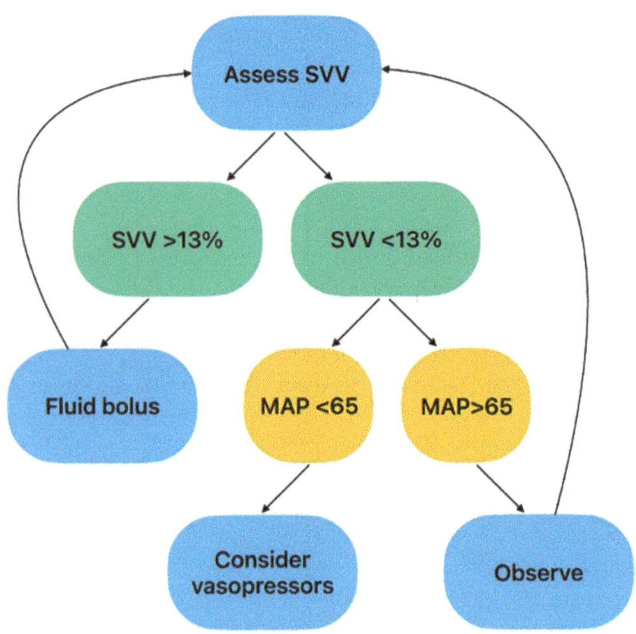

Fig. 18.6 Sample algorithm for goal directed fluid therapy with fluid administration guided by stroke volume variation. *SVV* Stroke volume variation, *MAP* Mean arterial pressure

highlight the heterogeneity of the studies, such as the devices, algorithms, hemodynamic targets, and fluid type, making it difficult to compare interventions and outcomes [76–78].

Fluid Management in Specific Patient Populations

Liver Disease and Hepatic Surgeries

Due to alterations in intravascular volume and fluid shifts, this population is highly susceptible to both hypervolemia and hypovolemia. Low albumin levels, malnutrition, and portal hypertension can further complicate volume status, resulting in the development of ascites and edema [79]. In general, a more restrictive fluid approach is preferred to avoid deleterious effects of hypervolemia. If possible, CVP and arterial line monitoring should be maintained through the perioperative period to continually assess volume status [80]. When massive volumes of ascites are surgically drained, reinfusion could be an option to minimize protein loss and hypovolemia. However, due to high levels of cytokines in the fluid and other mechanisms, fever and coagulopathy could be a danger.

Ideally ascites should be controlled with diuretics, in the preoperative period. The same tenants are generally followed for patients undergoing hepatic surgery, including transplantation, with CVP monitoring and SVV often used to guide fluid administration [81–83].

Cardiac Surgery

GDT has emerged as a recommended approach for fluid management [84]. GDT involves using advanced hemodynamic parameters such as cardiac index and mixed venous oxygenation to guide fluid therapy during the perioperative period. Furthermore, GDT can help prevent overzealous fluid administration, which can lead to fluid overload, impaired organ function, and increased morbidity and mortality. Notably the use of GDT in cardiac surgery has been associated with reduced incidence of acute kidney injury [16, 85]. Some groups advocate measuring kidney stress biomarkers, and restricting GDT to positive cases. Such would avoid extra fluid administration to those patients that do not need them.

Thoracic Surgery

In patients undergoing lung resection surgery, fluid management is challenging as diseased lungs, surgical exposure, and other factors can lead to interstitial and alveolar edema. Additionally, use of dynamic parameters for GDT may be less reliable during one lung ventilation. Again, a restrictive fluid strategy is defended with euvolemia being the goal, with special attention to avoid organ dysfunction, particularly kidney injury. ERAS guidelines support the use of balanced crystalloids over normal saline in these patients [15].

References

1. Bellamy MC. Wet, dry or something else? Br J Anaesth. 2006;97(6):755–7.
2. Doherty M, Buggy DJ. Intraoperative fluids: how much is too much? Br J Anaesth. 2012;109(1):69–79.
3. Holte K. Pathophysiology and clinical implications of peroperative fluid management in elective surgery. Dan Med Bull. 2010;57(7):B4156.
4. Jacob M, Chappell D, Rehm M. The 'third space'—fact or fiction? Best Pract Res Clin Anaesthesiol. 2009;23(2):145–57.
5. Voldby AW, Brandstrup B. Fluid therapy in the perioperative setting—a clinical review. J Int Care. 2016;4(1)
6. Luckey AE. Fluid and electrolytes in the aged. Arch Surg. 2003;138(10):1055.
7. Junghans T, Neuss H, Strohauer M, et al. Hypovolemia after traditional preoperative care in patients undergoing colonic surgery is underrepresented in conventional hemodynamic monitoring. Int J Color Dis. 2006;21(7):693–7.
8. Chappell D, Jacob M, Hofmann-Kiefer K, Conzen P, Rehm M. A rational approach to perioperative fluid management. Anesthesiology. 2008;109(4):723–40.
9. Jozwiak M, Monnet X, Teboul JL. Prediction of fluid responsiveness in ventilated patients. Ann Transl Med. 2018;6(18):352.
10. Danielsson EJD, Lejbman I, Åkeson J. Fluid deficits during prolonged overnight fasting in young healthy adults. Acta Anaesthesiol Scand. 2019;63(2):195–9.
11. Mendelson CL. The aspiration of stomach contents into the lungs during obstetric anesthesia. Am J Obstet Gynecol. 1946;52:191–205.
12. Brady M, Kinn S, Stuart P. Preoperative fasting for adults to prevent perioperative complications. Cochrane Database Syst Rev. 2003;(4):CD004423.
13. Anonymous. Practice guidelines for preoperative fasting and the use of pharmacologic agents to reduce the risk of pulmonary aspiration: application to healthy patients undergoing elective procedures: an updated report by the American Society of Anesthesiologists Task Force on preoperative fasting and the use of pharmacologic agents to reduce the risk of pulmonary aspiration. Anesthesiology. 2017;126(3):376–93.
14. Smith I, Kranke P, Murat I, et al. Perioperative fasting in adults and children: guidelines from the European Society of Anaesthesiology. Eur J Anaesthesiol. 2011;28(8):556–69.
15. Batchelor TJP, Rasburn NJ, Abdelnour-Berchtold E, et al. Guidelines for enhanced recovery after lung surgery: recommendations of the Enhanced Recovery After Surgery (ERAS®) Society and the European Society of Thoracic Surgeons (ESTS). Eur J Cardiothorac Surg. 2019;55(1):91–115.
16. Engelman DT, Ben Ali W, Williams JB, et al. Guidelines for perioperative care in cardiac surgery: enhanced recovery after surgery society recommendations. JAMA Surg. 2019;154(8):755–66.
17. Gustafsson UO, Scott MJ, Hubner M, et al. Guidelines for perioperative care in elective colorectal surgery: Enhanced Recovery After Surgery (ERAS). World J Surg. 2019;43(3):659–95.
18. Ljungqvist O, Scott M, Fearon KC. Enhanced recovery after surgery: a review. JAMA Surg. 2017;152(3):292–8.
19. Nelson G, Bakkum-Gamez J, Kalogera E, et al. Guidelines for perioperative care in gynecologic/oncology: Enhanced Recovery After Surgery (ERAS) Society recommendations-2019 update. Int J Gynecol Cancer. 2019;29(4):651–68.

20. Joshi GP, Abdelmalak BB, Weigel WA, et al. 2023 American Society of Anesthesiologists Practice Guidelines for preoperative fasting: carbohydrate-containing clear liquids with or without protein, chewing gum, and pediatric fasting duration-a modular update of the 2017 American Society of Anesthesiologists Practice Guidelines for preoperative fasting. Anesthesiology. 2023;138(2):132–51.
21. Thomas M, Morrison C, Newton R, Schindler E. Consensus statement on clear fluids fasting for elective pediatric general anesthesia. Paediatr Anaesth. 2018;28(5):411–4.
22. Morrison CE, Ritchie-McLean S, Jha A, Mythen M. Two hours too long: time to review fasting guidelines for clear fluids. Br J Anaesth. 2020:S0007-0912(19)31004-9.
23. Reithner L, Johansson H, Strouth L. Insensible perspiration during anaesthesia and surgery. Acta Anaesthesiol Scand. 1980;24(5):362–6.
24. Lamke LO, Nilsson GE, Reithner HL. Water loss by evaporation from the abdominal cavity during surgery. Acta Chir Scand. 1977;143(5):279–84.
25. Marik PE, Cavallazzi R. Does the central venous pressure predict fluid responsiveness? An updated meta-analysis and a plea for some common sense. Crit Care Med. 2013;41(7):1774–81.
26. Vincent JL, Weil MH. Fluid challenge revisited. Crit Care Med. 2006;34(5):1333–7.
27. Guerin L, Monnet X, Teboul JL. Monitoring volume and fluid responsiveness: from static to dynamic indicators. Best Pract Res Clin Anaesthesiol. 2013;27(2):177–85.
28. Michard F, Teboul JL. Using heart-lung interactions to assess fluid responsiveness during mechanical ventilation. Crit Care. 2000;4(5):282–9.
29. Marik PE, Cavallazzi R, Vasu T, Hirani A. Dynamic changes in arterial waveform derived variables and fluid responsiveness in mechanically ventilated patients: a systematic review of the literature. Crit Care Med. 2009;37(9):2642–7.
30. Shi R, Monnet X, Teboul JL. Parameters of fluid responsiveness. Curr Opin Crit Care. 2020;26(3):319–26.
31. Kumar N, Malviya D, Nath SS, et al. Comparison of the efficacy of different arterial waveform-derived variables (pulse pressure variation, stroke volume variation, systolic pressure variation) for fluid responsiveness in hemodynamically unstable mechanically ventilated critically ill patients. Indian J Crit Care Med. 2021;25(1):48–53.
32. Mathis MR, Schechtman SA, Engoren MC, et al. Arterial pressure variation in elective non-cardiac surgery: identifying reference distributions and modifying factors. Anesthesiology. 2017;126(2):249–59.
33. Hadian M, Kim HK, Severyn DA, Pinsky MR. Cross-comparison of cardiac output trending accuracy of LiDCO, PiCCO, FloTrac and pulmonary artery catheters. Crit Care. 2010;14(6):R212.
34. Pinsky MR, Cecconi M, Chew MS, De Backer D, Douglas I, Edwards M, Hamzaoui O, Hernandez G, Martin G, Monnet X, Saugel B, Scheeren TWL, Teboul JL, Vincent JL. Effective hemodynamic monitoring. Crit Care. 2022;26(1):294.
35. Zhang Z, Lu B, Sheng X, Jin N. Accuracy of stroke volume variation in predicting fluid responsiveness: a systematic review and meta-analysis. J Anesth. 2011;25(6):904–16.
36. Myatra SN, Prabu NR, Divatia JV, Monnet X, Kulkarni AP, Teboul JL. The changes in pulse pressure variation or stroke volume variation after a "tidal volume challenge" reliably predict fluid responsiveness during low tidal volume ventilation. Crit Care Med. 2017;45(3):415–21.
37. Chu H, Wang Y, Sun Y, Wang G. Accuracy of pleth variability index to predict fluid responsiveness in mechanically ventilated patients: a systematic review and meta-analysis. J Clin Monit Comput. 2016;30(3):265–74.
38. Cannesson M, Desebbe O, Rosamel P, et al. Pleth variability index to monitor the respiratory variations in the pulse oximeter plethysmographic waveform amplitude and predict fluid responsiveness in the operating theatre. Br J Anaesth. 2008;101(2):200–6.
39. Liu T, Xu C, Wang M, Niu Z, Qi D. Reliability of pleth variability index in predicting preload responsiveness of mechanically ventilated patients under various conditions: a systematic review and meta-analysis. BMC Anesthesiol. 2019;19(1):67.
40. Monnet X, Teboul JL. Passive leg raising: five rules, not a drop of fluid! Crit Care. 2015;19(1):18.

41. Dave C, et al. Dynamic assessment of fluid responsiveness in surgical ICU patients through stroke volume variation is associated with decreased length of stay and costs: a systematic review and meta-analysis. J Intensive Care Med. 2020;35(1):14–23.
42. Gavelli F, Teboul JL, Monnet X. The end-expiratory occlusion test: please, let me hold your breath! Crit Care. 2019;23(1):274.
43. Gavelli F, Shi R, Teboul JL, Azzolina D, Monnet X. The end-expiratory occlusion test for detecting preload responsiveness: a systematic review and meta-analysis. Ann Int Care. 2020;10(1):65.
44. Wang J, Zhou D, Gao Y, Wu Z, Wang X, Lv C. Effect of VTILVOT variation rate on the assessment of fluid responsiveness in septic shock patients. Medicine (Baltimore). 2020;99(47):e22702.
45. Blanco P. Rationale for using the velocity-time integral and the minute distance for assessing the stroke volume and cardiac output in point-of-care settings. Ultrasound J. 2020;12(1):21.
46. Long E, Oakley E, Duke T, Babl FE, (PREDICT) PRiEDIC. Does respiratory variation in inferior vena cava diameter predict fluid responsiveness: a systematic review and meta-analysis. Shock. 2017;47(5):550–9.
47. Ciozda W, Kedan I, Kehl DW, Zimmer R, Khandwalla R, Kimchi A. The efficacy of sonographic measurement of inferior vena cava diameter as an estimate of central venous pressure. Cardiovasc Ultrasound. 2016;14(1):33.
48. Antequera Martin AM, Barea Mendoza JA, Muriel A, et al. Buffered solutions versus 0.9% saline for resuscitation in critically ill adults and children. Cochrane Database Syst Rev. 2019;7:CD012247.
49. Gottlieb M, Petrak V, Binkley C. Are balanced crystalloid solutions better than Normal saline solution for the resuscitation of children and adult patients? Ann Emerg Med. 2020;75(4):532–4.
50. Self WH, Semler MW, Wanderer JP, et al. Balanced crystalloids versus saline in noncritically ill adults. NEJM. 2018;378(9):819–28.
51. Finfer S, Micallef S, Hammond N, et al. Balanced multielectrolyte solution versus saline in critically ill adults. NEJM. 2022;386(9):815–26.
52. Young P, Bailey M, Beasley R, et al. Effect of a buffered crystalloid solution vs saline on acute kidney injury among patients in the intensive care unit: the SPLIT randomized clinical trial. JAMA. 2015;314(16):1701–10.
53. Zampieri FG, Machado FR, Biondi RS, et al. Effect of intravenous fluid treatment with a balanced solution vs 0.9% saline solution on mortality in critically ill patients: the BaSICS randomized clinical trial. JAMA. 2021;326(9):1–12.
54. Semler MW, Self WH, Wanderer JP, et al. Balanced crystalloids versus saline in critically ill adults. NEJM. 2018;378(9):829–39.
55. Pfortmueller CA, Faeh L, Muller M, et al. Fluid management in patients undergoing cardiac surgery: effects of an acetate-versus lactate-buffered balanced infusion solution on hemodynamic stability (HEMACETAT). Crit Care. 2019;23(1):159.
56. He H, Liu D, Ince C. Colloids and the microcirculation. Anesth Analg. 2018;126(5):1747–54.
57. Lewis SR, Pritchard MW, Evans DJ, et al. Colloids versus crystalloids for fluid resuscitation in critically ill people. Cochrane Database Syst Rev. 2018;8(8):CD000567.
58. Finfer S, Bellomo R, Boyce N, et al. A comparison of albumin and saline for fluid resuscitation in the intensive care unit. NEJM. 2004;350(22):2247–56.
59. Myburgh J, Cooper DJ, Finfer S, et al. Saline or albumin for fluid resuscitation in patients with traumatic brain injury. NEJM. 2007;357(9):874–84.
60. Caironi P, Tognoni G, Masson S, et al. Albumin replacement in patients with severe sepsis or septic shock. NEJM. 2014;370(15):1412–21.
61. Frenette AJ, Bouchard J, Bernier P, et al. Albumin administration is associated with acute kidney injury in cardiac surgery: a propensity score analysis. Crit Care. 2014;18(6):602.
62. Kingeter AJ, Raghunathan K, Munson SH, et al. Association between albumin administration and survival in cardiac surgery: a retrospective cohort study. Can J Anaesth. 2018;65(11):1218–27.
63. Evans L, Rhodes A, Alhazzani W, et al. Surviving sepsis campaign: international guidelines for management of sepsis and septic shock 2021. Crit Care Med. 2021;49(11):e1063–143.

64. Brandstrup B, Tønnesen H, Beier-Holgersen R, et al. Effects of intravenous fluid restriction on postoperative complications: comparison of two perioperative fluid regimens: a randomized assessor-blinded multicenter trial. Ann Surg. 2003;238(5):641–8.
65. Tambyraja AL, Sengupta F, MacGregor AB, Bartolo DC, Fearon KC. Patterns and clinical outcomes associated with routine intravenous sodium and fluid administration after colorectal resection. World J Surg. 2004;28(10):1046–51.
66. Grass F, Lovely JK, Crippa J, et al. Potential association between perioperative fluid management and occurrence of postoperative ileus. Dis Colon Rectum. 2020;63(1):68–74.
67. Kubo Y, Tanaka K, Yamasaki M, et al. The impact of perioperative fluid balance on postoperative complications after esophagectomy for esophageal cancer. J Clin Med. 2022;11(11):3219.
68. Shin CH, Long DR, McLean D, et al. Effects of intraoperative fluid management on postoperative outcomes: a hospital registry study. Ann Surg. 2018;267(6):1084–92.
69. Myles PS, Bellomo R, Corcoran T, et al. Restrictive versus liberal fluid therapy for major abdominal surgery. NEJM. 2018;378(24):2263–74.
70. Messina A, Robba C, Calabrò L, et al. Perioperative liberal versus restrictive fluid strategies and postoperative outcomes: a systematic review and metanalysis on randomised-controlled trials in major abdominal elective surgery. Crit Care. 2021;25(1):205.
71. Melloul E, Lassen K, Roulin D, et al. Guidelines for perioperative care for pancreatoduodenectomy: Enhanced Recovery After Surgery (ERAS) recommendations 2019. World J Surg. 2020;44(7):2056–84.
72. Corcoran T, Rhodes JE, Clarke S, Myles PS, Ho KM. Perioperative fluid management strategies in major surgery: a stratified meta-analysis. Anesth Analg. 2012;114(3):640–51.
73. Benes J, Giglio M, Brienza N, Michard F. The effects of goal-directed fluid therapy based on dynamic parameters on post-surgical outcome: a meta-analysis of randomized controlled trials. Crit Care. 2014;18(5):584.
74. Pearse RM, Harrison DA, MacDonald N, et al. Effect of a perioperative, cardiac output-guided hemodynamic therapy algorithm on outcomes following major gastrointestinal surgery: a randomized clinical trial and systematic review. JAMA. 2014;311(21):2181–90.
75. Messina A, Robba C, Calabrò L, et al. Association between perioperative fluid administration and postoperative outcomes: a 20-year systematic review and a meta-analysis of randomized goal-directed trials in major visceral/noncardiac surgery. Crit Care. 2021;25(1):43.
76. Jessen MK, Vallentin MF, Holmberg MJ, et al. Goal directed haemodynamic therapy during general anaesthesia for noncardiac surgery: a systematic review and meta-analysis. Br J Anaesth. 2022;128(3):416–33.
77. Wrzosek A, Jakowicka-Wordliczek J, Zajaczkowska R, et al. Perioperative restrictive versus goal-directed fluid therapy for adults undergoing major non-cardiac surgery. Cochrane Database Syst Rev. 2019;12:CD012767.
78. Ebm CC, Sutton L, Rhodes A, Cecconi M. Cost-effectiveness in goal-directed therapy: are the dollars spent worth the value? J Cardiothorac Vasc Anesth 2014;28(6):1660–6.
79. Sun Y, Yang Z, Tan H. Perioperative nutritional support and fluid therapy in patients with liver diseases. Hepatobiliary Surg Nutr. 2014;3(3):140–8.
80. Muilenburg DJ, Singh A, Torzilli G, Khatri VP. Surgery in the patient with liver disease. Med Clin North Am. 2009;93(5):1065–81.
81. Morkane CM, Sapisochin G, Mukhtar AM, et al. Perioperative fluid management and outcomes in adult deceased donor liver transplantation—a systematic review of the literature and expert panel recommendations. Clin Transpl. 2022;36(10):e14651.
82. Carrier FM, Chassé M, Wang HT, et al. Restrictive fluid management strategies and outcomes in liver transplantation: a systematic review. Can J Anaesth. 2020;67(1):109–27.
83. Yoshino O, Perini MV, Christophi C, Weinberg L. Perioperative fluid management in major hepatic resection: an integrative review. Hepatobiliary Pancreat Dis Int. 2017;16(5):458–69.
84. Osawa EA, Rhodes A, Landoni G, et al. Effect of perioperative goal-directed hemodynamic resuscitation therapy on outcomes following cardiac surgery: a randomized clinical trial and systematic review. Crit Care Med. 2016;44(4):724–33.
85. Romagnoli S, Rizza A, Ricci Z. Fluid status assessment and management during the perioperative phase in adult cardiac surgery patients. J Cardiothorac Vasc Anesth. 2016;30(4):1076–84.

Chapter 19
Perioperative Fluid Administration and Complications in Emergency Gastrointestinal Surgery

Birgitte Brandstrup and Ann Merete Møller

Introduction

The patients needing surgery in the emergency setting differ from the patients in the elective setting in several ways: They are often in a septic state; they might have massive blood, fluid, and/or electrolyte imbalances; surgery is life-saving and might need to be performed as fast as possible and at least within a few hours.

The literature on emergency surgery is often difficult to interpret, because "emergency surgery" covers a wide range of very different diagnoses and surgical procedures. Many national databases include surgery for abscesses, appendicitis, and cholecystitis in the statistical analysis, giving better survival percentages. Nowadays, the risk of death from acute appendicitis or cholecystitis is close to zero. The mortality following surgery for bowel obstruction is also relatively low (up to 10% after 30 days [1, 2]) as is the risk of death from a bleeding ulcer [3, 4], while the mortality following perforations of the intestinal tract regardless whether the perforation is of the stomach or the colon continues to be high (30–40% after

B. Brandstrup (✉)
Department of Surgery, Holbæk Hospital, Part of Copenhagen University Hospitals, Holbæk, Denmark

Institute for Clinical Medicine, Faculty of Health, University of Copenhagen, Copenhagen N, Denmark
e-mail: bbrn@regionsjaelland.dk

A. M. Møller
Institute for Clinical Medicine, Faculty of Health, University of Copenhagen, Copenhagen N, Denmark

Department of Anesthesia, Herlev University Hospital, Herlev, Denmark
e-mail: ann.moeller@regionh.dk

© The Author(s), under exclusive license to Springer Nature Switzerland AG 2024

J. Faintuch, S. Faintuch (eds.), *Recent Strategies in High Risk Surgery*,
https://doi.org/10.1007/978-3-031-56270-9_19

30 days [2, 5, 6]). A condition with an even higher mortality is the patients with a proximal thrombosis of the superior mesenteric artery, causing infarction of the entire small bowel and the right side of the colon. Often it is impossible to save the lives of these patients.

The inclusion or exclusion of these different patient categories and differences in the ratios between them is vital for the comparison of results—a fact that is rarely taken into account when comparing survival numbers between countries or institutions.

Furthermore, national differences are present. This has many reasons ranging from differences in distances to medical aid, the number of hospitals/health staff per capita, to whether or not healthcare is free of charge or not. All these factors are important because patients may give up beforehand to seek help, and the general health of the patients might be very different. Good access to healthcare influences whether co-existing medical conditions are well treated or not. In many first-world countries, on the other hand, the population is getting older, and the patients often have multiple comorbidities—with a surgical emergency on top of it all.

Another very important factor differing between countries and regions is the presence of multi resistant bacteria in the environment. The surgical intervention needed for perforations of the colon illustrates this. In Denmark, even medium sized perforations of the colon are well treated with laparoscopic lavage and drainage only [7–9], while this is sometimes insufficient in other regions [10, 11]. Scandinavian countries have a very low presence of multi-resistant bacteria in the environment, rendering low-toxicity antibiotics to be effective treatment.

Correcting Preoperative Fluid and Electrolyte Imbalances

In a perfect world, fluid and electrolyte imbalances are corrected before the surgery. However, in emergency surgical situations, one must carefully weigh the risks of delaying the surgery against the risks associated with anesthesia and surgery in the presence of imbalances. In such circumstances, it may be necessary to initiate preoperative- and continue intraoperative correction of the condition. Especially in patients with chronic electrolyte imbalances, one has no other choice than to do the surgery and anesthesia with the imbalance present, because fast corrections are more hazardous.

Patients with bowel obstruction have combined hypovolemia and dehydration. Both can be corrected preoperatively relatively quickly. The correction of hypovolemia with isotonic fluids has priority, but often a hypotonic fluid containing glucose to correct the dehydration benefits the patient as well.

Hypovolemia

Hypovolemia remains a common cause of intraoperative death, and hypovolemia should therefore be corrected preoperatively whenever possible. In subacute surgical conditions, correction of hypovolemia is usually unproblematic as it can be corrected relatively quickly. This goes for patients with bowel obstruction without risk of intestinal ischemia. Here the surgery can often be postponed several hours, if the correction of fluid and/or electrolyte imbalances have priority. This illustrates why the decision to operate immediately or later is a team effort between surgeons and anesthetists, and why common decision-making is superior.

In cases of acute ongoing bleeding, the situation is challenging because volume administration can never replace surgical hemostasis. Both procedures often need to be performed simultaneously. Trauma centers prioritize to stabilize the patient's circulatory condition to the extent that vital functions are just maintained, allowing for the patient to be transferred to the operating room (with systolic blood pressure of 90 mmHg or higher) [12, 13]. Cerebral perfusion continues at lower pressures in supine patients [14].

Intensive Prehospital Treatment

In certain circumstances it increases both the complication rate and mortality, nominally in thoracic gunshot wounds [15]. A likely explanation is that volume replacement increases blood pressure, thus "flushing out" clots from the blood vessels and causing re-bleeding before surgical hemostasis is achieved. In addition, both dilution of coagulation factors and fluid overload may contribute to the observed harmful effect.

Likewise, research suggests blood pressure should not be raised to normal values in patients with a ruptured aortic aneurysm (after animal experiments, a threshold of systolic BP <95 mmHg has been set [16]) to avoid re-bleeding, however the evidence is low [17]. Re-bleeding can occur in the adventitia of the vessels (in dissecting aortic aneurysms), pericardium, thorax, or retroperitoneum, depending on the location of the aneurysm. Bleeding into the pericardium carries a risk of cardiac tamponade.

It is likely that intravenous fluid therapy, which increases blood pressure, can cause similar re-bleeding in other conditions (pelvic fractures, liver injuries, etc.) even if temporary hemostasis has been achieved. The rule is that the higher the blood pressure, the greater the blood loss during ongoing bleeding, and the greater the risk of re-bleeding in conditions with uncertain or inadequate hemostasis.

Such an effect is *not* seen in trauma cases where hemostasis is possible, for example, in extremity injuries with the application of effective hemostatic pressure (placement of a tourniquet).

All this circumstances notwithstanding, uncontrolled shock can rapidly lead to organ failures and death; therefore, early fluid administration is standard care for patients who have lost massive amounts of blood or other fluids and display markedly depressed hemodynamic findings. A mean arterial pressure of 50–65 mmHg should be the general aim.

Management of Acute Ongoing Bleeding

Administration of fluids during acute major bleeding should be guided by thromboelastography (TEG) or thromboelastometry (ROTEM) [18]. TEG- or ROTEM-guided transfusion strategies may reduce the need for blood products and improve morbidity in patients with ongoing hemorrhage.

In acute bleeding, crystalloids are administered while waiting for blood products. Artificial colloids such as hydroxyethyl starch are not recommended as they might worsen dilutional coagulopathy by their adverse effects on fibrin polymerization and platelet aggregation.

Subsequently, blood loss is replaced with either whole blood or "blood component packs," with regional variations in the ratio. In our routine the number of units is

$$\text{Red blood cells } 3 : \text{Fresh frozen plasma} \left(\text{FFP}\right) 3 : \text{Platelet concentrate } 1,$$

equivalent to whole blood transfusion.

In addition to the TEG/ROTEM, treatment is monitored using hemoglobin, international normalized ratio (INR), activated partial thromboplastin time (APTT), fibrinogen, and platelet concentration.

We recommend giving platelets immediately, while erythrocytes and FFP are given in separate IV lines. The strategy for replacement of blood loss during surgery is summarized in Table 19.1.

Table 19.1 Replacement of blood loss [19][a]

Loss in % of blood volume	Loss in mL (70–80 kg person)	Replacement	Volume
0–20%	0–1000 mL	Lactated or Acetated Ringers solution	500–3000 mL
20–40%	1000–2000 mL	Supplemental Human Albumin (HA)	1000 mL
40–80%	2000–4000 mL	Supplemental paced red blood cells (RBC) and HA	3–4 portions RBC (1000 mL) 1000 mL (HA)
Thereafter	For every 500 mL	Supplemental RBC And fresh frozen plasma (FFP)	1 portion (ca. 300 mL) 1 portion (ca. 250 mL)
		Platelets	1 for every 3 RBC and FFP

[a]Human albumin should be used at the physician's discretion. Current recommendations, such as Clinical Guidelines for Human Albumin Use (https://www.nppeag.scot.nhs.uk/wp-content/uploads/2020/07/2018-Albumin-Guideline.pdf), emphasize that no studies have convincingly shown that human albumin confers survival advantages for conventional volume expansion

Anemia

Anemia is corrected both preoperatively and intraoperatively. Typically, a blood hemoglobin level of >4.3 mmol/L (7 g/L) is aimed for in "healthy" individuals, and >5.6 mmol/L (9 g/L) in patients with severe heart/lung disease [20].

If significant blood loss is expected during the operation, a higher preoperative hemoglobin level may be appropriate, but there is a lack of evidence supporting this. In many institutions, transfusion is chosen when the intraoperative hemoglobin level falls below 6 mmol/L (9.6 g/L), as operative bleeding is considered severe acute bleeding.

Meeting the Basic Fluid and Electrolyte Requirements of the Body

The basic needs of patients undergoing surgery differ from those in normal conditions in three aspects:

1. Patients are instructed to fast.
2. Patients may experience trauma, inflammation, or metabolic stress, leading to the release of stress hormones, including aldosterone, which causes salt and water retention. In turn cytokines in the same setting could be natriuretic, such as TNF-alpha.
3. Patients are artificially ventilated with 100% humidified air, thus water loss from the airways are diminished.

Insensible perspiration is water loss through the skin and respiratory tract and is the only pure water loss from the body. Approximately two-thirds of the volume comes from the skin, while one-third comes from the respiratory tract [21]. Thus, in patients on mechanical ventilation with 100% humidified air, the insensible perspiration from the respiratory tract is reduced by approximately one-third. Otherwise the insensible perspiration is not much influenced by surgery [22].

The insensible perspiration is dependent on the skin surface. However, calculating skin surface may not be practical in the daily clinical setting. Therefore an approximation to body weight is made. This is introducing the mistake of underestimating the insensible perspiration for persons with a great skin surface relative to body weight (children) and overestimating in the opposite context (persons with a bodyweight >150 kg). Knowing these limitations, the insensible perspiration is in temperate climate very consistent [21] (10 mL/kg/day), and if the patient is on a ventilator using humidified air, 6.6 mL/kg/day.

If the patient is not on a ventilator, an increase in body temperature (fever) leads to an elevated respiratory frequency, however, the impact is minimal.

Sensible perspiration refers to visible sweat, which consists of salt and water and is always hypotonic compared to extracellular fluid. Exercise, elevated environmental temperature, and severe disease can increase sensible perspiration. Patients in emergency surgical conditions (such as sepsis or shock) may experience significant sensible perspiration.

Diuresis

The production of urine is approximately 1 L per day for a healthy individual with normal body weight, food- and fluid intake. In *elderly patients*, normal volumes of urine may not indicate sufficient diuresis. Assessing the adequacy of diuresis for each individual patient requires understanding their osmotic load and the kidney's ability to concentrate urine.

The glomerular filtration rate (GFR), which reflects kidney function, is approximately 140 mL/min/1.73 m^2 in young, healthy adults. It decreases by about 8 mL/min/1.73 m^2 every 10 years after the age of 40 [23]. Elderly patients generally have lower muscle mass, resulting in decreased creatinine production. As a result, the creatinine concentration may remain normal despite a reduced GFR [23, 24]. Aging is associated with a significant decline in the kidney's ability to both concentrate and dilute urine, as well as perform free water clearance [25].

In young, healthy male volunteers, urinary osmolality under different conditions is as follows:

500–950 mosm/kg after overnight fasting [26, 27].
Approximately 1100 mosm/kg after 24 h of fasting [27].
Maximum 1420 mosm/kg after fasting for 4 days [28].

In elderly healthy male volunteers (67–75 years of age), values reduce to around 700 mosm/kg following overnight fasting, and approximately 950 mosm/kg urine after fasting for 24 h [27].

For an 80-year-old person, urinary osmolality following 12 h of fasting can be as low as 400–600 mosm/kg urine [25].

Furthermore, plasma sodium levels increased significantly in elderly male volunteers, compared to volunteers aged 20–31. Despite the elevated plasma sodium, elderly participants do not consume as much water as younger individuals, resulting in sustained elevation of plasma sodium and osmolality for more than five days [27].

The corresponding information for women is unknown; therefore gender corrections are not currently adopted.

Sodium Excretion

It represents only a small fraction of total urine osmolality. With no pharmacological interference, urinary excretion of Na^+ can vary between less than 0.1% and no more than 3% of the filtered load (H_2O can vary between 0.3 and 15% of the intake)

[28]. In healthy young male volunteers given a dietary salt load (tablets) of up to 32 g/day, the maximum sodium excretion reached 300 mmol/L urine [29].

This explains why drinking seawater is unwise. The salt concentration in seawater is approximately 600 mmol/L, and considering the kidneys' maximum ability to concentrate 300 mmol of sodium in 1 L of urine (in young males), drinking seawater would provide the body with salt instead of water. Indeed regular consumption of just moderate excess of salinity in drinking water is already associated with arterial hypertension [29].

Classically the hormonal stress response in emergency surgical disease and after surgery tends to retain salt and water in the body, even though there are exceptions, such as severe spinal cord injury [30, 31]. Therefore, the formation of edema in surgical patients should not always be attributed to excessive hydration, even though this is relatively common. The presence of an osmotically active substance, namely sodium, is usually required to retain water. More accurately, postoperative edema formation can be seen as "over salting," and providing water to facilitate salt excretion, along with the administration of the diuretic furosemide (which promotes excretion of sodium), can help reduce edema.

Lactated or acetated Ringer's solutions have a sodium content at 130 mmol per liter, not significantly different from normal saline with 154 mmol per liter. However, lactate is metabolized into CO_2 and water by the cellular metabolism, making these fluids slightly hypotonic, thus providing the kidneys with slightly more water to excrete the salts.

It is important to note that without adequate water intake, all synthetic colloids will form a gel in the kidney tubules, potentially leading to kidney injury. Even in the absence of water deprivation, kidney damage is more likely with these artificial plasma expanders than with crystalloids.

The daily requirements can be summarized as follows for an 80 kg person (body surface of 1.85 m^2) with normal kidney function [19]:

Sodium: 75–150 mmol
Potassium: 60–100 mmol
Glucose: 850 mmol = 150 g (the brains basal requirement)
Water: 2000–3000 mL

Therefore, 2–3 L of a solution containing approximately 40 mmol of sodium, 20–30 mmol of potassium, and 50 mmol of glucose will meet the daily requirements.

Fluid Therapy During Preoperative Fasting

In an emergency setting, the emptying of the stomach is often slowed down by the underlying disease, and the patient may be dehydrated and/or hypovolemic. Several studies have demonstrated that preoperative administration of sugar-containing fluids (oral or intravenous) improves well-being, reduces hunger and thirst, enhances muscle strength, and decreases postoperative insulin resistance in elective abdominal surgical patients [32–34]. However, no evidence exist on the role of glucose-containing fluids in emergency surgical patients [35]; therefore the parenteral route is preferred.

In elective surgical patients, fluid and electrolyte loss during fasting will be normal, and if intravenous fluid supplementation is necessary, choosing a fluid that replaces normal losses is the logical approach, such as a solution containing K-Na-Glucose or Glucose 5%. In emergency surgical patients without hypovolemia the same choice of fluid seems rational, depending on the patients' blood glucose levels that might be elevated due to the emergency disease. In circumstances of hypovolemia or electrolyte disturbances, fluids correcting these conditions are a better choice.

During Surgery

Emergency surgical patients may experience blood loss, ascites formation, or prolonged ileus; however, basal fluid and electrolyte losses are not increased.

Is There a "Third Space" Compartment?

The historical non-anatomical third-space loss described a transfer of extracellular volume (ECV), resulting in a decreased total ECV. It was believed that the surgical trauma in itself or severe hemorrhagic shock caused a redistribution of body fluid compartments, leading to a reduction in ECV by several liters. The fluid was not found in the ECV, and later studies showed that it was not found in the intracellular volume (ICV) either, leading to speculation that there must be a yet unidentified "third space."

This decrease in ECV was recommended to be treated with intravenous fluids (0.9% NaCl or Ringer's solution), according to generous algorithms. However, there is a lack of evidence for the occurrence of this ECV loss [36], and it has not been shown that the administration of additional intravenous fluids has any beneficial effect for the patient. On the contrary, the prognosis of abdominal surgical patients is significantly worsened by this "replacement." [37] We have therefore totally abandoned the entire concept.

Effects of Intestinal Manipulation and Surgical Trauma

The surgical trauma itself and manipulation of the intestines during surgery can cause cellular damage and result in mild edema formation. Experimental studies have shown that the formation of a small bowel anastomosis increases the water content in the surrounding tissue by 5–10% [38]. If the same occurs in humans and the weight of the anastomosis is similar to that of a stoma removed during the reversal of the Hartmann's procedure (50 g) [39], the amount of fluid "lost to the traumatized tissue" is estimated to be approximately 2.5–5 g or 2.5–5 mL.

Intravenous fluid therapy exacerbates this edema formation and destabilizes the bowel anastomosis. When administered at a rate of 15 mL/kg/h, the local water content more than doubles to 10–20%, and the stability of the anastomosis decreases, making it more prone to bursting under lower pressure [40]. Additionally, inflammation around the anastomosis increases [41]. These findings are consistent with the research by Jacob et al. [42], who describe how fluid overload can disrupt the endothelial glycocalyx, leading to inflammation and fluid leakage into the interstitial space.

Exudation and Blood Loss

During open surgery, fluid may seep from the wound and intestines. Often, this ascitic fluid is contained in a suction bottle or/and absorbed by surgical dressings, and its volume is estimated.

In abdominal surgery where the viscera are exteriorized, the surgeon can use a plastic bag to collect and measure the fluid loss more accurately. The exudate typically contains albumin, and manipulation of the intestines can increase the albumin content. In patients treated by open abdomen, the protein content was estimated as 2 g of nitrogen per liter of abdominal fluid output [43].

Unless the patient is experiencing significant visible bleeding or occult blood loss (such as from a bleeding ulcer in the intestines), blood loss can be measured fairly accurately by assessing the content in suction bottles and monitoring changes in the weight of the surgical dressings.

The perspiration from the open abdomen is usually so small that it often needs no consideration. However, during maximal eventration about 1 mL/kg/h can be eliminated [44, 45]. Probably most of the fluid deficit in such circumstances stems from bowel edema [44, 45]. Placing the viscera in a plastic bag can ameliorate evaporation.

Intraoperative hypothermia is more common than previously estimated, both during open and laparoscopic interventions, even though the contribution of water evaporation is incompletely known [46].

The extent of evaporative fluid loss during laparoscopic surgery has been calculated as <1 mL/h only, when dry CO_2 is insufflated, and thus insignificant [47].

Conventional Protocols

Epidural Analgesia

The administration of epidurals blocks both sensory and sympathetic fibers in the affected area of the spinal cord, resulting in a reduction in heart rate (in cases of high blocks) and vasodilation, leading to a decrease in arterial blood pressure. Early studies suggested that a fluid bolus of 500 mL of colloid or 1000 mL of crystalloid could counteract this decrease in blood pressure [48, 49]. However, subsequent randomized clinical trials have failed to validate these findings. In fact, they have demonstrated that intravenous fluid administration alone is ineffective in treating the blood pressure decline caused by epidural dilation, and overall cardiac output remains largely unchanged [50–56]. Epidural and spinal anesthesia are effectively an iatrogenic sympathectomy. As a consequence, moderate fluid therapy should be combined with vasopressors, and various pharmacologic regimens are currently available [50].

Goal-Directed Fluid Therapy (GDT)

GDT has been implemented in various clinical trials, although there is inconsistency in defining the specific goals that characterize a trial as "goal directed," as indicated in published reviews.

Initially, the trials employed *a pressure-controlled* approach, focusing on parameters like blood pressure and central vein pressure [57, 58]. Most accepted goals now revolve around optimizing stroke volume (SV) or stroke volume variation (SVV), which can be considered as a form of *flow-controlled fluid therapy*.

Additionally, the concept of "zero fluid balance" or restricted fluid therapy has been included in the goal-directed fluid therapy approach [59], resembling a *balance-controlled strategy*. Some trials have explored biochemical markers such as lactate or central venous oxygen tension as targets for a *biochemical-controlled therapy* [60–64].

Combining multiple of the above goals is likely the most effective approach.

Henceforth, GDT refers to the administration of a fluid (colloid) to achieve near-maximal SV.

In elective abdominal surgical procedures, some investigations demonstrated benefits [65–70], whereas others did not [62, 71–73]. Notably, only a few trials measured the volume of intravenous fluids administered postoperatively, and those that did only measured fluid intake for the remainder of the surgery day [62, 65, 69, 72]. Interestingly, large amounts of crystalloid fluids were administered alongside colloid-based stroke volume optimization. This could be interpreted in two ways: either the crystalloid acted as a temporary fluid overload that quickly left the circulation (as typically observed in normovolemic individuals), or crystalloids are ineffective in increasing stroke volume. Another intriguing finding is that colloid solutions, including hydroxyethyl starch (HES), appeared to have positive effects on outcomes in elective bowel surgery without the side effects observed in septic patients [74].

Restricted Fluid Therapy Approach (Near Zero Fluid Balance)

It is believed that GDT (based on a near zero balance principle) is not superior to restricted fluid therapy [75–80]. In comparative studies, generally the group receiving the smallest fluid volume achieves the best outcomes. Still perioperative fluid therapy in major abdominal surgery requires finding the appropriate balance. In a study conducted by Warrillow et al. in 2010 [81], patients in their institution received a median of 4.2 L of intravenous fluid intraoperatively and 6.3 L postoperatively, resulting in a total of 10.5 L. They observed that 21% developed pulmonary edema, 12% experienced anastomotic leaks, and the overall complication rate was 57%, with 32% being major complications.

In our trial published in 2003 [37], fluid overload with saline and the subsequent increase in body weight (4 kg) were detrimental. By avoiding fluid overload, we have significantly reduced the incidence of postoperative atrial fibrillation, pulmonary congestion, edema, and acute respiratory distress syndrome (ARDS).

The benefit of restricted or near zero-balance fluid volumes has been confirmed in patients undergoing gastrointestinal [37, 63], urologic [82], pulmonary [83], cardiac [84], vascular [85], and mixed [63] surgical procedures, as well as in surgical patients in the intensive care unit [86]. The findings were consistent across these studies: there are adverse consequences associated with fluid overload.

The largest trial to date comparing restricted versus liberal fluid therapy was conducted by Myles et al., involving 3000 patients [87]. The median body weight increase was 0.3 kg in the restricted group versus 1.6 kg in the liberal group 24 h after surgery, indicating that both approaches were fairly restricted. Although no difference was found regarding one-year disability-free survival, more patients in the restricted fluid group experienced renal failure. However, it is worth noting that the restricted group did not have a protocol for administering fluids in cases of postoperative oliguria, suggesting that the restricted regimen may have been excessively restrictive and thus caused harm. The trial itself has several limitations [88], and it is possible that an optimal fluid strategy lies somewhere between the two treatment arms.

Weaknesses

Clinical randomized trials involving fluid therapy in general possess inherent weaknesses. It is challenging to blind such trials as fluid administration leads to observable changes in body weight, urinary output, and the formation of subcutaneous edema. Using length of stay (LoS) as an endpoint also poses challenges. The introduction of fast-track surgery has highlighted that patient and physician expectations play a crucial role in determining the LoS. Patients tend to remain in the hospital for the duration they are advised to stay.

Furthermore, controlling for other potential confounding factors is not always successful, such as laparoscopic or open surgery, the use of drains and tubes, the allowance for patients to resume oral fluid and food intake, and the type of postoperative analgesia administered. For instance, the occurrence of postoperative nausea and vomiting (PONV) is heavily influenced by the use of opiates.

The Emergency Surgical Setting

One trial of emergency surgical patients showed, that a multimodal treatment including fast CT-scan, early preoperative treatment of hypovolemia with goal-directed fluid therapy to near-maximal stroke volume achieved with bolus infusions of HES (Voluven®), and fast surgical intervention (<3 h from arrival to hospital) improved the outcome with reduced mortality compared with a historic control group [89].

Especially in Great Britain fellow researchers have argued that the lack of superiority of GDT can be attributed to the overall good health of the patients included in the trials of elective surgery. To meet this, we did a clinical randomized trial of the sickest patients we could think of, namely patients with gastrointestinal perforation or bowel obstruction needing emergency surgery. Up until now this is the only clinical randomized trial of fluid therapy specifically focusing on emergency abdominal surgical patients [2]. However, even for this patient population, we found no significant benefits in outcomes with GDT fluid therapy compared to restricted fluid therapy. On the contrary, the restricted fluid group had a shorter length of hospital stay (LoS).

A retrospective study of patients having emergency surgery for bowel obstruction or GI-perforation found a U-shaped relationship between the development of complications and fluid balance. The frequency of cardiopulmonary complications was lowest at a balance of 0–1000 mL, while the frequency of renal complications was lowest at approximately 0–2000 mL [90]. This trial, however, may suffer from indication-induced bias. In synthesis, even the emergency surgical patients are best treated following the principles of "restricted fluid therapy."

Recommendations for Pre- and Intraoperative Fluid Therapy

We recommend that fluid be replaced quantitatively (in volume) and qualitatively (with similar electrolyte content), starting preoperatively (upon admission) and only as needed, possibly guided by central hemodynamic values, exceeding measured losses by no more than +1–2 L.

1. Fasting: Give 80 mL per hour of fasting. Use Ringer's fluid or a glucose-containing fluid. Note that glucose may have contraindications in women giving birth and be aware of blood glucose.
2. Epidural preloading: There is no need for preloading. If fluid is administered, consider it as replacing the fasting deficit or as early replacement for expected blood loss.
3. Insensible perspiration and evaporation from open surgical wounds is small and usually need no consideration. Medical water in antibiotics, etc. is sufficient to replenish these losses unless the surgery is prolonged.
4. Drainage of pathological fluid: If ascites is drained, it does not need to be replaced. However record it in the intraoperative fluid chart. Note that postoperative reaccumulation of such fluid may lead to hypovolemia.
5. Bleeding and exudation: Replace blood loss with Ringer's fluid at a ratio of 1:2–3. Monitor hemoglobin (Hb) levels. Administer red blood cells to maintain Hb levels above 4.5 mmol/L (7 g/L) in young, healthy patients and above 5.6 mmol/L (9 g/L) in elderly patients with cardiopulmonary conditions. Refer to Table 19.1 for specific recommendations.
6. Continuous blood loss: Close control with TEG/ROTEM. After 6 units of red blood cells are transfused, administer fresh frozen plasma. Initiate platelet supplementation.
7. Emergency ongoing bleeding: Utilize "transfusion packages" with the ratio of 4 units of erythrocytes, 4 units of plasma, and 1 unit of platelets (similar to full blood).
8. Urine output: Intraoperative urinary loss does not need to be replaced. Low diuresis during surgery can be due to factors other than fluid deficit. If hypovolemia is ruled out, a reduced intraoperative diuresis is acceptable.
9. Maintain a background infusion rate of no more than 2 mL/kg/h and closely monitor blood loss to achieve these objectives.

Postoperative Fluid Therapy

In brief, we recommend the following postoperative fluid therapy:

1. Hypotonic fluid to meet their daily water, sodium, potassium, and glucose requirements (see above).
2. Replace pathological fluid losses with a fluid in similar volume and containing similar electrolyte content as the loss.
3. The electrolyte content in the different GI-fluid losses can be found in reference [91].
4. Maintain postoperative urinary output at 0.5–1 mL/kg/h.
5. Examine all patients with oliguria or hypotension and treat them accordingly. If hypovolemia is the cause, give additional IV crystalloid. In cases of epidural analgesia overdose, reduce the dose.

6. Address dehydration by providing additional water or IV-glucose.
7. Initiate feeding as soon as possible after surgery.
8. Avoid a weight increase >1–2 kg.

Enhanced Recovery After Surgery (ERAS)

Recommendations for fluid therapy in ERAS programs advocate for a zero fluid balance with no more than a 2–2.5 kg body weight gain [92]. Specialized ERAS programs for elderly individuals are available and highly recommended.

We recommend that patients be allowed to drink and eat freely after surgery, whenever tolerated. Intravenous fluid therapy should be considered if oral intake is insufficient, the patient has paralytic ileus, high output stoma, or complications have occurred.

References

1. Barrow E, Anderson ID, Varley S, et al. UK practice in emergency laparotomy. Ann R Coll Surg Engl. 2013;95:599–603.
2. Aaen AA, Voldby AW, Storm N, et al. Goal-directed fluid therapy in emergency abdominal surgery: a randomised multicentre trial. Br J Anaesth. 2021;127:521–31.
3. Mönig SP, Lübke T, Baldus SE, et al. Early elective surgery for bleeding ulcer in the posterior duodenal bulb. Own results and review of the literature. Hepato-Gastroenterology. 2002;49:416–8.
4. Stanley AJ, Laine L. Management of acute upper gastrointestinal bleeding. BMJ. 2019;364:1536.
5. Watt DG, Wilson MSJ, Shapter OC, et al. 30-Day and 1-year mortality in emergency general surgery laparotomies: an area of concern and need for improvement? Eur J Trauma Emerg Surg. 2015;41:369–74.
6. Møller MH, Vester-Andersen M, Thomsen RW. Long-term mortality following peptic ulcer perforation in the PULP trial. A nationwide follow-up study. Scand J Gastroenterol. 2013;48:168–75.
7. Azhar N, Johanssen A, Sundström T, et al. Laparoscopic lavage vs primary resection for acute perforated diverticulitis: long-term outcomes from the Scandinavian Diverticulitis (SCANDIV) randomized clinical trial. JAMA Surg. 2021;156:121–7.
8. Kohl A, Rosenberg J, Bock D, et al. Two-year results of the randomized clinical trial DILALA comparing laparoscopic lavage with resection as treatment for perforated diverticulitis. Br J Surg. 2018;105:1128–34.
9. Angenete E, Thornell A, Burcharth J, et al. Laparoscopic lavage is feasible and safe for the treatment of perforated diverticulitis with purulent peritonitis: the first results from the randomized controlled trial DILALA. Ann Surg. 2016;263(1):117–22.
10. Penna M, Markar SR, Mackenzie H, et al. Laparoscopic lavage versus primary resection for acute perforated diverticulitis: review and meta-analysis. Ann Surg. 2018;267:252–8.
11. Vennix S, Musters GD, Mulder IM, et al. Laparoscopic peritoneal lavage or sigmoidectomy for perforated diverticulitis with purulent peritonitis: a multicentre, parallel-group, randomised, open-label trial. Lancet. 2015;386:1269–77.
12. Wiles MD. Blood pressure management in trauma: from feast to famine? Anaesthesia. 2013;68:445–9.

13. Kolarik M, Roberts E. Permissive hypotension and trauma: can fluid restriction reduce the incidence of ARDS? J Trauma Nurs. 2017;24:19–24.
14. Tran A, Yates J, Lau A, et al. Permissive hypotension versus conventional resuscitation strategies in adult trauma patients with hemorrhagic shock: a systematic review and meta-analysis of randomized controlled trials. J Trauma Acute Care Surg. 2018;84:802–8.
15. Bickell WH, Wall MJ Jr, Pepe PE, et al. Immediate versus delayed fluid resuscitation for hypotensive patients with penetrating torso injuries. N Engl J Med. 1994;331:1105–9.
16. Roberts K, Revell M, Youssef H, et al. Hypotensive resuscitation in patients with ruptured abdominal aortic aneurysm. Eur J Vasc Endovasc Surg. 2006;31:339–44.
17. Moreno DH, Cacione DG, Baptista-Silva JC. Controlled hypotension versus normotensive resuscitation strategy for people with ruptured abdominal aortic aneurysm. Cochrane Database Syst Rev. 2018;6(6):CD011664.
18. Wikkelsø A, Wetterslev J, Møller AM, Afshari A. Thromboelastography (TEG) or thromboelastometry (ROTEM) to monitor haemostatic treatment versus usual care in adults or children with bleeding. Cochrane Database Syst Rev. 2016;8:CD007871.
19. Brandstrup B, Faber T, Engquist A. Rationel væske-og elektrolytbehandling (Rational fluid and electrolyte management). Denmark, Munksgaard: København; 2020.
20. National klinisk retningslinje om blodtransfusion (National clinical guideline on blood transfusion), 2014. 2023. Denmark, The Danish national board of health. https://www.app.magicapp.org/#/guideline/7035. Accessed 29 Aug 2023.
21. Cox P. Insensible water loss and its assessment in adult patients: a review. Acta Anesthesiol Scand. 1987;31:771–6.
22. Baumber CD, Clark RG. Insensible water loss in surgical patients. Br J Surg. 1974;61:53–6.
23. Weinstein JR, Anderson S. The aging kidney: physiological changes. Adv Chronic Kidney Dis. 2010;17:302–7.
24. Beck LH. Perioperative renal, fluid and electrolyte management. Clin Geriatric Med. 1990;6:557–69.
25. Musso CG, Alvarez Gregori J, Jauregui JR, Macías Núñez JF. Creatinine, urea, uric acid, water and electrolytes renal handling in the healthy oldest old. World J Nephrol. 2012;1(5):123–6.
26. Drummer C, Gerzer R, Heer M, et al. Effect of an acute saline infusion on fluid and electrolyte metabolism in humans. Am J Phys. 1992;262:F744–54.
27. Phillips PA, Rolls BJ, Ledingham JGG, et al. Reduced thirst after water deprivation in healthy elderly men. N Engl J Med. 1984;311:753–9.
28. Greger R. Physiology of renal sodium transport. Am J Med Sci. 2000;319(1):51–62.
29. Talukder MRR, Rutherford S, Phung D, Islam MZ, Chu C. The effect of drinking water salinity on blood pressure in young adults of coastal Bangladesh. Environ Pollut. 2016;214:248–54.
30. Kogawa R, Kinoshita K, Tanjoh K. Increase in urinary sodium excretion in spinal cord injury patients in the emergency department. Eur J Trauma Emerg Surg. 2016;42(1):61–6.
31. Kudoh A, Ishihara H, Matsuki A. Renin-aldosterone system and atrial natriuretic peptide during anesthesia in orthopedic patients over 80 years of age. J Clin Anesth. 1999;11:101–7.
32. Henriksen MG. Effects of preoperative oral carbohydrates and peptides on postoperative endocrine response, mobilization, nutrition and muscle function in abdominal surgery. Acta Anesthesiol Scand. 2003;47:191–9.
33. Ljungqvist O, Thorell A, Gutniak M, et al. Glucose infusion instead of preoperative fasting reduces postoperative insulin resistance. J Am Coll Surg. 1994;178:329–36.
34. Nygren J, Soop M, Thorell A, et al. Preoperative oral carbohydrates and postoperative insulin resistance. Clin Nutr. 1999;18:117–20.
35. Peden CJ, Aggarwal G, Aitken RJ, et al. Guidelines for perioperative Care for Emergency Laparotomy Enhanced Recovery After Surgery (ERAS) society recommendations: part 1—preoperative: diagnosis, rapid assessment and optimization. World J Surg. 2021;45:1272–90.
36. Brandstrup B, Svendsen C, Engquist A. Hemorrhage and operation cause a contraction of the extra cellular space needing replacement—evidence and implications? A systematic review. Surgery. 2006;139:419–32.

37. Brandstrup B, Tønnesen H, Beier-Holgersen R, et al. Effects of intravenous fluid restriction on postoperative complications: comparison of two perioperative fluid regimens. A randomized assessor blinded multi Centre trial. Ann Surg. 2003;238:641–8.
38. Chan STF, Kapadia CR, Johnson AW, et al. Extracellular fluid volume expansion and third space sequestration at the site of small bowel anastomoses. Br J Surg. 1983;70:36–9.
39. Brandstrup B. Restricted intravenous fluid therapy in colorectal surgery, results of a clinical randomised multi centre trial; 2003. https://www.researchgate.net/publication/279931470_Restricted_intravenous_fluid_therapy_in_colorectal_surgery_Results_of_a_clinical_randomised_multi_centre_trial/link/559e9b0508aea946c06a3671/download. Accessed 28 Aug 2023.
40. Marjanovic G, Villain C, Juettner E, et al. Impact of different crystalloid volume fluid regimens on intestinal anastomotic stability. Ann Surg. 2009;249:181–5.
41. Kulemann B, Timme S, Sifert G, et al. Intraoperative crystalloid overload leads to substantial inflammatory infiltration of intestinal anastomosis—a histomorphological analysis. Surgery. 2013;154:596–603.
42. Jacob M, Chappel D, Rehm M. The third space—fact or fiction? Best Pract Res Clin Anaesthesiol. 2009;23:145–57.
43. Cheatham ML, Safcsak K, Brzezinski SJ, Lube MW. Nitrogen balance, protein loss, and the open abdomen. Crit Care Med. 2007;35(1):127–31.
44. Rehm M, Hulde N, Kammerer T, Meidert AS, Hofmann-Kiefer K. State of the art in fluid and volume therapy : a user-friendly staged concept. Anaesthesist. 2019;68(Suppl 1):1–14.
45. Burlew CC. The open abdomen: practical implications for the practicing surgeon. Am J Surg. 2012;204(6):826–35.
46. Cumin D, Fogarin J, Mitchell SJ, Windsor JA. Perioperative hypothermia in open and laparoscopic colorectal surgery. ANZ J Surg. 2022;92(5):1125–31.
47. Biegner AR, Anderson D, Olson RL, et al. Quantification of insensible water loss associated with insufflation of nonhumidified CO2 in patients undergoing laparoscopic surgery. J Laparoendosc Adv Surg Tec A. 1999;9:325–9.
48. Clark RB, Thompson DS, Thompson CH. Prevention of spinal hypotension associated with cesarean section. Anesthesiology. 1976;45:670–4.
49. Fanelli G, Casati A, Berti M, et al. Incidence of hypotension and bradycardia during integrated epidural/general anaesthesia. An epidemiologic observational study on 1200 consecutive patients. Italian Study Group on Integrated Anaesthesia. Minerva Anesthesiol. 1998;64:313–9.
50. Massoth C, Töpel L, Wenk M. Hypotension after spinal anesthesia for cesarean section: how to approach the iatrogenic sympathectomy. Curr Opin Anaesthesiol. 2020;33(3):291–8.
51. Kinsella SM, Pirlet M, Mills MS, et al. Randomized study of intravenous fluid preload before epidural analgesia during labour. Br J Anaesth. 2000;85:311–3.
52. Kubli M, Shennan AH, Seed PT, et al. A randomised controlled trial of fluid pre-loading before low dose epidural analgesia for labour. Int J Obstet Anesth. 2003;12:256–60.
53. Nishimura N, Kajimoto Y, Kabe T, et al. The effect of volume loading during epidural analgesia. Resuscitation. 1985;13:31–9.
54. Jackson R, Reid JA, Thorburn J. Volume preloading is not essential to prevent spinal-induced hypotension at caesarean section. Br J Anaesth. 1995;75:262–5.
55. Park GE, Hauch MA, Curlin F, et al. The effects of varying volumes of crystalloid administration before cesarian delivery on maternal hemodynamics and colloid osmotic pressure. Anesth Analg. 1996;83:299–303.
56. Rout CC, Rocke DA, Levin J, et al. A reevaluation in the role of crystaloid preload in the prevention of hypotension associated with spinal anesthesia for elective cesarean section. Anesthesiology. 1993;79:262–9.
57. Rivers E, Nguyen B, Havstad S, et al. Early goal-directed therapy in the treatment of severe sepsis and septic shock. N Engl J Med. 2001;345:1368–77.
58. Shoemaker WC, Appel PL, Kram HB, et al. Prospective trial of supranormal values of survivors as therapeutic goals in high risk surgical patients. Chest. 1987;94:1176–86.

59. Navarro LH, Bloomstone JA, Auler JO Jr, et al. Perioperative fluid therapy: a statement from the international Fluid Optimization Group. Perioper Med. 2015;4:1–20.
60. Jones AE, Shapiro NI, Trzeciak S, et al. Emergency Medicine Shock Research Network (EMShockNet) Investigators. Lactate clearance vs central venous oxygen saturation as goals of early sepsis therapy: a randomized clinical trial. JAMA. 2010;303:739–46.
61. Wilms H, Mittal A, Haydock MD, et al. A systematic review of goal directed fluid therapy: rating of evidence for goals and monitoring methods. J Crit Care. 2014;29:204–9.
62. Forget P, Lois F, de Kock M. Goal-directed fluid management based on the pulse oximeter-derived pleth variability index reduces lactate levels and improves fluid management. Anesth Analg. 2010;111:910–4.
63. Lobo SM, Lobo FR, Polachini CA, et al. Prospective, randomized trial comparing fluids and Doputamine optimization of oxygen delivery in high-risk surgical patients. Crit Care. 2006;10:R72.
64. Lobo SMA, Salgado PF, Castillo VGT, et al. Effects of maximizing oxygen delivery on morbidity and mortality in high-risk surgical patients. Crit Care Med. 2000;28:3396–404.
65. Benes J, Chytra I, Altmann P, et al. Intraoperative fluid optimization using stroke volume variation in high risk surgical patients: results of prospective randomized study. Crit Care. 2010;14:1–15.
66. Gan TJ, Soppitt A, Maroof M, et al. Goal-directed intraoperative fluid administration reduces length of hospital stay after major surgery. Anesthesiology. 2002;97:820–6.
67. Lopes MR, Olivera MA, Pereira VOS, et al. Goal-directed fluid management based on pulse pressure variation monitoring during high-risk surgery: a pilot randomized controlled trial. Crit Care. 2007;11:R100.
68. Mayer J, Boldt J, Mengistu AM, et al. Goal-directed intraoperative therapy based on autocalibrated arterial pressure waveform analysis reduces hospital stay in high-risk surgical patients: a randomized, controlled trial. Crit Care. 2010;14:1–9.
69. Salzwedel C, Puig J, Carstens A, et al. Perioperative goal-directed hemodynamic therapy based on radial arterial pulse pressure variation and continuous cardiac index trending reduces postoperative complications: a multi-center, prospective, randomized study. Crit Care. 2013;17:1–11.
70. Wakeling HG, McFall MR, Jenkins CS, et al. Intraoperative oesophageal Doppler guided fluid management shortens postoperative hospital stay after major bowel surgery. Br J Anaesth. 2005;95:634–42.
71. Buettner M, Schummer W, Huetttemann E, et al. Influence of systolic-pressure-variation-guided intraoperative fluid management on organ function and oxygen transport. Br J Anaesth. 2008;101:194–9.
72. Challand C, Struthers R, Sneyd JR, et al. Randomized controlled trial of intraoperative goal-directed fluid therapy in aerobically fit and unfit patients having major colorectal surgery. Br J Anaesth. 2012;108:53–62.
73. Conway DH, Mayall R, Abdul-Latif MS, et al. Randomised controlled trial investigating the influence of intravenous fluid titration using oesophageal Doppler monitoring during bowel surgery. Anaesthesia. 2002;57:845–9.
74. Perner A, Haase N, Guttormsen AB, et al. Hydroxyethyl starch 130/0.42 versus Ringer's acetate in severe sepsis. N Engl J Med. 2012;367:124–34.
75. Zheng H, Guo H, Ye J, et al. Goal-directed fluid therapy in gastrointestinal surgery in older coronary heart disease patients: randomized trial. World J Surg. 2013;37:2820–9.
76. Srinivasa S, Taylor MH, Singh PP, et al. Randomized clinical trial of goal-directed fluid therapy within an enhanced recovery protocol for elective colectomy. Br J Anaesth. 2013;100:66–74.
77. Phan TD, D'Sousa B, Rattray MJ, et al. A randomised controlled trial of fluid restriction compared to oesophageal Doppler-guided goal-directed fluid therapy in elective major colorectal surgery within an Enhanced Recovery After Surgery program. Anaesth Intensive Care. 2014;42:752–60.

78. Brandstrup B, Svendsen PE, Rasmussen M, et al. Which goal for fluid therapy during colorectal surgery is followed by the best outcome: near maximal stroke volume or zero fluid balance? A clinical randomized double blinded multi centre trial. Eur J Anaesth. 2010;27:4.
79. Wrzosek A, Jakowicka-Wordliczek J, Zajaczkowska R, et al. Perioperative restrictive versus goal-directed fluid therapy for adults undergoing major non-cardiac surgery. Cochrane Database Syst Rev. 2019;12:CD012767.
80. Colantonio L, Claroni C, Fabrizi L, et al. A randomized trial of goal directed vs. standard fluid therapy in cytoreductive surgery with hyperthermic intraperitoneal chemotherapy. J Gastrointest Surg. 2015;19:722–9.
81. Warrillow SJ, Weinberg L, Parker F, et al. Perioperative fluid prescription, complications and outcomes in major elective open gastrointestinal surgery. Anaesth Intensive Care. 2010;38:259–65.
82. Wuethrich PY, Burchard FC, Thalmann GN, et al. Restrictive deferred hydration combined with preemptive norepinephrine infusion during radical cystectomy reduces postoperative complications and hospitalization time: a randomized clinical trial. Anesthesiology. 2014;120:365–77.
83. National Heart and Blood Institute Acute Respiratory Distress Syndrome (ARDS) Clinical Trials Network. Comparison of two fluid management strategies in acute lung injury. N Engl J Med. 2006;354:2564–75.
84. Bhaskaran K, Arumugam G, Kumar PV. A prospective randomized comparison study on effect of perioperative use of chloride liberal intravenous fluids versus chloride restricted intravenous fluids on postoperative acute kidney injury in patients undergoing off-pump coronary artery bypass grafting surgeries. Ann Card Anaesth. 2018;21:413–8.
85. McArdle GT, McAuley DF, McKinley A, et al. Preliminary results of a prospective randomized trial of restrictive versus standard fluid regime in elective open abdominal aortic aneuriysm repair. Ann Surg. 2009;250:28–34.
86. Stewart RM, Park PK, Hunt JP, et al. Less is more: improved outcomes in surgical patients with conservative fluid administration and central venous catheter monitoring. J Am Coll Surg. 2009;208:725–37.
87. Myles PS, Bellomo R, Corcoran T, et al. Restrictive versus liberal fluid therapy for major abdominal surgery. N Engl J Med. 2018;378:2263–74.
88. Brandstrup B. Finding the right balance. N Engl J Med. 2018;378:2335–6.
89. Tengberg LT, Bay-Nielsen M, et al. Multidisciplinary perioperative protocol in patients undergoing acute high-risk abdominal surgery. Br J Surg. 2017;104:463–71.
90. Voldby AW, Aaen AA, Loprete R, et al. Perioperative fluid administration and complications in emergency gastrointestinal surgery—an observational study. Perioper Med. 2022;11:9.
91. Brandstrup B, Møller AM. The challenge of perioperative fluid management in elderly patients. Curr Anesthesiol Report. 2019;9:406–13.
92. ERAS Society. ERAS programs; 2019. https://www.erassociety.org/guidelines/list-of-guidelines/. Accessed 28 Aug 2023.

Chapter 20
The Surgical Critically Ill Patients: A Focus on Deresuscitation Strategy

Martin Ruste, Jean-Luc Fellahi, and Matthias Jacquet-Lagrèze

Preliminary Concepts

Fluid Overload

The definition of fluid overload is heterogeneous in the literature and *originates in* the association of a daily positive cumulative fluid balance (the difference between total fluid intake and total fluid outputs, usually adjusted in percentage of body weight) with a worse prognosis. From a statistical approach, it is usually described as an all-or-nothing phenomenon, ranging from 5% to 10% of the patient's body weight, without discriminating intravascular and extravascular compartments nor characterizing the related damaged end-organ [1–3]. Such an approach is questionable as:

- there is no identified threshold effect between cumulative fluid balance and prognosis and each 1% of body weight or positive Liter in cumulative fluid balance is associated with an increase in morbimortality [4, 5];
- the various measurement methods of the cumulative fluid balance are not accurate nor interchangeable with body weight variation [6–8];
- peripheral edema may coexist with intravascular hypo or hypervolemia [9];

M. Ruste (✉) · J.-L. Fellahi · M. Jacquet-Lagrèze
Service d'anesthésie-réanimation, Hôpital Louis Pradel, Hospices Civils de Lyon, Bron Cedex, France

Faculté de Médecine Lyon Est, Université Claude Bernard Lyon 1, Lyon Cedex 08, France

Laboratoire CarMeN, Inserm UMR 1060, Université Claude Bernard Lyon 1, Lyon, France
e-mail: martin.ruste@chu-lyon.fr; jean-luc.fellahi@chu-lyon.fr; matthias.jacquet-lagreze@chu-lyon.fr

© The Author(s), under exclusive license to Springer Nature Switzerland AG 2024
J. Faintuch, S. Faintuch (eds.), *Recent Strategies in High Risk Surgery*,
https://doi.org/10.1007/978-3-031-56270-9_20

– the evaluation of the fluid overload impact on end-organ function may serve as a therapeutic trigger and/or target [10].

Recently, experts proposed new definitions for the "fluid accumulation," related to a pathologic state of overhydration whatever intravascular status and the "fluid accumulation syndrome" as the association between the fluid accumulation and impact on end-organ function [10].

Deresuscitation or De-escalation

A four-phase strategy of fluid management was first described 10 years ago in septic shock [11]. The first "salvage" or "rescue" phase consists of an aggressive therapy to restore organ perfusion at the very early management of shock state, which is then tightly promoted during the first hours (optimization phase). The following stabilization phase aims to maintain homeostasis by the way of organ support, titration of fluids and vasoactive medications and to initiate a late conservative fluid management inducing a slight negative fluid balance. Initially described as de-escalation, the fourth phase consists of achieving a net negative fluid balance after circulatory shock resolution to counteract the side effects of fluid accumulation. The term "deresuscitation" is suggested by other authors as a more "active" strategy of fluid removal [10]. This strategy involves fluid intake restriction with a forced diuresis or the application of net ultrafiltration to remove a large amount of fluid over several days (Fig. 20.1). There are no widely admitted nor accurate definitions of the beginning and end of each phase.

If this four-phase approach of fluid therapy fits well to the global intensive care trajectory for a large part of critically ill patients, a myriad of situations is encountered in clinical practice. For example, fluid overload may exist without or precede any circulatory shock (congestive cardiopathy, liver or renal failure, iatrogenia…) or may develop after initial resuscitation.

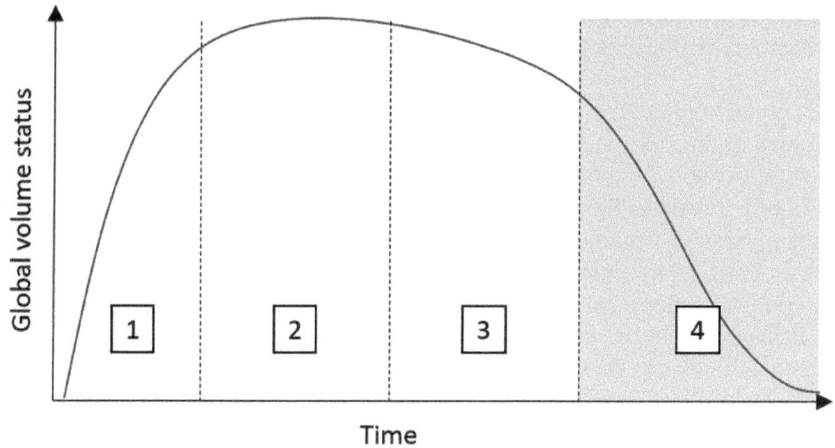

Fig. 20.1 Four-phase fluid management strategy of shock state 1. Salvage or Rescue Phase (Minutes to Hours) Lifesaving measures to restore a minimal arterial pressure and organ perfusion (aggressive fluid therapy, early introduction of Norepinephrine, blood transfusion) 2. Optimization Phase (Hours to Days) Personalized fluid therapy (fluid responsiveness assessment), catecholamine administration (echocardiography) and perfusion maximization (clinical and biological assessment) 3. Stabilization Phase (Days) Providing organ support and initiate their progressive weaning: decrease in catecholamine support, slight decrease in fluid balance to promote weaning from mechanical ventilation, venous congestion evaluation and treatment. Minimizing complications 4. De-escalation or deresuscitation phase (days to weeks) Correction of fluid accumulation: fluid intake restriction associated with fluid removal by the way of diuretics or ultrafiltration

Pathophysiology of Fluid Overload

Physiologically, fluid overload may be defined as a "pathologic accumulation of water and electrolytes in the body beyond that seen in healthy individuals" [12]. This accumulation originates in an inadequacy between the fluid intake and the outputs, largely mediated by a patient-physician interaction [12]. For example, if a crystalloid administration is temporarily efficient to increase plasma volume, only 20% of the initially administrated volume persists in intravascular compartment 30 min after the administration, with a re-distribution to the extravascular space followed by an elimination phase. Such transfers are moreover highly dependent on hemodynamic parameters and patient's related factors (i.e. context sensitive) [13, 14]. The extravasation is reinforced in systemic inflammatory state, where the endothelial glycocalyx and tight junction deterioration impaired the regulation of fluid and electrolytes movements across the capillary membrane [15, 16], promoting a high capillary permeability clinically traducing by the so-called capillary leak syndrome. There are reasons to believe that it is associated with a quasi-ubiquitarian impact on end-organ function [17, 18].

Following the four-phase concept of fluid management and clinicians' beliefs [19], fluid overload is inherent to the initial salvage phase responsible for a large amount of intravenous fluid and sodium intake. However, recent findings challenge this assumption as volume and sodium overload during the ICU stay are mainly driven by fluid creep (unintentional administration for vehiculate intravenous, oral or enteral medication) and maintenance fluids, much more than resuscitation fluids [20]. It may explain the progressive development of fluid overload in the case of inadequate diuresis as shown in patients with acute kidney injury [5].

Inadequate elimination of fluids administrated to critically ill patients is probably multifactorial. The end-organ implied in hydro-electrolytic balance may be impaired because of tissue injury, hemodynamic impairment or hormonal perturbations. At the ICU admission, 25% of patients were reported to present oliguria in the first 24 h, and this oliguria persists during the whole ICU stay in almost two out of three of them [21]. Among patients admitted for sepsis, almost one out of two have diastolic dysfunction [22] and one out of six a reduced left ventricular ejection fraction (<40%) [23]. Secondary acquired liver injury could concern as many as one out of three patients in the ICU [24]. Furthermore, several local factors promote the persistence of interstitial edema. The glycocalyx degradation is not rapidly reversible after the aggression. The extracellular matrix distortion decreases the interstitial pressure. The lymphatic dysfunction reduces the capacity for vascular refilling, which is the main determinant of edema resolution in the low filtration-low resorption revised Starling principle of microvascular fluid exchange [25]. All these phenomena are responsible for a vicious circle [26], making the spontaneous resolution of fluid accumulation unlikely or tardy. In this context, "active" fluid removal may decrease the intensity and the exposure duration to fluid overload and thus be considered as a full therapeutic tool to enhance organ recovery and prevent complications' occurrence.

In the particular context of the surgical critically ill patient, various factors predisposing for fluid overload may be encountered in the operating room: goaled-directed therapy improves prognosis but requires intravenous fluid therapy, hemorrhage may require blood product administration, surgical trauma or ischemia-reperfusion induce systemic inflammatory response, fluid creep may be related to medications or the priming of cardiopulmonary bypass. After the surgery, postoperative organ dysfunction (renal, cardiac or liver failures) may be responsible for inadequate outputs, and postoperative complications may require fluid creep, maintenance or resuscitation fluids. Data are scarce concerning this population specifically, but fluid overload >5% could concern more than 10% of the patients admitted in ICU after surgery [27] and capillary leak syndrome was recently reported in 50% of a cohort of surgical critically ill patients [28]. A positive cumulative fluid balance is associated with a worse prognosis after cardiac [29, 30] and non-cardiac surgery [27, 31, 32].

Fluid Removal: Tolerance and Targets

In deresuscitation strategy, fluid removal consists of an intravascular volume withdrawal by the way of diuretics or net ultrafiltration. Thus, whether the intravascular volume will keep constant or decrease depends on the vascular refilling rate, which in critically ill patients, as previously discussed, is probably low. Such an assumption is reinforced by the J-shaped association between net ultrafiltration intensity and prognosis in patients with continuous renal replacement therapy reported by several cohort studies [33]. On the one hand, in patients with intravascular hypervolemia, targeting a decrease in circulating blood volume makes sense. Indeed, it may participate in reducing venous congestion and thus improve end-organ function as the kidney or the liver [34]. But, on the other hand, in patients without intravascular hypervolemia, decreasing intravascular volume exposes to iatrogenic hypovolemia and hypoperfusion [33]. In this situation, the adequacy between the vascular refilling rate and the fluid removal rate is probably the cornerstone of hemodynamic tolerance during deresuscitation. However, such an approach remains simplistic regarding the complexity of the interaction between intravascular volume status and hemodynamic. Various strategies have been proposed to safely guide the fluid removal: passive leg raising predicts arterial hypotension during intermittent hemodialysis with high rate ultrafiltration [35] and peripheral perfusion index during continuous renal replacement therapy [36]; central venous pressure and cardiac output may be associated to estimate both efficiency and tolerance [37]; clinical and biological peripheral perfusion monitoring allows a more efficient fluid removal without sign of harm [38]. In any event, an individualization of the fluid removal rate associated with a frequent re-assessment of its tolerance reaches consensus [39, 40].

If applying fluid withdrawal to decrease the side effect of fluid accumulation raises the question of how to do it safely, the targets also remain unclear. The dry weight, an already challenging concept in patients with chronic hemodialysis, may look like a pipe dream in critically ill patients. Non-accurate or unavailable baseline weight measures, multifactorial and quick loss of muscle mass and imprecision of the measure during the ICU stay do not encourage to use it alone. A rigorous cumulative fluid balance estimation may help to quantitatively estimate the efficiency of the fluid removal strategy. Bio-electrical impedance analysis is a promising non-invasive and easy-to-use method to determine body composition at the bedside. Several of its derived parameters oriented to estimate fluid accumulation are associated with prognosis [41–44]. However, its sensibility seems to be low, the multi-compartmental models available are heterogenous, the estimation of the fluid status is not well validated in critically ill patients, a lot of research angles persist and no interventional study has demonstrated its impact on outcome [43, 45]. An end-organ approach may be used as a trigger and/or a target to guide fluid removal. Fluid removal decreases intraabdominal pressure and extravascular lung water [46], helps to decrease left and right ventricular filling pressure accelerating the mechanical ventilation weaning [47, 48], could improve renal venous congestion and decrease worsening kidney failure in acute heart failure [49, 50] and may participate to postoperative microcirculation improvement [51]. These factors may be estimated routinely with more or less invasive monitoring as pulmonary artery catheter, transpulmonary thermodilution, point of care ultrasound evaluation [52, 53] or noninvasive sublingual device.

Fluid Removal: with what tools?

Diuretics

A diuretic is a substance that increases the flow of urine, mainly by the way of a kidney action, allowing the removal of water and electrolytes. A recent large database cohort study reported an exposition to diuretics in nearly one out of two critically ill patient. The use was particularly important in patients with a history of heart failure, under mechanical ventilation or in postoperative care after cardiac surgery. Loop diuretic was by far the most frequently administrated class and diuretic combinations that concern less than one out of four patients receiving diuretics [54]. The continuous infusion of loop diuretics rather than an intermittent administration and their association with carbonic anhydrase inhibitors or thiazides could be more efficient to decrease cumulative fluid balance but are associated with more metabolic complications. However, the combination of loop diuretics with a thiazide decreases the risk for hypernatremia, and the administration of potassium sparing diuretics may help to avoid hypokalemia at the cost of decreasing diuresis [55]. These four pharmacological classes of diuretics are detailed in Table 20.1. Acute kidney injury and norepinephrine administration should probably not be impediments to diuretic prescription as it did not alter the outcome for the former [56] and worsen the prognosis for the latter [57].

Ultrafiltration

Extracorporeal ultrafiltration consists of the removal of water, electrolytes and molecules from the plasma below a certain weight mediated by hydrostatic pressure applied across a dedicated semi-permeable membrane. It is carried out with a double lumen central venous catheter, continuously or intermittently, and most of the time in association with renal replacement therapy (rather than isolated). Isolated ultrafiltration has no significant impact on plasma electrolytes, small solutes and proteins, whereas during renal replacement therapy, it contributes to the exchanges required to maintain homeostasis. In this case, the ultrafiltrate is totally

Table 20.1 Diuretics for deresuscitation

	Loop diuretics	Thiazides	Carbonic Anhydrase inhibitors	Potassium sparing diuretics
Site of action	NKCC-2 (Loop of Henle)	NCC (Distal convoluted tubule)	Carbonic anhydrase (Proximal convoluted tubule)	ENaC or mineralocorticoid receptor (Distal convoluted tubule, connecting tubule, collecting tubule)
Main effects	Loss of water +++ Natriuretic + Kaliuretic ++ Calciuretic	Loss of water + Natriuretic ++ Kaliuretic + Ca^{2+} reabsorption	Loss of water + Natriuretic ++ Kaliuretic +	Loss of water + Natriuretic + K^{+} reabsorption +
Molecules	Furosemide Bumetanide Torsemide	Hydrochlorothizide Indapamide Metolazone	Acetazolamide	Amiloride Spironolactone Aldactone
Main adverse events	Metabolic alkalosis Hypo/hypernatremia Hypokaliemia Ototoxicity	Metabolic alkalosis Hyponatremia Hypokaliema	Metabolic acidosis Hypokaliemia	Metabolic acidosis Hyperkaliemia
Cautions for usage	Resistance Dysnatremia Alkalosis Hypokaliemia Prefer continuous infusion	Hyponatremia Hypokaliemia	Tolerance after 48 h Respiratory acidosis Advance liver disease Hyponatremia Hypokaliemia	Shock state Hyperkaliemia (particularly if renal failure)
Main interests for combination with loop diuretics		Efficiency to decrease cumulative fluid balance Avoiding hypernatremia	Efficiency to decrease cumulative fluid balance	Avoiding hypokaliemia

or not compensated by fluid replacement, and the volume subtracted during renal replacement therapy is called the "net ultrafiltration" [33]. One of the theoretical advantages of ultrafiltration over diuretics is the lack of induced metabolic disorders as frequently observed with the former, and the easy-to-use and precise characteristics of the method. However, independently from the hemodynamic impact of fluid removal per se, renal replacement therapy is not devoid of side effects [58, 59], and some of them, such as complications related to catheter or blood-membrane interactions, probably exist in isolated ultrafiltration. Moreover, recent findings highlighted the advantages of delayed renal replacement therapy in critically ill patients [60], which does not promote early initiation of renal replacement therapy for fluid removal. In continuous renal replacement therapy, a net ultrafiltration between 1 and 1.75 mL/kg/h is associated with a better prognosis [33]. Targeting a net ultrafiltration of 2 mL/kg/h provides a significant decrease in fluid balance (if fluid intake is restrictive) and seems safe, provided a strict hemodynamic monitoring [38]. In chronic intermittent hemodialysis, a net ultrafiltration over 10 mL/kg/h is associated with increased mortality [61]; hence, it seems reasonable to use lower net ultrafiltration rate in critically ill patients. To this purpose, prolonged, more frequent sessions or isolated ultrafiltration may be carried out to induce a negative fluid balance [62]. Regarding the control of fluid balance, experts have suggested to not wean renal replacement if the diuresis is lower than 2 L/day with diuretics [63]. To finish, recent data indicates to avoid transition from continuous renal replacement therapy to intermittent hemodialysis if fluid accumulation persists, as it has shown as a marker of poor hemodynamic tolerance of intermittent hemodialysis [64].

Deresuscitation: Do Not Forget Fluid Intake

If restrictive strategies to initial resuscitation is beyond the scope of this focus, a tight control of fluid intake remains an integral part of deresuscitation strategy. A recent cohort emphasized that, in real-life, resuscitation fluids only count for 6.6% of the fluid intake during the ICU stay, whereas maintenance fluids count for 25%, nutrition for 33% and fluid creep (fluids administrated as a vehicle for medication or electrolytes) for 33%. Besides, resuscitation fluids' contribution to fluid balance decreases throughout the ICU stay, and the major determinants of the positive cumulative fluid balance, sodium and chloride burden are fluids of maintenance and fluid creep [20]. In this regard, the prescription of maintenance fluids and dilution for medication needs special attention as they largely participate to sodium and chloride load. As sodium-induced fluid retention and chloride-related renal vasoconstriction could be responsible for fluid accumulation themselves, maintenance fluids should preferably be orally administrated, hypotonic and for a total amount of intake without exceeding 25–30 mL/kg/day and 1 mmol/kg/day of sodium [65]. To this purpose, dissolving as many medications as possible in glucose 5% is efficient and probably safe [66].

Suggestions for daily clinical practice concerning deresuscitation are provided in Figs. 20.2 and 20.3.

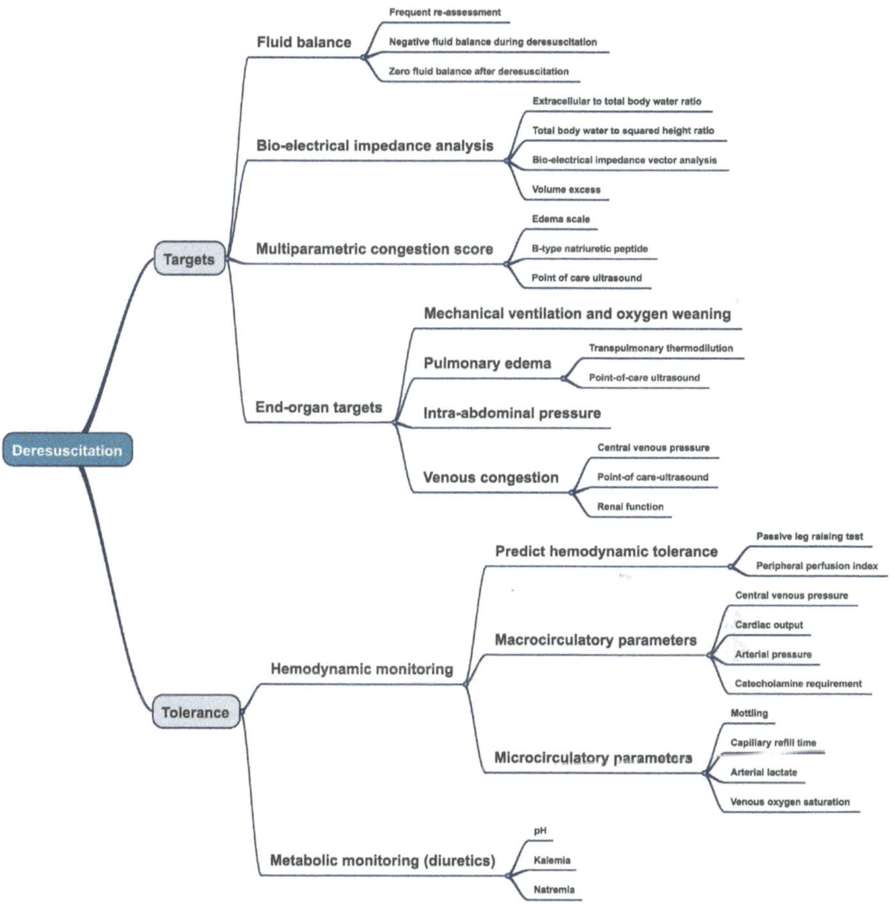

Fig. 20.2 Deresuscitation and monitoring

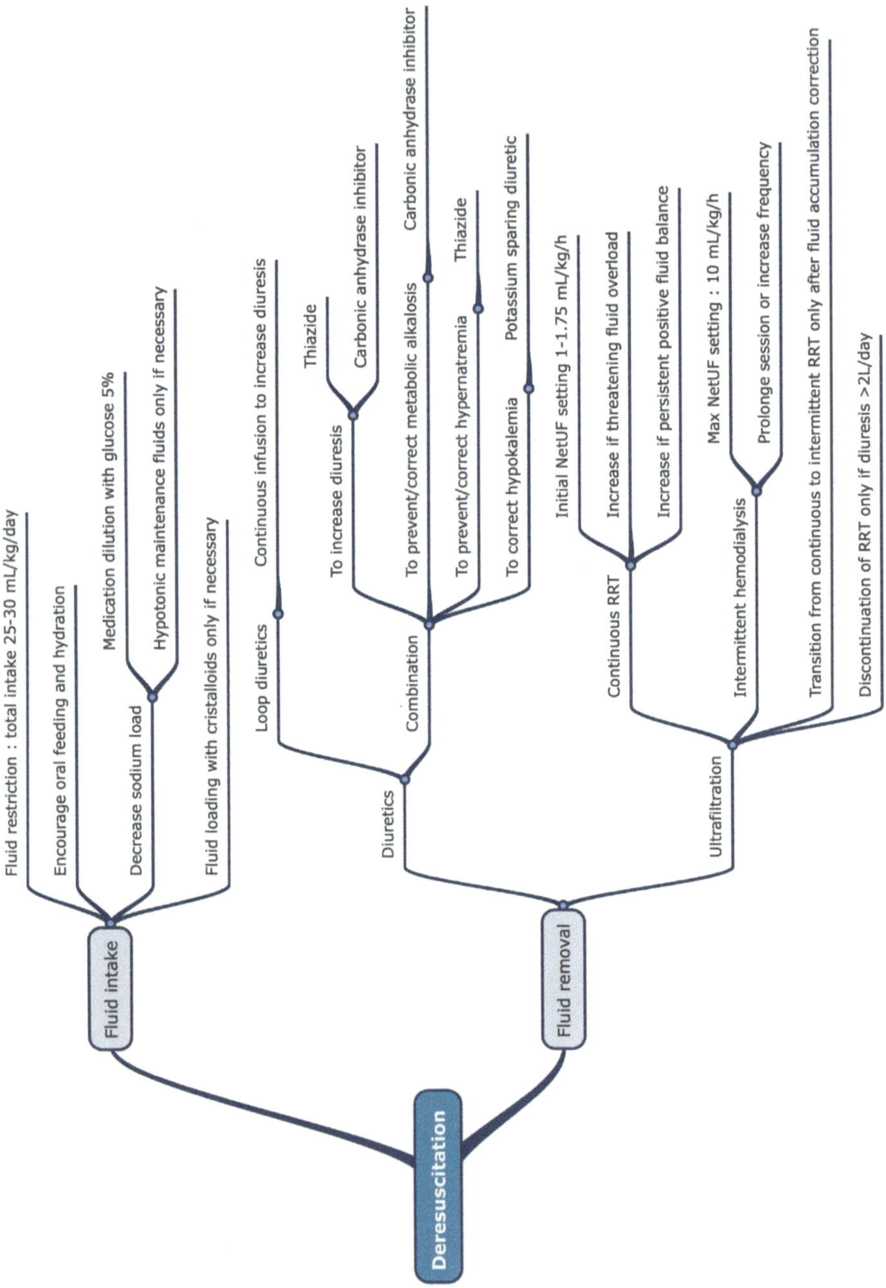

Fig. 20.3 Deresuscitation: suggestions for clinical practice. *RRT* Renal replacement therapy

Deresuscitation: Evidence-Based Patient-Centered Impact

If fluid overload was constantly associated with a worse prognosis, the causality link is not well-established. Thus, as a patient–physician interaction, fluid accumulation is probably in part inherent to pathological patient-related factors as capillary leakage and organ failure, which obviously participate in this worse prognosis. In this regard, interventional studies aiming to decrease fluid overload have shown relatively disappointing results. If restrictive strategies may help the mechanical ventilation weaning without improving mortality [67, 68], high-quality trials are scarce on deresuscitation strategy itself. They have shown difficulties to elaborate allowing a significant decrease in cumulative fluid balance and did not show any significant improvement in patients with sepsis outcomes [69]. A recent large randomized trial illustrates those difficulties: a protocol targeting a progressive weight decrease after day 2, using albumin, diuretics or ultrafiltration failed to decrease cumulative fluid balance compared to usual care [70]. Despite a complex dedicated design, the trial suffered from contamination between groups. Suboptimal protocol adherence was also reported and the strict safety criteria (suspension of the deresuscitation strategy if arterial hypotension, vasopressor requirement, renal function deterioration) may have induced undertreatment in the interventional group. However, to decrease cumulative fluid balance with deresuscitation strategy is not a quixotic goal as shown by two recent interventional or quasi-experimental studies [38, 71]. It must be noted that besides acute kidney injury and restrictive strategies in the peri-operative setting [72, 73] or cognitive dysfunction and restrictive strategy in acute respiratory distress syndrome [74], no sign of harm were suggested by studies on deresuscitation. It has to be modulated by the fact that data are scarce and originate from deresuscitation protocols with restrictive safety criteria applied to stabilized patients.

To conclude, if several experts support the concept of deresuscitation or de-escalation [40, 75], the lack of solid evidence-based demonstration of its clinical interest highlights the gap between physician practices and scientific knowledge. It may explain the heterogeneity in diagnosis and therapeutic interventions observed worldwide in several surveys on fluid overload and fluid removal [19, 76–78]. In this context, trials are urgently needed to determine the eligible population, the safety criteria, the targets and the means to "deresuscitate."

Acknowledgment Authors thank Lucie Bernigaud for help in manuscript preparation.

Conflict of Interest Statement The authors have no conflicts of interest related to the manuscript to declare.

Funding Sources No funding source.

Author Contributions Drafting of manuscript: *MR*.

Critical revision of the manuscript for important intellectual content: MR, **MJL, JLF.**

References

1. Messmer AS, Zingg C, Müller M, Gerber JL, Schefold JC, Pfortmueller CA. Fluid overload and mortality in adult critical care patients—a systematic review and meta-analysis of observational studies*. Crit Care Med. 2020;48(12):1862–70.
2. Zhang L, Chen Z, Diao Y, Yang Y, Fu P. Associations of fluid overload with mortality and kidney recovery in patients with acute kidney injury: a systematic review and meta-analysis. J Crit Care. 2015;30(4):860.e7–13.
3. Woodward CW, Lambert J, Ortiz-Soriano V, Li Y, Ruiz-Conejo M, Bissell BD, et al. Fluid overload associates with Major adverse kidney events in critically ill patients with acute kidney injury requiring continuous renal replacement therapy. Crit Care Med. 2019;47(9):e753–60.
4. Mele A, Cerminara E, Häbel H, Rodriguez-Galvez B, Oldner A, Nelson D, et al. Fluid accumulation and major adverse kidney events in sepsis: a multicenter observational study. Ann Intensive Care. 2022;12(1):62.
5. Garzotto F, Ostermann M, Martín-Langerwerf D, Sánchez-Sánchez M, Teng J, Robert R, et al. The Dose Response Multicentre Investigation on Fluid Assessment (DoReMIFA) in critically ill patients. Crit Care Lond Engl. 2016;20(1):196.
6. Schneider AG, Thorpe C, Dellbridge K, Matalanis G, Bellomo R. Electronic bed weighing vs daily fluid balance changes after cardiac surgery. J Crit Care. 2013;28(6):1113.e1–5.
7. Perren A, Markmann M, Merlani G, Marone C, Merlani P. Fluid balance in critically ill patients. Should we really rely on it? Minerva Anestesiol. 2011;77(8):802–11.
8. Davies H, Leslie G, Jacob E, Morgan D. Estimation of body fluid status by fluid balance and body weight in critically ill adult patients: a systematic review. Worldviews Evid Based Nurs. 2019;16(6):470–7.
9. Vincent JL, Pinsky MR. We should avoid the term « fluid overload ». Crit Care Lond Engl. 2018;22(1):214.
10. Malbrain MLNG, Martin G, Ostermann M. Everything you need to know about deresuscitation. Intensive Care Med. 2022;48:1781.
11. Vincent JL, De Backer D. Circulatory shock. N Engl J Med. 2013;369(18):1726–34.
12. O'Connor ME, Prowle JR. Fluid overload. Crit Care Clin. 2015;31(4):803–21.
13. Hahn RG. Understanding volume kinetics. Acta Anaesthesiol Scand. 2020;64(5):570–8.
14. Tatara T. Context-sensitive fluid therapy in critical illness. J Intensive Care. 2016;4(1):20.
15. Collins SR, Blank RS, Deatherage LS, Dull RO. The endothelial glycocalyx: emerging concepts in pulmonary edema and acute lung injury. Anesth Analg. 2013;117(3):664–74.
16. Lee WL, Slutsky AS. Sepsis and endothelial permeability. N Engl J Med. 2010;363(7):689–91.
17. Prowle JR, Echeverri JE, Ligabo EV, Ronco C, Bellomo R. Fluid balance and acute kidney injury. Nat Rev Nephrol. 2010;6(2):107–15.
18. Malbrain MLNG, Marik PE, Witters I, Cordemans C, Kirkpatrick AW, Roberts DJ, et al. Fluid overload, de-resuscitation, and outcomes in critically ill or injured patients: a systematic review with suggestions for clinical practice. Anaesthesiol Intensive Ther. 2014;46(5):361–80.
19. Silversides JA, McAuley DF, Blackwood B, Fan E, Ferguson AJ, Marshall JC. Fluid management and deresuscitation practices: a survey of critical care physicians. J Intensive Care Soc. 2020;21(2):111–8.
20. Van Regenmortel N, Verbrugghe W, Roelant E, Van den Wyngaert T, Jorens PG. Maintenance fluid therapy and fluid creep impose more significant fluid, sodium, and chloride burdens than resuscitation fluids in critically ill patients: a retrospective study in a tertiary mixed ICU population. Intensive Care Med. 2018;44(4):409–17.
21. For the ICON Investigators, Vincent JL, Ferguson A, Pickkers P, Jakob SM, Jaschinski U, et al. The clinical relevance of oliguria in the critically ill patient: analysis of a large observational database. Crit Care. 2020;24(1):171.
22. Sanfilippo F, Corredor C, Fletcher N, Landesberg G, Benedetto U, Foex P, et al. Diastolic dysfunction and mortality in septic patients: a systematic review and meta-analysis. Intensive Care Med. 2015;41(6):1004–13.

23. Dugar S, Sato R, Chawla S, You JY, Wang X, Grimm R, et al. Is left ventricular systolic dysfunction associated with increased mortality among patients with sepsis and septic shock? Chest. 2023:S0012369223001113.
24. Ruiz P, de Garibay A, Kortgen A, Leonhardt J, Zipprich A, Bauer M. Critical care hepatology: definitions, incidence, prognosis and role of liver failure in critically ill patients. Crit Care. 2022;26(1):289.
25. Jacob M, Bruegger D, Rehm M, Stoeckelhuber M, Welsch U, Conzen P, et al. The endothelial glycocalyx affords compatibility of Starling's principle and high cardiac interstitial albumin levels. Cardiovasc Res. 2007;73(3):575–86.
26. Prowle J, Mehta R. Fluid balance management during continuous renal replacement therapy. Semin Dial. 2021;34(6):440–8.
27. Oh TK, Song IA, Do SH, Jheon S, Lim C. Association of perioperative weight-based fluid balance with 30-day mortality and acute kidney injury among patients in the surgical intensive care unit. J Anesth. 2019;33(3):354–63.
28. Wollborn J, Hassenzahl LO, Reker D, Staehle HF, Omlor AM, Baar W, et al. Diagnosing capillary leak in critically ill patients: development of an innovative scoring instrument for non-invasive detection. Ann Intensive Care. 2021;11(1):175.
29. Stein A, de Souza LV, Belettini CR, Menegazzo WR, Viégas JR, Costa Pereira EM, et al. Fluid overload and changes in serum creatinine after cardiac surgery: predictors of mortality and longer intensive care stay. A prospective cohort study. Crit Care Lond Engl. 2012;16(3):R99.
30. Shen Y, Zhang W, Cheng X, Ying M. Association between postoperative fluid balance and acute kidney injury in patients after cardiac surgery: a retrospective cohort study. J Crit Care. 2018;44:273–7.
31. Miller TE, Mythen M, Shaw AD, Hwang S, Shenoy AV, Bershad M, et al. Association between perioperative fluid management and patient outcomes: a multicentre retrospective study. Br J Anaesth. 2021;126(3):720–9.
32. Silva JM, de Oliveira AMRR, Nogueira FAM, Vianna PMM, Pereira Filho MC, Dias LF, et al. The effect of excess fluid balance on the mortality rate of surgical patients: a multicenter prospective study. Crit Care Lond Engl. 2013;17(6):R288.
33. Murugan R, Bellomo R, Palevsky P, Kellum JA. Ultrafiltration in critically ill patients treated with kidney replacement therapy. Nat Rev Nephrol. 2020;17:262.
34. Marik PE. Iatrogenic salt water drowning and the hazards of a high central venous pressure. Ann Intensive Care. 2014;4(1):21.
35. Monnet X, Cipriani F, Camous L, Sentenac P, Dres M, Krastinova E, et al. The passive leg raising test to guide fluid removal in critically ill patients. Ann Intensive Care [Internet]. 2016;6(1):46. [cité 10 oct 2018] Disponible sur: http://annalsofintensivecare.springeropen.com/articles/10.1186/s13613-016-0149-1
36. Klijn E, Groeneveld ABJ, van Genderen ME, Betjes M, Bakker J, van Bommel J. Peripheral perfusion index predicts hypotension during fluid withdrawal by continuous Veno-venous hemofiltration in critically ill patients. Blood Purif. 2015;40(1):92–8.
37. Legrand M, Soussi S, Depret F. Cardiac output and CVP monitoring… to guide fluid removal. Crit Care Lond Engl. 2018;22(1):89.
38. Ruste M, Sghaier R, Chesnel D, Didier L, Fellahi JL, Jacquet-Lagrèze M. Perfusion-based deresuscitation during continuous renal replacement therapy: a before-after pilot study (the early dry cohort). J Crit Care. 2022;72:154169.
39. Rosner MH, Ostermann M, Murugan R, Prowle JR, Ronco C, Kellum JA, et al. Indications and management of mechanical fluid removal in critical illness. Br J Anaesth. 2014;113(5):764–71.
40. De Backer D, Cecconi M, Chew MS, Hajjar L, Monnet X, Ospina-Tascón GA, et al. A plea for personalization of the hemodynamic management of septic shock. Crit Care. 2022;26(1):372.
41. Samoni S, Vigo V, Bonilla Reséndiz LI, Villa G, De Rosa S, Nalesso F, et al. Impact of hyperhydration on the mortality risk in critically ill patients admitted in intensive care units: comparison between bioelectrical impedance vector analysis and cumulative fluid balance recording. Crit Care. 2016;20(1):95.

42. Rhee H, Jang KS, Shin MJ, Lee JW, Kim IY, Song SH, et al. Use of multifrequency bioimpedance analysis in male patients with acute kidney injury who are undergoing continuous Veno-venous Hemodiafiltration. PLoS One. 2015;10(7):e0133199.
43. Moonen HPFX, Van Zanten ARH. Bioelectric impedance analysis for body composition measurement and other potential clinical applications in critical illness. Curr Opin Crit Care. 2021;27(4):344–53.
44. Cleymaet R, Scheinok T, Maes H, Stas A, Malbrain L, De Laet I, et al. Prognostic value of bioelectrical impedance analysis for assessment of fluid overload in ICU patients: a pilot study. Anaesthesiol Intensive Ther. 2021;53(1):10–7.
45. Madsen JM, Wichmann S, Bestle MH, Itenov TS. Bioimpedance as a measure of fluid status in critically ill patients: a systematic review. Acta Anaesthesiol Scand. 2021;65(9):1155–67.
46. De Laet I, Deeren D, Schoonheydt K, Van Regenmortel N, Dits H, Malbrain ML. Renal replacement therapy with net fluid removal lowers intra-abdominal pressure and volumetric indices in critically ill patients. Ann Intensive Care. 2012;2(Suppl 1):S20.
47. Goudelin M, Champy P, Amiel JB, Evrard B, Fedou AL, Daix T, et al. Left ventricular overloading identified by critical care echocardiography is key in weaning-induced pulmonary edema. Intensive Care Med. 2020;46(7):1371–81.
48. National Heart, Lung, and Blood Institute Acute Respiratory Distress Syndrome (ARDS) Clinical Trials Network, Wiedemann HP, Wheeler AP, Bernard GR, Thompson BT, Hayden D, et al. Comparison of two fluid-management strategies in acute lung injury. N Engl J Med. 2006;354(24):2564–75.
49. Wallbach M, Valentova M, Schroeter MR, Alkabariti A, Iraki I, Leha A, et al. Intrarenal Doppler ultrasonography in patients with HFrEF and acute decompensated heart failure undergoing recompensation. Clin Res Cardiol [Internet]. 2023; [cité 22 mai 2023]; Disponible sur: https://link.springer.com/10.1007/s00392-023-02184-6
50. Aronson D, Abassi Z, Allon E, Burger AJ. Fluid loss, venous congestion, and worsening renal function in acute decompensated heart failure. Eur J Heart Fail. 2013;15(6):637–43.
51. Uz Z, Ince C, Guerci P, Ince Y, Araujo RP, Ergin B, et al. Recruitment of sublingual microcirculation using handheld incident dark field imaging as a routine measurement tool during the postoperative de-escalation phase—a pilot study in post ICU cardiac surgery patients. Perioper Med. 2018;7(1):18.
52. Deschamps J, Denault A, Galarza L, Rola P, Ledoux-Hutchinson L, Huard K, et al. Venous Doppler to assess congestion: a comprehensive review of current evidence and nomenclature. Ultrasound Med Biol. 2023;49(1):3–17.
53. Guinot PG, Bahr PA, Andrei S, Popescu BA, Caruso V, Mertes PM, et al. Doppler study of portal vein and renal venous velocity predict the appropriate fluid response to diuretic in ICU: a prospective observational echocardiographic evaluation. Crit Care. 2022;26(1):305.
54. McCoy IE, Chertow GM, Chang TIH. Patterns of diuretic use in the intensive care unit. PLoS One. 2019;14(5):e0217911.
55. Côté JM, Bouchard J, Murray PT, Beaubien-Souligny W. Diuretic strategies in patients with resistance to loop-diuretics in the intensive care unit: a retrospective study from the MIMIC-III database. J Crit Care. 2021;65:282–91.
56. Joannidis M, Druml W, Forni LG, Groeneveld ABJ, Honore PM, Hoste E, et al. Prevention of acute kidney injury and protection of renal function in the intensive care unit: update 2017: expert opinion of the working group on prevention, AKI section, European Society of Intensive Care Medicine. Intensive Care Med. 2017;43(6):730–49.
57. Shahn Z, Lehman LWH, Mark RG, Talmor D, Bose S. Delaying initiation of diuretics in critically ill patients with recent vasopressor use and high positive fluid balance. Br J Anaesth. 2021;127(4):569–76.
58. Douvris A, Zeid K, Hiremath S, Bagshaw SM, Wald R, Beaubien-Souligny W, et al. Mechanisms for hemodynamic instability related to renal replacement therapy: a narrative review. Intensive Care Med. 2019;45(10):1333–46.
59. Benichou N, Gaudry S, Dreyfuss D. The artificial kidney induces acute kidney injury: yes. Intensive Care Med. 2020;46(3):513–5.
60. Gaudry S, Hajage D, Benichou N, Chaïbi K, Barbar S, Zarbock A, et al. Delayed versus early initiation of renal replacement therapy for severe acute kidney injury: a system-

atic review and individual patient data meta-analysis of randomised clinical trials. Lancet. 2020;395(10235):1506–15.
61. Assimon MM, Wenger JB, Wang L, Flythe JE. Ultrafiltration rate and mortality in maintenance hemodialysis patients. Am J Kidney Dis. 2016;68(6):911–22.
62. Gaudry S, Palevsky PM, Dreyfuss D. Extracorporeal kidney-replacement therapy for acute kidney injury. Ingelfinger JR, éditeur. N Engl J Med. 2022;386(10):964–75.
63. Wald R, Beaubien-Souligny W, Chanchlani R, Clark EG, Neyra JA, Ostermann M, et al. Delivering optimal renal replacement therapy to critically ill patients with acute kidney injury. Intensive Care Med. 2022;48(10):1368–81.
64. Beaubien-Souligny W, Yang Y, Burns KEA, Friedrich JO, Meraz-Muñoz A, Clark EG, et al. Intra-dialytic hypotension following the transition from continuous to intermittent renal replacement therapy. Ann Intensive Care. 2021;11(1):96.
65. Van Regenmortel N, Moers L, Langer T, Roelant E, De Weerdt T, Caironi P, et al. Fluid-induced harm in the hospital: look beyond volume and start considering sodium. From physiology towards recommendations for daily practice in hospitalized adults. Ann Intensive Care. 2021;11(1):79.
66. Bihari S, Prakash S, Potts S, Matheson E, Bersten AD. Addressing the inadvertent sodium and chloride burden in critically ill patients: a prospective before-and-after study in a tertiary mixed intensive care unit population. Crit Care Resusc J Australas Acad Crit Care Med. 2018;20(4):285–93.
67. Silversides JA, Major E, Ferguson AJ, Mann EE, McAuley DF, Marshall JC, et al. Conservative fluid management or deresuscitation for patients with sepsis or acute respiratory distress syndrome following the resuscitation phase of critical illness: a systematic review and meta-analysis. Intensive Care Med. 2017;43(2):155–70.
68. Reynolds PM, Stefanos S, MacLaren R. Restrictive resuscitation in patients with sepsis and mortality: a systematic review and META-ANALYSIS with trial sequential analysis. Pharmacother J Hum Pharmacol Drug Ther. 2023;43(2):104–14.
69. Messmer AS, Dill T, Müller M, Pfortmueller CA. Active fluid de-resuscitation in critically ill patients with septic shock: a systematic review and meta-analysis. Eur J Intern Med. 2023;109:89–96.
70. Bollaert PE, Monnier A, Schneider F, Argaud L, Badie J, Charpentier C, et al. Fluid balance control in critically ill patients: results from POINCARE-2 stepped wedge cluster-randomized trial. Crit Care. 2023;27(1):66.
71. Silversides JA, McMullan R, Emerson LM, Bradbury I, Bannard-Smith J, Szakmany T, et al. Feasibility of conservative fluid administration and deresuscitation compared with usual care in critical illness: the Role of Active Deresuscitation After Resuscitation-2 (RADAR-2) randomised clinical trial. Intensive Care Med. 2022;48(2):190–200.
72. Chiu C, Fong N, Lazzareschi D, Mavrothalassitis O, Kothari R, Chen LL, et al. Fluids, vasopressors, and acute kidney injury after major abdominal surgery between 2015 and 2019: a multicentre retrospective analysis. Br J Anaesth. 2022;129(3):317–26.
73. Myles PS, Bellomo R, Corcoran T, Forbes A, Peyton P, Story D, et al. Restrictive versus liberal fluid therapy for major abdominal surgery. N Engl J Med. 2018;378(24):2263–74.
74. Mikkelsen ME, Christie JD, Lanken PN, Biester RC, Thompson BT, Bellamy SL, et al. The adult respiratory distress syndrome cognitive outcomes study: long-term neuropsychological function in survivors of acute lung injury. Am J Respir Crit Care Med. 2012;185(12):1307–15.
75. Malbrain MLNG, Langer T, Annane D, Gattinoni L, Elbers P, Hahn RG, et al. Intravenous fluid therapy in the perioperative and critical care setting: Executive summary of the International Fluid Academy (IFA). Ann Intensive Care. 2020;10(1):64.
76. Murugan R, Ostermann M, Peng Z, Kitamura K, Fujitani S, Romagnoli S, et al. Net ultrafiltration prescription and practice among critically ill patients receiving renal replacement therapy: a multinational survey of critical care practitioners. Crit Care Med. 2020;48(2):e87–97.
77. Lumlertgul N, Murugan R, Seylanova N, McCready P, Ostermann M. Net ultrafiltration prescription survey in Europe. BMC Nephrol. 2020;21(1):522.
78. Zeuthen E, Wichmann S, Schønemann-Lund M, Järvisalo MJ, Rubenson-Wahlin R, Sigurðsson MI, et al. Nordic survey on assessment and treatment of fluid overload in intensive care. Front Med. 2022;9:1067162.

Chapter 21
Extracorporeal Membrane Oxygenation

Sasa Rajsic, Benedikt Treml, and Robert Breitkopf

Introduction

Extracorporeal membrane oxygenation (ECMO, extracorporeal life support [ECLS]) presents a temporary life-saving technology used in patients with refractory cardiogenic shock or severe pulmonary failure. The main aim of ECMO is providing cardiac or respiratory support until the patient's heart or lungs recover. Moreover, it can bridge the time to organ transplantation or permanent organ assistance, such as mechanical circulatory support devices, ventricular assist devices, or total artificial heart.

The first reports on the use of a prolonged extracorporeal circuit and the beginning of ECMO support date from 1972 (Bramson-membrane heart-lung machine) [1]. Over the last two decades, the use of ECMO has expanded beyond severe cardiorespiratory failure, comprising an assortment of clinical presentations. Refractory cardiac arrest requiring prolonged resuscitation (i.e., refractory ventricular arrhythmias, local anesthetics intoxication, etc.) is an evolving indication for extracorporeal cardiopulmonary reanimation (eCPR). The successful use of ECMO support for out-of-hospital cardiac arrest is gaining popularity [2–5]. Moreover, ECMO support is increasingly used as bridge to heart and/or lung transplantation, rewarming of patients with deep hypothermia, or treating hypoxic respiratory failure triggered by trauma [6–10] or COVID-19 [11].

However, the overall survival after ECMO depends on many intrinsic variables of the patient, besides the interactions between extracorporeal circulation, circuit

S. Rajsic (✉) · B. Treml · R. Breitkopf
Medical University Innsbruck, Innsbruck, Austria
e-mail: sasa.rajsic@i-med.ac.at; benedikt.treml@i-med.ac.at; robert.breitkopf@tirol-kliniken.at

© The Author(s), under exclusive license to Springer Nature Switzerland AG 2024

J. Faintuch, S. Faintuch (eds.), *Recent Strategies in High Risk Surgery*,
https://doi.org/10.1007/978-3-031-56270-9_21

surface, hemostatic factors and blood components; generating complex coagulation and inflammatory reactions; and making the management of the critically ill more complex [12].

ECMO Physiology and Circuit

Homeostasis in critically ill patients, particularly those receiving ECMO support, is multifactorially compromised. Cardiac surgery or ECMO implantation (surgical trauma) and exposure of the patient's blood to the large surface of the circuit initiate and propagate an immediate inflammatory reaction and activation of the coagulation cascade [13]. Numerous cellular and humoral systems are involved in these complex inflammatory responses during ECMO support, resulting in a procoagulant state of the organism and the need for systemic anticoagulation. The balance between procoagulant factors and the iatrogenic coagulopathy is crucial to avoid severe adverse events (both hemorrhagic and/or thromboembolic), and for the patency of the circuit and its components [13].

The ECMO circuit is a closed system with a membrane-type gas-exchange technology. The main distinction between ECMO and a cardiopulmonary bypass is in the air–blood interface and the duration of support. In contrast to ECMO, venous reservoirs are integrated into cardiopulmonary bypass circuits for cardiotomy suction and venting of blood. Moreover, while cardiopulmonary bypass is usually used only for the surgery duration, ECMO support may be employed for weeks or even months [14].

The ECMO circuit comprises of inflow and outflow cannulas, a pump, an oxygenator, and heat exchanger (Fig. 21.1). The system components are connected by

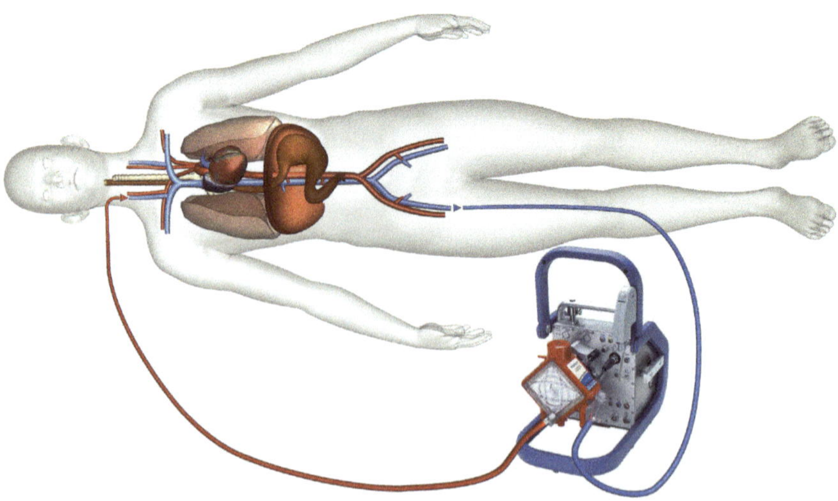

Fig. 21.1 Venovenous-ECMO circuit: cannulation of the internal jugular and femoral vein (Courtesy Getinge AB, Rastatt, Germany)

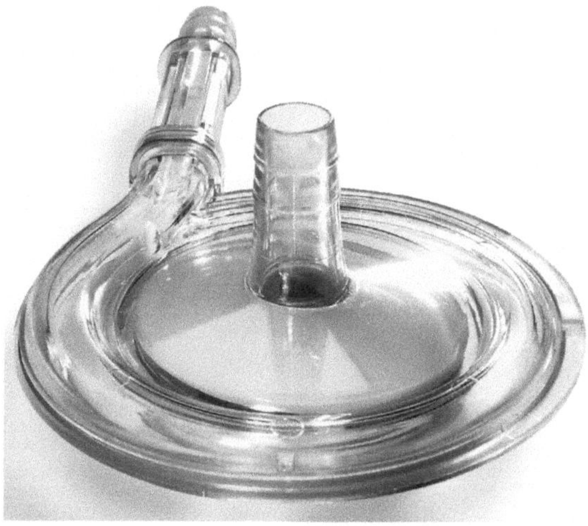

Fig. 21.2 Radial centrifugal blood pump (Courtesy Getinge AB, Rastatt, Germany)

a polyvinyl chloride tubing, usually coated with unfractionated heparin. The blood flow is controlled with magnetically actuated centrifugal pumps, replacing formerly used roller pumps, Fig. 21.2 [15, 16]. Due to a potentially developing negative pressure, a cautious approach is needed when inserting or removing indwelling catheters, or performing interventions which include the opening of blood vessels, as this could lead to aspiration of air by the ECMO system [14, 17].

Gas-exchange devices evolved from the direct air-blood contact systems to the membrane-based oxygenators, fulfilling the patient's need for oxygen supplementation and the carbon dioxide removal. Since the beginning of the twenty-first century, polymethylpentene hollow fiber membranes are gaining popularity, as gas is conveyed through bundles and the blood circulates around the hollow fibers (Fig. 21.3) [14, 18].

The portion of oxygen in the gas mixture is dosed depending on the patient's need and may be supplemented up to 100%. Increasing or decreasing of the sweep gas flow will increase or reduce the carbon dioxide clearance, not altering oxygenation. The gas-blood flow ratio is normally adjusted to maintain normal levels of carbon dioxide in the blood (normocapnia) [14]. Due to its structure, the oxygenator presents one of the most common locations for blood clots to form. Therefore, the regular check of the capacity and integrity of the oxygenator, including the search for clots, is obligatory in everyday practice.

Finally, the heat exchanger prevents circuit-related heat loss, giving the possibility of targeted temperature management (i.e., rewarming of accidental hypothermia, treatment of metabolic crisis, therapeutic hypothermia after cardiac arrest, etc.). It may be a separate component or integrated into the gas-exchange device, commonly based on hollow fiber bundles (nonpermeable) with circulating water (Fig. 21.3) [14].

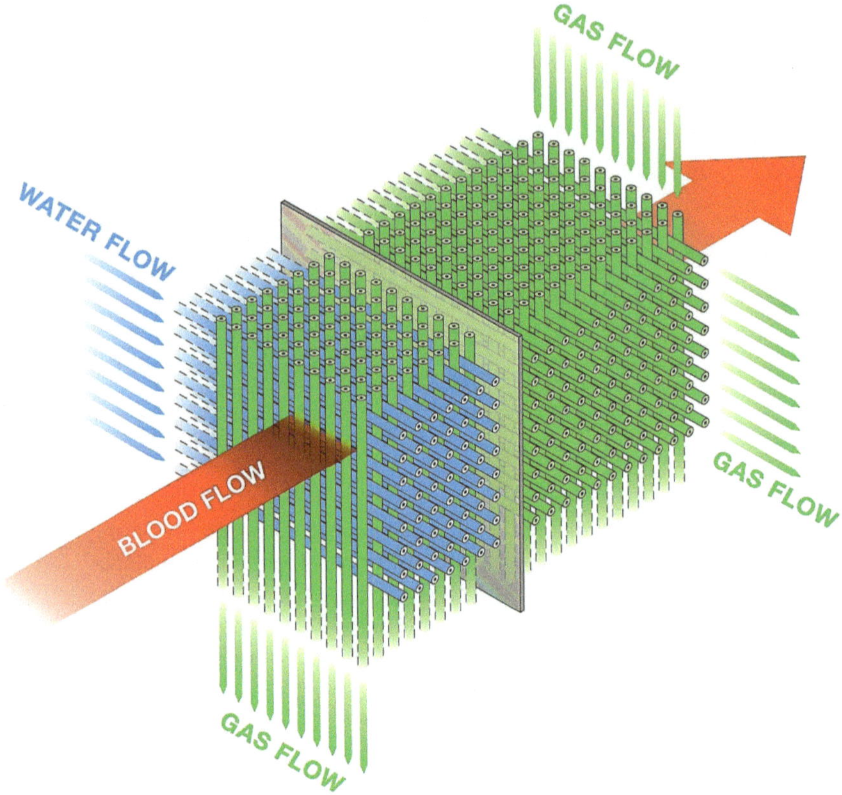

Fig. 21.3 Schematic presentation of a diffusion membrane showing blood flow between the gas and water-filled network of hollow fibers (Courtesy Getinge AB, Rastatt, Germany)

ECMO Indications and Configurations

According to the Extracorporeal Life Support Organization (ELSO), ECMO should be initiated in selected patients with cardiorespiratory failure when the mortality risk reaches 80%, and its initiation should be considered in cases with a high mortality risk (more than 50%) [14].

Two main configurations include the venoarterial (VA-ECMO) and venovenous ECMO (VV-ECMO). The VA-ECMO can be used as a mechanical circulatory support or a combination of both circulatory and pulmonary support. The VA-ECMO circuit consists of venous drainage to a circuit pump and an oxygenator, with the return of oxygenated blood to the arterial system. Cannulation can be central (i.e., failure to wean from cardiopulmonary bypass) or peripheral (i.e., eCPR). In the case of central cannulation, access is obtained by direct cannulation of the aorta and the right atrium. For peripheral cannulation, any large peripheral artery may be used with the femoral artery being the most common choice. For the venous drainage, at least one femoral catheter is advanced into the right atrium [19].

The main indications for VA-ECMO include postcardiotomy cardiac failure, myocardial infarction, acute-on-chronic heart failure, rewarming after accidental hypothermia, bridge to heart transplantation, myocarditis, pulmonary embolism, cardiac arrest, refractory ventricular arrhythmias, cardiac trauma, sepsis, ARDS with severe cardiac failure, or any other cause of a refractory cardiogenic shock [14].

The VV-ECMO can be used to support an isolated pulmonary failure, without any need for circulatory support. The circuit consists of venous drainage to a circuit pump and an oxygenator, with oxygenated blood returning to the venous system. The main indications include severe ARDS, severe air leak syndromes, resistant hypercapnia, bridge to lung transplantation, difficult airway management, or any other cause of acute hypoxemic respiratory failure unresponsive to conventional therapy [14].

Extended ECMO Indications and Contraindications

Extended ECMO indications present the use of extracorporeal life support in case of trauma, especially in cases of posttraumatic ARDS or transfusion-associated acute lung injury, high risk of airway compression (i.e., mediastinal masses), airway surgery, pulmonary thrombendarterectomy, accidental hypothermia, etc. [19]. Over the last years, even patients in septic shock could benefit from ECMO, if the hemodynamic compromise is mainly related to secondary myocardial dysfunction rather than distributive vasoplegia [20]. However, this option is reserved only for carefully selected patients. Another extended indication is rapid rewarming in case of cardiac instability due of accidental hypothermia. Finally, the use of ECMO in awake patients awaiting lung transplantation is being described increasingly, reducing the need for prolonged intubation, mechanical ventilation, and analgosedation.

Given the above, most contraindications for ECMO are rather relative than absolute, as age and size of patient or high risk of systemic bleeding under anticoagulation. Recent or expanding CNS hemorrhage, non-recoverable comorbidity, and disseminated malignancy remain contraindications for ECMO and have to be carefully weighed against possible benefits in terms of outcome [19, 21].

Anticoagulation Strategies During ECMO Support

The exposure of blood to artificial surfaces of the extracorporeal circuit and surgical trauma can initiate and propagate inflammatory and coagulation processes, leading to the need for therapeutic anticoagulation during ECMO support [12–14].

Systemic anticoagulation is considered the standard of care, crucial in the reduction of thrombosis risk and ECMO circuit components failure. Unfractionated heparin (UFH) is the primary anticoagulant [14, 22]. However, systemic anticoagulation carries a risk of serious bleeding, with the potential for permanent injury or even death [23–28]. On the other hand, thromboembolic events may occur as well, thus requiring careful therapeutic adjustments and follow-up [29–31].

In the case of the heparin-induced thrombocytopenia type II (HIT II) or heparin resistance, an alternative anticoagulation approach may be employed. When the HIT II is suspected, heparin should be stopped immediately, and heparin-coated components need to be removed. Furthermore, anticoagulation using direct thrombin inhibitors (i.e., argatroban, bivalirudin) or factor Xa inhibitors (i.e., rivaroxaban) should be considered [32]. Failure to continue anticoagulation in patients with HIT II could lead to a clinically significant thromboembolism, as this patient population is prone to thromboembolism [32].

In the last decade, evidence on the so-called anticoagulation-free ECMO support is emerging, with comparable incidences of thromboembolic events in anticoagulation-free ECMO patients compared to the standard ones [33]. Due to inconsistency in reporting, the authors could not draw any definitive conclusion in regard of hemorrhage [33]. The results of ongoing prospective studies (A-FREE ECMO-NCT04273607; SAFE-ECMO-NCT04997265; and RATE-NCT04536272) should help tailor future recommendations regarding anticoagulation.

Moreover, there is extensive research on the methods to reduce the need for systemic anticoagulation, including alternative approaches. Heparin-coated circuits are considered as the standard of care in many centers worldwide [34, 35]. However, the optimistic introduction of UFH-coated circuits did not lead to the omission or reduction of systemic anticoagulation. The use of citrate anticoagulation, as in continuous renal replacement therapy, is limited by the low clearance of citrate, restricting its use to blood flows below 200 mL/min, being significantly below the flow needed for ECMO.

Despite significant progress in the research on novel systemic anticoagulation therapies in the last two decades, the ideal anticoagulatory approach or drug are still not available. The ideal anticoagulant should have predictable anticoagulant effects and pharmacokinetics, with both oral and parenteral formulation, wide therapeutic range, eliminating the need for monitoring, with an available antidote and a rapid onset and offset of action, and lastly an affordable price [36]. Emerging preclinical data on novel anticoagulants and the role of antibodies targeting factors XI and XII showed good safety profiles and sufficient efficacy. However, there is still no evidence regarding their safe use in humans [37, 38].

Monitoring of Anticoagulation

Different in vitro modalities can aid anticoagulation monitoring and guidance.

The majority of centers employ serial measurements of the activated clotting time (ACT) and the activated partial thromboplastin time (aPTT), both being fast

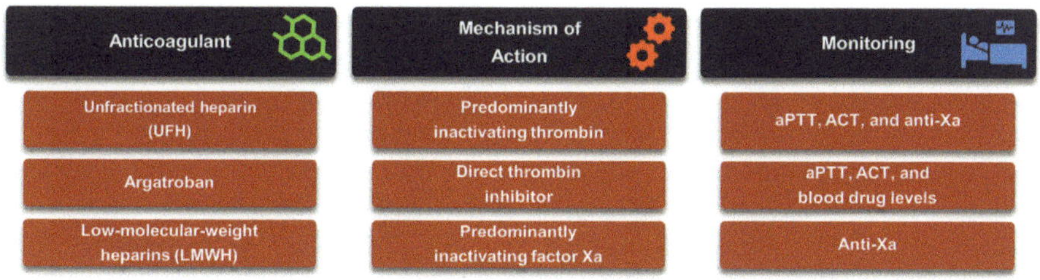

Fig. 21.4 Overview of the most commonly used anticoagulation agents during extracorporeal membrane oxygenation. aPTT: activated partial thromboplastin time; ACT: activated clotting time

and affordable methods [39]. Due to intrinsic limitations of both, ACT and aPTT, alternative methods as measurement of Anti-Xa levels and viscoelastic methods are being increasingly used (i.e., rotational thromboelastometry—ROTEM®, thromboelastography system-TEG®, viscoelastometry analyzer—ClotPro®, etc.) [13, 40]. An overview of the most commonly used anticoagulants with the mechanism of action and monitoring methods is presented in Fig. 21.4. Unfortunately the discordance between different methods is still common [13].

Complications and Mortality

Unfavorable outcomes are not unusual, generating debate about the real value of ECMO [22, 41–45]. Patient-related complications include acute renal failure, bleeding, thromboembolic events, sepsis, and pneumonia [22]. The circuit-related adverse events include formation of circuit clots and thrombi, with potentially devastating consequences. Finally, life-threatening acute mechanical failure, circuit fractures, or gas embolism are further, rather seldom circuit-related adverse events [19].

Within the patient-related complications, renal failure (51%) with the need for renal replacement therapy (44%) and hemorrhage (49%) are the most frequent adverse events during VA-ECMO support. Other frequently reported complications include pneumonia (24%), sepsis (18%), and thrombosis (13%) [22]. However, the approximate rates of complications are heterogeneously reported, making any systematization of the current evidence at least complex. Most of the reports originate from retrospective studies, with selection bias and potential underestimation as the main limitations [22].

Acute renal failure is commonly seen as a representation of a multiple organ failure, caused by a reduction in renal oxygen delivery and/or inflammatory kidney damage, with poor outcomes [46, 47]. Furthermore, bleeding presents one of the most common and serious ECMO complications, associated with an increased mortality. The identification of risk factors and predictors for adverse events during and shortly after ECMO support is subjected to intensive research, but strong evidence on potentially modifiable factors is still missing [19, 22, 23, 25, 27, 48, 49].

Depending on the selected population and bleeding definition, the reported rates of hemorrhage range from 16% to 46% [22]. Bleeding events occur mostly within the first 3 days of ECMO initiation, which is the reason why some centers employ a modified (reduced) anticoagulation protocol in the early ECMO phase. Given the above, early recognition of complications and their management, including anticoagulation monitoring, are crucial in the first days of ECMO support.

In regard to thromboembolic events, ECMO patients are at an increased risk independent of the modality (VA-ECMO vs. VV-ECMO) [31]. Patients receiving VA-ECMO are frequently postcardiotomy patients, with central cannulation and sternotomy. Therefore, the risk of bleeding may be increased due to the presence of surgical wounds. On the other hand, overcautious initiation of the anticoagulatory protocol may increase the risk of thrombosis. Moreover, patients with respiratory failure may suffer distinct thromboinflammation, a known procoagulant condition triggered by hyperinflammation [12, 50–54]. However, the reported incidence of thromboembolic events remains low, or underestimated due to unidentified thrombosis in asymptomatic patients. The majority of studies reporting on thrombosis are limited by their retrospective nature. Therefore, the true incidence of thromboembolic events remains unknown. Finally, the lack of standardized definitions for thromboembolic events, or outcomes in ECMO patients in general, makes the analysis of the available evidence complicated [31].

ECMO Mortality

Based on the data from more than 84,000 adult patients, ELSO reported an in-hospital mortality of 55% (VA-ECMO), and 42% (VV-ECMO). The highest rates of mortality (70%) are reported in case of eCPR [11].

Finally, in the CESAR trial, which compared conventional ventilatory support against ECMO support for severe ARDS, the survival without severe disability was significantly increased in the case of ECMO use [55]. However, a similar trial for patients suffering refractory cardiac failure is still lacking.

ECMO Weaning

Weaning from ECMO support should be guided by the daily clinical, echocardiographic, and hemodynamic evaluation of the cardiac and lung function recovery. The initial cause of cardiorespiratory failure should be resolved or at least corrected before the ECMO weaning trial is initiated.

Ensuing recovery of cardiac function, after at least of 24–48 h of VA-ECMO support, a weaning trial may be considered. In this phase, the arterial curve should show pulsatility, with a mean arterial blood pressure of at least 60 mmHg (with or without inotropic support), and all metabolic disturbances should be corrected according to the arterial blood gas measurements [56, 57]. In case of combined cardiorespiratory failure, before weaning initiation, the lung function should be evaluated. Otherwise, conversion to VV-ECMO may be considered.

The weaning strategy includes the gradual reduction of pump flow (0.5–1 L/min) over a period of hours, under hemodynamic and echocardiographic control. As the VA-ECMO circuit flow decreases, the preload will increase with consequent afterload reduction, supporting increase in cardiac ejection. If the cardiac function is successfully recovered to meet a satisfying organ and limb perfusion, further reduction of pump flow is warranted. However, due to flow reduction in the weaning phase, the increased risk of thrombosis should be considered [14].

Identification of predictors for successful weaning is still a subject of ongoing research, and consensus is missing. However, multidisciplinary approach with the repeated evaluation of cardiac function including the ejection fraction of at least 20%–25% are important factors for ECMO support weaning and decannulation [14, 57–61].

In case of VV-ECMO support, the recovery of lung function may take more time compared to cardiac failure. The improvement in patient chest radiography, reduced airway resistance, increased lung compliance, and improving oxygen saturation with lower ECMO blood and/or swap gas flows together with reduced venous oxygen saturation may indicate lung recovery.

In these cases ECMO weaning may be considered when a satisfying pulmonary gas exchange can be guaranteed under a lung protective ventilatory support (i.e., fraction of inspired oxygen of 30–60%, positive end expiratory pressure of 5–10 cmH_2O, peak inspiratory pressure of 25–30 cmH_2O) [14]. The monitoring during VV-ECMO weaning should include evaluation of respiratory mechanics, serial arterial blood gas measurements, and hemodynamics. If all criteria for ECMO weaning are met, pump flow is stopped, and the cannulas are clamped before decannulation.

Finally, there are diverse ECMO weaning approaches, and each center should implement a local operating procedure for ECMO weaning until the evidence from randomized trials is available.

Future Perspectives

Despite continuous research in this field, it remains difficult to identify modifiable factors. Hemorrhage or high disease severity scores may be important for timely intervention to prevent the occurrence of complications, potentially reducing morbidity and mortality.

The adaptation of systemic anticoagulation remains the most approachable factor; however, the ideal anticoagulant or monitoring tool are still lacking. Surface coating is promising; however, it neither eradicates the need for anticoagulation nor it reduces the risk of hemorrhage [13, 51, 52].

The use of aPTT as a main monitoring tool of systemic anticoagulation is increasingly questioned, and alternatives are being introduced. Validation for existing recommendations on the aPTT-guided protocol are still lacking [13, 62, 63]. Anti-factor-Xa for UFH monitoring is based on preliminary evidence [64–67].

The increasing use of ECMO for extended indications, reduction of contraindications, and patient individualized approach will lead to further popularization of this life support technology. Further adaptations and modifications of ECMO circuits and systems may lead to new indications, supporting the evolution of awake ECMO. Moreover, this will be accompanied by more sophisticated therapies, and older and sicker patients will be assessed for ECMO support. Therefore, meticulous weighting of the risks and benefits will become even more important in future.

Artificial Intelligence

Artificial intelligence in medicine is becoming an unavoidable tool for patient management, including a growing interest in the use for ECMO support. It can be useful in providing real-time data, prediction algorithms, and optimization of ECMO support management, with potential to reduce the risk of adverse events and consequently improving patient outcomes.

Algorithms using artificial intelligence can be built on large databases containing patient demographics, basic disease, comorbidities, medical history, and outcomes. This may be used to identify patterns and predict patients being at higher risk of poor outcome and thus further adjust the treatment for each patient's individual needs. Moreover, it could be used for the monitoring of patient's vital parameters (arterial blood pressure, blood oxygen saturation, or carbon dioxide levels), with algorithms analyzing real-time data. The prediction of worsening of vital parameters may facilitate and accelerate the adjustment of the ECMO support, for example, in case of constant decrease of the patient's oxygen saturation, or hypercapnia, such programs could alert the physician to adjust the ECMO system. This holds especially true in times of strained personal resources.

Finally, artificial intelligence has the potential to revolutionize the management of critically ill patients. Developed algorithms may identify patterns and predict outcomes, alerting health workers on potential optimization of care. With the constant development in the field of machine learning, we can expect significant benefits in critical care medicine of the future.

Conclusion

The use of ECMO support is becoming more common, and centers of excellence with higher volumes will present the safest places to indicate and manage this high-risk life support modality.

References

1. Hill JD, O'Brien TG, Murray JJ, Dontigny L, Bramson ML, Osborn JJ, Gerbode F. Prolonged extracorporeal oxygenation for acute post-traumatic respiratory failure (shock-lung syndrome). Use of the Bramson membrane lung. N Engl J Med. 1972;286:629–34. https://doi.org/10.1056/nejm197203232861204.
2. Bougouin W, Dumas F, Lamhaut L, Marijon E, Carli P, Combes A, Pirracchio R, Aissaoui N, Karam N, Deye N, et al. Extracorporeal cardiopulmonary resuscitation in out-of-hospital cardiac arrest: a registry study. Eur Heart J. 2020;41:1961–71. https://doi.org/10.1093/eurheartj/ehz753.
3. Downing J, Al Falasi R, Cardona S, Fairchild M, Lowie B, Chan C, Powell E, Pourmand A, Tran QK. How effective is extracorporeal cardiopulmonary resuscitation (ECPR) for out-of-hospital cardiac arrest? A systematic review and meta-analysis. Am J Emerg Med. 2022;51:127–38. https://doi.org/10.1016/j.ajem.2021.08.072.
4. Inoue A, Hifumi T, Sakamoto T, Kuroda Y. Extracorporeal cardiopulmonary resuscitation for out-of-hospital cardiac arrest in adult patients. J Am Heart Assoc. 2020;9:e015291. https://doi.org/10.1161/jaha.119.015291.
5. Scquizzato T, Bonaccorso A, Consonni M, Scandroglio AM, Swol J, Landoni G, Zangrillo A. Extracorporeal cardiopulmonary resuscitation for out-of-hospital cardiac arrest: a systematic review and meta-analysis of randomized and propensity score-matched studies. Artif Organs. 2022;46:755–62. https://doi.org/10.1111/aor.14205.
6. Kim H, Cho YH. Role of extracorporeal cardiopulmonary resuscitation in adults. Acute Crit Care. 2020;35:1–9. https://doi.org/10.4266/acc.2020.00080.
7. Morley D, Yamane K, O'Malley R, Cavarocchi NC, Hirose H. Rewarming for accidental hypothermia in an urban medical center using extracorporeal membrane oxygenation. Am J Case Reports. 2013;14:6–9. https://doi.org/10.12659/ajcr.883728.
8. Schechter MA, Ganapathi AM, Englum BR, Speicher PJ, Daneshmand MA, Davis RD, Hartwig MG. Spontaneously breathing extracorporeal membrane oxygenation support provides the optimal bridge to lung transplantation. Transplantation. 2016;100:2699–704. https://doi.org/10.1097/tp.0000000000001047.
9. Shekar K, Mullany DV, Thomson B, Ziegenfuss M, Platts DG, Fraser JF. Extracorporeal life support devices and strategies for management of acute cardiorespiratory failure in adult patients: a comprehensive review. Crit Care. 2014;18:219. https://doi.org/10.1186/cc13865.
10. Wang C, Zhang L, Qin T, Xi Z, Sun L, Wu H, Li D. Extracorporeal membrane oxygenation in trauma patients: a systematic review. World J Emerg Surg. 2020;15:51. https://doi.org/10.1186/s13017-020-00331-2.
11. Extracorporeal Life Support Organization (ELSO). Registry report on extracorporeal life support, international summary. https://www.elso.org/Registry/InternationalSummaryandReports/InternationalSummary.aspx. Accessed 19 Feb.
12. Millar JE, Fanning JP, McDonald CI, McAuley DF, Fraser JF. The inflammatory response to extracorporeal membrane oxygenation (ECMO): a review of the pathophysiology. Crit Care. 2016;20:387. https://doi.org/10.1186/s13054-016-1570-4.
13. Rajsic S, Breitkopf R, Jadzic D, Popovic Krneta M, Tauber H, Treml B. Anticoagulation strategies during extracorporeal membrane oxygenation: a narrative review. J Clin Med. 2022;11:5147.
14. MacLaren G, Peek G, Lorusso R, Brodie D, Thiagarajan R, Vercaemst L. Extracorporeal life support: the ELSO red book. 6th ed. Extracorporeal Life Support Organization; 2022.
15. Khan S, Vasavada R, Qiu F, Kunselman A, Undar A. Extracorporeal life support systems: alternative vs. conventional circuits. Perfusion. 2011;26:191–8. https://doi.org/10.1177/0267659110395060.
16. Palanzo D, Qiu F, Baer L, Clark JB, Myers JL, Undar A. Evolution of the extracorporeal life support circuitry. Artif Organs. 2010;34:869–73. https://doi.org/10.1111/j.1525-1594.2010.01127.x.

17. Diehl A, Pellegrino V, Sheldrake J. ECMO guideline. https://ecmo.icu/#menuRoot. Accessed 09 July.
18. Iwahashi H, Yuri K, Nosé Y. Development of the oxygenator: past, present, and future. J Artif Organs. 2004;7:111–20. https://doi.org/10.1007/s10047-004-0268-6.
19. Brogan TV, Lequier L, Lorusso R, MacLaren G, Peek GJ. Extracorporeal life support: the ELSO red book. 5th ed. Ann Arbor, MI: Extracorporeal Life Support Organization; 2017. p. 831.
20. Ling RR, Ramanathan K, Poon WH, Tan CS, Brechot N, Brodie D, Combes A, MacLaren G. Venoarterial extracorporeal membrane oxygenation as mechanical circulatory support in adult septic shock: a systematic review and meta-analysis with individual participant data meta-regression analysis. Crit Care. 2021;25:246. https://doi.org/10.1186/s13054-021-03668-5.
21. General guidelines for all ECLS cases; 2017.
22. Rajsic S, Treml B, Jadzic D, Breitkopf R, Oberleitner C, Popovic Krneta M, Bukumiric Z. Extracorporeal membrane oxygenation for cardiogenic shock: a meta-analysis of mortality and complications. Ann Intensive Care. 2022;12:93. https://doi.org/10.1186/s13613-022-01067-9.
23. Aubron C, DePuydt J, Belon F, Bailey M, Schmidt M, Sheldrake J, Murphy D, Scheinkestel C, Cooper DJ, Capellier G, et al. Predictive factors of bleeding events in adults undergoing extracorporeal membrane oxygenation. Ann Intensive Care. 2016;6:97. https://doi.org/10.1186/s13613-016-0196-7.
24. Levy JH, Staudinger T, Steiner ME. How to manage anticoagulation during extracorporeal membrane oxygenation. Intensive Care Med. 2022;48:1076–9. https://doi.org/10.1007/s00134-022-06723-z.
25. Rajsic S, Breitkopf R, Bukumiric Z, Treml B. ECMO support in refractory cardiogenic shock: risk factors for mortality. J Clin Med. 2022;11:6821.
26. Rajsic S, Breitkopf R, Oezpeker UC, Bukumirić Z, Dobesberger M, Treml B. The role of excessive anticoagulation and missing hyperinflammation in ECMO-associated bleeding. J Clin Med. 2022;11 https://doi.org/10.3390/jcm11092314.
27. Treml B, Breitkopf R, Bukumirić Z, Bachler M, Boesch J, Rajsic S. ECMO predictors of mortality: a 10-year referral centre experience. J Clin Med. 2022;11 https://doi.org/10.3390/jcm11051224.
28. Rajsic S, Breitkopf R, Oezpeker UC, Treml B. ECMO in cardiogenic shock: time course of blood biomarkers and associated mortality. Diagnostics (Basel). 2022;12:2963.
29. Abruzzo A, Gorantla V, Thomas SE. Venous thromboembolic events in the setting of extracorporeal membrane oxygenation support in adults: a systematic review. Thromb Res. 2022;212:58–71. https://doi.org/10.1016/j.thromres.2022.02.015.
30. Deshpande SR, Hastings S, Wagoner S, Ku D, Maher K. New insights into thrombosis in ECMO: circuits: where, how and why? J Heart Lung Transplant. 2015;34:S87–8. https://doi.org/10.1016/j.healun.2015.01.232.
31. Rajsic S, Breitkopf R, Rugg C, Bukumiric Z, Reitbauer J, Treml B. Thrombotic events develop in 1 out of 5 patients receiving ECMO support: an 11-year referral centre experience. J Clin Med. 2023;12:1082.
32. Pollak U. Heparin-induced thrombocytopenia complicating extracorporeal membrane oxygenation support: review of the literature and alternative anticoagulants. J Thromb Haemost. 2019;17:1608–22. https://doi.org/10.1111/jth.14575.
33. Olson SR, Murphree CR, Zonies D, Meyer AD, McCarty OJT, Deloughery TG, Shatzel JJ. Thrombosis and bleeding in extracorporeal membrane oxygenation (ECMO) without anticoagulation: a systematic review. ASAIO J. 2021;67:290–6. https://doi.org/10.1097/mat.0000000000001230.
34. de Vroege R, Huybregts R, van Oeveren W, van Klarenbosch J, Linley G, Mutlu J, Jansen E, Hack E, Eijsman L, Wildevuur C. The impact of heparin-coated circuits on hemodynamics during and after cardiopulmonary bypass. Artif Organs. 2005;29:490–7. https://doi.org/10.1111/j.1525-1594.2005.29083.x.

35. Sohn N, Marcoux J, Mycyk T, Krahn J, Meng Q. The impact of different biocompatible coated cardiopulmonary bypass circuits on inflammatory response and oxidative stress. Perfusion. 2009;24:231–7. https://doi.org/10.1177/0267659109351218.
36. Hirsh J, O'Donnell M, Weitz JI. New anticoagulants. Blood. 2005;105:453–63. https://doi.org/10.1182/blood-2003-12-4195.
37. DeLoughery EP, Olson SR, Puy C, McCarty OJT, Shatzel JJ. The safety and efficacy of novel agents targeting factors XI and XII in early phase human trials. Semin Thromb Hemost. 2019;45:502–8. https://doi.org/10.1055/s-0039-1692439.
38. Wallisch M, Lorentz CU, Lakshmanan HHS, Johnson J, Carris MR, Puy C, Gailani D, Hinds MT, McCarty OJT, Gruber A, et al. Antibody inhibition of contact factor XII reduces platelet deposition in a model of extracorporeal membrane oxygenator perfusion in nonhuman primates. Res Pract Thromb Haemost. 2020;4:205–16. https://doi.org/10.1002/rth2.12309.
39. Bembea MM, Annich G, Rycus P, Oldenburg G, Berkowitz I, Pronovost P. Variability in anticoagulation management of patients on extracorporeal membrane oxygenation: an international survey. Pediatr Crit Care Med. 2013;14:e77–84. https://doi.org/10.1097/PCC.0b013e31827127e4.
40. Rajsic S, Breitkopf R, Bachler M, Treml B. Diagnostic modalities in critical care: point-of-care approach. Diagnostics (Basel). 2021;11:2202.
41. Goldberg RJ, Spencer FA, Gore JM, Lessard D, Yarzebski J. Thirty-year trends (1975 to 2005) in the magnitude of, management of, and hospital death rates associated with cardiogenic shock in patients with acute myocardial infarction: a population-based perspective. Circulation. 2009;119:1211–9. https://doi.org/10.1161/circulationaha.108.814947.
42. Napp LC, Kühn C, Bauersachs J. ECMO in cardiac arrest and cardiogenic shock. Herz. 2017;42:27–44. https://doi.org/10.1007/s00059-016-4523-4.
43. Sayer GT, Baker JN, Parks KA. Heart rescue: the role of mechanical circulatory support in the management of severe refractory cardiogenic shock. Curr Opin Crit Care. 2012;18:409–16. https://doi.org/10.1097/MCC.0b013e328357f1e6.
44. Wilson-Smith AR, Bogdanova Y, Roydhouse S, Phan K, Tian DH, Yan TD, Loforte A. Outcomes of venoarterial extracorporeal membrane oxygenation for refractory cardiogenic shock: systematic review and meta-analysis. Ann Cardiothorac Surg. 2019;8:1–8. https://doi.org/10.21037/acs.2018.11.09.
45. Cheng R, Hachamovitch R, Kittleson M, Patel J, Arabia F, Moriguchi J, Esmailian F, Azarbal B. Complications of extracorporeal membrane oxygenation for treatment of cardiogenic shock and cardiac arrest: a meta-analysis of 1,866 adult patients. Ann Thorac Surg. 2014;97:610–6. https://doi.org/10.1016/j.athoracsur.2013.09.008.
46. Chen Y-C, Tsai F-C, Fang J-T, Yang C-W. Acute kidney injury in adults receiving extracorporeal membrane oxygenation. J Formos Med Assoc. 2014;113:778–85. https://doi.org/10.1016/j.jfma.2014.04.006.
47. Villa G, Katz N, Ronco C. Extracorporeal membrane oxygenation and the kidney. Cardiorenal Med. 2015;6:50–60. https://doi.org/10.1159/000439444.
48. Fisser C, Reichenbächer C, Müller T, Schneckenpointner R, Malfertheiner MV, Philipp A, Foltan M, Lunz D, Zeman F, Lubnow M. Incidence and risk factors for cannula-related venous thrombosis after venovenous extracorporeal membrane oxygenation in adult patients with acute respiratory failure. Crit Care Med. 2019;47:e332–9. https://doi.org/10.1097/ccm.0000000000003650.
49. Sohail S, Fan E, Foroutan F, Ross HJ, Billia F, Alba AC. Predictors of mortality in patients treated with veno-arterial ECMO for cardiogenic shock complicating acute myocardial infarction: a systematic review and meta-analysis. J Cardiovasc Transl Res. 2022;15:227–38. https://doi.org/10.1007/s12265-021-10140-w.
50. Connors JM, Levy JHJB. COVID-19 and its implications for thrombosis and anticoagulation. Blood. 2020;135:2033–40.

51. Lim MS, Mcrae S. COVID-19 and immunothrombosis: pathophysiology and therapeutic implications. Crit Rev Oncol Hematol. 2021;168:103529.
52. Ranucci M, Ballotta A, Di Dedda U, Baryshnikova E, Dei Poli M, Resta M, Falco M, Albano G, Menicanti L. The procoagulant pattern of patients with COVID-19 acute respiratory distress syndrome. J Thromb Haemost. 2020;18:1747–51. https://doi.org/10.1111/jth.14854.
53. Weir-McCall JR, Galea G, Mun Mak S, Joshi K, Agrawal B, Screaton N, Toshner M, Ruggiero A, Benedetti G, Brozik J, et al. Vascular thrombosis in severe COVID-19 requiring extracorporeal membrane oxygenation: a multicenter study. Crit Care Med. 2022;50:624–32. https://doi.org/10.1097/ccm.0000000000005322.
54. Yusuff H, Zochios V, Brodie D. Thrombosis and coagulopathy in COVID-19 patients requiring extracorporeal membrane oxygenation. ASAIO J. 2020;66:844–6. https://doi.org/10.1097/mat.0000000000001208.
55. Peek GJ, Mugford M, Tiruvoipati R, Wilson A, Allen E, Thalanany MM, Hibbert CL, Truesdale A, Clemens F, Cooper N, et al. Efficacy and economic assessment of conventional ventilatory support versus extracorporeal membrane oxygenation for severe adult respiratory failure (CESAR): a multicentre randomised controlled trial. Lancet (London, England). 2009;374:1351–63. https://doi.org/10.1016/s0140-6736(09)61069-2.
56. Pappalardo F, Pieri M, Arnaez Corada B, Ajello S, Melisurgo G, De Bonis M, Zangrillo A. Timing and strategy for weaning from Venoarterial ECMO are complex issues. J Cardiothorac Vasc Anesth. 2015;29:906–11. https://doi.org/10.1053/j.jvca.2014.12.011.
57. Aissaoui N, Luyt CE, Leprince P, Trouillet JL, Léger P, Pavie A, Diebold B, Chastre J, Combes A. Predictors of successful extracorporeal membrane oxygenation (ECMO) weaning after assistance for refractory cardiogenic shock. Intensive Care Med. 2011;37:1738–45. https://doi.org/10.1007/s00134-011-2358-2.
58. Cavarocchi NC, Pitcher HT, Yang Q, Karbowski P, Miessau J, Hastings HM, Hirose H. Weaning of extracorporeal membrane oxygenation using continuous hemodynamic transesophageal echocardiography. J Thorac Cardiovasc Surg. 2013;146:1474–9. https://doi.org/10.1016/j.jtcvs.2013.06.055.
59. Aissaoui N, El-Banayosy A, Combes A. How to wean a patient from veno-arterial extracorporeal membrane oxygenation. Intensive Care Med. 2015;41:902–5. https://doi.org/10.1007/s00134-015-3663-y.
60. Santise G, Panarello G, Ruperto C, Turrisi M, Pilato G, Giunta A, Sciacca S, Pilato M. Extracorporeal membrane oxygenation for graft failure after heart transplantation: a multidisciplinary approach to maximize weaning rate. Int J Artif Organs. 2014;37:706–14. https://doi.org/10.5301/ijao.5000353.
61. Ortuno S, Delmas C, Diehl JL, Bailleul C, Lancelot A, Naili M, Cholley B, Pirracchio R, Aissaoui N. Weaning from veno-arterial extra-corporeal membrane oxygenation: which strategy to use? Ann Cardiothorac Surg. 2019;8:E1–e8. https://doi.org/10.21037/acs.2018.08.05.
62. Rajsic S, Breitkopf R, Treml B, Jadzic D, Oberleitner C, Oezpeker UC, Innerhofer N, Bukumiric Z. Association of aPTT-guided anticoagulation monitoring with thromboembolic events in patients receiving V-A ECMO support: a systematic review and meta-analysis. J Clin Med. 2023;12:3224.
63. Rajsic S, Treml B, Jadzic D, Breitkopf R, Oberleitner C, Bachler M, Bösch J, Bukumiric Z. aPTT-guided anticoagulation monitoring during ECMO support: a systematic review and meta-analysis. J Crit Care. 2023;77:154332. https://doi.org/10.1016/j.jcrc.2023.154332.
64. Guervil DJ, Rosenberg AF, Winterstein AG, Harris NS, Johns TE, Zumberg MS. Activated partial thromboplastin time versus antifactor Xa heparin assay in monitoring unfractionated heparin by continuous intravenous infusion. Ann Pharmacother. 2011;45:861–8. https://doi.org/10.1345/aph.1Q161.

65. Swayngim R, Preslaski C, Burlew CC, Beyer J. Comparison of clinical outcomes using activated partial thromboplastin time versus antifactor-Xa for monitoring therapeutic unfractionated heparin: a systematic review and meta-analysis. Thromb Res. 2021;208:18–25. https://doi.org/10.1016/j.thromres.2021.10.010.
66. Willems A, Roeleveld PP, Labarinas S, Cyrus JW, Muszynski JA, Nellis ME, Karam O. Anti-Xa versus time-guided anticoagulation strategies in extracorporeal membrane oxygenation: a systematic review and meta-analysis. Perfusion. 2021;36:501–12. https://doi.org/10.1177/0267659120952982.
67. Zhang M, Pauls JP, Bartnikowski N, Haymet AB, Chan CHH, Suen JY, Schneider B, Ki KK, Whittaker AK, Dargusch MS, et al. Anti-thrombogenic surface coatings for extracorporeal membrane oxygenation: a narrative review. ACS Biomater Sci Eng. 2021;7:4402–19. https://doi.org/10.1021/acsbiomaterials.1c00758.

Part VI
Perioperative Surgical Challenges

Chapter 22
Damage Control Laparotomy

David Ray Velez and Anthony Joseph Duncan

Abbreviations

ATLS	Advanced Trauma Life Support
BAT	Blunt abdominal trauma
CT	Computerized tomography
DCL	Damage control laparotomy
DPL	Diagnostic peritoneal lavage
FAST	Focused Assessment with Sonography for Trauma
NPWT	Negative pressure wound therapy
PAT	Penetrating abdominal trauma
REBOA	Resuscitative Endovascular Balloon Occlusion of the Aorta

Introduction

History of the traumatic abdomen extends through antiquity. Although management has evolved over time, the traumatic abdomen in a crashing patient can still, as described by Hippocrates, "mortify imperatively."

Damage control is not a novel modality for therapeutic interventions. The term itself comes from the US Navy and refers to the ability of a ship to undergo damage

D. R. Velez (✉)
Department of Surgery, University of Nevada, Las Vegas, Las Vegas, NV, USA
e-mail: david.velez@unlv.edu

A. J. Duncan
University of North Dakota, Grand Forks, ND, USA
e-mail: Anthony.Duncan@ndus.edu

© The Author(s), under exclusive license to Springer Nature Switzerland AG 2024

J. Faintuch, S. Faintuch (eds.), *Recent Strategies in High Risk Surgery*,
https://doi.org/10.1007/978-3-031-56270-9_22

but still maintain mission integrity. The term was brought into the mainstream surgical community in 1993, when Rotondo et al. proposed it as an approach for managing penetrating abdominal injuries [1]. Before the adoption of damage control as a therapeutic intervention, several methodologies were implemented to reduce surgical time at the index procedure and improve outcomes of critically ill patients. These included peri-hepatic packing and Feliciano et al.'s rapid conservative operative techniques, which were published in 1993 [2, 3].

Damage control surgery is a surgical technique that involves a brief initial operation aimed at quickly controlling severe bleeding and/or contamination in critically ill patients [4]. Following the initial surgery, patients are admitted to the intensive care unit where their condition is stabilized with the objective of returning them to their pre-injury state before definitive repair can be carried out [4]. While advancements in technology have led to significant improvements in this technique over the years, the fundamental principles of damage control surgery have remained unchanged.

Epidemiology and Etiology

There are 5.8 million traumatic deaths every year across the globe [5]. Trauma is the third leading cause of death in the United States with 150,000 deaths per year [6]. Trauma is largely a disease of young males with over 50% between the ages of 10 and 24 years and over 66% male [7]. Trauma is the most common cause of death between ages 1 and 44 years [8].

The most common causes of traumatic death in the United States are motor vehicle collision (37,991 deaths/year), falls (37,455 deaths/year), and gunshot wounds with suicide (24,432 deaths/year) accounting for almost twice that of homicide (13,958 deaths/year) [9]. Blunt abdominal trauma (BAT) accounts for 90% of patients presenting but only 67% of those requiring laparotomy [10]. Penetrating abdominal trauma (PAT) accounts for only 10% of patients presenting but 33% of those requiring laparotomy [9, 10]. Of penetrating mechanisms, stab wounds are the most common, although gunshot wounds are approximately eight times more lethal [11].

Among patients with injury due to BAT, the most commonly injured organs are the spleen (40–55%), liver (35–45%), and small bowel (5–10%) [9]. The most common injuries after PAT are small bowel (50%), colon (40%), liver (30%), and vascular injury (25%) [9]. After the decision is made to proceed with trauma laparotomy, the most common procedures performed are enterectomy (23%), hepatorrhaphy (20%), enterorrhaphy (16%), splenectomy (16%), and colectomy (15%) [10]. Damage control procedures are used in 38% of cases [10]. Overall mortality is 21% which doubles to 46% in hypotensive patients [10]. Surprisingly, despite major advancements in the field of trauma, these high mortality rates have seen minimal change over the last two decades [10].

General Management of Abdominal Trauma

As with any trauma, abdominal trauma begins with a thorough primary and secondary survey [12]. Advanced Trauma Life Support (ATLS) algorithms start with the management of airway, breathing, circulation, disability, exposure, and then a head-to-toe injury inventory and exam [12]. Diagnosis then diverges depending on the patient's condition and mechanism of injury.

All patients with overt peritonitis or evisceration mandate trauma laparotomy [6, 13]. Regarding patients without peritonitis or evisceration, management will then differ by the mechanism of injury. In an unstable patient after PAT, a trauma laparotomy is mandated. In an unstable patient after BAT, the abdomen must first be confirmed as the source of instability by a Focused Assessment with Sonography for Trauma (FAST) prior to laparotomy. Some surgeons do elect for diagnostic peritoneal lavage (DPL), although it has almost entirely been replaced since the advent of FAST and is now primarily used when FAST results are equivocal. A positive FAST requires trauma laparotomy but a negative FAST should instead prompt further evaluation for other sources of instability with chest X-ray or computerized tomography (CT) scan as indicated. A stable patient allows more time for diagnosis in a comprehensive manner. As such, a stable patient after BAT should be evaluated by CT scan. A stable patient after PAT should undergo local wound exploration.

The primary goal of local wound exploration is to evaluate for violation of posterior fascia, not peritoneum. If no fascial violation is found in a PAT that is stable with no other indication for admission, the patient may be discharged home [13]. Fascial violation requires further evaluation to determine peritoneal violation or damage to intrabdominal structures. This can be accomplished by CT scan, FAST, DPL, or diagnostic laparoscopy dependent on surgeon preference. A patient without any evidence of peritoneal violation should be monitored for 24 h with serial clinical exams. Peritoneal violation mandates surgical evaluation with either laparotomy or diagnostic laparoscopy. Of note, when evaluating anterior abdominal stab wounds, only 50–75% will penetrate the peritoneum and of those, only 50–75% will require repair of intraabdominal injury [13].

Trauma Laparotomy: A Systematic Approach

Upon arrival in the operating room, skin should be prepped from chin to knees with arms extended allowing adequate access for the worst-case scenarios. Understand that sterility is a luxury in hemorrhagic shock. Rather than disappearing for a prolonged relaxing scrub, if necessary the surgeon should throw on gloves and dive-in if needed to save the patient's life.

The trauma laparotomy "Operative Sequence" was outlined by Hirshberg and Mattox in the book "Top Knife" published two decades ago in 2004 [14]. It follows four basic steps: access and exposure, temporary bleeding control, exploration, and then decision of definitive repair versus damage control [14]. There have been many descriptions of how to approach a trauma laparotomy, and although they do not always use the same terminology, they all at their core follow the same format [13–15].

Access and Exposure

The first steps of an efficient trauma laparotomy are access and exposure to facilitate the ensuing procedure. The typical access is through a long midline incision from xiphoid to pubis. However, every effort should be made to enter through virgin territory to avoid scars and internal adhesions. This may be accomplished by extending the incision superiorly or inferiorly if able. If unable, an alternative incision can be chosen such as the chevron incision which resembles the military chevron insignia just under the rib cage bilaterally. This is also known as a bilateral subcostal, double Kocher, or rooftop incision. For additional access, a Mercedes Incision can be made by adding a small midline extension toward the xiphoid from the chevron incision, therefore, resembling a Mercedes-Benz automobile emblem. Immediately upon entry into the abdomen, the bowel should be eviscerated early. Incision should be done rapidly but in a controlled manner as a major pitfall during this step would be iatrogenic injury to the liver, bowel, or bladder.

Temporary Bleeding Control

Once inside the abdomen, the first step should be temporary bleeding control. BAT begins with empiric packing. Packing should be placed over and under the liver, over and medial to the spleen, along the right gutter, along the left gutter, and in the pelvis. Although it will not arrest major hemorrhage, it will give time to organize efforts and systematically explore the abdomen. PAT begins by directly approaching the bleed. Although some have recommended empiric packing in all trauma laparotomies, the consensus appears to be in favor of directly approaching the bleed.

The exsanguinating patient should be approached by obtaining supraceliac control of the Aorta. This is done through division of the Gastrohepatic ligament. Although normally avascular, care should be taken to watch for a replaced left hepatic artery. The stomach and esophagus are then reflected to the left to allow access to the aorta. Division of the diaphragmatic crura may be required. The aorta can then be bluntly dissected and occluded. Aortic occlusion is typically with a vascular clamp although it can also be compressed against the spine either manually or with an aortic root compressor.

Other described methods for aortic control include suprahepatic control through the triangular ligaments, inframesocolic control through the inferior mesentery, or a left-sided medial visceral rotation (Mattox maneuver). These other methods, however, have fallen out-of-favor as suprahepatic control is technically more difficult, inframesocolic control does not halt bleeding supplied by the proximal aortic branches, and the Mattox maneuver, although providing more extensive exposure, takes more time and should be reserved for exploration after temporary bleeding control. A left anterolateral thoracotomy can also provide excellent control of the distal thoracic aorta. However, it may produce unnecessary morbidity if the aorta can instead be accessed directly from the abdomen. Resuscitative Endovascular Balloon Occlusion of the Aorta (REBOA) is another technique being utilized at some centers although its use is evolving and is not available in all centers.

Exploration

After bleeding has been temporarily controlled, time is allowed to systematically explore the abdomen for signs of injury. Newly identified sites of bleeding should be controlled with clamps or packing. Gastrointestinal perforations should be temporarily controlled with bowel, vascular, Babcock, or Allis clamps. The order of exploration is not as important as making sure that the surgeon performs the same steps the same way every time so that injuries are not missed. The most commonly described order starts with inframesocolic exploration followed by supramesocolic, lesser sac, and then finally retroperitoneum.

For inframesocolic exposure, the transverse colon is lifted cranially and the bowel is run from the ligament of Treitz down to the rectum. Each loop of bowel is systematically flipped between hands inspecting both sides as well as the associated mesentery. Notorious sites of missed injury include the proximal jejunum near the ligament of Treitz, posterior transverse colon, hepatic flexure, and splenic flexure. Once finished, the bladder and pelvis are inspected. The transverse colon is then pulled caudally for supramesocolic exposure. Typically, structures are inspected from the patient's right-to-left as if reading a book. First the liver and gallbladder are palpated, the right kidney is palpated, the stomach is evaluated from the gastroesophageal junction down through the duodenal loop, and then the spleen and left kidney are palpated. The gastroesophageal junction and retroperitoneal duodenum are also at higher risk for missed injury and should allocate special attention. Next the lesser sac is accessed by blunt dissection through the greater omentum, allowing inspection of the posterior stomach and pancreas.

Finally, the retroperitoneum is evaluated. Exploration should be kept targeted and limited based on missile trajectory and presence of hematoma. Hematoma exploration is based on the retroperitoneal zones. Zone I is midline between the kidneys from the aortic hiatus to the sacral promontory. Zone II exists lateral to the kidneys. Zone III encompasses the pelvis with everything inferior to the sacral promontory. All Zone I hematomas should be explored with risk for major vascular injury. Penetrating Zone II hematomas should be selectively explored. Blunt Zone II hematomas are further directed by associated structures. Peri-Colonic and Peri-Duodenal hematomas should all be explored [16]. Peri-Renal hematomas should be explored only if expanding, pulsatile or with active hemorrhage [16]. Exploration of Zone II should be kept limited to exclude injury with the first step being palpation of the contralateral kidney to determine the need for heroic measures. Needless exploration of Zone II may result in unnecessary loss of the kidney. All Zone III hematomas due to penetrating trauma should be explored. Zone III hematomas due to blunt trauma should be explored only if expanding, pulsatile, or with active hemorrhage. Unnecessary exploration of blunt Zone III hematomas can result in uncontrolled bleeding.

Retroperitoneal exposure is generally accomplished through any of four primary maneuvers: the Mattox Maneuver, inframesocolic division, Kocher Maneuver, or Cattell-Braasch Maneuver. In general, left-sided supramesocolic injuries should be approached by a Mattox Maneuver, while isolated left-sided inframesocolic injuries can be approached through an inframesocolic division. A right-sided suprarenal injury can be approached through a simple Kocher Maneuver, although a right-sided infrarenal injury would require a Cattell-Braasch Maneuver. These maneuvers, however, have significant overlap, and the exploration should be based on the patient's presentation, keeping it limited to avoid unnecessary morbidity yet extensive enough to allow adequate exposure.

A Mattox Maneuver, also known as a left-sided medial visceral rotation, allows for visualization of the entire abdominal aorta as well as the primary arterial branches. The descending colon is mobilized by incising along the Line of Toldt from the sigmoid colon up to the splenic flexure and then extending laterally around the spleen. A hand is then used to sweep from inferior to superior with the dissection plane directly against the posterior abdominal wall. All structures are then rotated medially. To visualize the left renal artery, the kidney may be left behind during the rotation. Major pitfalls to avoid would be injury to the spleen or risk for avulsion of the left descending lumbar vein as it connects to the renal vein.

Inframesocolic division allows visualization of the inframesocolic aorta. It is commonly used outside of trauma as the preferred operative approach for a transperitoneal open abdominal aortic aneurysm repair. Although a Mattox Maneuver allows visualization of the same structures, the inframesocolic division allows for a more targeted and limited dissection if access to the supramesocolic aorta is unnecessary. In practice the transverse mesocolon is reflected cephalad and the small bowel is eviscerated to the right. A retroperitoneal incision is then made starting at the Ligament of Treitz to the left of the aorta. Avoid injury to the inferior mesenteric vein with this initial cut. The incision is then carried inferiorly and should course to the right of the aortic midline preventing the major pitfall of injury to the inferior mesenteric artery or sigmoid mesentery.

The Kocher Maneuver provides visualization of the suprarenal inferior vena cava, right renal hilum, duodenum, and pancreas. It is performed by incising the posterior peritoneum lateral to the duodenum. A hand is then placed behind to retract the duodenum and pancreatic head medially. A major pitfall of this maneuver is injury to the right gonadal vein as it drains into the inferior vena cava.

The Cattell-Braasch Maneuver, also known as a right-sided medial visceral rotation, provides a panoramic view of the entire inframesocolic retroperitoneum. It is performed in three stages. First, a classic Kocher Maneuver is performed as previously described. The incision is then extended caudally along the Line of Toldt to fully mobilize the ascending colon. Finally, the incision is extended around the cecum and along the posterior peritoneum to the Ligament of Treitz while retracting the bowel up and to the right. These extensions are referred to as the "Extended Kocher Maneuver" and the "Super-Extended Kocher Maneuver," respectively. Care must be taken during this maneuver as the right colon will hang by its mesentery alone. A major pitfall would be avulsion of the right colic vein off the superior mesenteric vein after an inadvertent pull.

Decision: Definitive Repair Versus Damage Control

Once the injuries have been identified and the surgeon knows the state of the patient, the decision can be made to proceed with definitive repair or to elect for damage control with stabilization and delayed definitive repair. If damage control is required, the goals of the initial surgery are to arrest hemorrhage, limit contamination, maintain blood flow, and provide temporary abdominal closure. Operative time is limited to minimize further hypothermia, coagulopathy, and acidemia. Damage control procedures vary based on the injury but can include resection of necrotic bowel leaving in discontinuity, shunting, and simple packing.

The indications for damage control surgery are evolving and varied [4, 17–19]. General guidelines include the following:

- Severe Physiologic Insult
  - Acidosis (pH <7.2 or Base Deficit >15)
  - Hypothermia (Core Temperature <34 °C)
  - Coagulopathy (INR >1.5 or Clinical Evidence)
  - Lactate >5
  - Intraoperative Ventricular Arrhythmia
- Significant Blood Loss
  - Unable to Control Bleeding by Conventional Methods
  - Blood Loss >4 L
  - Blood Transfusion >10 U
- Significant Injury Pattern
  - Difficult to Assess Major Venous Injury
  - Major Liver or Pancreaticoduodenal Injury with Hemodynamic Instability

  - Combined Pancreaticoduodenal Injury with Massive Hemorrhage from the Pancreatic Head
  - Devascularization or Massive Disruption of the Duodenum, Pancreas or Pancreaticoduodenal Complex with Involvement of Ampulla or Ducts
- Need for Staged Reconstruction
  - Need to Reassess Bowel Viability
  - Unable to Close Abdominal Wall Without Tension
  - Signs of Abdominal Compartment Syndrome While Attempting Closure

Temporary Abdominal Closure

There are numerous methods available to the surgeon electing to proceed with temporary abdominal closure during a damage control laparotomy. The most common include negative pressure wound therapy, patch closure, Wittmann patch, Bogota bag, and a skin-only closure. However, even with many options for temporary abdominal closure, the goal should still be closure of the abdomen as soon as safe and feasible. Diaz et al. showed a decreased rate of complications if the abdomen was closed in less than 8 days [20].

Negative Pressure Wound Therapy (NPWT)

Over the past decade, NPWT has become the mainstream in many aspects of surgery. The NPWT closure provides temporary closure with an element of negative pressure. It helps with both the management of intrabdominal fluid and lateral forces on the abdominal wall. While this has been shown to have improved rates of fascial closure by some studies, it does come at a significantly increased cost [21]. It is becoming increasingly utilized and is now essentially available in one of two options.

The ABThera from KCI is commercially available. It is composed of an initial polyurethane foam covered with a film which is placed intraperitoneally. This film has perforations that allow fluid to be extracted while also keeping the bowel from adhesion formation. A second oval foam is then placed extraperitoneal to the level of the skin where an occlusive drape and suction can be applied. Negative pressure is then generated between 100 and 150 mmHg.

The other, less expensive option was first described by Barker's group [22]. It is similar to the ABThera VAC, but it is composed of materials already found within the operating room, thus limiting the cost. The first layer uses a perforated nonadherent polyethylene sheet which is placed between the peritoneum and visceral organs to prevent adhesions of the bowel. The perforations allow for reliable evacuation of fluid. Over the sheet, surgical towels or sponges are placed. Over these, drains are placed which give the ability to create the negative pressure. An adhesive dressing is then placed over the top to finish the seal.

Patch Closure

Many different options for use of a temporary abdominal closure have been described utilizing both permanent and absorbable mesh. Absorbable meshes are typically placed with the intent of allowing granulation tissue to form for a skin graft and eventual delayed ventral hernia repair. Non-absorbable meshes, however, can be used to help with serial approximation of the fascial edges. Both mesh options have reasonable delayed closure rates but non-absorbable have been quoted higher at almost 90% [23].

Wittmann Patch

When primary closure cannot be achieved in a timely manner, a Wittmann patch can be used. This is composed of two opposing sheets that, when pushed together, maintain force against lateral shear, similar to Velcro. The sheets will be attached to fascial edges and tightened every 24–48 h until a primary fascial closure can be performed. Benefits of the Wittmann patch are that it prevents loss of lateral abdominal domain; it is easily placed; and once the initial patch is in place, it requires no exchange of material, just serially tightening. Once the fascial edges are within a few centimeters, they can be closed primarily. This method can achieve primary closure in over 78%–100% of patients [24, 25].

Bogota Bag

Used in Bogota, Colombia for several decades, the Bogota Bag involves the use of hard intrabdominal plastic as a temporary layer. This was then described by Mattox after seeing its usage. The original description involved cutting a sterile IV bag into an oval shape and suturing or stapling it to the skin. Sterile moist towels would then be placed over it, followed by another iodine drape. While this allows for dressing changes to be performed at the bedside, which can be advantageous in certain clinical situations, it does not aid in preventing lateral abdominal wall retraction [26, 27]. Furthermore, the Bogota Bag is associated with higher rates of evisceration, sepsis, and lower primary closure rates. This limits its usage predominantly to areas that lack resources for other temporary abdominal closures [28]. Reported rates of closure after a Bogota Bag vary significantly between 12% and 80% [25, 28].

Skin-Only Closure

Perhaps the most rapid method for containing bowel intra-abdominally while minimizing heat and fluid loss can be accomplished with a skin-only closure. This can be achieved by several options, including towel clamps, staples, or a running suture. This closure should then be covered with a plastic drape to further decrease heat and fluid loss. While the skin closure can be done exceptionally fast, it does not provide any additional medial traction to the fascia in helping prevent loss of domain. Skin only closures are associated with higher rates of complications including evisceration, infection, and loss of skin. Because of increased rates of complications and other options, few situations call for a skin-only closure.

Vacuum-Assisted Wound Closure and Mesh-Mediated Fascial Traction (VAWCM)

Initially introduced in a small case series by Peterson et al., this technique serves as a promising hybrid between negative pressure wound therapy (NPWT) and the Wittmann patch [29]. The first step involves placement of a perforated plastic sheet within the peritoneum, followed by placement of a polypropylene mesh that is sutured to each fascial edge to provide constant medial traction. In between the plastic sheet and mesh, moist laparotomy pads and drains are carefully placed. Subsequently, the entire wound is covered with an occlusive dressing, and the drains are connected to suction with settings similar to those utilized in NPWT.

Regular evaluation of the patient for possible abdominal wall closure is necessary, which typically involves taking the patient to the operating room every few days or exchanging the laparotomy pads, if needed. Since its initial description, several additional authors have reported promising results with the use of this technique. Fascial closure rates have been cited as ranging from 60% to 89%, indicating its effectiveness in aiding wound healing and closure [30–32].

Outcomes and Complications

Damage control laparotomy (DCL) is an important surgical procedure that can help save the lives of critically ill patients. However, like all surgical operations, it is not without risks and complications. While it is clear that in true damage control situations, an expedited laparotomy is beneficial and can reduce mortality rates, studies have shown that there are increased rates of specific complications associated with an open abdomen. In fact, the mortality rate for patients who experience complications with an open abdomen can be as high as 25% [18].

Some of the complications that can occur with a delayed closure of the abdomen include ventral hernias, enterocutaneous or entero-atmospheric fistulas, loss of abdominal domain, ventilator-associated pneumonia, bacteremia, and sepsis. It has been found that the risk of these complications can be minimized if the abdomen is closed within 8 days from the index operation [20].

Despite the potential risks associated with DCL, there has been an increase in the number of these procedures being performed, with estimates suggesting that up to 40% of trauma patients may have an open abdomen [33, 34]. However, due to the lack of randomized controlled trials, identifying the appropriate indications for DCL has been left largely to expert opinion.

This has led some authors to suggest that DCL may be overused in situations where a definitive repair could be performed at the index procedure [18]. However, a recent matched trial conducted by George et al. found that there was no difference in mortality or major abdominal complications between patients who underwent a definitive laparotomy versus those who were left open and could have been closed at the index procedure. It should be noted, however, that the latter group did have a higher risk of fascial dehiscence [34].

Conclusion

The trauma laparotomy still follows the same "Operative Sequence" of access and exposure, temporary bleeding control, exploration, and then decision of definitive repair versus damage control as outlined by Hirshberg and Mattox over 15 years ago. As operative trauma cases are declining and are increasingly concentrated in a few centers, the need to maintain adequate surgical training is vital. Today, the trauma laparotomy serves as a life-saving intervention in the management of abdominal trauma. It is a tool that every graduating surgical resident and every surgeon taking trauma call should thoroughly understand and be prepared to utilize.

References

1. Rotondo MF, Schwab CW, McGonigal MD, Phillips GR 3rd, Fruchterman TM, Kauder DR, Latenser BA, Angood PA. 'Damage control': an approach for improved survival in exsanguinating penetrating abdominal injury. J Trauma. 1993;35(3):375–82; discussion 382–373.
2. Feliciano DV, Burch JM, Spjut-Patrinely V, Mattox KL, Jordan GL Jr. Abdominal gunshot wounds. An urban trauma center's experience with 300 consecutive patients. Ann Surg. 1988;208(3):362–70.
3. Ivatury RR, Nallathambi M, Gunduz Y, Constable R, Rohman M, Stahl WM. Liver packing for uncontrolled hemorrhage: a reappraisal. J Trauma. 1986;26(8):744–53.
4. Roberts DJ, Bobrovitz N, Zygun DA, Ball CG, Kirkpatrick AW, Faris PD, Stelfox HT. Indications for use of damage control surgery and damage control interventions in civilian trauma patients: a scoping review. J Trauma Acute Care Surg. 2015;78(6):1187–96.

5. Violence and injury prevention. Injuries and violence—the facts. https://www.who.int/violence_injury_prevention/key_facts/en/
6. National Center for Health Statistics (NCHS). Mortality in the United States.
7. Feliciano DV. Abdominal trauma revisited. Am Surg. 2017;83(11):1193–202.
8. WISQARS. https://www.cdc.gov/injury/wisqars/index.html.
9. 10 Leading causes of injury deaths by age group highlighting unintentional injury deaths, United States. https://www.cdc.gov/injury/wisqars/LeadingCauses.html
10. Harvin JA, Maxim T, Inaba K, Martinez-Aguilar MA, King DR, Choudhry AJ, Zielinski MD, Akinyeye S, Todd SR, Griffin RL, et al. Mortality after emergent trauma laparotomy: a multi-center, retrospective study. J Trauma Acute Care Surg. 2017;83(3):464–8.
11. Sakran JV, Mehta A, Fransman R, Nathens AB, Joseph B, Kent A, Haut ER, Efron DT. Nationwide trends in mortality following penetrating trauma: are we up for the challenge? J Trauma Acute Care Surg. 2018;85(1):160–6.
12. Atls course administration and faculty guide, 10th ed. Chicago, IL: American College of Surgeons; 2017.
13. Asensio JA, Trunkey DD. Current therapy of trauma and surgical critical care. 2nd ed. Philadelphia, PA: Elsevier; 2016.
14. Hirshberg A, Mattox KL, Allen MK, Weldon S. Top knife: the art & craft of trauma surgery. Castle Hill Barns, Shrewsbury: TFM Publishing; 2005.
15. Kobayashi LM, Costantini TW, Hamel MG, Dierksheide JE, Coimbra R. Abdominal vascular trauma. Trauma Surg Acute Care Open. 2016;1(1):e000015.
16. Manzini N, Madiba TE. The management of retroperitoneal haematoma discovered at laparotomy for trauma. Injury. 2014;45(9):1378–83.
17. Roberts DJ, Bobrovitz N, Zygun DA, Ball CG, Kirkpatrick AW, Faris PD, Brohi K, D'Amours S, Fabian TC, Inaba K, et al. Indications for use of damage control surgery in civilian trauma patients: a content analysis and expert appropriateness rating study. Ann Surg. 2016;263(5):1018–27.
18. Roberts DJ, Bobrovitz N, Zygun DA, Kirkpatrick AW, Ball CG, Faris PD, Stelfox HT. Indications for trauma damage control surgery international study G: evidence for use of damage control surgery and damage control interventions in civilian trauma patients: a systematic review. World J Emerg Surg. 2021;16(1):10.
19. Bentin JM, Possfelt-Moller E, Svenningsen P, Rudolph SS, Sillesen M. A characterization of trauma laparotomies in a scandinavian setting: an observational study. Scand J Trauma Resusc Emerg Med. 2022;30(1):43.
20. Diaz JJ Jr, Dutton WD, Ott MM, Cullinane DC, Alouidor R, Armen SB, Bilanuik JW, Collier BR, Gunter OL, Jawa R, et al. Eastern Association for the Surgery of Trauma: a review of the management of the open abdomen—part 2 "Management of the open abdomen". J Trauma. 2011;71(2):502–12.
21. Montori G, Allievi N, Coccolini F, Solaini L, Campanati L, Ceresoli M, Fugazzola P, Manfredi R, Magnone S, Tomasoni M, et al. Negative pressure wound therapy versus modified Barker vacuum pack as temporary abdominal closure technique for open abdomen management: a four-year experience. BMC Surg. 2017;17(1):86.
22. Brock WB, Barker DE, Burns RP. Temporary closure of open abdominal wounds: the vacuum pack. Am Surg. 1995;61(1):30–5.
23. Regner JL, Kobayashi L, Coimbra R. Surgical strategies for management of the open abdomen. World J Surg. 2012;36(3):497–510.
24. Nemec HM, Benjamin Christie D, Montgomery A, Vaughn DM. Wittmann patch : superior closure for the open abdomen. Am Surg. 2020;86(8):981–4.
25. Mahoney EJ, Bugaev N, Appelbaum R, Goldenberg-Sandau A, Baltazar GA, Posluszny J, Dultz L, Kartiko S, Kasotakis G, Como J, et al. Management of the open abdomen: a systematic review with meta-analysis and practice management guideline from the Eastern Association for the Surgery of Trauma. J Trauma Acute Care Surg. 2022;93(3):e110–8.

26. Fernandez L, Norwood S, Roettger R, Wilkins HE 3rd. Temporary intravenous bag silo closure in severe abdominal trauma. J Trauma. 1996;40(2):258–60.
27. Manterola C, Moraga J, Urrutia S. Contained laparostomy with a Bogota bag. Results of case series. Cir Esp. 2011;89(6):379–85.
28. Muhammad Y, Gondal KM, Khan UA. Use of the "bogota bag" for closure of open abdominal wound after exploratory laparotomy—our experience at Mayo Hospital Lahore. J Pak Med Assoc. 2016;66(8):980–3.
29. Hadeed JG, Staman GW, Sariol HS, Kumar S, Ross SE. Delayed primary closure in damage control laparotomy: the value of the Wittmann patch. Am Surg. 2007;73(1):10–2.
30. Petersson P, Montgomery A, Petersson U. Vacuum-assisted wound closure and permanent onlay mesh-mediated fascial traction: a novel technique for the prevention of incisional hernia after open abdomen therapy including results from a retrospective case series. Scand J Surg. 2019;108(3):216–26.
31. Petersson P, Petersson U. Dynamic fascial closure with vacuum-assisted wound closure and mesh-mediated fascial traction (VAWCM) treatment of the open abdomen-an updated systematic review. Front Surg. 2020;7:577104.
32. Jakob MO, Schwarz C, Haltmeier T, Zindel J, Pinworasarn T, Candinas D, Starlinger P, Beldi G. Mesh-augmented versus direct abdominal closure in patients undergoing open abdomen treatment. Hernia. 2018;22(5):785–92.
33. Harvin JA, Wray CJ, Steward J, Lawless RA, McNutt MK, Love JD, Moore LJ, Wade CE, Cotton BA, Holcomb JB. Control the damage: morbidity and mortality after emergent trauma laparotomy. Am J Surg. 2016;212(1):34–9.
34. George MJ, Adams SD, McNutt MK, Love JD, Albarado R, Moore LJ, Wade CE, Cotton BA, Holcomb JB, Harvin JA. The effect of damage control laparotomy on major abdominal complications: a matched analysis. Am J Surg. 2018;216(1):56–9.

Chapter 23
Abdominal Compartment Syndrome and Emergency Decompressive Laparotomy

Sissy-Amelie Engelien and Dirk R. Bulian

Abbreviations

ACS	Abdominal compartment syndrome
ADH	Anti-diuretic hormone
DCL	Damage control laparotomy
DL	Decompressive laparotomy
ECMO	Extracorporeal membrane oxygenation
IAH	Intraabdominal hypertension
IAP	Intraabdominal pressure
ICU	Intensive care unit
IVC	Inferior vena cava
MODS	Multiple organ dysfunction syndrome
NPWT	Negative pressure wound therapy
PCD	Percutaneous drainage
RVEF	Right ventricular ejection fraction
WSACS	World Society of the Abdominal Compartment Syndrome

S.-A. Engelien
Department of Plastic Surgery, Hand Surgery, and Burn Center, Cologne-Merheim Medical Center (CMMC), Witten/Herdecke University, Cologne, Germany
e-mail: engelien@web.de

D. R. Bulian (✉)
Department of Abdominal, Tumor, Transplant and Vascular Surgery, Center for Interdisciplinary Visceral Medicine (CIV), Cologne-Merheim Medical Center (CMMC), Witten/Herdecke University, Cologne, Germany
e-mail: dirk.bulian@uni-wh.de

© The Author(s), under exclusive license to Springer Nature Switzerland AG 2024

J. Faintuch, S. Faintuch (eds.), *Recent Strategies in High Risk Surgery*,
https://doi.org/10.1007/978-3-031-56270-9_23

Introduction/Background

Intraabdominal hypertension (IAH) and especially the abdominal compartment syndrome (ACS) often describe inadequately diagnosed clinical entities accompanied by an increased morbidity and mortality.

Knowledge of these conditions is of major importance in both medical and surgical intensive care units (ICU), the emergency department, and the general ward. An adequate diagnosis and immediate therapy are necessary to improve the outcome. For the diagnosis, identifying risk factors and monitoring of the intraabdominal pressure play a key role [1–3].

Patients with abdominal diseases most frequently die from infectious complications: peritonitis, on the one hand, due to a primary inflammatory disease or ischemia of an abdominal organ with bacterial translocation or organ perforation; on the other hand, after complicative abdominal surgery with anastomotic insufficiency or bowel injury, but also from intraperitoneal hemorrhage or mechanical causes such as intestinal obstruction. Another abdominal cause of lethal disease progression is untreated abdominal compartment syndrome (ACS). It describes a mismatch of space required by the abdominal organs including their blood supply and the available abdominal volume. Especially in the case of both, an increased space requirement of abdominal or retroperitoneal organs and reduced space inside the abdominal cavity, the development of an ACS is more likely.

The abdominal wall is physiologically very distensible compared with other compartments such as the skull. An increase of intraabdominal volume can usually be tolerated for a certain period of time without a negative impact on organ function. However, this distensibility has its limits, especially when the volume increase occurs in a short period of time. Conservative therapeutic measures are usually insufficient making emergency decompression laparotomy (EDL) a rarely necessary but often life-saving procedure in visceral as well as in burn medicine.

IAH leads to organ dysfunction and even organ failure via disturbance of abdominal organ perfusion. Usually, the kidneys are the first to be affected. In addition, an increase of the intraabdominal pressure leads to a pathological diaphragmatic elevation, which culminates in ventilatory dysfunction and lung failure. These consequences have a relevant impact on the mortality of critically ill patients.

Since ACS can be seen as a consequence of other pathologies, EDL is only a symptomatic and not a causal therapy of the underlying disease. Moreover, EDL is part of the complication management, which, on the other hand, requires prolonged treatment for secondary abdominal wall closure and involves additional, severe complications such as enteroatmospheric fistulas. In this regard, the surgical technique and the EDL approach have a crucial influence on the EDL-associated complication rate and the secondary abdominal wall closure rate. EDL buys time for further therapy of the underlying disease by preventing a short-term lethal course due to multiorgan failure and improving organ function. Thereby, the overall outcome can be improved.

Definitions

A compartment syndrome describes an elevated pressure inside an inextensible anatomical space like the cranial, abdominal, and thoracic cavity, which leads to a compromitted tissue perfusion.

In a normal weight person, the physiological pressure in the abdominal cavity is 5 mmHg, whereas in highly obese patients, an increased baseline IAP of 9–14 mmHg can be found.

IAH is defined as an IAP >12 mmHg and subdivided into four Grades (Grade I IAP 12–15 mmHg, Grade II IAP 16–20 mmHg, Grade III IAP 21–25 mmHg, Grade IV IAP > 25 mmHg). The definition of ACS includes an IAP >20 mmHg combined with a newly emerging organ dysfunction or organ failure. Acute elevations in IAP have shown similar effects in obese patients, but the threshold IAP associated with organ dysfunction is assumed to be higher in this population [4–9].

Epidemiology

Concerning the epidemiology of IAH and ACS, data show significant differences. Causal may, on one hand, be the level of awareness among clinicians. In teaching hospitals, ACS is claimed to be diagnosed more often compared to district hospitals. On the other hand, the epidemiology depends on the studied population.

In general, critical patients show a higher risk in developing ACS than non-critical patients. Most studies focused on homogenous populations showing significant differences in concerning the incidence rate. So, an overall incidence of IAH and ACS cannot be numbered [7, 10].

Incidence

For IAH including ACS, the following incidences are described: aortic surgery, 39.7% (33.3% elective and 61.5% emergency surgery); liver transplant, 59.5%; severe and acute pancreatitis, 85.7%; major trauma, 58.8–72.8%; mixed ICU, 39–48.9%; and septic shock, 18.9–68%.

If we consider only ACS, the incidences are aortic surgery, 5.2%; liver transplant, 7.7%; mixed ICU, 2–6%; septic shock, 28%; and severe acute pancreatitis, 57% [6].

Due to advanced recognition and management of IAH as well as improved intensive care and perioperative treatment including fluid management optimization, critically ill patients progressively survive the initial phase. The incidence of IAH persists and is probable to increase, whereas the incidence of ACS lessens [6, 11].

Mortality

IAH is an independent predictor for mortality increasing the mortality in ICU patients from 1–11% to 6–30% and an inverse relation between IAH and the outcome is described. Concerning the underlying condition causing IAH, the mortality of a secondary IAH is higher than the mortality of primary IAH [6, 12].

In contrast to IAH, the overall mortality of ACS is higher than 60% with a 90-day mortality of 39%–76% depending on patient selection and management. Without any treatment, mortality is more than 90%, and despite treatment, conservative and surgical, mortality still lies between 25% and 75%. In patients undergoing decompressive laparotomy, mortality is 16–49.2%, which is described as a reduction of the mortality by decompressive laparotomy between 16% and 37% [3, 6, 13, 14].

IAH and ACS not only increase the mortality rate, but also the length of ICU stay and severity of organ failure. The underlying pathophysiology especially leads to impaired kidney and lung function, which in turn can lead to increased use of renal replacement therapy and prolonged mechanical ventilation [6].

Anatomy and Physiology

The abdominal cavity contains organs and major blood vessels supplying and draining them. Pressure can be transmitted among the intra- and retroperitoneal spaces as well as the anterior abdominal wall. By transmitting pressure among the intraabdominal structures, arterial blood supply and venous drainage of intra- and retroperitoneal organs may be impaired. Another parameter describing the abdominal conditions is the abdominal compliance pointing out the relationship between intraabdominal volume changes and changes in the IAP. Normal abdominal compliance is around 250–450 mL/mmHg and in male patients, a decreased abdominal compliance may be found. This parameter is not routinely used as its assessment is difficult. Its curvilinear relationship explains the effectiveness of abdominal drainage [5–7].

Terminology and Etiology

ACS results from a persistent IAH and can be characterized as primary and secondary. An ACS caused by a pathology located in the abdominal region, for example, an abdominal trauma or pancreatitis, is termed a primary ACS, whereas pathologies, anatomically not specifically located in the abdominal region, but leading to a fluid accumulation there, define a secondary ACS. Examples for pathologies leading to a secondary ACS are extensive fluid resuscitation and sepsis. Another subdivision of IAH can be made depicting the onset and course, which can be acute and chronic. Usually, ACS emerges from acute elevations in IAP. A chronic elevation of IAP can result from obesity or liver cirrhosis and lead to an increased compliance of the abdominal wall as well as compensatory mechanisms in the afflicted organ systems [2, 7, 10, 15].

Risk Factors

The risk factors for IAH and ACS can, on one hand, be divided into factors increasing the volume and thereby the pressure inside the abdominal cavity, putting pressure on the abdominal cavity from the outside, and factors decreasing the compliance of the abdominal wall.

For the latter, major abdominal trauma including burns, especially of 30% total body surface area, or abdominal surgery can be responsible, as well as an increased head of bed angle, a bent or prone body position, and a high body mass index [6, 8, 10, 15, 16].

A rising pressure inside the abdominal cavity can be aggravated by either an increased intraluminal content, like an ileus, or an increased intraabdominal content like an acute pancreatitis, a massive hernia repair, edema, ascites, hemoperitoneum or pneumoperitoneum, for example, following laparoscopy with excessive insufflation pressures. The extraperitoneal space can gain volume as well, for example, by bleedings from pelvic fractures or the rupture of an aortic aneurysm.

Volume shifts are in general known to potentially cause an elevated IAP. That includes massive fluid resuscitation, a positive fluid balance, polytransfusion, as well as sepsis, shock, and hypotension.

Mechanical ventilation, especially a PEEP >10 mmHg, or the before mentioned obesity apply pressure on the abdominal cavity from the outside [2, 8, 10, 15, 17–19].

On the other hand, factors like age, bacteremia, transplants (renal allograft compartment syndrome, RACS), extracorporeal membrane oxygenation (ECMO), and coagulopathy have been shown to potentially lead to IAH.

These risk factors can influence and aggravate each other. Like massive volume resuscitation not only leads to intraabdominal fluid excess, but it may also facilitate a reduced compliance of the abdominal wall by causing abdominal wall edema. IAP rises even more, the blood circulation wanes, and ischemia occurs affecting organs and the abdominal wall, which leads to a reduced compliance of the latter. This is just one partial aspect of the vicious circle induced [8, 10, 15, 20, 21] (Table 23.1).

Table 23.1 Causes of IAH and ACS

Primary ACS	Secondary ACS
Abdominal trauma	Positive fluid balance
Pancreatitis	Sepsis, shock, hypotension
Bleeding, i.e. rupture of an aneurysm, or pelvic fracture	Severe burn
Tumor	Polytransfusion
Surgery, e.g. massive hernia replacement	ECMO
Pneumoperitoneum	Bacteriemia
Ileus	Coagulopathy
Transplant	
Edema of intra–/retroperitoneal organs	
Ascites	
Peritonitis	
Postoperative complication, e.g. anastomosis leakage	

Pathophysiology

IAH may lead to compromises in several organ systems. Its pathophysiological impact on them resembles a state like sepsis. The vasomotor tone is lost, the glycocalyx is damaged, and intercellular junctions of the endothelium collapse. Consequently, the vascular permeability increases. In this scenario, fluid resuscitation is required to stabilize hemodynamics. That results in a vicious circle as fluid resuscitation leads to IAH and ACS and as IAH stimulates anti-diuretic hormone (ADH) release, the situation aggravates. In the critically ill, a correlation between IAP and extracellular water content is reported. Moreover, an elevated IAP may result in prodromal, sub-clinical organ dysfunction and can lead to multiple organ dysfunction syndrome (MODS). In the following, the effects of IAH and ACS on different organ systems are depicted [7, 12, 22].

Cardiovascular System

An elevation of IAP leads to a reduced cardiac preload by diminishing the venous return to the heart. This may be due to an absolute loss of volume or compression of the inferior vena cava (IVC). Furthermore, an increased IAP can influence the intrathoracic pressure. Pulmonary vascular resistance rises compromising the right ventricular ejection fraction (RVEF). This expedites a loss of left ventricular end-diastolic volume and a disturbed myocardial contractility while the cardiac afterload increases due to a mounting vascular resistance. These effects come along with a decreased cardiac output and arterial hypotension leading to tachycardia, which shortens the diastolic coronary blood flow [7, 12, 23].

Gastrointestinal System

Abdominal perfusion pressure (APP) is the difference between the mean arterial pressure (MAP) and the IAP (APP = MAP − IAP). In other words, an increase in IAP leads to capillary compression, a lowered APP, and thereby, intestinal hypoxia. Mesenteric vein compression makes matters worse. The decreased venous drainage facilitates intestinal edema and bacterial translocation [7, 8, 12].

Renal System

The impact of IAH on the renal system is also multifactual. The diminished cardiac output and therewith a reduced intravascular pressure come up against the raised pressure in the abdominal cavity. Not only a sufficient splanchnic, but also renal perfusion may not be retained. The microcirculatory flow and the glomerular filtration rate are reduced as the renal cortex and veins are compressed. The latter can be described as an increased renal venous pressure, which seems to play the most important role in renal failure in IAH.

The renin–angiotensin–aldosterone system (RAAS) is activated as renin is secreted when the renal blood flow is lowered. Blood pressure regulation, vascular resistance, as well as fluid and electrolyte balance are deranged. As IAH often affects the kidneys first, oliguria may be one of the earliest signs of ACS [7, 12, 23].

Respiratory

A raised pressure in the abdominal cavity elevates the diaphragm and the intrathoracic pressure increases. This causes both a decreased compliance and functional residual capacity.

Furthermore, compressive atelectasis occurs, as well as an increased alveolar dead space followed by a ventilation-perfusion mismatch and hypoxic bronchial artery vasoconstriction. Accessory breathing muscles come into use, while the chest wall compliance is reduced and breathwork increases. Consequently, in mechanically ventilated patients, this necessitates an elevated inspiratory peak pressure and end expiratory pressure. Hypercapnia as well as a decline in PaO_2/FiO_2 ratio may be observed [7, 12, 23].

Central Nervous System

The high intrapleural pressure caused by ACS raises a functional compression of the jugular veins. Venous drainage of the cranium is affected, intracranial pressure rises, and the cerebral perfusion pressure is decreased. The result is cerebral hypoxia, which leads to encephalopathy impairing among others the vital regulatory centers in the brain and homeostatic mechanisms are compromised [7, 12].

Poly-Compartment Syndrome

Poly-compartment syndrome describes a simultaneously increased pressure in two or more body compartments. It is a rare but life-threatening condition. By a pressure relief of one of the affected compartments, the outcome can be improved [12].

Symptoms

As ACS is mostly seen in critically ill and not always addressable patients, the determination of clinical symptoms is limited. Some patients report abdominal pain, dyspnea, or other non-specific symptoms like fatigue and headache. Clinical hints for ACS may be progressive oliguria and respiratory distress. Hypotension and tachycardia can be observed as well as high jugular venous pressure, jugular venous distension, and peripheral oedema. In the clinical examination, signs of peritonism or hypoperfusion may be found, and some patients show a restlessness. In the blood gas analysis, inferences from metabolic acidosis about ACS can be drawn [10].

Diagnostics

Clinical Examination

Physical examination of the abdomen may give hints but fails to assuredly reveal an ACS. The palpatory findings may show a tense abdomen, but the sensitivity of abdominal palpation in this issue is only 40% [10, 24–26].

Imaging Techniques

In radiological examinations of the abdomen or thorax, especially a CT scan, hints of an ACS can be found like compression of the IVC, infiltration of the retroperitoneum, and an increased ratio of anteroposterior-to-transverse abdominal diameter (positive round belly sign). Furthermore, bowel wall thickening with enhancement and bilateral inguinal herniation may be pictured [7, 27, 28].

An adjuvant usage of ultrasound may give more information on possible dysfunctions: a smaller IVC section area and an increased resistive index of the renal arteries may be hints for an early hemodynamic impairment. Via echocardiography a reduced preload or ventricular dysfunctions can possibly be detected. Furthermore, ultrasound can be used to show the bowel activity qualitatively and quantitatively, large bowel contents or free intrabdominal fluid.

Even if imaging techniques can reveal pathologies associated with IAH, they are insufficient for an early and accurate diagnosis, and IAP measurements are recommended [8, 29–31].

IAP Measurement

There are many techniques described to measure IAP. In general, it can be measured directly and indirectly. Direct measurement via an intraabdominal catheter is the most sensitive but also most invasive method and thereby potentially complicative. It is, for example, used during laparoscopy when the abdomen is insufflated with gas. Indirect measurements use hollow organs in the abdominal cavity and include intragastric, intraintestinal (colon, rectum), intravaginal, and intravesical. Moreover, intravenous measurements (IVC) can be helpful.

But despite these numerous options, the standard method for IAP measurement is via the bladder using an instillation volume of maximal 25 mL of sterile saline after zeroing the transducer at the level of the midaxillary line. The wall of the bladder is considered to function as a membranous pressure transducer, but only when containing 25 mL of liquid. Compared to the simple catheterization of the bladder, intravesical pressure monitoring does not increase the risk of urinary tract infection.

An IAP measurement is recommended in critical patients with (the above-mentioned) risk factors for IAH. Measurements are recommended every 4–6 h and the development of protocols for IAP measurement is endorsed.

Continuous and real-time IAP monitoring is viable, but it is not standard practice. Therefore, a three-way vesical catheter is needed to provide a steady flow of 25 mL saline solution [3, 6, 8, 24, 32–34].

Advice on Intravesical Measurement of IAP

IAP should be measured at end-expiration in the supine position. As described previously, an increased head of bed angle is known to be a risk factor for IAP and ACS. For a head of the bed angle of 30°, the average increase of IAP is 4 mmHg and for 45°, it is 9 mmHg. The absence of abdominal muscle contractions should be checked in advance [5, 6, 8, 35].

Prevention

To prevent IAH and ACS, some aspects can be taken care of in patients at risk, such as the before-mentioned patient's body position with a recommended low head of the bed angle. A positive fluid balance can increase IAP, so after the acute resuscitation of the critically ill, further fluid overload should be avoided and a protocol can help to do so. Moreover, the use of enhanced ratios of plasma to red blood cells is recommended. In general, an optimal pain and anxiety relief should be aimed, and to prevent malperfusion, an APP of a minimum of 50 mmHg should be aimed in critically ill patients [7, 8, 36].

Therapy of IAH and ACS

Conservative Treatment

In general, the soonest possible initiation of an adequate therapy is of major concern. A stepwise application of interventions is recommended to maintain an IAP below 15 mmHg considering the etiology of IAH or ACS in the patient as well as the clinical situation [8].

Evacuate Intraluminal Content

Gastroenteral decompression with nasogastric or rectal tubes can contribute to pressure relief in a dilated stomach or colon. To evacuate intraluminal contents, the use of prokinetic agents is also recommended. If these actions are not sufficient, enteral nutrition should be minimized and enemas should come to use. A further escalation is a discontinuation of enteral feeding, and a colonoscopic decompression should be considered [6, 8].

Evacuate Intraabdominal Space Occupying Lesions/Fluid

In suspicion of intraabdominal space occupying lesions, ultrasound should be used for the detection in the first place. If ultrasound is not informative, a computed tomography is recommended. To evacuate fluid, percutaneous catheter drainage should be performed firstly, if technically possible, before considering surgical treatment. That drainage of intraabdominal fluid is a safe as well as effective therapy. The efficiency of draining a few hundred milliliters in significantly lowering IAP as well as partially avoiding EDL has been demonstrated, especially in severely burned patients [8, 37–40].

Improve Abdominal Wall Compliance

The first step to improve abdominal wall compliance is to ensure an adequate analgesia and sedation and remove constrictive dressings. The head of the bed angle should be lowered. If these actions are not sufficient, a reverse Trendelenburg position may be supportive. Brief trials of neuromuscular blockade as further, temporary interventions are suggested [5, 6, 8, 35].

Optimize Fluid Administration

In the case of an elevated IAP, excessive fluid resuscitation must be avoided and after initial stabilization of the patient, a zero to negative fluid balance by day three should be targeted. The use of hypertonic fluids and colloids as an escalation of therapy can be considered. Moreover, diuretics may be used. If these therapies are depleted, hemodialysis and ultrafiltration come into question [6, 8].

Optimize Systemic/Regional Perfusion

For an optimized systemic or regional perfusion, a goal-directed fluid resuscitation guided by hemodynamic monitoring is endorsed [8].

However, if there is insufficient success by the conservative therapy with development of organ dysfunction or failure and progressive IAH or an existing intraabdominal focus as a trigger for IAH, EDL is necessary. In the latter case, the combination of pressure relief and simultaneous focal treatment is crucial.

Surgical Treatment

The correct and, above all, timely indication of EDL is a decisive factor for patient outcome. An unnecessary EDL can worsen the patient's outcome just as much as a delayed EDL. EDL should be performed immediately at the onset of ACS and after the failure of the above-mentioned interventions. This should be at least within the first 24 h but can then reduce mortality by almost 10% [41].

Persistent hypotension, acidosis, hypothermia, and coagulopathy associated with IAH indicate the need for EDL. If correctly indicated, an improvement in oxygenation and a reduction in ventilatory pressures occur immediately. Furthermore, a resumption of urine output or an increase in diuresis usually arises within a few hours [42]. This is also a positive predictive value for patient survival.

In the case of an unstable patient, we prefer a damage control approach. A primary resection of the ischemic, perforated, or severely injured bowel segments with respective blind closure using a stapler and secondary anastomotic creation in a second procedure after intensive care stabilization of the patient would be exemplary. In the case of mesenteric ischemia, the indication for damage control is very generous, even if indocyanine green perfusion control of the bowel is used [43, 44] since secondary resection is more frequently necessary.

Surgical Technique

Incision Pattern

Even though transverse incisions, also with leaving the peritoneum intact, are described, we prefer the median laparotomy. In our opinion, the cranial extent should be limited as much as possible, especially in the case of an acute costal arch angle, since here a later, secondary fascial closure may become impossible even with minor fascial dehiscence due to the fixation of the abdominal wall fascia at the costal arch.

After the abdomen has been opened, the entire intraabdominal content should always be explored first. Surprising findings, especially perfusion disturbances of the intestine or previously unknown hernias, can possibly be detected and must be treated properly. As a next step, the underlying disease of the ACS, for example, an acute, necrotizing, and infected pancreatitis, must be addressed according to the findings. An infectious focus underlying the ACS should be treated following general standards of care, if possible.

Technique of Temporary Abdominal Wall Closure

After completion of the focus control and thorough irrigation of the abdomen, the first question is whether the abdominal wall can be definitively and completely closed again. This is usually not possible without risking a recurrence of IAH or persistent ACS. Multiple procedures with varying degrees of complexity and cost have been described. For example, we would like to mention the skin only or silo closure [45], the inexpensive Bogota bag [46], the use of a so-called Wittman patch [47], and the use of a commercial abdominal Negative Pressure Wound Therapy (NPWT) set, which we prefer (Fig. 23.1). The NPWT seems to improve the survival rate of the patients undergoing open abdomen therapy, even if the mechanism is still unclear [48].

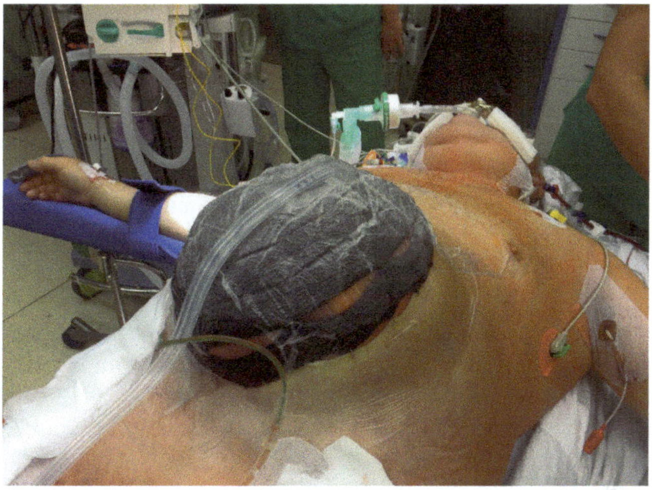

Fig. 23.1 Commercial abdominal Negative Pressure Wound Therapy (NPWT) set

Open Abdomen

In our opinion, the second question is whether an open abdomen is necessary in the longer term or whether a definitive abdominal closure already seems realistic a few days later, after one or if need be two revisions. The fascial edges of the laparotomy wound retract if laparostomy is necessary in the longer term, making definitive secondary abdominal wall closure more difficult or impossible. This is why we take a different approach here to counteract fascial retraction in this case.

In the case of an open abdomen expected only for a short time or in a damage control procedure, we recommend repositioning the intestine and the omentum majus, if present, and completely covering the intraabdominal organ volume with a large visceral protective layer (VPL). The omentum majus should be stretched as far as possible to cover the small intestine, as it provides protection and is easy to detach during revision. The VPL must always be placed far laterally into the paracolic gutters as well as cranially and caudally so that the bowel is not in contact with the anterior and lateral abdominal wall.

To place the foil far cranially, the ligamentum teres et falciforme hepatis must be cut. If a stoma is present, the foil must be slit and placed far laterally around the stoma on both sides. Then a polyurethane sponge, cut according to the size of the remaining abdominal wall defect, is placed on the VPL in the defect and the defect is taped with a foil, which is overlapping several inches. Any contact between the sponge and the intestine must be absolutely avoided. A small hole is cut in the adhesive foil, the suction foot is attached and, after the connection to a pump, a negative pressure of approximately 75 mmHg is applied. However, the level of suction possibly needs to be adjusted, especially lowered in the presence of a coagulopathy and increased risk of rebleeding. This procedure takes only a few minutes, which is particularly advantageous in the context of damage control.

NPWT promotes granulation of the adjacent subcutaneous tissue and reduction of tissue edema of the abdominal organs. If completely sealed, the nursing effort with the dressing, other than changing pump canisters and periodically checking the set suction, is minimal, as well as the risk of contamination of the abdomen. The commercial pumps control the set suction and give an alarm in case of problems like obstruction or leakage, which should be corrected promptly.

However, if one assumes that the abdomen will have to remain open for a longer period of time due to a further increasing edema of the abdominal organs, a retroperitoneal mass as in pancreatitis or hemorrhage, or a questionable perfusion situation of the organs, the incipient retraction of the fascial edges should be prevented. Again, various techniques are described for this, but we prefer the so-called Koblenz model, a combination of a visceral protective layer, negative-pressure wound therapy, and dynamic closure techniques [49]. Here, after insertion of the VPL, a polyglactin mesh inlay is sewn into the fascial defect with continuous suturing using 2-0 polyglactin circumferentially in the sense of continuous (mesh-mediated) fascial traction before the polyurethane sponge is inserted and the dressing is completed with a negative pressure of 75 mmHg.

At the next revision, the adhesive sheet and sponge are then removed and the polyglactin mesh is subtotally cut along its longitudinal axis and the abdomen is explored after removal of the VPL. Subtotal cutting of the mesh simplifies re-sutured closure of the mesh. At the end of this procedure, the mesh slit is closed again by a continuous suture using 2-0 polyglactin. In this process, the size of the mesh can be diminished at each revision according to the local findings to approximate the fascial edges (Fig. 23.2a, b). Of course, this would also be possible with bridging fascial sutures, but these increase the risk for fascial defects and soft tissue necrosis with every procedure (Fig. 23.3).

In the "Koblenz model" the fascia is only damaged twice, by the mesh fixation suture and the final fascial suture, which is simplified in this technique. In any case, the combination of VPL, NPWT, and continuous (mesh-mediated) fascial traction guarantees a maximized definitive abdominal closure rate.

Another new, alternative technique to prevent fascial retraction in the case of long-term open abdomen is the use of the Fasciotens Abdomen, for which the first promising experience reports also exist for this indication [50]. However, this technique is more complex and also cost-intensive.

Revisions

In our opinion, a meticulous adhesiolysis of the entire small intestine should be performed in every revision; otherwise, block formation will occur, which will massively complicate or impede a later complication treatment by, for example, stoma

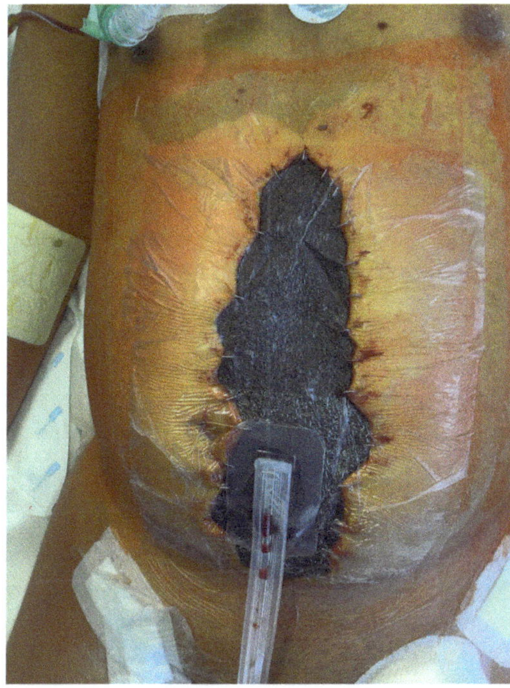

Fig. 23.2 (**a**, **b**) Approximating the fascial edges

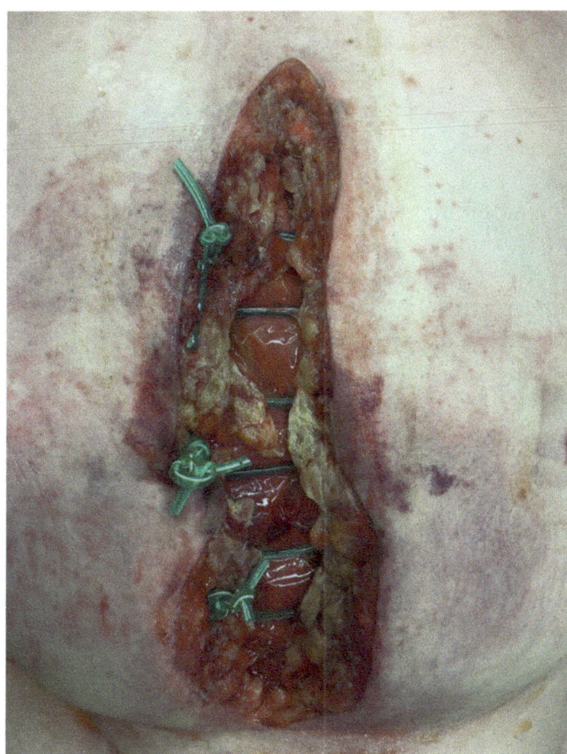

Fig. 23.3 Soft tissue necrosis after bridging fascial sutures

creation. We strongly recommend the implementation of all procedures on one patient by the same surgical team. The accomplishment of revisions after the elective program by the surgeon on duty leads, in our opinion, to more complications and a delayed definitive abdominal closure and consequently a prolonged open abdomen therapy, due to the ignorance of previous findings. The interval between revisions depends on the patient's condition and should not exceed 72 h. Even if some colleagues disagree, in sepsis-related unstable patients as well as in the absence of evidence of an intraabdominal focus, we tend to wait one more day until the patient has recovered. In the case of any suspicion, immediate revision is indicated.

Definitive abdominal closure should be performed as early as possible and as late as necessary, but depends on several factors, especially intraabdominal findings and volume (abdominal organ edema). The requirements for definitive abdominal closure are an adequate minus balance after control of septic or trauma stress response, resolution of septic capillary leak with consecutive anasarca, secure focal control, an ensured vitality of the bowel, no need for surgical re-exploration, and no evidence of persistent abdominal compartment syndrome. General, intensive care treatment recommendations such as fluid balance, avoidance of hypothermia, coagulation management, substitution for coagulopathy, adapted catecholamine administration, and nutritional support can have a positive impact on early definitive abdominal wall closure.

Nutritional Replenishment

Sufficient enteral nutrition, including oral nutrition if tolerated, should be provided immediately when possible due to nitrogen loss through the open abdomen and preferred to parenteral nutrition. Contraindications to this are only a lack of bowel continuity after damage control surgery, signs of intestinal obstruction, and high enteroatmospheric fistulae, where enteral nutrition via transfistular access to aboral positioning is not possible. Within such circumstances, parenteral feeding will be required. Sedation and ventilation are dependent on the patient's intensive care status and not on the presence of an open abdomen.

Technique of Definitive Abdominal Wall Closure

In definitive abdominal closure, complete fascial suture should be aimed. In this regard, fascial suture is possible with or without mesh reinforcement.

Without the use of mesh reinforcement, fascial suture is performed as a direct suture or with the Ramirez component separation technique if complete approximation of the fascia is not primarily possible but can thereby be achieved [51]. Fascia suturing is possible continuously or with interrupted sutures. We prefer the former with a very slowly absorbable monofilament elastic thread (poly-4-hydroxybutyrate).

In any of these cases, the skin should be closed; otherwise, a vacuum therapy kit should be applied subcutaneously. Another alternative is the combination of component separation with the implantation of a (partially resorbable) mesh in the sublay position, which potentially can reduce the risk of hernia in the future.

If approximation of the fascia and closing of the skin is not achievable by this either, granulation and mesh graft coverage of the remaining defect is an inappropriate solution and should be avoided. It results in a thin covering of the abdominal organs that is barely protective, hardly mechanically resilient, and thereby bulging due to the positive intraabdominal pressure. This is often referred to as a hernia mistakenly, but this is not correct, since there is no hernia sac. Therefore, it generally leads to the need for tertiary abdominal wall reconstruction after 6–12 months with again a high morbidity and mortality.

It requires excision of the epithelium covering the defect, complete adhesiolysis, and abdominal wall reconstruction, usually with component separation. To achieve this, pretreatment with Botox injections into the oblique abdominal muscles is usually required 4–6 weeks beforehand [52].

An alternative bridging of a remaining fascial defect can be done with a mesh in inlay technique. In this case, synthetic meshes should be avoided if possible due to wound contamination and the associated risk of infection. At best, biological meshes should be used, which in turn are quite costly. Polyglactin meshes offer a comparable but only short-term benefit. They are considerably less expensive, but are also absorbed much more quickly, which means that the redressing effect is quickly eliminated.

Complications of EDL and Further Treatment with Open Abdomen Therapy

As a result of open abdomen therapy, enteroatmospheric fistulas and frozen abdomen may develop. The potential impossibility of a secondary abdominal wall closure with a persistent laparostoma (by definition not a hernia) and, if necessary, skin-graft coverage has already been described above.

Open abdomen management therefore means keeping an eye on early, secondary abdominal wall closure and the avoidance of secondary complications right from the beginning, that is, already when performing the EDL.

Treatment for Enteroatmospheric Fistula

Due to shear forces, especially in the case of adhesions of the intestine to the ventral abdominal wall at the wound edge of the dehiscent fascia, a defect of the intestinal wall may occur, resulting in an enteroatmospheric fistula. The incidence of fistula is approximately 10% [53, 54]. Sometimes, due to pathogenesis, more than one fistula occurs at the same time.

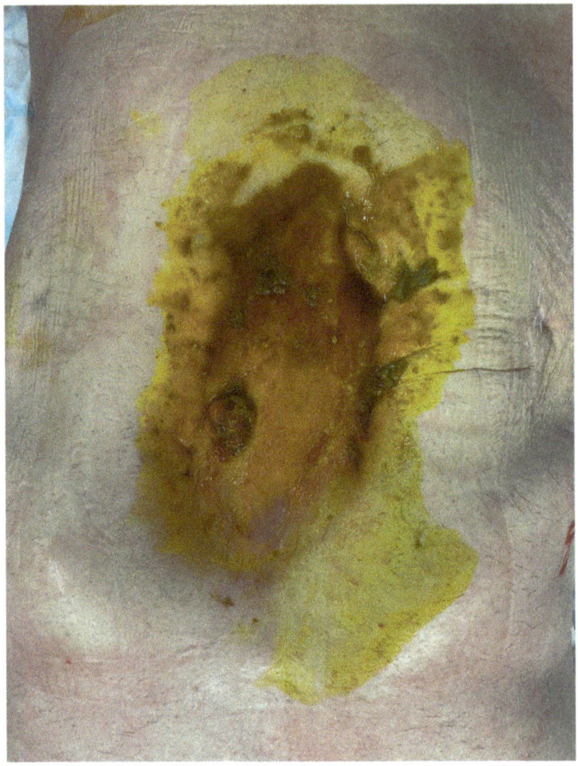

Fig. 23.4 Enteroatmospheric fistula

The hazards of these fistulas are bleeding, uncontrollable loss of fluids, electrolytes, and bile acids, which must be replaced accordingly, as well as the impossibility of enteral nutrition and a leaky coverage of the laparostoma with subsequent dermatitis even of the adjacent healthy skin (Fig. 23.4).

In this case, wound dressings no longer adhere here and the resulting skin erosion and dermatitis worsen. Repeated suturing of the fistula should not be performed in our opinion, because it regularly leads to an enlargement of the defect. It should be preferred to establish a funnel directly over the fistula and to attach an ostomy bag in a notch of the abdominal vacuum therapy kit covering the rest of the wound for passive drainage and fistula stabilization (Fig. 23.5).

Commercial items also exist for this purpose. The fistula secretion can then passively drain into the stoma bag via the funnel, protecting the surrounding wound surface from the irritating intestinal secretion. In some cases, it is also possible to feed the patient enterally via a catheter inserted into the aboral branch of the fistula. However, this should only be done after exclusion of a passage obstruction aborally of the fistula, for example, by means of CT with contrast medium via the aboral fistula branch. To make the vacuum dressing tight, additional stoma paste can be applied to the wound edge. We also recommend early skin-graft coverage of the surrounding granulation tissue so that an ostomy bag can then be tightly adhered to

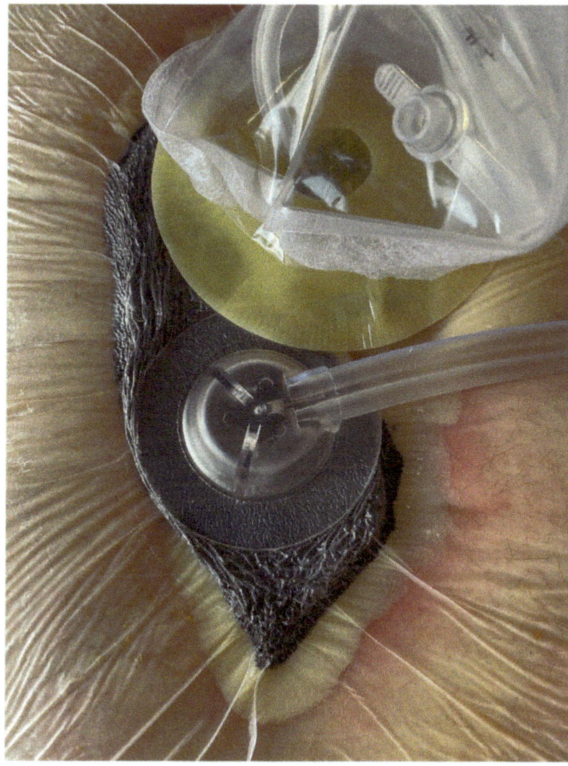

Fig. 23.5 Dressing for an enteroatmospheric fistula

the skin surrounding the fistula. Abdominal wall reconstruction in the presence of an enteroatmospheric fistula is otherwise almost impossible in the primary setting. Skin grafting on the surrounding granulation tissue succeeds more frequently than thought, despite the frequent initial fecal contamination.

More than half of enterocutaneous fistulas close with conservative therapy, although this is successful in about 75% in the upper gastrointestinal tract and in only about 35% in the lower gastrointestinal tract [55]. However, after open abdomen, the spontaneous closure rate is only 37% [56]. Conservative therapy is complex and consists of fluid and electrolyte replacement, pharmacotherapy, nutrition, adequate therapy for sepsis, as well as skin protection and wound care.

The definitive therapy for enteroatmospheric fistulas in case of failed conservative treatment is surgical and consists of a combination of complete adhesiolysis, resection of the fistula-bearing bowel loop with anastomosis, and abdominal wall reconstruction, possibly with prior bilateral Botox infiltration into the oblique abdominal muscles, and possibly with Ramirez component separation. We avoid the use of mesh for reinforcement in these cases because of the risk of infection due to bacterial contamination. Alternatively, a two-staged procedure with secondary abdominal wall reconstruction can be performed by a component separation according to Ramirez with implantation of a partially absorbable mesh in sublay position.

This should be performed approximately 7 days after primary adhesiolysis, bowel resection, anastomosis, and temporary abdominal wall closure, for example, according to the "Koblenz model"for temporary fascial approximation.

Alternatively, the Fasciotens Abdomen can be used, even if this significantly limits the patient's mobilization during the treatment [50].

We consider the use of biologic meshes, which is recommended as an ultima ratio in cases of a contaminated situs, because of so far not convincing results. However, surgical revision of the fistula with the intention of repairment and reconstruction of the abdominal wall should only be performed after 6–12 months at the earliest, as long as the patient has recovered and is able to bear sufficient physical strain for this major intervention by then. In the meantime, the patient should receive adequate enteral and/or parenteral nutrition to optimize the patient's nutritional and immunologic status, which eventually leads to a decrease in the complication.

Preventing Enteroatmospheric Fistulas

The simplest thing to do is to prevent the formation of enteroatmospheric fistulas. In this regard, we believe that complete adhesiolysis of the entire small bowel at each revision to prevent severe adhesions that could later be resolved only at the risk of intestinal wall lesions and extensive insertion of the VPL, as described above, are the key points of treatment [57]. Adhesiolysis should be avoided only if the intestinal loops are severely inflamed and edematous, as manipulation could backfire and result in additional fistulas. However, these alterations are usually due to inadequate adhesiolysis in the previous procedures, which underlines the importance of having the same team manage the patient every time.

Acknowledgments The authors would like to thank Arnulf G. Willms, Sebastian Schaaf, and all other members of the Open Abdomen Group within the European Registry of Abdominal Wall Hernia (EuraHS) for their support in the field of this topic.

References

1. Leon M, Chavez L, Surani S. Abdominal compartment syndrome among surgical patients. World J Gastrointest Surg. 2021;13:330–9.
2. Luckianow GM, Ellis M, Governale D, Kaplan LJ. Abdominal compartment syndrome: risk factors, diagnosis, and current therapy. Crit Care Res Pract. 2012;2012:908169.
3. Popescu GA, Bara T, Rad P. Abdominal compartment syndrome as a multidisciplinary challenge. A literature review. J Crit Care Med (Targu Mures). 2018;4:114–9.
4. Paduraru DN, Andronic O, Musat F, Bolocan A, Dumitrascu MC, Ion D. Abdominal compartment syndrome-when is surgical decompression needed? Diagnostics (Basel). 2021;11
5. De Keulenaer BL, De Waele JJ, Powell B, Malbrain ML. What is normal intra-abdominal pressure and how is it affected by positioning, body mass and positive end-expiratory pressure? Intensive Care Med. 2009;35:969–76.

6. Smit M, van Meurs M, Zijlstra JG. Intra-abdominal hypertension and abdominal compartment syndrome in critically ill patients: a narrative review of past, present, and future steps. Scand J Surg. 2022;111:14574969211030128.
7. Sanda RB. Abdominal compartment syndrome. Ann Saudi Med. 2007;27:183–90.
8. Kirkpatrick AW, Roberts DJ, De Waele J, Jaeschke R, Malbrain ML, De Keulenaer B, Duchesne J, Bjorck M, Leppaniemi A, Ejike JC, Sugrue M, Cheatham M, Ivatury R, Ball CG, Reintam Blaser A, Regli A, Balogh ZJ, D'Amours S, Debergh D, Kaplan M, Kimball E, Olvera C. Intra-abdominal hypertension and the abdominal compartment syndrome: updated consensus definitions and clinical practice guidelines from the World Society of the Abdominal Compartment Syndrome. Intensive Care Med. 2013;39:1190–206.
9. Malbrain ML, De Keulenaer BL, Oda J, De Laet I, De Waele JJ, Roberts DJ, Kirkpatrick AW, Kimball E, Ivatury R. Intra-abdominal hypertension and abdominal compartment syndrome in burns, obesity, pregnancy, and general medicine. Anaesthesiol Intensive Ther. 2015;47:228–40.
10. Maffongelli A, Fazzotta S, Palumbo VD, Damiano G, Buscemi S, Maione C, Lo Monte AI. Abdominal compartment syndrome: diagnostic evaluation and possible treatment. Clin Ter. 2020;171:e156–60.
11. De Waele JJ, Malbrain ML, Kirkpatrick AW. The abdominal compartment syndrome: evolving concepts and future directions. Crit Care. 2015;19:211.
12. Jacobs R, Wise RD, Myatchin I, Vanhonacker D, Minini A, Mekeirele M, Kirkpatrick AW, Pereira BM, Sugrue M, De Keulenaer B, Bodnar Z, Acosta S, Ejike J, Tayebi S, Stiens J, Cordemans C, Van Regenmortel N, Elbers PWG, Monnet X, Wong A, Dabrowski W, Jorens PG, De Waele JJ, Roberts DJ, Kimball E, Reintam Blaser A, Malbrain M. Fluid management, intra-abdominal hypertension and the abdominal compartment syndrome: a narrative review. Life (Basel). 2022;12
13. Schachtrupp A, Jansen M, Bertram P, Kuhlen R, Schumpelick V. Abdominal compartment syndrome: significance, diagnosis and treatment. Anaesthesist. 2006;55:660–7.
14. McNelis J, Soffer S, Marini CP, Jurkiewicz A, Ritter G, Simms HH, Nathan I. Abdominal compartment syndrome in the surgical intensive care unit. Am Surg. 2002;68:18–23.
15. Saggi BH, Sugerman HJ, Ivatury RR, Bloomfield GL. Abdominal compartment syndrome. J Trauma. 1998;45:597–609.
16. Malbrain ML, Chiumello D, Pelosi P, Wilmer A, Brienza N, Malcangi V, Bihari D, Innes R, Cohen J, Singer P, Japiassu A, Kurtop E, De Keulenaer BL, Daelemans R, Del Turco M, Cosimini P, Ranieri M, Jacquet L, Laterre PF, Gattinoni L. Prevalence of intra-abdominal hypertension in critically ill patients: a multicentre epidemiological study. Intensive Care Med. 2004;30:822–9.
17. Karkos CD, Menexes GC, Patelis N, Kalogirou TE, Giagtzidis IT, Harkin DW. A systematic review and meta-analysis of abdominal compartment syndrome after endovascular repair of ruptured abdominal aortic aneurysms. J Vasc Surg. 2014;59:829–42.
18. Rajasurya V, Surani S. Abdominal compartment syndrome: often overlooked conditions in medical intensive care units. World J Gastroenterol. 2020;26:266–78.
19. Zong ZW, Bao QW, Liu HY, Shen Y, Zhao YF, Hua X, Guo QS, Zhang LY, Chen H. Diagnosis and treatment of rare complications of pelvic fractures. Chin J Traumatol. 2016;19:199–205.
20. Damiano G, Maione C, Maffongelli A, Ficarella S, Carmina L, Buscemi S, Palumbo VD, De Luca S, Spinelli G, Lo Monte AI, Buscemi G. Renal allograft compartment syndrome: is it possible to prevent? Transplant Proc. 2016;48:340–3.
21. Schulz SA, Schaefer S, Richards DC, Karagiannidis C, Thomaidis P, Heiss MM, Bulian DR. The need for emergency laparotomy with open abdomen therapy in the course of ECMO-A retrospective analysis of course and outcome. Front Surg. 2020;7:63.
22. Dąbrowski W, Kotlinska-Hasiec E, Jaroszynski A, Zadora P, Pilat J, Rzecki Z, Zaluska W, Schneditz D. Intra-abdominal pressure correlates with extracellular water content. PLoS One. 2015;10:e0122193.
23. Copur S, Berkkan M, Hasbal NB, Basile C, Kanbay M. Abdominal compartment syndrome: an often overlooked cause of acute kidney injury. J Nephrol. 2022;35:1595–603.

24. Malbrain ML. Different techniques to measure intra-abdominal pressure (IAP): time for a critical re-appraisal. Intensive Care Med. 2004;30:357–71.
25. Sugrue M, Bauman A, Jones F, Bishop G, Flabouris A, Parr M, Stewart A, Hillman K, Deane SA. Clinical examination is an inaccurate predictor of intraabdominal pressure. World J Surg. 2002;26:1428–31.
26. Cheatham ML, Malbrain ML, Kirkpatrick A, Sugrue M, Parr M, De Waele J, Balogh Z, Leppäniemi A, Olvera C, Ivatury R, D'Amours S, Wendon J, Hillman K, Wilmer A. Results from the international conference of experts on intra-abdominal hypertension and abdominal compartment syndrome. II Recommendations. Intensive Care Med. 2007;33:951–62.
27. Pickhardt PJ, Shimony JS, Heiken JP, Buchman TG, Fisher AJ. The abdominal compartment syndrome: CT findings. AJR Am J Roentgenol. 1999;173:575–9.
28. Zissin R. The significance of a positive round belly sign on CT. AJR Am J Roentgenol. 2000;175:267–8.
29. Cavaliere F, Cina A, Biasucci D, Costa R, Soave M, Gargaruti R, Bonomo L, Proietti R. Sonographic assessment of abdominal vein dimensional and hemodynamic changes induced in human volunteers by a model of abdominal hypertension. Crit Care Med. 2011;39:344–8.
30. Mahjoub Y, Plantefeve G. Cardiac ultrasound and abdominal compartment syndrome. Acta Clin Belg. 2007;62(Suppl 1):183–9.
31. Pereira BM, Pereira RG, Wise R, Sugrue G, Zakrison TL, Dorigatti AE, Fiorelli RK, Malbrain M. The role of point-of-care ultrasound in intra-abdominal hypertension management. Anaesthesiol Intensive Ther. 2017;49:373–81.
32. Cheatham ML, Sagraves SG, Johnson JL, White MW. Intravesicular pressure monitoring does not cause urinary tract infection. Intensive Care Med. 2006;32:1640–3.
33. Kron IL, Harman PK, Nolan SP. The measurement of intra-abdominal pressure as a criterion for abdominal re-exploration. Ann Surg. 1984;199:28–30.
34. De Waele J, Pletinckx P, Blot S, Hoste E. Saline volume in transvesical intra-abdominal pressure measurement: enough is enough. Intensive Care Med. 2006;32:455–9.
35. Vasquez DG, Berg-Copas GM, Wetta-Hall R. Influence of semi-recumbent position on intra-abdominal pressure as measured by bladder pressure. J Surg Res. 2007;139:280–5.
36. Rahouma M, Kamel M, Jodeh D, Kelley T, Ohmes LB, de Biasi AR, Abouarab AA, Benedetto U, Guy TS, Lau C, Lee PC, Girardi LN, Gaudino M. Does a balanced transfusion ratio of plasma to packed red blood cells improve outcomes in both trauma and surgical patients? A meta-analysis of randomized controlled trials and observational studies. Am J Surg. 2018;216:342–50.
37. Parra MW, Al-Khayat H, Smith HG, Cheatham ML. Paracentesis for resuscitation-induced abdominal compartment syndrome: an alternative to decompressive laparotomy in the burn patient. J Trauma. 2006;60:1119–21.
38. Corcos AC, Sherman HF. Percutaneous treatment of secondary abdominal compartment syndrome. J Trauma. 2001;51:1062–4.
39. Latenser BA, Kowal-Vern A, Kimball D, Chakrin A, Dujovny N. A pilot study comparing percutaneous decompression with decompressive laparotomy for acute abdominal compartment syndrome in thermal injury. J Burn Care Rehabil. 2002;23:190–5.
40. Cheatham ML, Safcsak K. Percutaneous catheter decompression in the treatment of elevated intraabdominal pressure. Chest. 2011;140:1428–35.
41. Muresan M, Muresan S, Brinzaniuc K, Voidazan S, Sala D, Jimborean O, Hussam AH, Bara T Jr, Popescu G, Borz C, Neagoe R. How much does decompressive laparotomy reduce the mortality rate in primary abdominal compartment syndrome?: a single-center prospective study on 66 patients. Medicine (Baltimore). 2017;96:e6006.
42. De Waele JJ, Kimball E, Malbrain M, Nesbitt I, Cohen J, Kaloiani V, Ivatury R, Mone M, Debergh D, Bjorck M. Decompressive laparotomy for abdominal compartment syndrome. Br J Surg. 2016;103:709–15.

43. Joosten JJ, Longchamp G, Khan MF, Lameris W, van Berge Henegouwen MI, Bemelman WA, Cahill RA, Hompes R, Ris F. The use of fluorescence angiography to assess bowel viability in the acute setting: an international, multi-Centre case series. Surg Endosc. 2022;36:7369–75.
44. Karampinis I, Keese M, Jakob J, Stasiunaitis V, Gerken A, Attenberger U, Post S, Kienle P, Nowak K. Indocyanine green tissue angiography can reduce extended bowel resections in acute mesenteric ischemia. J Gastrointest Surg. 2018;22:2117–24.
45. Tremblay LN, Feliciano DV, Schmidt J, Cava RA, Tchorz KM, Ingram WL, Salomone JP, Nicholas JM, Rozycki GS. Skin only or silo closure in the critically ill patient with an open abdomen. Am J Surg. 2001;182:670–5.
46. Myers JA, Latenser BA. Nonoperative progressive "Bogota bag" closure after abdominal decompression. Am Surg. 2002;68:1029–30.
47. Wittmann DH, Aprahamian C, Bergstein JM. Etappenlavage: advanced diffuse peritonitis managed by planned multiple laparotomies utilizing zippers, slide fastener, and Velcro analogue for temporary abdominal closure. World J Surg. 1990;14:218–26.
48. Roberts DJ, Zygun DA, Grendar J, Ball CG, Robertson HL, Ouellet JF, Cheatham ML, Kirkpatrick AW. Negative-pressure wound therapy for critically ill adults with open abdominal wounds: a systematic review. J Trauma Acute Care Surg. 2012;73:629–39.
49. Willms A, Gusgen C, Schaaf S, Bieler D, von Websky M, Schwab R. Management of the open abdomen using vacuum-assisted wound closure and mesh-mediated fascial traction. Langenbeck's Arch Surg. 2015;400:91–9.
50. Hees A, Willeke F. Prevention of fascial retraction in the open abdomen with a novel device. Case Rep Surg. 2020;2020:8254804.
51. Ramirez OM, Ruas E, Dellon AL. "Components separation" method for closure of abdominal-wall defects: an anatomic and clinical study. Plast Reconstr Surg. 1990;86:519–26.
52. Timmer AS, Claessen JJM, Atema JJ, Rutten MVH, Hompes R, Boermeester MA. A systematic review and meta-analysis of technical aspects and clinical outcomes of botulinum toxin prior to abdominal wall reconstruction. Hernia. 2021;25:1413–25.
53. Willms A, Muysoms F, Gusgen C, Schwab R, Lock J, Schaaf S, Germer C, Richardsen I, Dietz U. The Open Abdomen Route by EuraHS: introduction of the data set and initial results of procedures and procedure-related complications. Hernia. 2017;21:279–89.
54. Coccolini F, Ceresoli M, Kluger Y, Kirkpatrick A, Montori G, Salvetti F, Fugazzola P, Tomasoni M, Sartelli M, Ansaloni L, Catena F, Negoi I, Zese M, Occhionorelli S, Shlyapnikov S, Galatioto C, Chiarugi M, Demetrashvili Z, Dondossola D, Ioannidis O, Novelli G, Nacoti M, Khor D, Inaba K, Demetriades D, Kaussen T, Jusoh AC, Ghannam W, Sakakushev B, Guetta O, Dogjani A, Costa S, Singh S, Damaskos D, Isik A, Yuan KC, Trotta F, Rausei S, Martinez-Perez A, Bellanova G, Fonseca V, Hernandez F, Marinis A, Fernandes W, Quiodettis M, Bala M, Vereczkei A, Curado R, Fraga GP, Pereira BM, Gachabayov M, Chagerben GP, Arellano ML, Ozyazici S, Costa G, Tezcaner T, Porta M, Li Y, Karateke F, Manatakis D, Mariani F, Lora F, Sahderov I, Atanasov B, Zegarra S, Gianotti L, Fattori L, Ivatury R. Open abdomen and entero-atmospheric fistulae: an interim analysis from the International Register of Open Abdomen (IROA). Injury. 2019;50:160–6.
55. Quinn M, Falconer S, McKee RF. Management of enterocutaneous fistula: outcomes in 276 patients. World J Surg. 2017;41:2502–11.
56. Fischer PE, Fabian TC, Magnotti LJ, Schroeppel TJ, Bee TK, Maish GO 3rd, Savage SA, Laing AE, Barker AB, Croce MA. A ten-year review of enterocutaneous fistulas after laparotomy for trauma. J Trauma. 2009;67:924–8.
57. Schaaf S, Schwab R, Wohler A, Muysoms F, Lock JF, Sorelius K, Fortelny R, Keck T, Berrevoet F, Stavrou GA, von Websky M, Tartaglia D, Bulian D, Willms A. Use of a visceral protective layer prevents fistula development in open abdomen therapy: results from the European Hernia Society Open Abdomen Registry. Br J Surg. 2023;110:1607.

Chapter 24
Post-Operative Complications After Emergency Laparotomy

Zi Qin Ng and Dieter Weber

Introduction

Emergency laparotomy (EL) has an important role in modern surgical practice. This role remains relevant, even though minimally invasive surgery and advances in non-operative care have fundamentally changed the care of these patients in recent years. EL forms a significant part of acute general surgery for various pathologies such as incarcerated hernia, perforated viscus, intestinal obstruction, haemorrhage and sepsis.

Historically, considerable mortality and morbidity are associated with EL. A recent systematic review found that the one-year mortality following EL is up to 20% [1]. Since the initiative of National Emergency Laparotomy (NELA) in the UK in 2012, there have been significant efforts in reducing the mortality rates following EL. The concept of risk stratification pre-operatively has been adopted across continents [2–4].

In Australia, the introduction of ANZELA-QI has been modelled upon the NELA concept [5, 6]. The hospitals across Australia and New Zealand are encouraged to participate in prospective data collection on the emergency laparotomy on indices

---

Consent: The authors have obtained consent from the individual patients for the use of clinical photographs or cross-sectional imaging for submission and publication.

Z. Q. Ng (✉)
Department of General Surgery, Royal Perth Hospital, Perth, WA, Australia
e-mail: ziqin.ng@health.wa.gov.au

D. Weber
Department of General Surgery, Royal Perth Hospital, Perth, WA, Australia

School of Surgery, University of Western Australia, Nedlands, WA, Australia
e-mail: dieter.weber@health.wa.gov.au

© The Author(s), under exclusive license to Springer Nature Switzerland AG 2024

J. Faintuch, S. Faintuch (eds.), *Recent Strategies in High Risk Surgery*,
https://doi.org/10.1007/978-3-031-56270-9_24

that could impact on outcomes such as: time seen by the consultant, sub-specialty of the surgical team, the lactate level on arrival, time to access computed tomography (CT) scan and theatre, the most senior surgical and anasthesiology staff members, admission to critical care unit, unplanned return to theatre or intensive care unit, post-operative complications and mortality and discharge destination. Each individual hospital will receive an annual report on its performance against national standards.

Apart from NELA, other scoring systems such as P-POSSUM and ACS-NSQIP have been studied with varying sensitivity and specificity [2, 7, 8]. Some studies have combined these clinical scores with CT-derived parameters such as psoas density to predict the post-operative complications following EL [7, 9]. In association with these developments, significant shifts in clinical management have also occurred: implementation of sepsis bundles, early theatre access, involvement of consultant surgeon and anaesthetist in decision-making and post-operative admission to intensive care unit [10], are strategies, which among others, continue to push for the better care of the emergency general surgery patient.

Despite the efforts to better patient selection and early discussion of ceiling of care, clinicians are expected to face patients with more complex comorbidities and poorer physiological reserves. This chapter focuses on the common post-operative complications following EL and strategies to manage and prevent them. The authors also illustrate some examples of the management of complications and potential pitfalls post-EL.

Post-operative Complications

Haemorrhage

Post-operative haemorrhage refers to excessive bleeding that occurs after a surgical procedure. It is a potentially serious complication that can range from minor bleeding to severe and life-threatening blood loss. Haemorrhage can occur at the surgical site, or at sites distant to the surgery in situations of coagulopathy.

Post-operative haemorrhage is usually accompanied by pain, deranged physiology by the hypovolaemia and reduced urine output. The haemoglobin level drop may lag time. In younger patients, the initial response may be just compensatory tachycardia due to the physiological reserves. If there is any suggestion of post-operative haemorrhage, it is imperative to take the patient back to theatre to control the bleed. In certain cases, where there has been a drain placed, the clinician should not be reassured by the lack of blood in the drain as it can easily be clogged. Often, during the takeback, there is no active bleeding but rather generalized ooze. Intraoperative check of the rotational thromboelastometry or thromboelastometry can guide product replacement to aid haemostasis. In patients with an underlying coagulation deficiency, a consultation with the haematologist can assist in the management with replacement of specific factors, fresh frozen plasma and/or

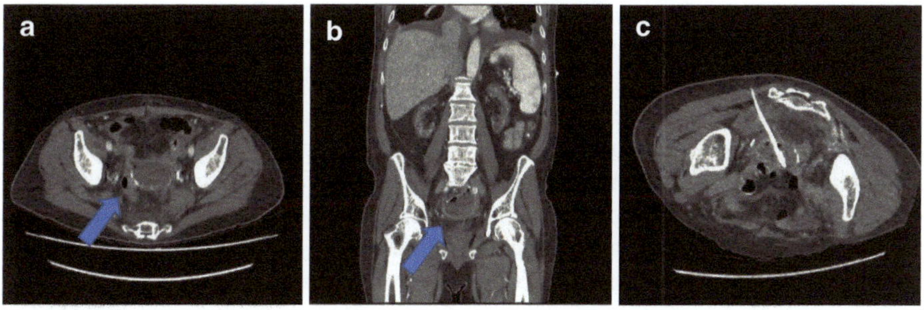

Fig. 24.1 This patient has a history of chronic kidney failure on haemodialysis presented with large bowel obstruction secondary to perforated sigmoid diverticulitis. The patient underwent emergency Hartmann's procedure. Two weeks post-surgery, the patient presented with per rectal bleeding and lower abdominal pain. CT scan (**a**, **b**) showed a rim-enhancing collection at the pelvis adjacent to the staple-line of the rectal stump likely an infected haematoma. The interventional radiology placed a percutaneous drain into the collection (**c**)

cryoglobulin. Certain groups of patients may be at a higher risk of bleeding due to the underlying use of antiplatelets or anticoagulants for various cardiovascular indications or underlying chronic kidney disease with dysfunctional platelets. Often, due to the urgency of the intra-abdominal sepsis, the EL has to proceed without the wearing off of medication therapeutic effect with time. Energy device such as ultrasonic shears and bipolar can be used with good effect. Careful suture ligation of the vessels should be performed. Various adjunct topical haemostatic agents such as oxidized regenerated cellulose (Surgicel™), haemostatic matrix containing thrombin (SURGIFLO™), haemostatic matrix containing both thrombin and fibrinogen (Tisseel) can be applied in cases with generalized ooze.

In cases of delayed presentation a few days post-EL and patient remaining haemodynamically stable, a CT angiogram can be performed to locate the source of the haemorrhage. Depending on the location, the interventional radiologist may be able to access with view of performing embolization of the targeted bleeding vessel.

In certain cases, it may manifest as an infected haematoma when a cross-sectional imaging is performed a few days post-EL for investigation of a septic source. Depending on the clinical status of the patient, size and location of the infected haematoma, percutaneous drainage by the interventional radiologist can be considered (Fig. 24.1).

Surgical Site Infection

EL and some risk factors such as obesity, immunocompromised, diabetes mellitus, smoking and perforated viscus with gross contamination increase the risk of wound infections. It will be difficult to optimize these risk factors in an emergency setting. Nevertheless, a few approaches can be employed to mitigate the risk of wound infections: using a wound protector and ensuring the wounds are protected by packs when performing intestinal resections with potential spillage of enteric contents and use saline and/or betadine wash of the wound.

Most cases are superficial wound infections and are characterized by the presence of erythema around the incision site, tenderness and a bulge (from the underlying pus). They occur around day 5–7 post-EL. Occasionally, it is detected on cross-sectional imaging with the presence of fluid collection and air at the incision site. It should be corresponded with the clinical findings. The infected wound site can be opened and drained at bedside with simple daily dressing change. If there is a suggestion of a deeper infective collection, it is advisable to perform in theatre under a general anaesthetic for proper washout of the wound and ensure the fascia closure remains intact. A vacuum assisted closure can be applied.

There is recent evidence to show that prophylactic use of negative pressure wound dressings can reduce the incidence of wound infections in contaminated wounds [11, 12]. Different commercial products such as Prevena, PICO dressings can be applied. These negative pressure dressings are applied for a period of 5–7 days and removed. It is important to inspect the underlying wound site of the negative pressure wound dressing if there is suggestion of an undiagnosed infective source.

Certain surgical site infections may be deep and manifest as intra-abdominal abscess. The causes of it need to be investigated to ensure it is not secondary to an anastomotic leak. The management of anastomotic leak is discussed later. Most cases can be managed non-operatively with intravenous antibiotics and/or percutaneous drainage by the interventional radiologist (Fig. 24.2).

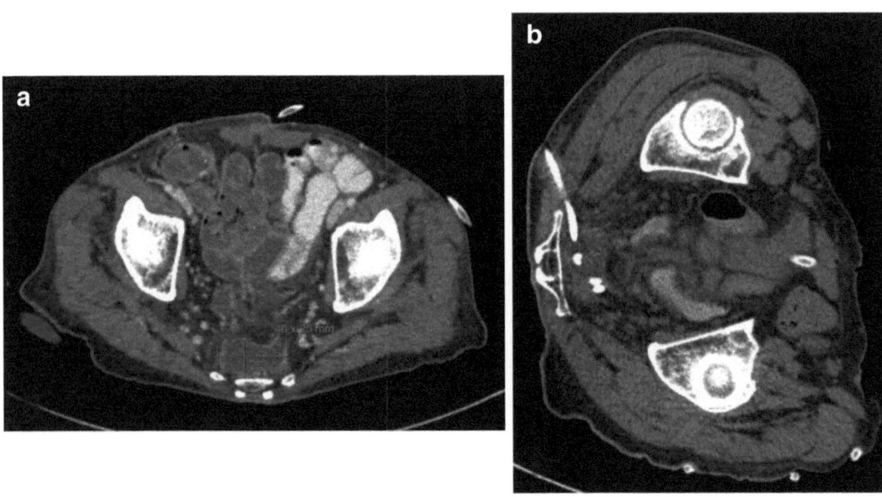

Fig. 24.2 This was an elderly man that underwent an emergency ultralow Hartmann's procedure for perforated stercoral colitis at the rectosigmoid junction with an underlying mid rectal tumour. On post-operative day 7, he developed some febrile episodes. A CT scan performed showed a pelvic rim-enhancing collection as the most likely source of infection (**a**). Percutaneous drainage under CT guidance was done with success (**b**)

Pain Control

Following EL, post-operative pain control is crucial to prevent the development of complications [13]. The techniques have advanced over the last decade. The planning of pain control commences prior to the EL. Spinal or epidural anaesthesia can be considered but may not always be feasible in the unwell or haemodynamically unstable patient. Bilateral transabdominis plane blocks with catheters for continuous infusion post-operatively function well [14]. The placement of the catheters in the correct anatomical plane is important [15]. Its use can help to reduce opioid requirements. Other strategies should be based on the WHO analgesia ladder: paracetamol, non-steroidal anti-inflammatory, slow-release opioids. In cases where oral intake or return of gastrointestinal tract function is expected to be delayed, the use of patient-controlled analgesia with opioids or ketamine can be used. Dedicated Acute Pain Service (APS) is valuable to assist the clinicians in adjustment of the different regimes based on the assessment of daily visual analogue scores.

Atelectasis

It is a common post-operative complication post-EL. It is usually addressed by encouraging patients to sit out of bed and mobilize early. Adequate analgesia is vital to allow early mobilization. Routine physiotherapist assessment post-EL should be part of the daily practice [16, 17].

Post-operative Ileus

Post-operative ileus is defined based on clinical and/or radiological findings [18, 19]: when patient develops two or more symptoms of the following five criteria on post-operative day 4 onwards:

- Nausea or vomiting over the preceding 12 h
- Inability to tolerate an oral diet over the prior 24 h
- Absence of flatus over the prior 24 h
- Abdominal distension (increased abdominal girth with tympany on percussion)
- Radiological findings: gastric distention, presence of air-fluid levels, dilated small or large bowel loops without a transition point.

Its incidence has been reported ranging from 10–30% following abdominal surgery [20]. In the elective setting, various perioperative measures can be optimized to prevent its occurrence. It is usually multifactorial [18]. In the emergency setting, certain measures such as the amount of fluids administered can be difficult due to the initial sepsis [13]. The goal-directed fluid resuscitation via the measurement of the urine output perhaps is most realistic.

Management of post-operative ileus is supportive [19] with nasogastric decompression, replacement and maintenance of fluid and electrolytes losses, reduction in the use of opioid analgesia, use of prokinetic agents such as metoclopramide and mobilization. In certain cases where there was gross peritonitis in the index operation, a CT scan should be organized to ensure there is no underlying infective collection or an anastomotic leak that has contributed to the post-operative ileus. It is also useful to differentiate with small bowel obstruction which may require surgical intervention.

The duration of post-operative ileus can be unpredictable which range from days to weeks. It is important to support the nutritional requirements with parenteral nutrition.

Small Bowel Obstruction

Its presentation can be similar to post-operative ileus. In patients who have been treated as ileus initially but are not progressing clinically, a CT abdomen should be performed. Most cases are adhesive in nature [21] which will resolve with non-operative management. A water-soluble oral contrast can be administered which has both diagnostic and therapeutic values. A follow-up abdominal X-ray 6-h post administration is performed to appreciate if the contrast has reached the large intestine. Very rarely, it could be due to small bowel incarceration from an internal hernia resulting from the unclosed mesentery from bowel resection which will require a return to theatre. It is usually more common in laparoscopic cases but certainly can occur in open bowel resections [22]. A high index of suspicion is needed to diagnose on the CT scan.

Aspiration Pneumonia

It could happen on presentation or on anaesthetic induction in patients presenting with bowel obstruction. It is important to have nasogastric tube decompression early on to prevent repeated vomiting. When dealing with the intra-abdominal pathology intraoperatively, communication with anaesthetics team is vital before milking the small bowel content proximally to prevent the content entering the lungs. Suction should be connected to the nasogastric tube.

It is also common in the post-operative period when the patient goes into post-operative ileus. It is manifested with reduced oxygen saturation with increasing oxygen needs and tachypnea clinically. Blood tests might show rising inflammatory markers and a plain chest X-ray film will typically show haziness in the right lower lobe. Other information on the chest X-ray might show atelectasis, dilated stomach and small bowel loops indicating ileus (Fig. 24.3).

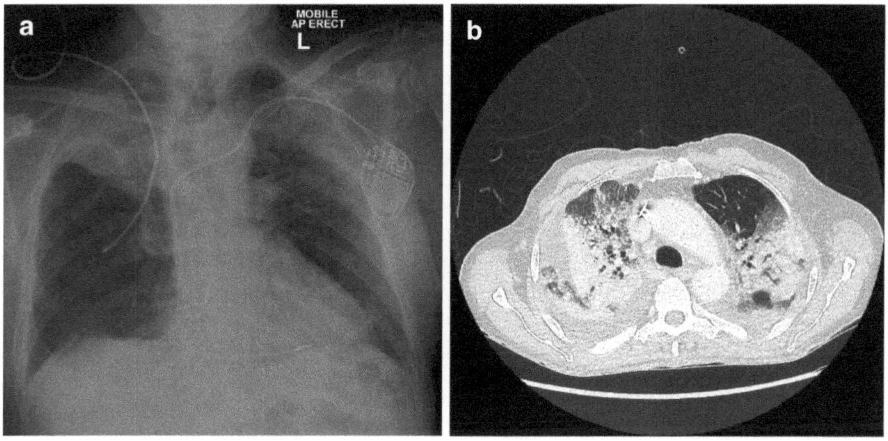

Fig. 24.3 This elderly patient underwent an emergency laparotomy with small bowel resection for ischemic bowel secondary from band adhesion. The surgery was uneventful. Post-operatively, the patient suffered from delirium and was given anti-psychotic medication and led to drowsiness. As a result, the patient aspirated and developed significant aspiration pneumonia (**a** and **b**—chest X-ray and CT chest showing significant bilateral upper lobes aspiration pneumonia). This led a vicious cycle of sepsis and further delirious episodes. The patient later succumbed to increasing need of respiratory support

Management is mainly supportive with nasogastric decompression, fluid resuscitation and electrolytes optimization to resolve the post-operative ileus. Broad spectrum intravenous antibiotics to cover the anaerobic microorganism should be given. Aggressive chest physiotherapy should be encouraged [16, 17]. In severe cases, the patient may require respiratory support in the critical care unit.

Anastomotic Leak

A significant proportion of EL is performed for pathologies associated with the small and large bowels [23]. Anastomotic leak is the most feared complication as its impact can have a devastating effect on the quality of life of patients.

The decision to perform an anastomosis depends on a few factors [23–25]: patient's comorbidities, nutritional state, location of the bowel resection, degree of peritoneal contamination, intraoperative haemodynamic status, and presence of vasopressor/inotropic support. In the presence of these factors, the clinician should consider the safest option that is construction of a stoma upfront.

The options of the type of stoma are summarized below:

- Distal small bowel resection/right hemicolectomy/extended right hemicolectomy/subtotal colectomy—end ileostomy alone, Abcarian end ileostomy, end ileostomy with venting distal colostomy

- Left sided segmental colectomy—end colostomy with a short distal stump, double-barrel colostomy, end colostomy with a long distal stump sutured below the fascia or as a mucous fistula

A practical way of management is based on the International Study Group of Rectal Cancer grading system. Most of the anastomotic leaks present during the first few days post-EL. It can be subtle with rising inflammatory markers of white cell count and c-reactive protein. Clinically, the patient may have febrile episodes, increasing abdominal pain and distention. With that, it prompts an urgent CT abdomen/pelvis with intravenous and oral contrast or rectal contrast (for left sided colonic anastomosis) (Fig. 24.4). The considerations for the management of the anastomotic leak are [26]:

(a) The location and degree of the anastomotic leak (contained vs free)
(b) The haemodynamic status of the patient

In cases with a contained anastomotic leak and clinically patient remains well, a period of intravenous antibiotics and nil by mouth may be adequate. In cases with a local abscess adjacent to the anastomosis, percutaneous drainage via interventional radiology should be considered. In cases where patients are unwell, they should be taken back to the theatre for re-exploration and washout. Depending on the integrity of the anastomosis, a few options can be explored:

1. pinhole anastomotic leak without significant contamination—oversew the defect and perform a proximal defunctioning loop ileostomy.

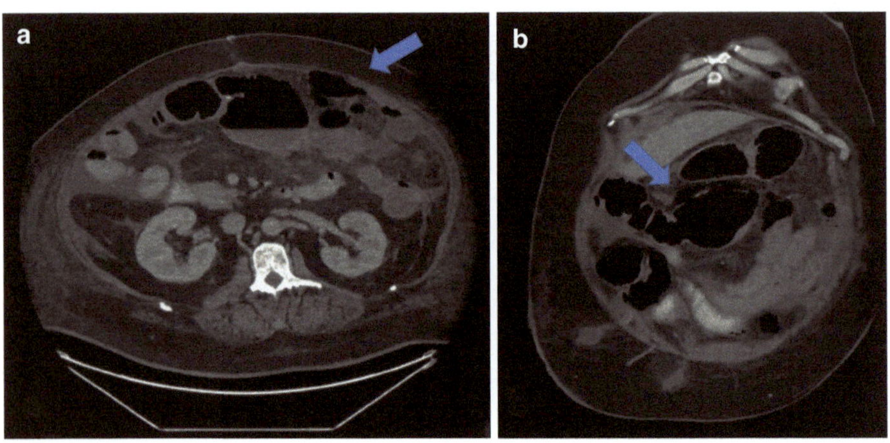

Fig. 24.4 This patient presented with perforated proximal transverse colon cancer. He underwent an emergency laparotomy and extended right hemicolectomy. On post-operative day 9, his inflammatory markers of white cell count and c-reactive protein were rising despite relatively asymptomatic clinically
A CT scan showed free gas locules adjacent to the anastomosis, representing anastomotic leak (**a**, **b**). The patient was taken back to theatre. The ileocolic anastomosis was resected, and an end ileostomy was performed

2. a large defect or disintegration of the anastomosis—
   (a) Ileocolic anastomosis: resection of the anastomosis and perform an end ileostomy. Alternatively, an Abcarian end ileostomy or double-barrel stoma can be performed depending on the distal colonic conduit.
   (b) Colorectal anastomosis: resection of the anastomosis and perform and end colostomy.
3. small bowel anastomotic leak—the principles are similar to the above. Nevertheless, the location of the proximity of the stoma should be considered as it is certain that high output stoma which will subject the patient being reliant on parenteral nutrition till its reversal.

In the presence of intra-abdominal sepsis, the bowel is generally dilated and oedematous. To create the stomal trephine, it is important to ensure it is wide enough to allow the construct of the stoma without tension. The use of a wound protector such as Alexis allows smooth delivery of the stoma. Another option would be to perform an end loop stoma.

In cases where there is insufficient space to accommodate the distal efferent limb, it can be sutured to the midline fascia as a mucus fistula if blowout occurs.

Enterocutaneous Fistula (ECF)

It is often a sequela of anastomotic leak or iatrogenic injury to the intestine. Often, it presents in the early post-operative period. Depending on the location of the intestinal injury, the content could be biliary-type (small intestine) or faeculent-type (large intestine) through the drain or the wounds (Fig. 24.5).

In early detection (<7 days), the patient should be taken back to the theatre for a relook. The bowel should be handled gently to avoid further serosal injury or enterotomies/colotomies. The identified enterotomy can be either primarily repaired or resected depending on the size of the defect.

There are situations where a takeback is not feasible due to delayed presentation, significant malnutrition, and risk of further injuries due to hostile abdomen.

The principles of management are [27]:

(a) Controlling the sepsis—percutaneous drainage of any collection or a controlled fistula. The output of the ECF can be high (>500 mL/24 h) and irritating to the surrounding skin. Appropriate wound care with appliances is important.
(b) The patients are in a catabolic state and nutritionally depleted. To control the ECF output, the patient is kept nil orally initially. Total parenteral nutrition is administered with careful replacement of electrolyte losses.

With these fundamental approaches, certain ECFs will likely resolve with non-operative management, provided there is no distal obstruction or discontinuity of the intestine (Fig. 24.6).

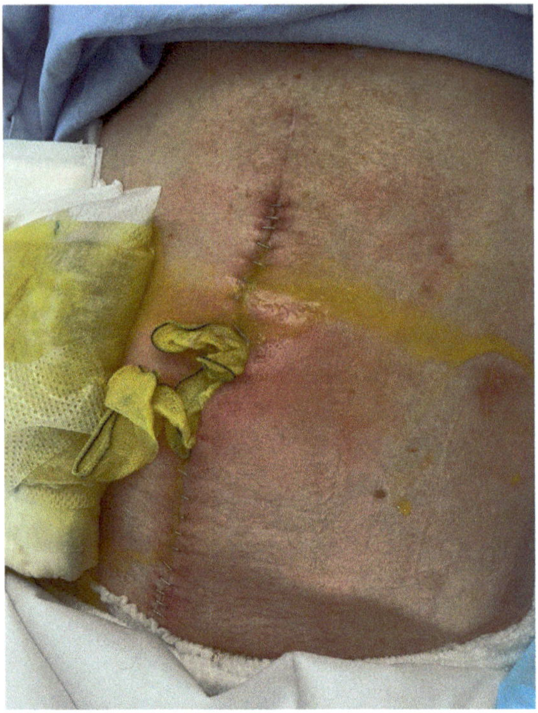

Fig. 24.5 This was a case of small bowel ischemia secondary to superior mesenteric thrombosis. The patient underwent an exploratory laparotomy and small bowel resection of the gangrenous small bowel at a peripheral hospital prior to transfer. The patient was left with 80 cm of small bowel from the duodenal-jejunal flexure and 10 cm of distal terminal ileum from the ileocecal valve. On the arrival at the tertiary centre, the patient was taken back to theatre for a relook laparotomy. A thrombectomy was performed at the superior mesenteric artery and the abdomen was left open with view of return the following day. The subsequent relook laparotomy found viable remaining small intestine albeit mild degree of ischemia at the distal terminal ileum. A handsewn end-to-end small bowel anastomosis was performed. At post-operative day 7, the midline laparotomy wound looked erythematous with signs of infection. The staples were removed, and enteric content discharged. A CT scan performed showed anastomotic leak leading to ECF. The patient was managed with non-operative strategies (kept nil orally, intravenous proton pump inhibitor, subcutaneous octreotide, wound care with dressing changes and total parenteral nutrition). The ECF output reduced in the following days and resolved. This is a case to demonstrate the difficulty of returning to theatre in the setting of ECF as it would have not been survivable with the length of jejunum left as a jejunostomy

In cases with continuous high output ECF, multiple ECFs, discontinuity of intestine, patience in the management is key. This group of patients will require multidisciplinary care: wound care, outpatient administration and monitoring of the total parenteral nutrition and physiotherapy due to deconditioning.

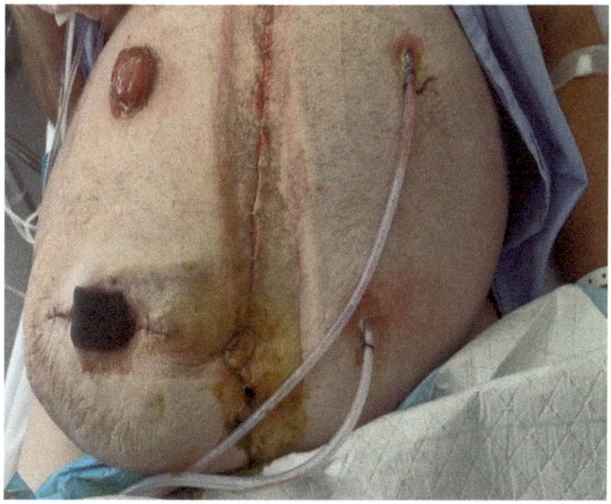

Fig. 24.6 This patient has a previous prolonged history of total colectomy with end ileostomy for large bowel obstruction secondary to sigmoid cancer. The patient presented with small bowel obstruction that failed to resolve with non-operative management. The initial operation found ischemic small bowel 40 cm proximal to the end ileostomy, requiring small bowel resection. Unfortunately, there was an anastomotic leak on post-operative day 4. The patient was taken back to theatre. The end ileostomy was fully mobilized and the anastomosis was resected. The neo end ileostomy was fashioned on the upper abdomen. Given the contamination, a prophylactic negative pressure wound dressing was placed on the wound. Following that, on day 3, the negative pressure wound dressing was removed and there was evidence of bile staining on the midline wound, consistent with ECF. The patient was managed with the abovementioned strategies successfully. The ECF resolved

Prior to any reintervention, adequate time of at least 6 months should be allowed with optimization of all modifiable factors. Planning of the anatomy of the ECFs can be performed with CT with oral contrast and/or sinogram.

These patients should be referred to a centre with expertise in managing complex ECFs or entero-atmospheric fistula with abdominal wall reconstruction.

Stoma-Related Complications

In the emergency setting, when a stoma is formed, it can be associated with a range of mild to severe complications. We describe the most common complications encountered as the followings:

High Output Stoma

It is defined as an output of more than 1.2–1.5 L/24 h recorded in the ileostomy. In the event where it is not secondary to anatomical proximity of the ileostomy, the majority of cases will resolve in a few weeks with intestinal adaptation. A small proportion of patients will require medication to reduce the intestinal transit time.

Multidisciplinary management is crucial [28, 29]. The accurate recording of the oral intake and stoma output helps to determine the necessary management. Any fluids and electrolytes losses should be replaced intravenously. Any potential factors such as infections (*Clostridium difficile*), use of prokinetics (metoclopramide, domperidone) or metformin should be carefully reviewed. Introduction of certain foods can help to thicken up the consistency of the output. Different types of rehydration solution can be given to the patients; St Mark's solution (consisting of glucose, sodium bicarbonate and sodium chloride) can be easily prepared by patients themselves in the outpatient setting [30].

Proton pump inhibitors such as pantoprazole 40 mg once a day is used to reduce gastric secretions. Loperamide is usually given 30 min before the meals. It is important to make sure that the capsule is opened. The doses can be titrated according to the output. Codeine can be added on top to slow the intestinal transit. It should be used with caution in patients with chronic renal failure as it can lead to drowsiness from its retained metabolites.

In cases with significant high output, keeping nil orally initially helps to control the output. Total parenteral nutrition is usually provided till oral intake is re-established. The use of somatostatin analogue which reduces pancreatic secretions can be trialled for a short term. The authors' experience is that if it makes a difference to the stoma output, a long-acting somatostatin analogue can be used.

In certain cases, despite optimal medical management, the patients may still require replacement of intravenous fluids and electrolytes daily. This could be carried out in the outpatient setting with same principles of patients on home parenteral nutrition.

A protocol/guideline adopted in the authors' institute is illustrated in Fig. 24.7.

Stoma Retraction

It is often a difficult problem to manage with mucocutaneous separation and stoma retraction [31]. The faecal content seeps into the parastomal space leading to wound infection that requires drainage and dressings (Fig. 24.8). Regular stoma therapist review with regular dressing change in the parastomal space is needed. Mild stomal retraction can be managed with specific stoma appliances. In cases with severe retraction, it is likely to require revision.

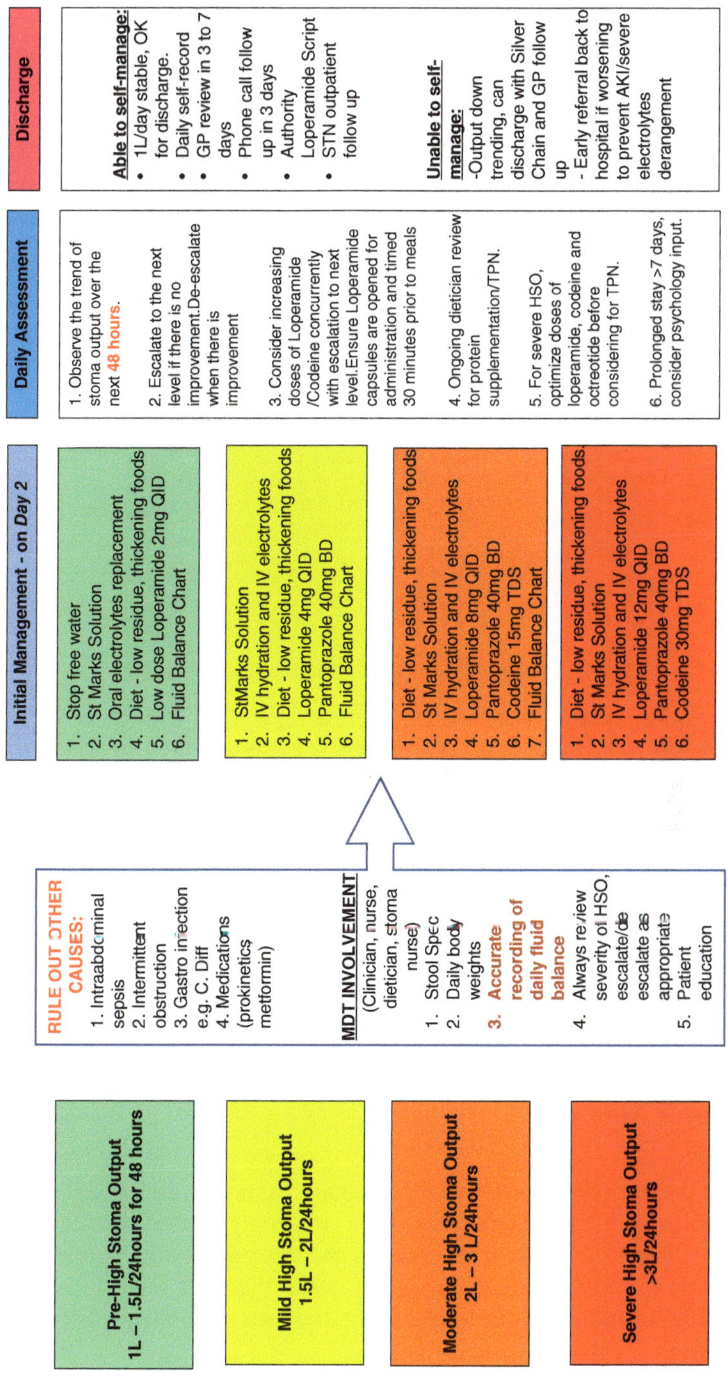

Fig. 24.7 Classification of severity of high output stoma with management strategy in the author's institution

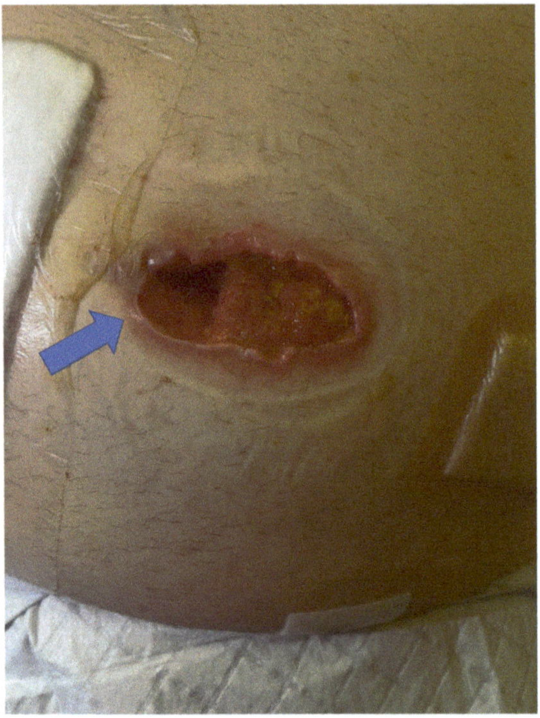

Fig. 24.8 This patient was morbidly obese with history of chronic renal failure on peritoneal dialysis. The patient initially presented with abdominal sepsis thought to be secondary to infected peritoneal dialysis catheter. A CT scan showed localized perforated sigmoid diverticulitis which failed to respond to intravenous antibiotics. He underwent a Hartmann's procedure. The colonic conduit was difficult to bring through due to the thick abdominal wall and the surrounding epiploic appendages were thickened due to long-term peritoneal dialysis despite large stomal trephine created and mobilization of the proximal colon. It became apparent there was mild degree of stomal retraction and mucocutaneous separation on post-operative day 5. The parastomal mucocutaneous separation at the medial aspect was filled with feculent content with wound infection. It was a challenging problem to perform frequent dressing change and the constant feculent contamination. A CT scan performed ruled out any deeper collection. With the assistance of the stoma therapist, the parastomal wound was carefully managed with modified stomal appliances and resolved

The Ischemic Stoma

This is often apparent on day 1 post-EL, ranging from mild ischemia to complete gangrene/necrosis [31]. Most cases stem from colostomy. In cases of mild ischemia, usually it is managed with close observation and the majority of cases do not need any intervention. Supportive care from the stoma therapist with different stoma appliances usually suffice. In the longer term, there is a possibility of stomal stenosis which requires revision.

In cases with complete gangrene and necrosis, the extent of it usually goes beyond the fascia level. It will require a return to theatre to determine the extent

(Fig. 24.8). The stoma along with the colonic conduit needs to be mobilized until it is tension free with good marginal blood supply. In obese patients with a thick abdominal wall, it is advisable to position the stoma in the upper quadrant of the abdomen (which has a thinner abdominal wall) and ensure adequate trephine size.

Wound Dehiscence/Burst Abdomen

It is no longer a frequent complication post-EL but can still occur. Often, it is due to a combination of factors from patient factors (diabetes, smoking, obesity, recti diastasis, and sarcopenia) [32–35] to technical aspect and post-operative superficial or deep surgical site infections and ileus/intestinal obstruction. To reduce the risk of long-term incisional hernia, recent evidence recommends the suture to be of smaller calibre and bites [36]. The pitfall with that technique is junior surgical trainees may not completely grasp the adequate fascia for closure [37].

In acute burst abdomen, the evisceration of the intra-abdominal organs is obvious (Fig. 24.9). Sterile large packs soaked in saline should be placed on top and covered with Ioban while awaiting return to theatre. In return to theatre, the fascial

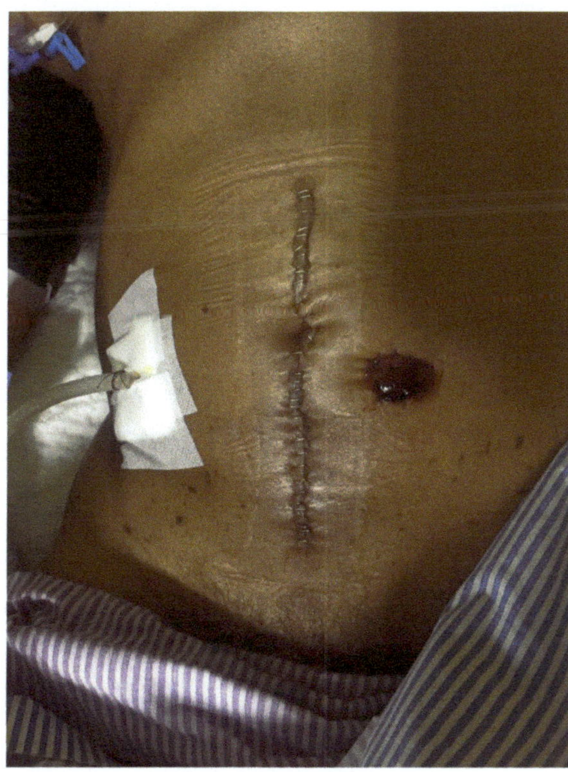

Fig. 24.9 This was a middle-aged male patient that underwent an emergency Hartmann's procedure for obstructing sigmoid cancer
On post-operative day 1, it was apparent that the stoma looked ischemic with some degree of gangrene. The patient was taken back to theatre which found the ischemic stoma extended proximally beyond the fascia level. The proximal colonic conduit was fully mobilized including the splenic flexure to ensure no tension and good marginal blood supply prior to refashioning a new end colostomy

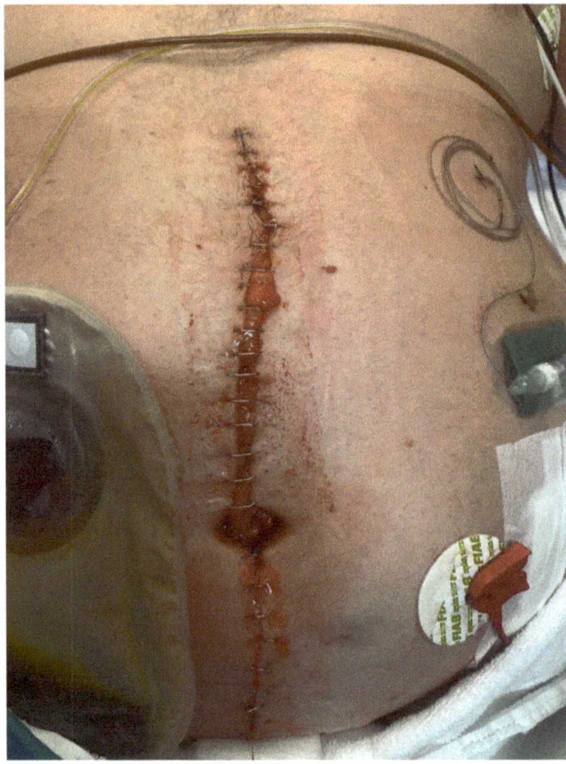

Fig. 24.10 This patient underwent a laparotomy for perforated Meckel's diverticulitis. Intraoperatively, there was also significant sigmoid diverticulitis where the Meckel's was adherent to. An en-bloc small bowel resection with anterior resection was performed. Given the significant contamination, an Abcarian end ileostomy was performed. On post-operative day 1, the patient had a large cough with a deep wound dehiscence as evident by the presence to omentum on view. He was taken back to theatre to close the fascia. The fascia closure was reinforced with interrupted figure of "8" sutures

closure is redone, and additional interrupted stitches can be placed at equal intervals (Fig. 24.10).

Any attempt to perform component separation should be considered carefully as it may impact on future hernia repair if there is an occurrence of incisional hernia. There is some evidence to suggest that prophylactic placement of mesh in the midline incision is safe and effective in preventing incisional hernia [38]. Nevertheless, there is no firm recommendation from the European Hernia Society currently [39]. The authors have not needed to perform that frequently as the incidence of burst abdomen and incisional hernia is low.

Venous Thromboembolism (VTE)

The incidence of VTE is reported up to 2% after EL. VTE represents a spectrum of conditions ranging from deep vein thrombosis to pulmonary embolism [40]. Preventative strategies commence prior to EL. Compressive stockings and calf compression pumps are applied prior to the EL and continue post-operatively. Post-operatively, early mobilization is encouraged. Unless there is a contraindication for chemical VTE prophylaxis, patients should receive either subcutaneous Heparin or low molecular weight Heparin (Enoxaparin). There is Cochrane evidence in 2019 that in major abdominal surgery, extended period of VTE prophylaxis up to 28 days should be given [41]. However, this practice is variable and dependent on the institution. The authors' practice is selective based on patient's previous history of VTE events and likelihood of remaining immobile.

Deep vein thrombosis usually manifests with lower limb swelling and tenderness at the calf. A duplex ultrasound is performed to confirm its location and extent. Advice from the haematologist should be sought for choice of anticoagulation. In recent times, the novel oral anticoagulants of either Rivaroxaban, Apixaban or Dabigatran can be prescribed. Alternatively, subcutaneous injection with Enoxaparin either once a day (1.5 mg/kg) or twice a day (1 mg/kg) can be given.

Another common scenario where VTE is presented. There is unexplained ongoing sinus tachycardia. Pulmonary embolism needs to be excluded with a CT pulmonary angiogram. If pulmonary embolism is diagnosed, similar advice from a Haematologist should be sought in view of therapeutic anticoagulation. Very rarely, therapeutic anticoagulation is contraindicated due to risk of bleeding. The use of inferior vena cava filters should be considered to prevent further propagation of clots.

A rare VTE complication of portomesenteric vein thrombosis can occur post-EL especially if there is intestinal resection or significant manipulation of the mesentery [42]. It is usually difficult to diagnose based on clinical assessment. A CT scan with intravenous contrast will demonstrate the extent of the thrombosis and any associated complications that will require surgical intervention. In the absence of haemodynamic instability and pneumatosis coli, therapeutic anticoagulation usually suffices.

ERAS in Emergency Laparotomy

The practice of enhanced recovery after surgery (ERAS) is well established in the elective setting with focus on 24-items in the pre-, intra- and post-operative period to minimize the morbidity associated with the procedure. There is increasing interest for the application of ERAS in the emergency surgery setting [43, 44]. A few trials showed that a modified ERAS protocol can be safely applied in the setting of small bowel resection, colonic surgery, and perforated peptic ulcer disease [45–47].

It is likely that the current practice in most centres is based on a modified ERAS concept with certain aspects achieving high agreement such as: selective use of nasogastric tube or early removal of nasogastric tube, goal-directed fluid resuscitation, use of opioid-sparing analgesia methods, avoidance of drain placement or early removal of drain, early removal of indwelling urinary catheter, early mobilization, use of prophylactic DVT measures and early introduction of enteral feeding as tolerated.

Continuous education and audits are important for the medical and allied health staff members to ensure the ongoing improvement on the practice of ERAS.

Miscellaneous Complications and Perioperative Physician

Some of these complications may seem mild but often interconnected and can lead to a vicious cycle and cascade of other complications.

- Urinary tract infection—early removal of indwelling urinary catheter is important. In patients with suspected sepsis, a urine sample is collected for microscopy and culture to direct targeted antimicrobial treatment.
- Acute kidney injury—it is manifested by the rise in creatinine level from baseline. Most of the cases are pre-renal in origin from intravascular volume depletion. In patients with underlying cardiac failure, input from cardiology colleagues is useful to prevent the cardiorenal syndrome.
- Delirium—it is not infrequent in the geriatric patients following EL [48]. Sometimes, it is unavoidable following a general anaesthetic despite avoiding certain medications with the potential for delirium. To tackle this, identify any underlying cause (i.e. sepsis), avoid any use of sedatives or anti-psychotics for behavioural management, place the patients in a less-stimulating environment.

The patient population continues to age and is medically more complex. The perioperative management will benefit from the collaboration of a physician with special interest in this field. This has been evident in the reduction of mortality in orthogeriatric patients from the lessons learnt from fracture neck of femur [49]. This service has been trialled in various subspecialties with good success [50].

The authors' institution has a perioperative physician (geriatrician by training) involved in the care of patients above the age of 65 in the various medical conditions and coordinate the need of rehabilitation [51]. It has helped to proactively prevent and manage any medical complications instead of the traditional model of care [52].

Recommendations/Future Research

The occurrence of complications following emergency laparotomy often has an impact on the patients. Nevertheless, the long-term effect especially on quality of life is unknown. Future research should focus on the quality of life following all the common complications following emergency laparotomy.

Acknowledgements The authors would like to thank Dr. Jih Huei Tan for his contribution in providing some clinical photos.

References

1. Ng ZQ, Weber D. One-year outcomes following emergency laparotomy: a systematic review. World J Surg. 2022;46(3):512–23.

2. Lai CPT, Goo TT, Ong MW, Prakash PS, Lim WW, Drakeford PA. A comparison of the P-POSSUM and NELA risk score for patients undergoing emergency laparotomy in Singapore. World J Surg. 2021;45(8):2439–46.
3. Broughton K, Soukhin E, Moot AR, Griffiths B. The time has come for New Zealand to improve outcomes after emergency laparotomy. N Z Med J. 2019;132(1488):55–61.
4. Lasithiotakis K, Kritsotakis EI, Kokkinakis S, Petra G, Paterakis K, Karali GA, et al. The Hellenic Emergency Laparotomy Study (HELAS): a prospective multicentre study on the outcomes of emergency laparotomy in Greece. World J Surg. 2023;47(1):130–9.
5. Party A-QW, James Aitken R, Griffiths B, Van Acker J, O'Loughlin E, Fletcher D, et al. Two-year outcomes from the Australian and New Zealand emergency laparotomy audit-quality improvement pilot study. ANZ J Surg. 2021;91(12):2575–82.
6. Tran ET, Ho KM. Utility of the National Emergency Laparotomy Audit prognostic model in predicting outcomes in an Australian health system. Anaesth Intensive Care. 2023;51(1):51–8.
7. Ming YJ, Howley P, Holmes M, Gani J, Pockney P. Sarcopenia 'made simple' and outcomes from emergency laparotomy. ANZ J Surg. 2022;92(12):3198–203.
8. Vaid S, Bell T, Grim R, Ahuja V. Predicting risk of death in general surgery patients on the basis of preoperative variables using American College of Surgeons National Surgical Quality Improvement Program data. Perm J. 2012;16(4):10–7.
9. Ng ZQ, Cohen R, Misur P, Weber DG. Poorer outcomes associated with sarcopenia following emergency laparotomy: a systematic review and meta-analysis. ANZ J Surg. 2022;92(12):3145–53.
10. Ong MW, Goh SSN, Tung WMJ, Lim WW, Hu HH, Lim CY, et al. Initial emergency laparotomy outcomes following a transdisciplinary perioperative care pathway in Singapore. Acute Med Surg. 2021;8(1):e702.
11. Meyer J, Roos E, Abbassi Z, Buchs NC, Ris F, Toso C. Prophylactic negative-pressure wound therapy prevents surgical site infection in abdominal surgery: an updated systematic review and meta-analysis of randomized controlled trials and observational studies. Clin Infect Dis. 2021;73(11):e3804–e13.
12. Lakhani A, Jamel W, Riddiough GE, Cabalag CS, Stevens S, Liu DS. Prophylactic negative pressure wound dressings reduces wound complications following emergency laparotomies: a systematic review and meta-analysis. Surgery. 2022;172(3):949–54.
13. Foss NB, Kehlet H. Challenges in optimising recovery after emergency laparotomy. Anaesthesia. 2020;75(Suppl 1):e83–e9.
14. Desai N, El-Boghdadly K, Albrecht E. Epidural vs. transversus abdominis plane block for abdominal surgery—a systematic review, meta-analysis and trial sequential analysis. Anaesthesia. 2021;76(1):101–17.
15. Tran DQ, Bravo D, Leurcharusmee P, Neal JM. Transversus abdominis plane block: a narrative review. Anesthesiology. 2019;131(5):1166–90.
16. Boden I, Sullivan K, Hackett C, Winzer B, Hwang R, Story D, et al. Intensive physical therapy after emergency laparotomy: pilot phase of the incidence of complications following emergency abdominal surgery get exercising randomized controlled trial. J Trauma Acute Care Surg. 2022;92(6):1020–30.
17. Katsura M, Kuriyama A, Takeshima T, Fukuhara S, Furukawa TA. Preoperative inspiratory muscle training for postoperative pulmonary complications in adults undergoing cardiac and major abdominal surgery. Cochrane Database Syst Rev. 2015;2015(10):CD010356.
18. Wells CI, Milne TGE, Seo SHB, Chapman SJ, Vather R, Bissett IP, et al. Post-operative ileus: definitions, mechanisms and controversies. ANZ J Surg. 2022;92(1–2):62–8.
19. Gero D, Gie O, Hubner M, Demartines N, Hahnloser D. Postoperative ileus: in search of an international consensus on definition, diagnosis, and treatment. Langenbeck's Arch Surg. 2017;402(1):149–58.
20. Sugawara K, Kawaguchi Y, Nomura Y, Suka Y, Kawasaki K, Uemura Y, et al. Perioperative factors predicting prolonged postoperative ileus after major abdominal surgery. J Gastrointest Surg. 2018;22(3):508–15.

21. Smolarek S, Shalaby M, Paolo Angelucci G, Missori G, Capuano I, Franceschilli L, et al. Small-bowel obstruction secondary to adhesions after open or laparoscopic colorectal surgery. JSLS. 2016;20(4):e2016.00073.
22. Portale G, Popescu GO, Parotto M, Cavallin F. Internal hernia after laparoscopic colorectal surgery: an under-reported potentially severe complication. A systematic review and meta-analysis. Surg Endosc. 2019;33(4):1066–74.
23. Sakr A, Emile SH, Abdallah E, Thabet W, Khafagy W. Predictive factors for small intestinal and colonic anastomotic leak: a multivariate analysis. Indian J Surg. 2017;79(6):555–62.
24. Alves A, Panis Y, Trancart D, Regimbeau JM, Pocard M, Valleur P. Factors associated with clinically significant anastomotic leakage after large bowel resection: multivariate analysis of 707 patients. World J Surg. 2002;26(4):499–502.
25. Awad S, El-Rahman AIA, Abbas A, Althobaiti W, Alfaran S, Alghamdi S, et al. The assessment of perioperative risk factors of anastomotic leakage after intestinal surgeries; a prospective study. BMC Surg. 2021;21(1):29.
26. Thomas MS, Margolin DA. Management of Colorectal Anastomotic Leak. Clin Colon Rectal Surg. 2016;29(2):138–44.
27. Gribovskaja-Rupp I, Melton GB. Enterocutaneous fistula: proven strategies and updates. Clin Colon Rectal Surg. 2016;29(2):130–7.
28. Baker ML, Williams RN, Nightingale JM. Causes and management of a high-output stoma. Color Dis. 2011;13(2):191–7.
29. Arenas Villafranca JJ, Lopez-Rodriguez C, Abiles J, Rivera R, Gandara Adan N, Utrilla NP. Protocol for the detection and nutritional management of high-output stomas. Nutr J. 2015;14:45.
30. Medlin S. Nutritional and fluid requirements: high-output stomas. Br J Nurs. 2012;21(6):S22–5.
31. Tsujinaka S, Tan KY, Miyakura Y, Fukano R, Oshima M, Konishi F, et al. Current management of intestinal stomas and their complications. J Anus Rectum Colon. 2020;4(1):25–33.
32. Kvist M, Burcharth J, Nielsen YW, Jensen TK. Abdominal subcutaneous obesity and the risk of burst abdomen: a matched case-control study. Langenbeck's Arch Surg. 2022;407(8):3719–26.
33. Kvist M, Henriksen NA, Burcharth J, Nielsen YW, Jensen TK. Rectus diastasis increases risk of burst abdomen in emergency midline laparotomies: a matched case-control study. Hernia. 2022;27:353.
34. Waqar SH, Malik ZI, Razzaq A, Abdullah MT, Shaima A, Zahid MA. Frequency and risk factors for wound dehiscence/burst abdomen in midline laparotomies. J Ayub Med Coll Abbottabad. 2005;17(4):70–3.
35. Jensen TK, Nielsen YW, Gogenur I, Tolstrup MB. Sarcopenia is associated with increased risk of burst abdomen after emergency midline laparotomy: a matched case-control study. Eur J Trauma Emerg Surg. 2022;48(5):4189–96.
36. Israelsson LA, Millbourn D. Prevention of incisional hernias: how to close a midline incision. Surg Clin North Am. 2013;93(5):1027–40.
37. Israelsson LA. Abdominal incision closure: small but important bites. Lancet. 2015;386(10000):1216–8.
38. Bravo-Salva A, Argudo-Aguirre N, Gonzalez-Castillo AM, Membrilla-Fernandez E, Sancho-Insenser JJ, Grande-Posa L, et al. Long-term follow-up of prophylactic mesh reinforcement after emergency laparotomy. A retrospective controlled study. BMC Surg. 2021;21(1):243.
39. Muysoms FE, Antoniou SA, Bury K, Campanelli G, Conze J, Cuccurullo D, et al. European hernia society guidelines on the closure of abdominal wall incisions. Hernia. 2015;19(1):1–24.
40. Dobaria Bs V, Hadaya J, Ebrihiminan S, Verma A, Sanaiha Y, Benharash P. Impact of venous thromboembolism on readmissions and resource use following emergency general surgery. Am Surg. 2022;88(10):2436–9.
41. Felder S, Rasmussen MS, King R, Sklow B, Kwaan M, Madoff R, et al. Prolonged thromboprophylaxis with low molecular weight heparin for abdominal or pelvic surgery. Cochrane Database Syst Rev. 2019;8(8):CD004318.

42. Robinson KA, O'Donnell ME, Pearson D, Kriegshauser JS, Odeleye M, Kalkbrenner K, et al. Portomesenteric venous thrombosis following major colon and rectal surgery: incidence and risk factors. Surg Endosc. 2015;29(5):1071–9.
43. Burcharth J, Abdulhady L, Danker J, Ekeloef S, Jorgensen T, Lauridsen H, et al. Implementation of a multidisciplinary perioperative protocol in major emergency abdominal surgery. Eur J Trauma Emerg Surg. 2021;47(2):467–77.
44. Ceresoli M, Biloslavo A, Bisagni P, Ciuffa C, Fortuna L, La Greca A, et al. Implementing enhanced perioperative care in emergency general surgery: a prospective multicenter observational study. World J Surg. 2023:1–9.
45. Pathrikar SG, Jadhav GS, Adhikari GR. The application of enhanced recovery after surgery protocols in patients with perforated duodenal ulcer. Cureus. 2023;15(3):e35760.
46. Lohsiriwat V, Jitmungngan R. Enhanced recovery after surgery in emergency colorectal surgery: review of literature and current practices. World J Gastrointest Surg. 2019;11(2):41–52.
47. Vinas X, Macarulla E, Brugiotti C, Ramirez JM, Pedregosa A, Sanchez S, et al. Feasibility and effects of enhanced recovery vs. conventional care after emergency colon surgery for patients with left colon perforation. Sci Rep. 2020;10(1):7346.
48. Loran DB, Hyde BR, Zwischenberger JB. Perioperative management of special populations: the geriatric patient. Surg Clin North Am. 2005;85(6):1259–66. xi
49. Middleton M, Wan B, da Assuncao R. Improving hip fracture outcomes with integrated orthogeriatric care: a comparison between two accepted orthogeriatric models. Age Ageing. 2017;46(3):465–70.
50. Eamer G, Taheri A, Chen SS, Daviduck Q, Chambers T, Shi X, et al. Comprehensive geriatric assessment for older people admitted to a surgical service. Cochrane Database Syst Rev. 2018;1(1):CD012485.
51. Aitken RM, Partridge JSL, Oliver CM, Murray D, Hare S, Lockwood S, et al. Older patients undergoing emergency laparotomy: observations from the National Emergency Laparotomy Audit (NELA) years 1-4. Age Ageing. 2020;49(4):656–63.
52. Joughin AL, Partridge JSL, O'Halloran T, Dhesi JK. Where are we now in perioperative medicine? Results from a repeated UK survey of geriatric medicine delivered services for older people. Age Ageing. 2019;48(3):458–62.

Chapter 25
Open Abdomen as an Effective Therapy for Abdominal Sepsis, Bedside Assistance for the Surgeon

Thijs Cornette and Frederik Berrevoet

Introduction

Abdominal sepsis is, after pulmonary sepsis, the second most common cause of sepsis that needs intensive care management and has a high morbidity and mortality rate. It can arise from many different pathologies, both infectious and non-infectious. However, even when the "obvious" focus in a patient with SIRS is non-infectious, an infectious origin must be excluded. Age, smoking, immunosuppression (e.g., cancer, corticosteroids), diabetes mellitus, morbid obesity, acute renal failure, and dialysis are all predisposing factors that result in higher complication rates [1].

Contained infections result in the formation of an intra-abdominal abscess, whereas uncontained infection can lead to local or diffuse peritonitis. The etiology of primary peritonitis is not well understood, but is defined as a spontaneous, diffuse peritoneal infection with or without intra-abdominal source. Although it can occur at any age, it is more frequently observed in children. Possible routes of infection are hematogenous, lymphatic, gastrointestinal, and genital/fallopian tubes (females). Urinary tract and intra-abdominal foreign body are other possible routes of infection. If peritonitis follows intra-abdominal lesions such as gastrointestinal perforations, ischemia or infected necrosis associated with severe acute pancreatitis, we define it as a secondary peritonitis. Tertiary peritonitis refers to a persistent or

T. Cornette
Faculty of Medicine and Health Sciences, Ghent University, Ghent, Belgium

Department of General and HPB Surgery and Liver Transplantation, Ghent University Hospital, Ghent, Belgium

F. Berrevoet (✉)
Department of General and HPB Surgery and Liver Transplantation, Ghent University Hospital, Ghent, Belgium
e-mail: Frederik.Berrevoet@UGent.be

© The Author(s), under exclusive license to Springer Nature Switzerland AG 2024
J. Faintuch, S. Faintuch (eds.), *Recent Strategies in High Risk Surgery*,
https://doi.org/10.1007/978-3-031-56270-9_25

recurring infection with organisms of low or high virulence. It is seen after multiple operative attempts to treat secondary peritonitis, particularly in circumstances of open abdomen, fistula formation, and gut dysfunction [2].

Sepsis and Septic Shock

In 2016 new definitions for sepsis and septic shock were proposed by Singer et al. [3]. The systemic inflammatory response syndrome or SIRS term can still be used to describe a systemic response to a sterile hit or an infection. However, there is an insight that sepsis does not follow a continuum from infection and sepsis to shock. Severe sepsis is a term that is no longer used, as it caused confusion. Sepsis is now defined as a life-threatening organ dysfunction caused by a dysregulated host response to infection. Septic shock entails higher mortality, demanding vasopressors (>65 mmHg), or exhibiting a lactate > 2 mmol/L after hypovolemia was excluded [3].

Organ Dysfunction

It can be quantified by the Sequential Organ Failure Assessment (SOFA) score [4] for screening purposes, to assess severity, to predict outcomes, and as follow-up in the intensive care unit/ICU (Table 25.1). It has higher specificity than the previous SIRS criteria, but lower sensitivity [5]. The q-SOFA score is an abbreviated score for patients outside the ICU [6]. It focusses on low blood pressure (SBP (≤100 mmHg)), high respiratory rate (≥22/min), or altered mentation (GCS ≤ 14). Fulfilling two of the three criteria in the q-SOFA score is an indication for ICU hospitalization. For surgeons, however, the SIRS criteria (Sepsis-2) remain the most important tool for detecting a septic patient, as it has the highest sensitivity for early detection of inflammation and infection, both crucial for early treatment [1]. To fulfill the SIRS criteria the patient must have two out of the four criteria:

- Body temperature over 38 °C or under 36 °C
- Heart rate >90/min
- Respiratory rate >20/min or partial pressure CO_2 < 32 mmHg
- Leukocyte count > 12,000 or less than 4000/mL or over 10% immature forms

Patients with abdominal sepsis often require standard surgical exploration as a crucial component of their management, although multiple minimally invasive procedures seem to achieve the same target with less morbidity [2, 7].

Table 25.1 Sequential (sepsis related) organ failure assessment (SOFA) score. (Gyawali et al.) [4]

System	Score				
	0	1	2	3	4
Respiration					
P_aO_2/FIO_2 mmHg (kPa)	≥400 (53.3)	<400 (53.3)	<300 (40)	<200 (26.7) with respiratory support	<100 (13.3) with respiratory support
Coagulation platelets, $\times 10^3\ \mu L^{-1}$	≥150	<150	<100	<50	<20
Liver bilirubin, mg dL^{-1}	<1.2 (20)	1.2–1.9 (20–32)	2.0–5.9 (33–101)	6.0–11.9 (102–204)	>12.0 (204)
Cardiovascular	MAP ≥70 mmHg	MAP <70 mmHg	Dopamine <5 or dobutamine (any dose)[a]	Dopamine 5.1–15 or epinephrine ≤0.1 or norepinephrine ≤0.1[a]	Dopamine >15 or epinephrine >0.1 or norepinephrine 0.1[a]
Central Nervous system (CNS)					
Glasgow Coma Scale scare[b]	15	13–14	10–12	6–9	<6
Renal Creatinine, mg dL^{-1} ($\mu mol\ L^{-1}$)	<1.2 (110)	1.2–1.9 (110–170)	2.0–3.4 (171–299)	3.5–4.9 (300–440)	>5.0 (440)
Urine output, mL per day				<500	<200

FIO_2 fraction of inspired oxygen, *MAP* mean arterial pressure, PaO_2 partial pressure of oxygen

[a]Catecholamine doses are given as $\mu g\ kg^{-1}\ min^{-1}$ for at least 1 h

[b]Glasgow Coma Scale scores range from 3 to 15: higher score indicates better neurological function

Key Surgical Steps

Identification of the source: It may not be apparent or diagnostic imaging techniques are inconclusive.

Source control: Draining an abscess, resecting a diseased or perforated organ, repairing an anastomotic leak, or removing necrotic tissue are typical maneuvers. By addressing the source, surgeons aim to eliminate or minimize ongoing contamination, preventing the further spread of infection and allowing the body's immune system to better combat the sepsis.

Debridement: Removal of infected or necrotic tissue is commonly performed. This helps eliminate bacteria, toxins, and debris, promoting wound healing and reducing the risk of recurrent infection. Debridement also aids in removing potential sources of ongoing sepsis and contributes to the overall management of the patient. Irrigation has been routinely used in the past; however, it is not recommended anymore. At least in the context of trauma, even with heavy contamination, outcomes are not improved and new abscess may appear [7].

Evaluation of complications: Exploration allows surgeons to assess peritonitis, abscesses, and adhesions; provide appropriate treatment; and determine the need for additional interventions or specialized care.

Damage and Source Control Surgery

Damage control surgery (DCS) is a surgical intervention with rapid termination when a good level of control is achieved over a life-threatening bleeding or contamination. It is surgery to keep the patient alive rather than correct anatomy. If adequate stabilization is obtained, a more profound resuscitation on the ICU is performed and physiology is corrected. Closure of the abdominal wall can be further delayed if necessary [8]. Surgical source control consists of debridement of necrotic or infected tissues, drainage of abscesses or infected fluid collections, and definite control over the source of contamination. The sequence for damage control in the septic abdomen is slightly altered from the trauma procedure. The first phase, ground zero, can be longer to accommodate a good level of resuscitation until a safe induction of anesthesia can be performed. The urgency to operate can be evaluated by the SOFA score, the presence of shock, and the severity of organ system involvement.

Role of Relaparotomies in Septic Patients

Relaparotomies are frequently needed and should eventually be planned in circumstances of extensive and incompletely controlled abdominal sepsis. In some patients, peritoneal infection can deteriorate quickly to an excessive inflammatory response

(SIRS), causing organ failure. An early reintervention with evacuation of toxic content and inflammatory cytokines may be crucial for stopping the septic cascade [9].

The origin of secondary peritonitis and perioperative findings at emergency laparotomy tend to be poor indicators for early relaparotomy, whereas signs of progressive or persistent organ failure in the early postoperative phase seem more reliable. A proposed model by Kiewiet et al. showed a significant correlation when six variables are combined, that is heart rate, hemoglobin level, body temperature, no defecation, the extent of contamination found at initial laparotomy, and the need for inotropic medication. This model is then combined with CT scan findings [10]. The development of elevated intra-abdominal pressure (IAP) during the early postoperative period is associated with increased risk of prolonged postoperative peritonitis and could be used as a predictor of early relaparotomy [11].

Intra-abdominal Hypertension (IAH) and Abdominal Compartment Syndrome (ACS)

According to severity, IAP can be classified as Grade I: IAP 12–15 mmHg; Grade II: IAP 16–20 mmHg; Grade III: IAP 21–25 mmHg; and Grade IV: IAP > 25 mmHg [12]. Hyperacute forms exist, representing elevations in IAP that last only a few seconds or minutes as a result of laughing, straining, coughing, sneezing, defecation, or physical activity. They have limited surgical interest. The acute modality corresponds to IAH developing over a period of hours and is seen primarily in surgical patients as a result of trauma or intra-abdominal hemorrhage. Subacute cases occur over a period of days and are the most encountered form in medical patients. Chronic examples evolve along months (i.e., pregnancy) or years (i.e., morbid obesity, intra-abdominal tumor, peritoneal dialysis, chronic ascites, or cirrhosis). Intrinsically they don't represent emergencies; however, they may place patients at risk for developing either acute or subacute IAH when critically ill [13].

Diagnosis

When undetected, ACS is an independent predictor of mortality [14–16]. The exact clinical symptoms that define ACS are not well defined. Abdominal distention can be observed, but is not sensitive, nor specific to diagnose ACS, as well as respiratory complications or urine output due to renal non-perfusion. The surgeon must always be aware of the possibility of developing ACS) and has to exclude it actively from the differential diagnosis in critically ill patients.

The Open Abdomen Treatment

The open abdomen has to be distinguished from a "burst abdomen" after primary closure of a laparotomy incision where the fascial dehiscence is unintended and unforeseen [17]. Here we deal with an abdominal wall defect when it is impossible or not desired to fully close the wound after surgery. Temporary Abdominal Closure (TAC) devices are easily placed and removed, resulting in a quick re-access when necessary.

Three well-described scenarios can lead to the creation of an open abdomen: surgical packing to control coagulopathy with massive bleeding, and to achieve the shortest possible time to get back to the ICU [18]; severe abdominal compartment syndrome demanding decompression of the internal organs [12]; selected cases of severe peritonitis, to accommodate possible swelling due to edema of the internal organs, or when subsequent laparotomies are envisaged to treat intra-abdominal infection and complications [19].

Modalities of Open Abdomen

Björk et al. proposed a classification system for open abdomen in 2009 that was revised in 2016 (Table 25.2) [20, 21]. This clarification, aside from bringing uniformity in description, allows to describe the evolution of the open abdomen during treatment. There is a numerical triage of 1–4, with Grade 1 having no adherences between bowel and abdomen or no lateralization. Grade 2 where fixation is being developed as opposed to Grade 3 where there is a frozen abdomen. When an entero-atmospheric fistula is already established it is categorized as Grade 4 and considered as a continuous enteric leak into the open abdomen. The numerical value is combined with a letter, where A is clean, B is contaminated, and C is when an enteric leak is present in Grade 1–3 [21].

Mentula et al. showed a significant decrease in mortality in a small retrospective series of 26 patients with an abdominal compartment syndrome following severe acute pancreatitis. The overall mortality was 46%, but patients who received an

Table 25.2 Open abdomen classification, amended by Björk et al. [21]

1A	Clean, no fixation
1B	Contaminated, no fixation
1C	Enteric leak, no fixation
2A	Clean, developing fixation
2B	Contaminated, developing fixation
2C	Enteric leak, developing fixation
3A	Clean, frozen abdomen
3B	Contaminated, frozen abdomen
4	Established enteroatmospheric fistula, frozen abdomen

early open abdomen within 4 days of disease onset were less at risk (18%) in comparison to patients who underwent surgery after 5 days or more who suffered 100% mortality [22]. Controversies remain concerning timing and actual benefits of open abdomen in this setting, given the risks of infection, fluid and protein deficit, entero-atmospheric fistulas, and ischemia-reperfusion syndrome.

The Role of Open Abdomen in Sepsis

Current guidelines do not recommend routine use of open abdomen management for secondary peritonitis, in the light of the alluded to risks, notably enteroatmospheric fistula and fascial dehiscence, despite the benefits of preventing ACS and providing rapid and easy relaparotomies [1]. It should however be considered for patients with secondary peritonitis in which a high risk for ACS development is estimated, or when a number of relaparotomies is to be expected [17].

Surgical Techniques for Open Abdomen Management

Fascial closure has to prevent evisceration without pressure building up. Abdominal fluid accumulations need to be evacuated to decrease volume (pressure) and to prevent bacterial proliferation due to fluid stasis. Fistula formation should be prevented by means of gut protection from exposure, drying, ischemia, and friction with rough surfaces. With an eye on future closure, which is a similarly essential component of surgical planning, the technique must also preserve the fascia from lateral retraction so as to facilitate easy primary fascial closure.

These criteria can be met by different techniques and closure devices involving both static and dynamic measures (Fig. 25.1). In 2018 the European Hernia Society published their Guidelines on the management of open and burst abdomen. Looking at the existing evidence there is a clear advantage in using dynamic fascial closure techniques compared to static options. The pooled fascial closure rate results comparing static (33.9%) versus dynamic techniques (75.9%) were clearly in favor of the dynamic techniques [23].

Static Management

Static open abdomen management does not facilitate sequential tightening of the abdominal wall in-between operations. Such encompassed the Bogota bag [24], which is still popular in certain low-income countries due to its availability and low cost, in the face of lack of resources. A temporary absorbable mesh or Gore-Tex mesh was sutured to both fascial edges (inlay); however, this technique seems

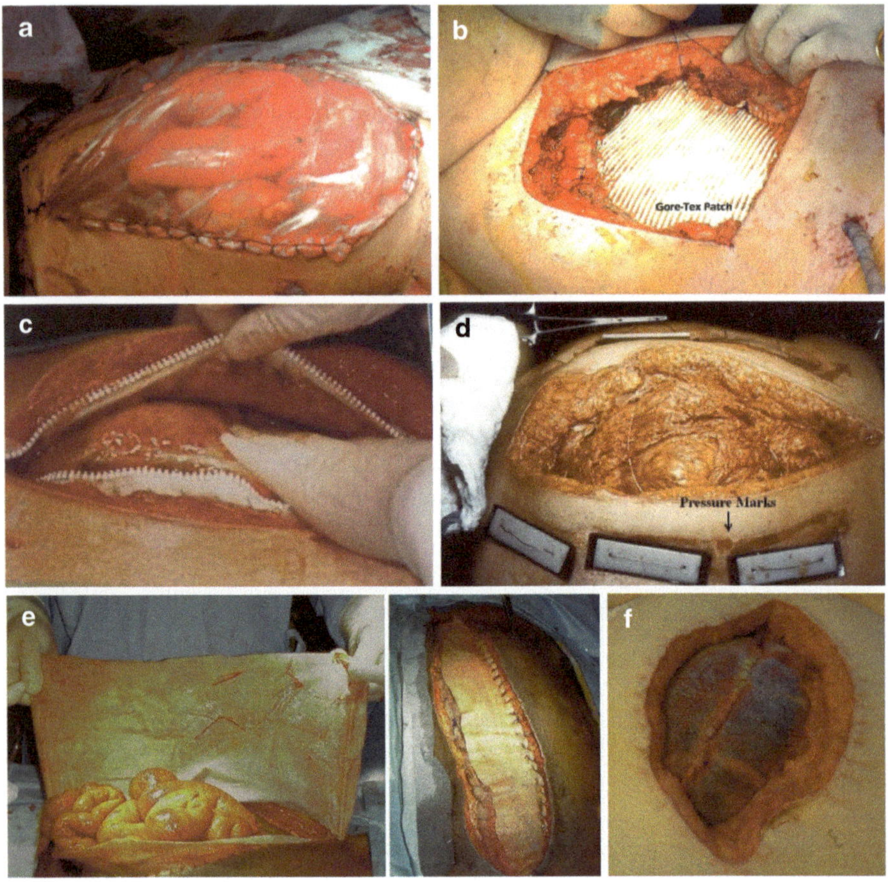

Fig. 25.1 (**a**) Bogota bag; (**b**) Gore-Tex mesh; (**c**) zipper mesh; (**d**) Ventrofil™; (**e**) Wittmann patch™; (**f**) mesh-mediated fascial traction

associated with a higher incidence of fistula formation [25, 26]; A mesh with a zipper for easy re-access to the abdominal cavity; however, similar dangers [27] to the previous one; Ventrofil™ (B.Braun, Melsungen, Germany) plates, to relieve strain on wounds and prevent infection [28]; Even negative pressure wound therapy (NPWT) is also considered a static measure as it does not prevent fascial retraction. It consists of a bowel protecting layer, a soft spongy material, followed by an adhesive bandage with a small opening for drain connection to continuous suction [29].

Dynamic Management

Dynamic techniques combine the temporary closure of the abdominal cavity with active fascial traction: They are represented by a number of devices and resources. The Wittmann patch™ (Starsurgical, Burlington, WI, USA) is a velcro-like device for re-approximating the abdominal wall and bridging for future abdominal entries. It consists of two sheets respectively with hooks and loops, which are pressed together to form a secure closure, but easily peeled apart for re-entry surgery. The overlap is adjusted to get the desired tension and allow accommodation for swelling [30]. Dynamic retention sutures anchored to the skin on the outside of both wound sides have been used in the past [31, 32]. Although sometimes effective, they may incur some risks namely pain, hernia, and infections. Moreover the effectiveness in preventing wound dehiscence is debated.

NPWT and Mesh-Mediated Fascial Traction (MMFT)

This combination is now considered the gold standard, with fascial closure rates up to 90% [33–36]. A mesh is sewed in at both sides of the open fascia on which tension is applied and covered by NPWT [33, 34]. Treatment should begin as early as possible, preferably within 24–48 h after open abdomen management has started. This was studied by Berrevoet et al. in a cohort of 152 patients, in which early MMFT and NPWT had a significantly better fascial closure rate compared to patients who started three or more days later ($p < 0.001$) [34] (Fig. 25.1).

How to Perform NPWT + MMFT

Under sterile conditions a visceral protective layer (VPL), either a commercial type or a self-made coverage, is placed deep to the anterior abdominal wall as a protective barrier between the abdominal content and the overlying mesh, aiming to reduce the frequency of enteroatmospheric fistula formation [37, 38]. In case there is a need for a temporary protective ostomy a poor location should meticulously be avoided, as it can make future OA management and NPWT or TAC placement a real challenge. They should be placed as laterally as possible to allow maximal medial mobility of the abdominal wall during closing [39].

A heavyweight polypropylene mesh is sewn to the fascia by overlapping 2–2.5 cm, using a non-absorbable monofilament 2/0 suture. When using MMFT technique it is advised to use a small pore mesh for traction. Large pore meshes are not suitable for heavy traction as they are too elastic and will be torn during the process [34]. The mesh is then divided down the middle to introduce the VPL. The negative pressure wound therapy system (NPWT) can be applied when no recent anastomoses are present and preferably no bile leak or active bleeding either. Next to drainage, the NPWT increases granulation and angiogenesis by stimulating cell reproduction and proliferation [34] (Fig. 25.2).

It is important to drape the VPL as lateral as possible circumferentially, reaching the paracolic gutters as well as the subdiaphragmatic space, to achieve best fluid drainage out of the abdominal cavity and to prevent fluid collection formation and abscesses. Traction is then applied on the level of the mesh when suturing the two

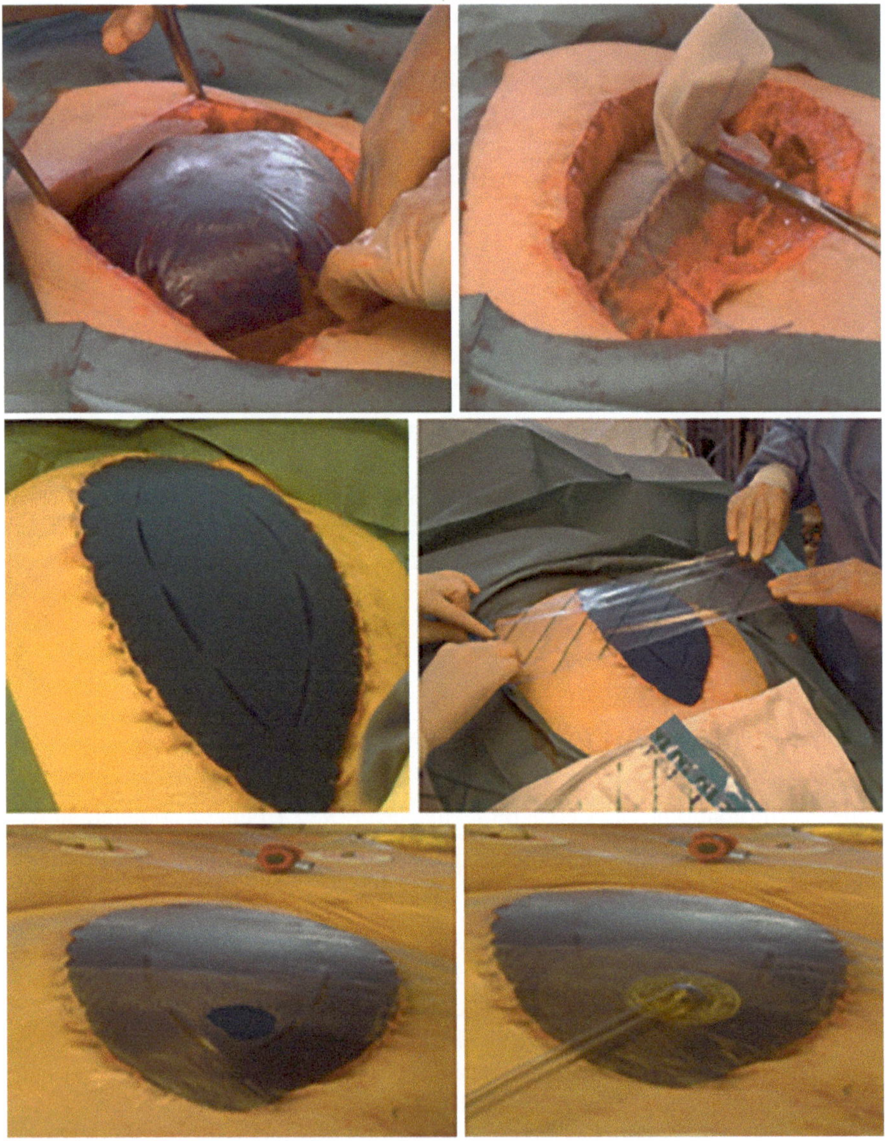

Fig. 25.2 Mesh-mediated fascial traction with negative pressure therapy

halves together with a continuous non-absorbable monofilament 2/0 suture [40]. After applying traction ventilatory pressures should be checked by the anesthesiologist to exclude significant rise in intra-abdominal pressure. On top of the mesh a layer of extra foam is positioned to cover the mesh, and the procedure is then finalized by draping over the sponge, connecting the suction cap and applying negative pressure (−125 mmHg) (Fig. 25.3).

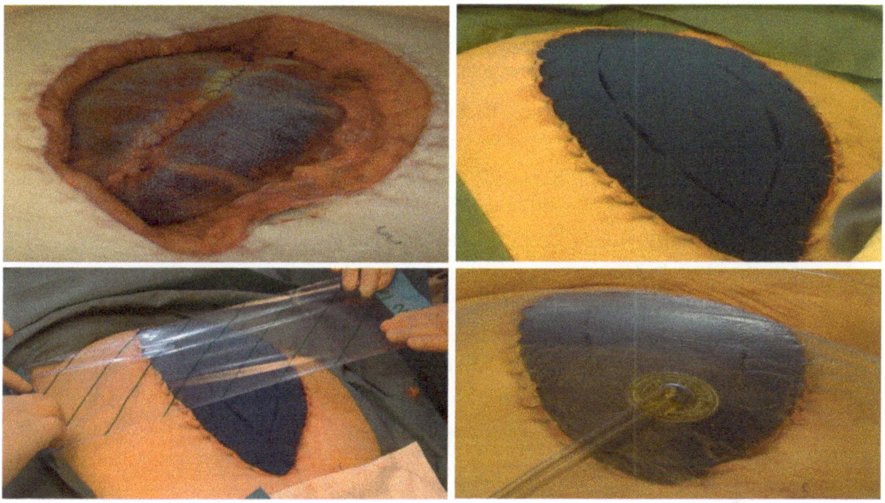

Fig. 25.3 Step by step application of mesh-mediated traction and intra-abdominal negative pressure therapy

Patients should return to the operating room every 3–4 days to change the NPWT dressing and further increase the tension on the abdominal wall, by trimming the mesh and re-suturing it at the midline. Ideally, complete fascial closure will be achieved after 7–14 days. At the time of complete fascial closure, the subcutaneous tissue might receive further NPWT for several days to decrease wound morbidity [34].

Results and Complications

At the ICU, hypothermia and fluid loss are common and need to be addressed all the time. Heat loss and evaporation occur due to the large abdominal defect. When the core temperature drops it causes coagulopathy and bleeding problems, which impact metabolic acidosis, thus this lethal triad must be corrected.

In 2014 worldwide mortality rates in septic patients were as high as 36.5% [41]. The Closed or Open after Source Control Laparotomy for Severe Complicated Intra-Abdominal Sepsis (COOL trial) is currently including patients in a RCT and could be a benchmark for assessing its benefits [42]. Whenever OA is used for a septic abdomen, early fascial closure should be obtained as soon as the damage or source control has been performed according to the guidelines of both the World Society of Emergency Surgery and the guidelines of the European Hernia Society early fascial closure, because it results in lower complications ratios and mortality [9, 23].

A small retrospective study of 25 patients reported a significantly lower mortality incidence after the use of open abdomen management in septic patients (30–35% mortality rate found in the literature to only 4%) [43]. However, another recent study by Prete et al., found no clear difference and reported a mortality rate of 32% in OA patients, in line with the non-OA mortality for sepsis [44]. The international registry of open abdomen reported a lower mortality of 20% during OA treatment, but mortality after closure was not included. The Apache II score was the only predictor of in-hospital mortality in their analysis [45].

The reported morbidity rate of surviving patients in these two studies is similar: 58.3% by Inukai et al. and 58.8% by Prete et al. [43, 44]. The study by Inukai et al. reported surgical site infections (SSI) as the main complication (24%). Fistulae were less observed when early fascial closure could be obtained and risk factors for development of complications were age over 70 years old, diabetes mellitus, OA duration more than 3 days, and initial operative time more than 60 min [43].

Enteroatmospheric Fistula

This is the most feared surgical complication. It can be caused by anastomotic leakage or serosal damage during previous surgery. The bowel itself is more fragile during OA, due to evaporation and accompanying dried out serosa. Attempts to seal the fistula are usually unsuccessful, and the common approach is to conduct the contents of the fistula to the exterior. Recent literature suggests two new methods to drain the fistula efficiently [46, 47]. A Foley catheter and a special donut (covered vacuum sponge) can be introduced to exclude the fistula site from the rest of the abdomen under NPWT. Another possibility is the off-label use of Flexi-Seal (Convatec, Reading, UK) to divert the fistula to outside the patient.

The data of the international register of open abdomen show for sepsis, trauma, and IAH/ ACS similar rates of definitive fascial closure rates and fistula formation [45]. In a study by Kritayakirana et al. the mortality rate in abdominal sepsis patients using OA was practically equal to IAH, respectively (35% and 31%), whereas in trauma patients it was lower (11%) [48].

Optimizing the Outcome After Open Abdomen Management

As fascial closure should be obtained as quickly as possible to improve outcomes, several options are recently suggested to increase the primary fascial closure rate. Specifically in abdominal sepsis, severe necrotizing pancreatitis or stiff abdominal wall due to critical illness and generalized edema, the use of NPWT + MMFT might still not be enough to achieve primary fascial closure.

Botulinum Toxin A

Closing complex and open abdomens when fascial retraction has already occurred is still very challenging. Not all patients can be primarily closed without a mesh bridging the defect. Botulinum toxin A (BTA) can be injected in all three muscles of the abdominal wall (external oblique, internal oblique, and transversus abdominis) using ultrasound guidance. BTA acts as a long-term muscle relaxant, allowing better approximation of the fascia. Doses of 200–300 IU per patient, dispersed into three points on each side of the abdominal wall, or 35–50 IU per injection site (±11–17 IU per muscle layer) seem safe and well-tolerated [49–51]. The optimal effect is late, 2–3 weeks after injection, yet in a cohort of 18 patients with OA, 89% underwent primary fascial closure if BTA was administered within 24 h before surgery [52]. Nevertheless conflicting results have been announced, and the debate goes on [53, 54]

Fasciotens™

This vertical traction device (Fasciotens, Essen, Germany) might show potential benefit in early closure of the open abdomen [55]. The idea is counteracting the natural muscle traction and attenuating fascial retraction, while simultaneously allowing pressure release with the open abdomen. The current devices can only accommodate one or the other at the same time. The technique consists of sewing a double layered mesh to each fascial margin when there was a midline or transverse laparotomy. The mesh is then connected through surgical sutures to a common suspension with adjustable traction force. Such force is implemented in a routine of 5 h high tension interspersed with 1 h of tension release. Fasciotens™ must be repositioned every time to its indicated original place, namely the pubis bone and sternum, avoiding soft tissue pressure. It is crucial to monitor the patient continuously for pressure wounds caused by the device, as the involved pulling forces are high. This device is primarily being indicated in patients under mechanical ventilation in the intensive care unit [56].

Available evidence suggests reduction in fascia-to-fascia distance.

Conflict of Interest All authors declare that they have no conflict of interest.

References

1. Hecker A, et al. Intra-abdominal sepsis: new definitions and current clinical standards. Langenbeck's Arch Surg. 2019;404(3):257–71.
2. Leppäniemi A, et al. Management of abdominal sepsis—a paradigm shift? Anaesthesiol Intensive Ther. 2015;47(4):400–8.

3. Singer M, et al. The third international consensus definitions for sepsis and septic shock (sepsis-3). JAMA. 2016;315(8):801–10.
4. Gyawali B, Ramakrishna K, Dhamoon A. Sepsis: the evolution in definition, pathophysiology, and management. SAGE Open Med. 2019;7:205031211983504.
5. Vermassen J, et al. Characteristics of Sepsis-2 septic shock patients failing to satisfy the Sepsis-3 septic shock definition: an analysis of real-time collected data. Ann Intensive Care. 2021;11(1):154.
6. Shahsavarinia K, et al. qSOFA score for prediction of sepsis outcome in emergency department. Pak J Med Sci. 2020;36(4):668–72.
7. Mashbari H, Hemdi M, Chow KL, Doherty JC, Merlotti GJ, Salzman SL, Singares ES. A randomized controlled trial on intra-abdominal irrigation during emergency trauma laparotomy; time for yet another paradigm shift. Bull Emerg Trauma. 2018;6(2):100–7.
8. Ordoñez CA, et al. Evolution of damage control surgery in non-traumatic abdominal pathology: a light in the darkness. Colombia Medica (Cali, Colombia). 2021;52(2):e4194809.
9. Sartelli M, Abu-Zidan FM, Ansaloni L, Bala M, Beltrán MA, Biffl WL, Catena F, Chiara O, Coccolini F, Coimbra R, Demetrashvili Z, Demetriades D, Diaz JJ, Di Saverio S, Fraga GP, Ghnnam W, Griffiths EA, Gupta S, Hecker A, Karamarkovic A, Kong VY, Kafka-Ritsch R, Kluger Y, Latifi R, Leppaniemi A, Lee JG, McFarlane M, Marwah S, Moore FA, Ordonez CA, Pereira GA, Plaudis H, Shelat VG, Ulrych J, Zachariah SK, Zielinski MD, Garcia MP, Moore EE. The role of the open abdomen procedure in managing severe abdominal sepsis: WSES position paper. World J Emerg Surg. 2015;10:35.
10. Kiewiet JJS, et al. A decision rule to aid selection of patients with abdominal sepsis requiring a relaparotomy. BMC Surg. 2013;13(1):28.
11. Basu A, Pai DR. Early elevation of intra-abdominal pressure after laparotomy for secondary peritonitis: a predictor of relaparotomy? World J Surg. 2008;32(8):1851–6.
12. Kirkpatrick AW, et al. Intra-abdominal hypertension and the abdominal compartment syndrome: updated consensus definitions and clinical practice guidelines from the World Society of the Abdominal Compartment Syndrome. Intensive Care Med. 2013;39(7):1190–206.
13. Papavramidis TS, et al. Intra-abdominal pressure alterations after large pancreatic pseudocyst transcutaneous drainage. BMC Gastroenterol. 2009;9(1):42.
14. Cheatham ML, et al. Abdominal perfusion pressure: a superior parameter in the assessment of intra-abdominal hypertension. J Trauma. 2000;49(4):621–6. discussion 626-7
15. Kirkpatrick AW, et al. Intra-abdominal hypertension and abdominal compartment syndrome after abdominal wall reconstruction: quaternary syndromes? Scand J Surg. 2017;106(2):97–106.
16. Rajasurya V, Surani S. Abdominal compartment syndrome: often overlooked conditions in medical intensive care units. World J Gastroenterol. 2020;26(3):266–78.
17. Poortmans N, Berrevoet F. Dynamic closure techniques for treatment of an open abdomen: an update. Hernia. 2020;24(2):325–31.
18. Stone HH, Strom PR, Mullins RJ. Management of the major coagulopathy with onset during laparotomy. Ann Surg. 1983;197(5):532–5.
19. Sartelli M, et al. WSES/GAIS/SIS-E/WSIS/AAST global clinical pathways for patients with intra-abdominal infections. World J Emerg Surg. 2021;16(1):49.
20. Björck M, et al. Classification—important step to improve management of patients with an open abdomen. World J Surg. 2009;33(6):1154–7.
21. Björck M, et al. Amended classification of the open abdomen. Scand J Surg. 2016;105(1):5–10.
22. Mentula P, et al. Surgical decompression for abdominal compartment syndrome in severe acute pancreatitis. Arch Surg (Chicago, IL: 1960). 2010;145(8):764–9.
23. López-Cano M, et al. EHS clinical guidelines on the management of the abdominal wall in the context of the open or burst abdomen. Hernia. 2018;22(6):921–39.
24. Muhammad Y, Gondal KM, Khan UA. Use of the "bogota bag" for closure of open abdominal wound after exploratory laparotomy—our experience at Mayo Hospital Lahore. J Pak Med Assoc. 2016;66(8):980–3.

25. Prichayudh S, et al. Management of open abdomen with an absorbable mesh closure. Surg Today. 2011;41(1):72–8.
26. Dayton MT, et al. Use of an absorbable mesh to repair contaminated abdominal-wall defects. Arch Surg. 1986;121(8):954–60.
27. Hedderich GS, et al. The septic abdomen: open management with Marlex mesh with a zipper. Surgery. 1986;99(4):399–408.
28. Bayraktar B, et al. A retrospective analysis of early and late term complications in patients who underwent application of retention sutures for gastrointestinal tract malignancies. Ulusal cerrahi dergisi. 2015;31(1):15–9.
29. Kirkpatrick AW, et al. Active negative pressure peritoneal therapy after abbreviated laparotomy: the intraperitoneal vacuum randomized controlled trial. Ann Surg. 2015;262(1):38–46.
30. Nemec HM, et al. Wittmann patch: superior closure for the open abdomen. Am Surg. 2020;86(8):981–4.
31. Fortelny RH, et al. Delayed closure of open abdomen in septic patients is facilitated by combined negative pressure wound therapy and dynamic fascial suture. Surg Endosc. 2014;28(3):735–40.
32. Hofmann AT, et al. Delayed closure of open abdomen in septic patients treated with negative pressure vacuum therapy and dynamic sutures: a 10-years follow-up on long-term complications. Front Surg. 2020;7:611905.
33. Petersson P, Petersson U. Dynamic fascial closure with vacuum-assisted wound closure and mesh-mediated fascial traction (VAWCM) treatment of the open abdomen-an updated systematic review. Front Surg. 2020;7:577104.
34. Berrevoet F, et al. Early initiation of a standardized open abdomen treatment with vacuum assisted mesh-mediated fascial traction achieves best results. Front Surg. 2020;7:606539.
35. Cristaudo A, et al. Complications and mortality associated with temporary abdominal closure techniques: a systematic review and meta-analysis. Am Surg. 2017;83(2):191–216.
36. Acosta S, et al. Multicentre prospective study of fascial closure rate after open abdomen with vacuum and mesh-mediated fascial traction. Br J Surg. 2011;98(5):735–43.
37. Schaaf S, et al. Use of a visceral protective layer prevents fistula development in open abdomen therapy: results from the European Hernia Society Open Abdomen Registry. Br J Surg. 2023;
38. Willms AG, et al. The significance of visceral protection in preventing enteroatmospheric fistulae during open abdomen treatment in patients with secondary peritonitis: a propensity score-matched case-control analysis. Ann Surg. 2021;273(6):1182–8.
39. Coccolini F, et al. The open abdomen in trauma and non-trauma patients: WSES guidelines. World J Emerg Surg. 2018;13(1):7.
40. Jacobs R. We asked the experts: modified mesh-mediated fascial traction in the management of the open abdomen. World J Surg. 2023;47(1):103–5.
41. Sartelli M, et al. Complicated intra-abdominal infections worldwide: the definitive data of the CIAOW Study. World J Emerg Surg. 2014;9:37.
42. Kirkpatrick AW, et al. Closed or open after source control laparotomy for severe complicated intra-abdominal sepsis (the COOL trial): study protocol for a randomized controlled trial. World J Emerg Surg. 2018;13:26.
43. Inukai K, et al. Open abdominal management for perforative peritonitis with septic shock: a retrospective analysis on usefulness of a standardized treatment protocol. Eur J Trauma Emerg Surg. 2021;47(1):93–8.
44. Prete F, et al. Retrospective study of indications and outcomes of open abdomen with negative pressure wound therapy technique for abdominal sepsis in a tertiary referral centre. Antibiotics (Basel, Switzerland). 2022;11(11)
45. Coccolini F, et al. IROA: International Register of Open Abdomen, preliminary results. World J Emerg Surg. 2017;12:10.
46. Di Saverio S, et al. Classification, prevention and management of entero-atmospheric fistula: a state-of-the-art review. Langenbeck's Arch Surg. 2016;401(1):1–13.

47. Pereira B, et al. Entero-atmospheric fistula migration: a new management alternative for complex septic open abdomen. Anaesthesiol Intensive Ther. 2020;52(1):56–62.
48. Kritayakirana K, et al. Outcomes and complications of open abdomen technique for managing non-trauma patients. J Emerg Trauma Shock. 2010;3(2):118–22.
49. Lim EC, Seet RC. Botulinum toxin: description of injection techniques and examination of controversies surrounding toxin diffusion. Acta Neurol Scand. 2008;117(2):73–84.
50. Zendejas B, et al. Outcomes of chemical component paralysis using botulinum toxin for incisional hernia repairs. World J Surg. 2013;37(12):2830–7.
51. Soltanizadeh S, Helgstrand F, Jorgensen LN. Botulinum toxin a as an adjunct to abdominal wall reconstruction for incisional hernia. Plastic Reconstruct Surg Global Open. 2017;5(6):e1358.
52. Zielinski MD, et al. Chemical components separation with botulinum toxin A: a novel technique to improve primary fascial closure rates of the open abdomen. Hernia. 2013;17(1):101–7.
53. Laurens JR, Foster A, Hardley A. Closing difficult laparostomies with the aid of botulinum toxin A: an audit of 12 cases. Cureus. 2021;13(3):e14066.
54. Zielinski MD, et al. Botulinum toxin A-induced paralysis of the lateral abdominal wall after damage-control laparotomy: a multi-institutional, prospective, randomized, placebo-controlled pilot study. J Trauma Acute Care Surg. 2016;80(2):237–42.
55. Fung S, et al. Vertical traction device prevents abdominal wall retraction and facilitates early primary fascial closure of septic and non-septic open abdomen. Langenbeck's Arch Surg. 2022;407(5):2075–83.
56. Eickhoff R, et al. A new device to prevent fascial retraction in the open abdomen—proof of concept in vivo. BMC Surg. 2019;19(1):82.

Chapter 26
Acute Mesenteric Ischaemia: Imaging and Intervention

Lucy Rose Howroyd, Ben Hawthorn, Nirav Patel, and Lakshmi Ratnam

Abbreviations

AF	Atrial fibrillation
AMI	Acute mesenteric ischaemia
CMI	Chronic mesenteric ischaemia
CT	Computed tomography
CTA	Computed tomography angiography
DVT	Deep vein thrombus
FMD	Fibromuscular dysplasia
IMA	Inferior mesenteric artery
MAE	Mesenteric arterial embolism
MAT	Mesenteric arterial thrombus
MRA	Magnetic resonance angiography
MRI	Magnetic resonance imaging
MVT	Mesenteric venous thrombus
NOMI	Non-occlusive mesenteric ischaemia
PE	Pulmonary embolus
ROMS	Retrograde open mesenteric stenting
SMA	Superior mesenteric artery

L. R. Howroyd · B. Hawthorn · N. Patel · L. Ratnam (✉)
Department of Radiology, St George's University Hospitals NHS Foundation Trust, London, UK
e-mail: rose.howroyd@nhs.net; b.hawthorn@nhs.net; nirav.patel@stgeorges.nhs.uk; lakshmi.ratnam@stgeorges.nhs.uk

© The Author(s), under exclusive license to Springer Nature Switzerland AG 2024

J. Faintuch, S. Faintuch (eds.), *Recent Strategies in High Risk Surgery*,
https://doi.org/10.1007/978-3-031-56270-9_26

Introduction

Acute Mesenteric Ischaemia (AMI) is a clinical emergency in which there is a sudden and significant reduction of blood flow to the bowel, leading to ischaemic injury, risking infarction and intestinal necrosis. Irrespective of the cause of the reduced intestinal blood flow, without adequate arterial blood supply the bowel will infarct, with potentially catastrophic consequences, leading to bowel perforation, septic shock and ultimately death.

Whilst AMI is not common, accounting for approximately 0.09–0.2% of acute admissions to emergency departments [1], and around 1% of patients with an acute abdomen [2], it is a highly morbid condition. The prevalence of AMI increases with age, significant co-morbidities and a poorer baseline performance status [3–5] AMI has been cited as the cause of an acute abdomen in up to 10% of patients over 70 [2].

Despite improvement in diagnosis and treatment options in recent decades, the reported mortality rates can reach up to 50% [4], and it is ranked as the fifth most common cause of death globally in patients presenting with emergency surgical conditions [6]. Mortality approaches 100% if treatment is delayed by more than 24 h [2, 7, 8].

Aetiologies of Ischaemia

In the obstructive cases, there is a blockage in either the artery supplying or vein draining the affected segment of bowel. Examples include mesenteric arterial embolism (MAE), mesenteric arterial thrombus (MAT) or mesenteric venous thrombosis (MVT). In the absence of a physical occlusion, it arises instead because of prolonged and severe mesenteric arterial spasm, or as a consequence of diminished regional blood flow. This entity is called non-occlusive mesenteric ischaemia (NOMI) and whilst the pathophysiology is poorly understood, it is a well-recognised complication of severe systemic illness.

Normal Arterial and Venous Anatomy

The coeliac artery arises anteriorly from the abdominal aorta just below the diaphragm at the T12 level. It supplies the stomach and duodenum to the level of the ampulla of Vater in the second segment. It also supplies the liver, gallbladder, spleen, pancreas, greater and lesser omentum. Although not directly involved with the intestine, it can supply some flow by means or arcades and collateral vessels (Fig. 26.1a).

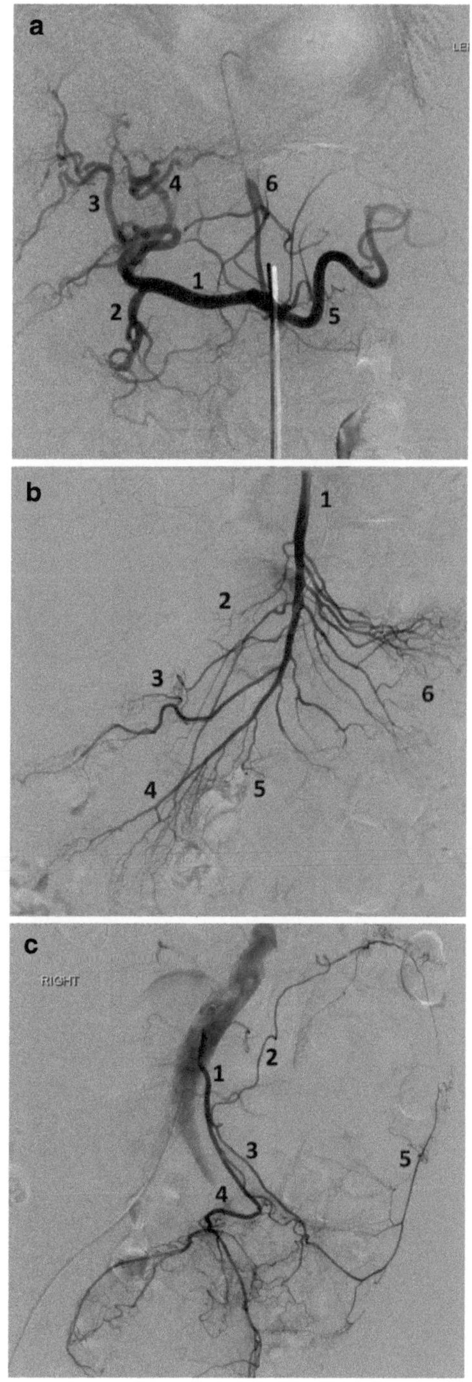

Fig. 26.1 Mesenteric arterial anatomy. (**a**) Selective digital subtraction angiogram of celiac axis. 1. Common hepatic artery. 2. Gastroduodenal artery. 3. Right hepatic artery. 4. Left hepatic artery. 5. Splenic artery. 6. Left gastric artery. (**b**) Selective digital subtraction angiogram of superior mesenteric artery. 1. Proximal superior mesenteric artery. 2. Middle colic artery. 3. Right colic artery. 4. Ileocolic artery. 5. Ileal branches. 6. Jejunal branches. (**c**) Selective digital subtraction angiogram of inferior mesenteric artery. 1. Proximal inferior mesenteric artery. 2. Left colic artery. 3. Sigmoid arteries. 4. Superior rectal artery. 5. Marginal artery of Drummond

The SMA arises anteriorly from the abdominal aorta, just below the coeliac artery, at around the level of L1. It has the widest calibre of the three arteries and its downwards sloping angle of origin makes it the most susceptible to embolic occlusion. The SMA supplies the duodenum from the ampulla of Vater to the distal third of the transverse colon. Numerous branches arise from the SMA to supply the bowel, and these form anastomotic arcades in the mesentery. From these arcades, the vasa recta arise which directly supply the ileal and jejunal walls. There are fewer jejunal arterial arcades, making the jejunum more vulnerable to ischaemic injury compared to the ileum (Fig. 26.1b).

The IMA has the smallest calibre of the three major arteries and arises from the anterior abdominal aorta at the level of L3. It supplies the distal two-thirds of the transverse colon, the descending and sigmoid colon, and supplies the upper two-thirds of the **rectum** (Fig. 26.1c). The marginal artery of Drummond along the large bowel can also be helpful in circumstances of embolism or stenoses.

Anatomical Variants

Both the SMA and coeliac artery can arise as a single trunk from the aorta (coeliacomesenteric trunk), or the SMA can arise from the common hepatic artery. The Arc of Riolan is a possibility for collateral flow in the event of occlusion, and in these cases, the splenic flexure can be spared [9].

Venous Anatomy

The portal venous system and the inferior vena cava should be considered. The portal venous system transports nutrient rich blood from the bowel to the liver for processing. At the level of the bowel, the veins are paired in the mesentery with the arteries. The SMV and splenic vein converge at the portovenous or portomesenteric confluence and form the portal vein.

General Pathophysiology of AMI

The development of AMI depends on several factors, including how many vessels are involved, the level at which the vascular occlusion occurs, the quality of the available arterial collateral network, and crucially, the duration of interrupted arterial supply. Ischaemic injury develops when there is insufficient delivery of oxygen and nutrients required to support cellular metabolism. The bowel is thought to be able to tolerate major reduction in mesenteric blood flow for up to 3 h without substantial injury [10, 11].

In the initial stages of hypoxic injury, the mucosa is affected first and if the vascular obstruction is relieved rapidly, injured cells may recover. If the hypoxia persists, the submucosa, muscularis propria and eventually serosa become involved, with oedema, haemorrhage and necrosis occurring. Once the muscularis is affected, the ischaemia is called transmural and is irreversible. This can occur in as little as 6 h in cases of complete vascular obstruction [12]. Once the bowel wall is infarcted, bacterial translocation leads to gangrene, peritonitis, sepsis and multi-organ failure.

The most important prognostic factor is the duration of inadequate blood supply [13]. Therefore rapid diagnosis and effective intervention are fundamental to an improved outcome.

General Management Principles

The management of AMI is primarily focussed on restoring adequate blood flow to the mesenteric vessels and treating any identifiable underlying causes. Adequate resuscitation and anticoagulation if appropriate are early steps in any case.

With the advent and continuing evolution of image-guided endovascular procedures, the open surgery is not obligatory anymore, as treatment options are expanding.

Mesenteric Arterial Embolism (MAE)

This is the most common cause of AMI, accounting for approximately 33–50% of cases [4, 14]. The most common origin of the emboli is cardiac, with around 50% of patients presenting with MAE having atrial fibrillation (AF) [8]. Related risk factors include recent myocardial infarct, known cardiac thrombi, mitral valve disease and previous embolic disease.

Pathophysiology

Due to its wide calibre and narrow take off angle from the aorta, the SMA is particularly vulnerable to embolic events. Usually, the embolus lodges in the proximal SMA approximately 3–10 cm beyond the vessel origin as it tapers in calibre at around the level of the middle colic artery branch [15–17]. When this occurs, the proximal branches of the SMA remain patent and therefore the proximal jejunum remains partially perfused, whereas the distal jejunum and ileum are vulnerable to ischaemia [18, 19].

Clinical Presentation

The typical presentation is with sudden and severe abdominal pain. Nausea, vomiting, tachycardia and hypotension may ensue. Abdominal guarding and rebound tenderness suggest that bowel gangrene is already occurring.

Mesenteric Arterial Thrombus (MAT)

Accounts for approximately 25–30% of cases [4, 5], often in association with coronary artery disease, peripheral arterial disease, or diabetic arteriopathy.

Due to the chronic nature of the underlying cause, there is usually a well-established collateral arterial supply, and ischaemia usually only develops when two of the three major mesenteric arteries suffer severe stenosis or occlusion (usually the coeliac artery and SMA).

Alternatively, ischaemia can develop in the absence of complete occlusion in the setting of generalised reduction in blood flow to the bowel, for example, in states of hypotension or low cardiac output.

Given that the patients with MAT tend to be older, with multiple co-morbidities, and a larger portion of the bowel is affected, the prognosis of MAT is worse when compared to MAE [5].

Clinical Presentation

As there is a sudden obstruction to an already stenosed artery, the typical presentation is that of an acute exacerbation of pain on a background of longstanding abdominal angina. However previous angina is not obligatory, and new onset of pain can be the only evidence of the trouble.

Mesenteric Venous Thrombosis (MVT)

Incidence and Risk Factors

MVT accounts for 5–11% of cases [4, 5]. Of all the causes of AMI detailed here, this has the youngest peak age of onset. In up to 75% of these patients a background derangement is present [20].

Approximately 50% of patients have a history of previous venous thrombus, that is a deep vein thrombus (DVT) or pulmonary embolus (PE) [21]. Risk factors for venous thromboembolism in general are risk factors for MVT, such as oral contraceptive pill use and pregnancy [22]. Portal hypertension, hypercoagulable states (e.g. inherited diseases such as Factor V Leiden and antiphospholipid syndrome), intraabdominal infection, intraabdominal inflammation (e.g. pancreatitis), malignancy, and abdominal trauma or recent surgery are all common risk factors.

Pathophysiology

Propensity to thrombosis is classically attributed to a combination of Virchow's triad (stagnant flow, hypercoagulability and endothelial damage). The above risk factors/secondary causes can all be understood within this framework. Thrombosis starts in the intramural venules, vasa recta and venous arcades [20]. The SMV and ileal loops it drains are most affected, with the IMV and colon rarely affected, thought in part due to collateral flow in the pelvic systemic veins making the IMV less vulnerable.

Bowel wall oedema and luminal distention in the affected bowel are the consequence. The oedema and distention lead to increased tissue pressure and the arterial inflow is compromised, thus leading to ischaemia. MVT may not necessarily cause intestinal infarction, instead collateral venous drainage can form. Chronic venous thrombosis can lead to raised portal venous pressures (portal hypertension) and dilated venous collaterals, prone to bleeding.

Clinical Presentation

Typically, there is a subacute presentation with abdominal pain over a period of days to weeks.

Non-occlusive Mesenteric Ischaemia

NOMI accounts for 15–20% of cases of AMI [4, 5].It classically occurs in critically unwell or physiologically vulnerable patients. Notably, it complicates 0.5–1% of all cardiac operations [23] and heart failure is a strong risk factor. Cocaine use has also been identified in younger patients presenting with NOMI [24].

Pathophysiology

NOMI used to be attributed to prolonged and severe mesenteric arterial spasm; however, hypoperfusion with no spasm seems to be the major driver. This is a poorly understood phenomenon typically occurring in critically ill patients with deranged tissue perfusion. The combination of the often vulnerable physiological state of the patient with the difficulties in identifying and treating NOMI effectively lead to a mortality rate of NOMI of around 50% [25, 26].

Presentation

NOMI is difficult to identify as patients are usually already very unwell or post surgical, and as such are likely intubated and ventilated, unable to communicate any symptoms, and the signs can be masked. It should be suspected in any critically unwell patient with a sudden and unexpected deterioration. If the patient is conscious, this may be in the form of nonspecific pain, bloating and nausea and acute confusion. If the patient is sedated, the warning signs include an unexplained metabolic acidosis and need for more inotropic support.

Other Causes of AMI

Arterial Dissection

Approximately 5% of patients with an aortic dissection develop AMI [4, 27].

Fibromuscular Dysplasia (FMD)

FMD is a rare but well-recognised cause of CMI which can develop into MAT. If the patient is not known to have FMD the appearances on imaging are the same as in the more common renal artery manifestation of the disease, with a classically described 'string of beads' appearance to the affected arteries [28].

Inflammatory

Takayasu's arteritis and Ehlers Danlos syndrome have both been reported as causes for AMI [29, 30]. Cases of trauma, retroperitoneal fibrosis, abdominal coarctation, neurofibromatosis and post irradiation arteritis have all been identified as possible causes for AMI [27].

Diagnostic Imaging

Double or Triple-Phase CT with CT Angiography

CT can distinguish between AMI and other causes of abdominal pain, as well as demonstrate specific features of causes of AMI. Furthermore, CT is key in establishing potential options for management, in planning endovascular procedures, or identifying irreversible damage which will indicate that the situation cannot be rectified by simply restoring mesenteric blood flow and will require open surgical resection.

Contrast-Enhanced Phases

The contrast given in CT contains iodine, which absorbs X-rays differently to tissues in the body and appears denser or brighter on the acquired images, acting to highlight the vessels or organ it is in. Altering the time delay between when the contrast is given intravenously and when the CT is then acquired gives different phases of imaging.

Arterial Phase

A time delay of 20–40 s will result in an arterial phase scan, where the contrast is mainly in the abdominal aorta and mesenteric arteries. This is often known as a CT Angiogram (CTA) and in AMI will enable assessment for intravascular filling defects. In cases of AMI the sensitivity for CTA alone is as much as 93.3% and the specificity 95.9% [31].

Portal Venous Phase

If the interval between contrast administration and image acquisition is delayed to 60–90 s, the contrast bolus has had time to pass through the capillary beds and is within the mesenteric venous system. This phase provides information about end-organ perfusion and allows for assessment of venous patency.

Enteric Contrast Administration

Administration of oral or per rectum contrast has no role in suspected cases of AMI. High-density contrast in the lumen of the bowel can mask features of ischaemia.

Unenhanced/Non-contrast Phase

A possible pitfall with contrast-enhanced images is differentiating structures that are inherently dense, like calcium in atherosclerotic plaque, with iodine contrast. To differentiate between contrast and pre-existing densities, an unenhanced scan before any contrast is given is necessary. In AMI, this enables detection of vascular calcification or high-density intravascular thrombus that may be masked by contrast administration.

If these three phases are acquired in the same study, non-contrast or unenhanced, arterial and portal venous phases, this is known as a triple-phase study. The downside is that the three phases require three separate acquisitions through the scanner, and so the dose of ionising radiation is greater. Techniques such as dual-energy CT and iodine mapping can further increase accuracy in diagnosis of AMI [32].

In suspected cases of AMI, a clinical conversation with the radiologist in the vetting process facilitates appropriate protocolling of the study. A decision can be made about whether a single phase, for example, just an arterial (i.e., just a CTA) or just a portal venous phase study is sufficient to make the diagnosis, or whether a triple phase will enable more detailed conclusions to be drawn.

CT in AMI

General CT Features

Bowel wall thickening is the most common finding in AMI representing mural oedema, haemorrhage, or infection but this is not specific to AMI and is seen in other scenarios such as inflammation [33]. Importantly, not all causes of AMI result in bowel wall thickening. Indeed, in cases of complete arterial occlusion, the bowel wall can be thinned [34]. Wall thickening is most prominent in cases of MVT, and in cases of MAE and MAT wall thickening is usually only seen once the perfusion has been restored. [35]

Bowel wall enhancement patterns are variable. High density on the unenhanced phase is indicative of intramural haemorrhage. High density on the contrast-enhanced images is indicative of congestion or reperfusion. A target or halo appearance is the classical description.

Reduced bowel wall enhancement is specific, but not sensitive for ischaemia [36]. In arterial causes, decreased enhancement will occur early and is not necessarily indicative of irreversible ischaemia. Conversely, in venous causes decreased enhancement occurs late and is more indicative of irreversible ischaemia [37].

The presence of mesenteric stranding is also variable and does not correlate with the severity of ischaemia. Stranding is more prominent in MVT and NOMI, and if present in arterial causes of occlusion, it is a later sign and may indicate more advanced irreversible ischaemia [34].

Features of Advanced Ischaemia

An important role of CT is in identifying advanced and likely irreversible ischaemia. Imaging features of this are ileus, with bowel wall dilatation being the best predictor of transmural necrosis in arterial occlusions [38]. Thinning of the bowel wall indicative of muscular and neurological ischaemia is highly specific [37]. Late signs are intramural gas (pneumatosis intestinalis) and portal venous gas. Free intraperitoneal air is another late sign signifying perforation (Fig. 26.2).

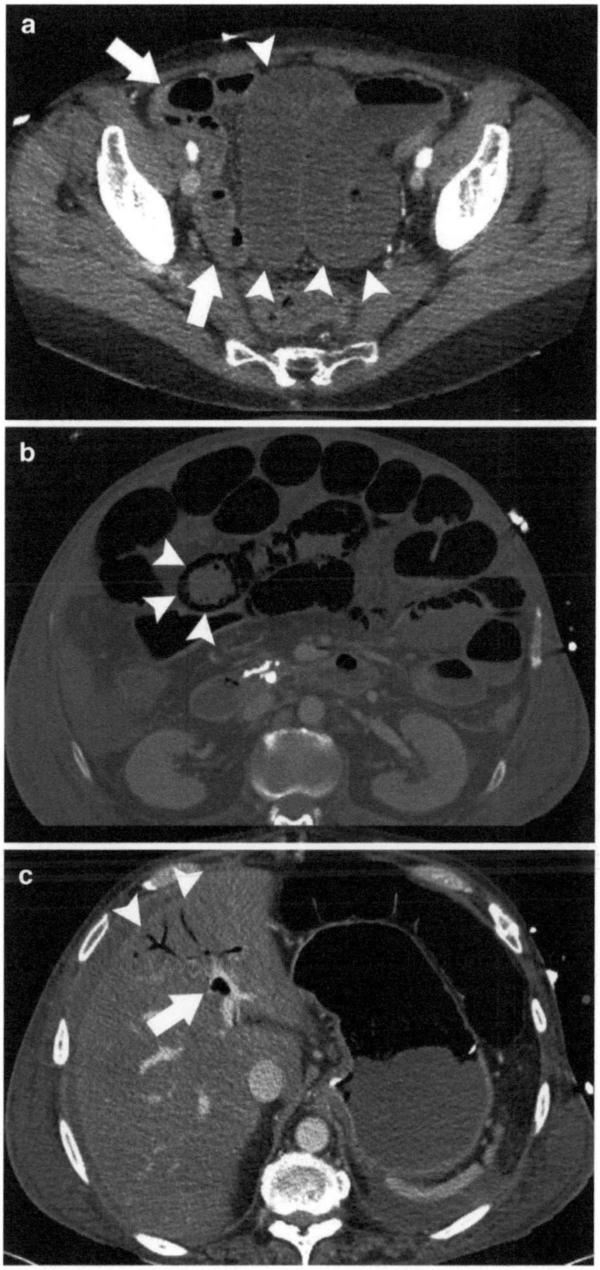

Fig. 26.2 Features of advanced mesenteric ischemia. (**a**), (**b**) and (**c**) are contrast-enhanced axial CT images. (**a**) Distended, fluid-filled small bowel loops indicating adynamic ileus (white arrowheads). These loops show absent mural enhancement and paper-thin bowel wall. Note non-distended small bowel loops in the right hemipelvis showing normal bowel wall thickness and enhancement (white arrows). (**b**) Circumferential small bowel pneumatosis (white arrowheads). (**c**) A large locule of gas within the left portal vein (white arrow) with gas-filled peripheral portal vein branches in the anterior liver (white arrowheads)

Specific Features of the Subtypes of AMI

MAE: emboli may be visualised as high-density material within the arterial lumen on the unenhanced CT, or as either luminal filling defects or an abrupt transition to completely non-opacified artery on the arterial phase CT. As described above, the SMA is the most affected vessel due to its anatomy. CT in these patients may reveal further emboli elsewhere, such as the peripheral arteries causing limb ischaemia, or in solid abdominal organs—causing hepatic, splenic, or renal infarcts. The vascular territory affected will determine the segments of bowel that are affected (Fig. 26.3).

MAT: Calcification at the ostia of the major splanchnic vessels is typical in atherosclerotic disease and can point towards MAT as a potential underlying cause. Arterial stenosis or occlusion is well-visualised in arterial phase imaging. However acute and chronic occlusion can look identical and can only be reliably distinguished if there are bowel or mesenteric changes suggestive of acute ischaemia. Additionally, the clinical picture must be considered when differentiating the two (Fig. 26.4).

MVT: In >90% of cases [39] a filling defect is evident in the portal venous system on a portal venous phase CT. Additional features include mural rim enhancement in the wall of the vein at the site of thrombus, mesenteric engorgement and ascites. Prominent bowel wall thickening reflecting marked mural oedema is not uncommon (Fig. 26.5).

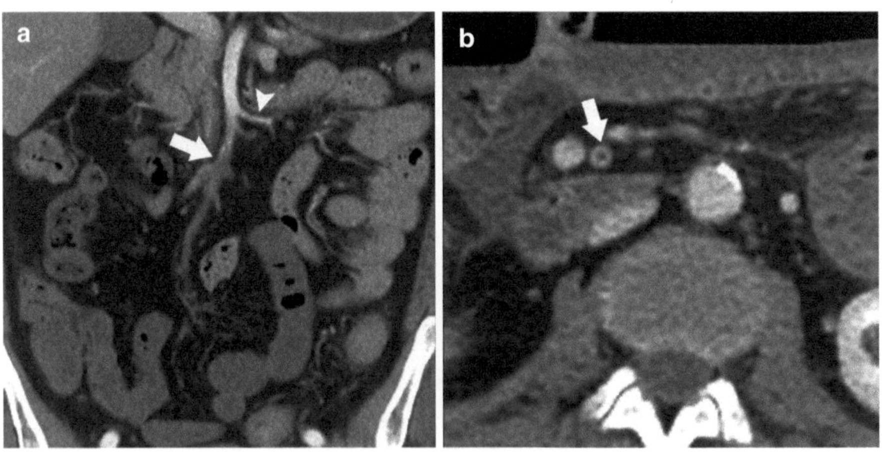

Fig. 26.3 Features of mesenteric arterial embolism. (**a**) Coronal arterial phase CT showing an occlusive filling defect within the SMA lodged at the orifice of the middle colic artery (white arrow) with poorly enhancing ileal loops in the right lower abdomen. Note that the proximal jejunal branches remain patent (white arrowhead) and the jejunal loops in the left upper abdomen have preserved normal enhancement. (**b**) Axial arterial phase CT shows a filling defect within the SMA with a characteristic peripheral rim of enhancement representing contrast between the embolus and the vessel wall (white arrow)

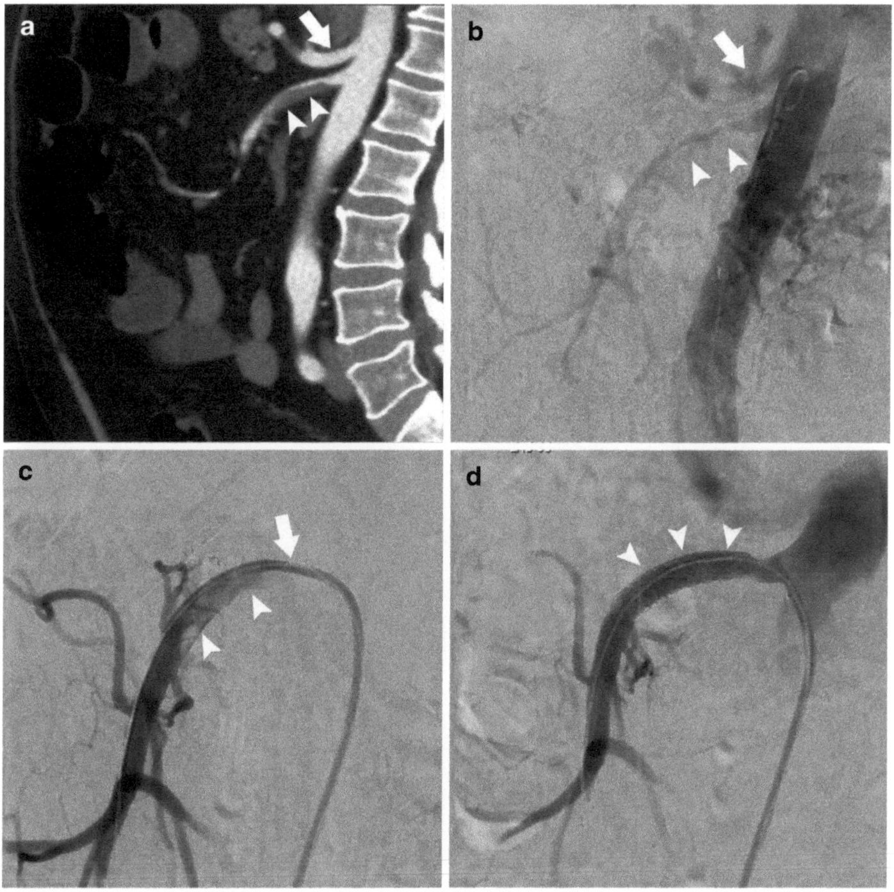

Fig. 26.4 Intervention for mesenteric arterial thrombus. (**a**) Sagittal arterial phase CT showing non-occlusive filling defect within the proximal SMA (white arrowheads). The origin of the coeliac axis is patent (white arrow). (**b**) Lateral projection digital subtraction angiogram performed via a flush catheter in the abdominal aorta. Proximal SMA non-occlusive thrombus is again demonstrated (white arrowheads). The proximal celiac axis is again shown to be patent (white arrow). (**c**) Angiogram performed after suction thrombectomy shows improved patency of proximal SMA and its branches but with residual vessel wall irregularity (white arrowheads) and an underlying stenosis in the proximal SMA (white arrow). (**d**) Completion angiogram performed following deployment of a balloon-expandable metal stent in the proximal SMA (white arrowheads) showing significantly improved vessel calibre and flow

NOMI: NOMI is a diagnosis of exclusion, and occlusive causes must be actively ruled out. Classically the distribution of the bowel ischaemia is segmental and discontinuous and there is no occlusive cause evident. Watershed areas tend to be affected first, and arterial diameters tend to be particularly small [5, 33, 34, 40].

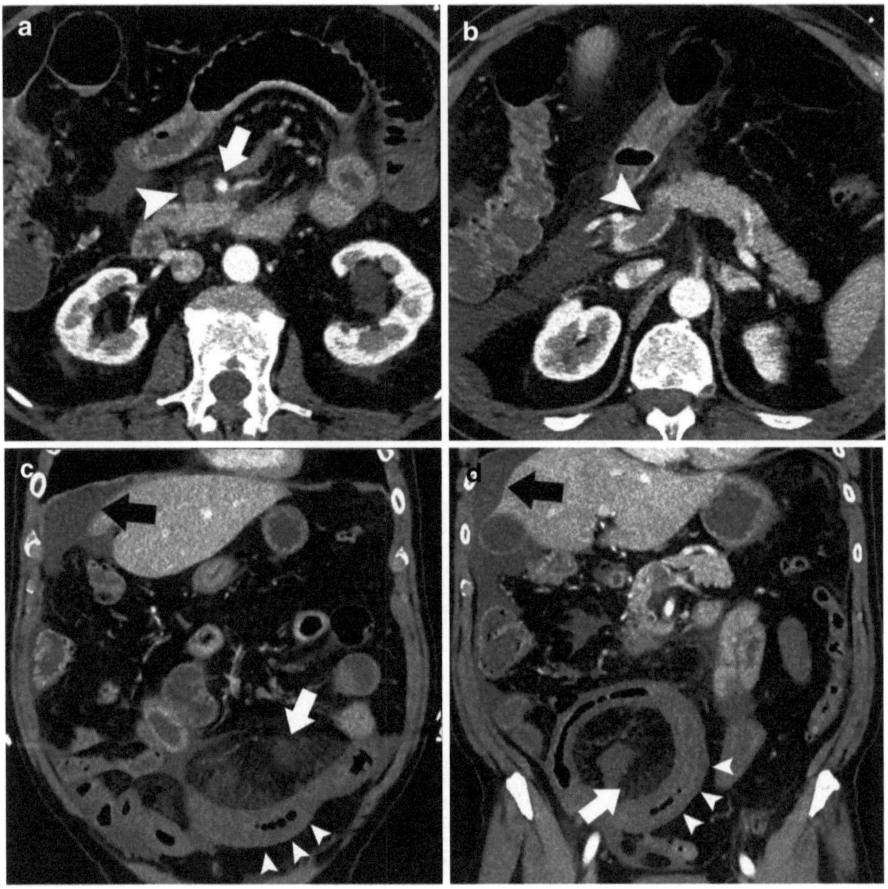

Fig. 26.5 Features of mesenteric venous thrombosis (**a**) and (**b**) are axial venous phase CT images showing filling defects within the superior mesenteric vein and portal vein (white arrowheads). Note that the SMV appears expanded when compared to the adjacent patent SMA (white arrow). (**c**) and (**d**) are coronal venous phase CT images showing prominent small bowel wall thickening with a target pattern of mural enhancement (white arrowheads). There is also extensive stranding of the mesentery and engorgement of the mesenteric veins (white arrows) and a small volume of perihepatic ascites (black arrows)

Ultrasound

Ultrasound can have a role in investigation of pregnant patients with suspected MVT (100% sensitivity, 93% specificity). [41]

Magnetic Resonance Imaging (MRI)

It can demonstrate arterial or venous occlusion with near 100% sensitivity and specificity [42, 43]. However, much of the support apparatus required for resuscitation and stabilisation of critically unwell patients cannot go into the MR scanner, the access to emergency MR imaging is limited in most centres, and the acquisition time (the time required to gather a complete set of images) is significantly longer than for CT.

There is a role in the acute management of pregnant women presenting with suspected MVT where ionising radiation (from CT) should be avoided, if possible, to protect the developing foetus [44]. However, there are some safety concerns from foetal exposure to magnetic fields with MRI.

Percutaneous Catheter Angiography

Catheter angiography is now only performed in cases in which a CT has already established that endovascular intervention is appropriate and can also be performed in suspected NOMI if there is diagnostic uncertainty.

MAE: angiograms classically show a filling defect with partial or complete occlusion of the artery (most commonly the SMA). A 'tram-track' sign can be seen where thin parallel lines of contrast are seen between the embolus and the vessel wall.

NOMI: Diffuse constriction of the mesenteric arterial branches, with a 'string of sausages' sign indicating alternate dilatation and narrowing seen in arterial spasm, is occasionally documented. Absence of any constriction is a frequent finding (Fig. 26.6).

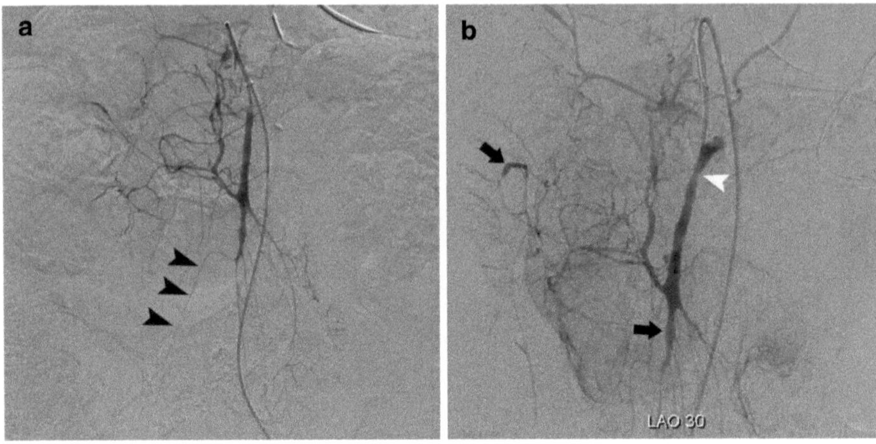

Fig. 26.6 Features of non-occlusive mesenteric ischaemia. (**a**) and (**b**) are selective digital subtraction angiograms of the SMA. There is diffuse constriction of the distal arterial branches (black arrowheads) with alternating dilatation and narrowing (black arrows) referred to as the 'string of sausages' sign. Note that there is spasm within the main SMA trunk (white arrowhead) but no gross occlusion is evident

Contribution of Interventional Radiology

Supportive Management

Initial care should include resuscitation with intravenous fluids, correction of acid-base status, pain management, nasogastric tube decompression and broad-spectrum antibiotics. Open surgery has ceased to be the first option in most circumstances. Should it be envisaged, anticoagulation with heparin is preferable, to enable easy reversal if required. In all circumstances where there is some hope of curative treatment, rapid and aggressive management is required to reduce mortality and morbidity [45].

Open Surgery or Endovascular Intervention?

The decision between open surgical approach and endovascular approach is typically governed by whether there is a suspicion that the bowel is viable or not, which is determined based on imaging findings and clinical signs of peritonism.

Open surgery has a high associated morbidity and mortality in these patients, and the patient must be fit for a general anaesthetic. Additionally, surgical embolectomy and revascularisation can be incredibly challenging in peripheral emboli and heavily calcified atherosclerotic vessels. If the patient has been anticoagulated, there is a risk of significant bleeding.

Endovascular Options

Endovascular treatments can be performed with local anaesthetic alone if necessary, although they often are performed under conscious sedation, meaning a general anaesthetic can be avoided in frail, comorbid, or physiologically compromised patients [45, 46]. It is important to be aware that if endovascular therapy is unsuccessful, the patient can always progress to having open surgery if necessary.

A survival of 89% in patients treated with endovascular therapy has been reported (with or without additional surgery) which is clearly a vast improvement.

The best results correspond to cases where the occlusion is less than 72 h old [47].

Technique

Endovascular treatments can be performed in the same sitting as diagnostic angiography. Digital subtraction aortography is followed by selective mesenteric angiography, including availability and patency of any collateral supply.

Direct Intra-Arterial Thrombolytic Therapy

A guidewire is manipulated across the occlusion and followed by a catheter placed into or usually just proximal to the thrombus/embolus. A bolus of thrombolytic agent can then be introduced directly through the catheter. After the initial bolus, the catheter is secured in a fixed position and a continuous infusion of thrombolytic agent is established. This requires close surveillance to ensure the catheter is not displaced and to identify any bleeding complications swiftly.

In addition to thrombolysis via the catheter, a heparin infusion is commonly administered via the arterial sheath in the groin. The rationale for this is that the systemic heparin infusion acts to treat small residual thrombi or distal embolic fragments within the more distal mesenteric arteries. Complete restoration of flow in all distal branches is not required, but rather the aim is to restore flow through enough distal vessels to ensure there is a sufficient perfusion to the bowel by the network of collaterals.

Arterial flow is rapidly re-established; however, somewhat longer treatment gives more complete clot dissolution. A limit of 48 h is widely accepted.

This is a relatively simple technique and as such often the approach chosen for frail patients in the early stages of AMI.

Risks and Complications

The main risk of any thrombolytic therapy is inadvertent bleeding. Contraindications to endovascular thrombolytic therapy are the same as in thrombolytic therapy for other thrombotic or embolic events, such as acute infarcts. Absolute contraindications include central nervous system tumours and recent haemorrhagic strokes. Relative contraindications include pregnancy, severe uncontrolled hypertension and recent major surgery.

In intra-arterial thrombolysis specifically, bleeding complications can occur at the percutaneous access site (usually the groin).

One of the most feared complications is haemorrhagic transformation of ischaemic bowel and catastrophic gastrointestinal haemorrhage. This is not common, and in fact has not been reported in SMA occlusion treatment, but gastrointestinal haemorrhage is a well-recognised complication in lower limb arterial occlusion thrombolysis [47, 48].

Another disadvantage of this technique is the long period of continuous infusion that is necessary. Reversible ischaemia may progress to irreversible ischaemia during the initial hours of therapy. Careful monitoring for peritonism is therefore advised.

It is important for the treating team to be aware that initiation of thrombolysis does not preclude surgery. If there is evidence of bowel gangrene thrombolysis can be discontinued, heparin reversed and laparotomy performed without significant delay.

Endovascular Embolectomy/Thrombectomy/Thrombo-Aspiration

An adjunct or alternative to intra-arterial thrombolytic therapy is mechanical thrombus fragmentation to reduce the embolic mass more rapidly and achieve arterial reperfusion more quickly (Fig. 26.4c).

The benefits of these approaches are that the dose and time necessary for the thrombolytic infusion is reduced, and thus the risk of bleeding complications are also reduced. After removal of the clot, treatment of any underlying stenosis can be performed in the same procedure.

Techniques

Techniques for fragmentation include use of a wire, using an angioplasty balloon and specialised thrombectomy devices which work via endovascular vacuum aspiration of the clot fragments.

Angioplasty and Stenting

Endovascular treatment should be the first line option in cases of MAT where there is an underlying vascular stenosis (provided there are no clinical or radiological features of irreversible ischaemia) [49, 50] (Fig. 26.4d).

Techniques

Following angiography, a guidewire is manipulated across the stenosis. Predilatation angioplasty using a balloon is usually performed, followed by deployment of a stent across the stenotic segment.

Retrograde Open Mesenteric Stenting (ROMS)

Heavy calcification of the aortic wall, origin of the mesenteric artery (e.g., SMA) and stenotic segment can sometimes mean attempts at recanalisation from an antegrade endovascular approach are not possible. In these cases, a surgical recanalisation can be considered. ROMS is a hybrid technique combining endovascular and open surgical approaches. Via a midline laparotomy, the SMA is exposed and punctured distally, retrograde angiography is performed, and a wire is used to cross the occlusion before a stent is deployed. In the same procedure, non-viable bowel can be resected.

Risks and Complications

Complications of these techniques include distal embolisation of thrombus fragments. Thrombo-aspiration and/or thrombolysis used as adjuncts may help to reduce the risk of distal embolisation. Other complications are those associated with any arterial manipulation (e.g. arterial dissection, rupture and occlusion) or those associated with any arterial stent use (e.g. stent migration, intimal hyperplasia and re-stenosis).

Direct Intra-Arterial Vasodilator Therapy (NOMI)

Following angiography, a wire and catheter are manipulated into the proximal segments of the affected artery (usually the SMA). A direct bolus of a vasodilator can then be injected through the catheter and a slow infusion initiated. This infusion runs for approximately 24 h. Vasodilator agents used for this include prostaglandin E1 and papaverine. Results in small studies suggest a significant reduction in mortality when compared to conservative management alone [51].

Venous Endovascular Techniques

In patients with MVT who deteriorate while on systemic anticoagulation, a more aggressive treatment may be necessary to restore the venous flow [52].

Techniques

Endovascular techniques to access the mesenteric veins include placement of a trans-jugular intrahepatic portosystemic shunt (TIPS) or percutaneous transhepatic access to a portal vein branch. Few groups advocate access via a surgically placed SMV catheter.

Once access is obtained to the mesenteric veins, mechanical thrombo-aspiration and thrombolysis can be combined to restore flow (in a similar way to the arterial techniques described above). Additionally, if there is any residual venous stenosis, this can be treated with balloon venoplasty, and even stenting if necessary. Another less-effective alternative is to administer indirect thrombolysis via an intra-arterial catheter (i.e. a catheter placed in the SMA).

Limitations to an Endovascular Approach

Specialist Knowledge and Logistics: To ensure the best management strategy is created for individual patients, a multidisciplinary approach is required, including input from vascular surgeons, general surgeons and interventional radiologists. Additionally, the specialised operating suites where endovascular procedures can be performed must be available. Smaller hospitals typically lack the facilities and the specialists.

Data Analysis: Caution is needed when comparing the outcomes in endovascular techniques and traditional open surgical techniques. There is no prospective randomised data comparing the two, and there is an inherent selection bias as endovascular revascularisation is suitable only for the patients without irreversible ischaemia.

Reperfusion Injury

Reperfusion injury is a worrying consequence of both open surgical and endovascular revascularisation. The exact mechanism is unclear but occurs when blood supply is restored to the bowel after a period of ischaemia. It involves release of free oxygen radicals and neutrophil activation causing additional cell injury and local inflammation. The consequences can be catastrophic, leading to bowel necrosis, pancreatitis and multi-organ failure [10, 53].

Reperfusion injury is difficult to distinguish from incomplete treatment and ongoing persistent ischaemia. Post procedural CT is recommended if there are any concerning clinical symptoms after revascularisation. These include abdominal pain and bloody diarrhoea—which could be indicative of persistent ischaemia or could be due to reperfusion injury. C-reactive protein levels rising post treatment have also been described as a sensitive (but not particularly specific) marker of reperfusion injury [54].

The CT features are thickened bowel wall, oedema of the submucosa, and fat stranding or free fluid adjacent to the affected bowel segment. Additional features are venous dilatation in the mesentery of the affected segment and luminal haemorrhage (seen best on the unenhanced phase).

Conclusions

Establishing dedicated tertiary centres offering multidisciplinary emergency revascularisation based on the stroke unit model has been shown to improve outcomes for patients [55].

Peritonitis is well-recognised as a clinical marker of bowel infarction in AMI, and currently used to differentiate whether a patient is suitable for endovascular therapy or open surgery. However, this may change in future guidelines, with one study showing that peritoneal irritation is not a significant predictive factor for irreversible necrosis in AMI [35], and another showing that up to 86% of patients with peritonitis on clinical examination had reversible ischaemia during their subsequent operation [56]. If imaging features alone are utilised, many more patients would initially undergo the less-invasive endovascular procedures which do not preclude surgical intervention if still required.

References

1. Bala M, Catena F, Kashuk J, De Simone B, Gomes CA, Weber D, Sartelli M, Coccolini F, Kluger Y, Abu-Zidan FM, Picetti E, Ansaloni L, Augustin G, Biffl WL, Ceresoli M, Chiara O, Chiarugi M, Coimbra R, Cui Y, Damaskos D, Di Saverio S, Galante JM, Khokha V, Kirkpatrick AW, Inaba K, Leppäniemi A, Litvin A, Peitzman AB, Shelat VG, Sugrue M, Tolonen M, Rizoli S, Sall I, Beka SG, Di Carlo I, Ten Broek R, Mircea C, Tebala G, Pisano M, van Goor H, Maier RV, Jeekel H, Civil I, Hecker A, Tan E, Søreide K, Lee MJ, Wani I, Bonavina L, Malangoni MA, Koike K, Velmahos GC, Fraga GP, Fette A, de'Angelis N, Balogh ZJ, Scalea TM, Sganga G, Kelly MD, Khan J, Stahel PF, Moore EE. Acute mesenteric ischemia: updated guidelines of the World Society of Emergency Surgery. World J Emerg Surg. 2022;17(1):1–54.
2. Klar E, Rahmanian PB, Bücker A, Hauenstein K, Jauch K, Luther B. Acute mesenteric ischemia: a vascular emergency. Deut Ärztebl Int. 2012;109(14):249–56.
3. Fuglseth H, Søreide K, Vetrhus M. Acute mesenteric ischaemia. Br J Surg. 2023;110(9):1030–4.
4. Tamme K, Reintam Blaser A, Laisaar K, Mändul M, Kals J, Forbes A, Kiss O, Acosta S, Bjørck M, Starkopf J. Incidence and outcomes of acute mesenteric ischaemia: a systematic review and meta-analysis. BMJ Open. 2022;12(10):e062846.
5. Hawthorn BR, Ratnam LA. Acute mesenteric ischaemia: imaging and intervention. Clin Radiol. 2020;75(5):398.e19.
6. Stewart B, Khanduri P, McCord C, Ohene-Yeboah M, Uranues S, Vega Rivera F, Mock C. Global disease burden of conditions requiring emergency surgery. Br J Surg. 2014;101(1):e9–e22.
7. Bordet M, Tresson P, Huvelle U, Long A, Passot G, Bergoin C, Lermusiaux P, Millon A, Della Schiava N. Natural history of asymptomatic superior mesenteric arterial stenosis depends on coeliac and inferior mesenteric artery status. Eur J Vasc Endovasc Surg. 2021;61(5):810–8.

8. Magnus L, Lejay A, Philouze G, Chakfe N, Collange O, Thaveau F, Georg Y. Mortality and delays of management of acute mesenteric ischemia: the need of a dedicated program. Ann Vasc Surg. 2022;
9. Silva NGO, Barbosa ABM, Silva NA, Araújo DN, Assis TO. Anatomical variations of the superior mesenteric artery and its clinical and surgical implications in humans. ABCD. 2020;33(2):e1508.
10. Strand-Amundsen RJ, Reims HM, Reinholt FP, Ruud TE, Yang R, Høgetveit JO, Tønnessen TI. Ischemia/reperfusion injury in porcine intestine—viability assessment. World J Gastroenterol. 2018;24(18):2009–23.
11. Clarysse M, Dubois A, Vanuytsel T, Pirenne J, Ceulemans LJ. Potential options to expand the intestinal donor pool: a comprehensive review. Curr Opin Organ Transplant. 2022;27(2):106.
12. Gonzalez LM, Stewart AS, Freund J, Kucera CR, Dekaney CM, Magness ST, Blikslager AT. Preservation of reserve intestinal epithelial stem cells following severe ischemic injury. Am J Physiol Gastrointest Liver Physiol. 2019;316(4):G482–94.
13. Luther B, Mamopoulos A, Lehmann C, Klar E. The ongoing challenge of acute mesenteric ischemia. Visceral Medicine. 2018;34(3):217–23.
14. Kärkkäinen JM. Acute mesenteric ischemia: a challenge for the acute care surgeon. Scand J Surg. 2021;110(2):150–8.
15. Gore RM, Yaghmai V, Thakrar KH, Berlin JW, Mehta UK, Newmark GM, Miller FH. Imaging in intestinal ischemic disorders. Radiol Clin North Am. 2008;46(5):845–75.
16. Herbert GS, Steele SR. Acute and chronic mesenteric ischemia. Surg Clin North Am. 2007;87(5):1115–34.
17. Schoots IG, Koffeman GI, Legemate DA, Levi M, van Gulik TM. Systematic review of survival after acute mesenteric ischaemia according to disease aetiology. Br J Surg. 2004;91(1):17–27.
18. Kärkkäinen JM. Acute mesenteric ischemia in elderly patients. Expert Rev Gastroenterol Hepatol. 2016;10(9):985–8.
19. Lawson RM. Mesenteric ischemia. Crit Care Nurs Clin North Am. 2018;30(1):29–39.
20. Demelo-Rodríguez P, Ordieres-Ortega L, Oblitas CM. Mesenteric venous thrombosis. Med Clin (Barc). 2023;160(9):400–6.
21. Cangemi JR, Picco MF. Intestinal ischemia in the elderly. Gastroenterol Clin North Am. 2009;38(3):527–40.
22. Ozturk G, Aydinli B, Atamanalp SS, Yildirgan MI, Özoğul B, Kısaoğlu A. Acute mesenteric ischemia in young adults. Wien Med Woch. 2012;162(15–16):349–53.
23. Bourcier S, Klug J, Nguyen LS. Non-occlusive mesenteric ischemia: diagnostic challenges and perspectives in the era of artificial intelligence. World J Gastroenterol. 2021;27(26):4088–103.
24. Veloso Costa A, Zhunus A, Hafeez R, Gupta A. Cocaine-induced mesenteric ischaemia requiring small bowel resection. BMJ Case Rep. 2021;14(1):e238593.
25. Yu H, Kirkpatrick IDC. An update on acute mesenteric ischemia. Can Assoc Radiol J. 2023;74(1):160–71.
26. Adaba F, Askari A, Dastur J, Patel A, Gabe SM, Vaizey CJ, Faiz O, Nightingale JMD, Warusavitarne J. Mortality after acute primary mesenteric infarction: a systematic review and meta-analysis of observational studies Colorec Dis. 2015;17(7):566–77.
27. Shih MP, Hagspiel KD. CTA and MRA in mesenteric ischemia: Part 1: Role in diagnosis and differential diagnosis. Am J Roentgenol. 2007;188(2):452–61.
28. Du S, Yang S, Jia K, Du P, Zhang L, Wang J. Fibromuscular dysplasia of mesenteric arteries: a rare cause of multiple bowel resections-a case report and literature review. BMC Gastroenterol. 2021;21(1):133.
29. Mehta R, Deepak JA, Shine R, Balakrishnan. Takayasu arteritis presenting as chronic mesenteric ischemia. Ind J Gastroenterol. 2004;23(2):73–4.
30. Skeik N, Smith J, Olson SL, Lohese OL, Mirza A, Manunga J. Mesenteric artery dissection and wall-thickening, case study and general review. Angiology. 2023;74(1):7–21.
31. Menke J. Diagnostic accuracy of multidetector CT in acute mesenteric ischemia: systematic review and meta-analysis. Radiology. 2010;256(1):93–101.

32. Lourenco PDM, Rawski R, Mohammed MF, Khosa F, Nicolaou S, McLaughlin P. Dual-energy CT iodine mapping and 40-keV monoenergetic applications in the diagnosis of acute bowel ischemia. Am J Roentgenol. 2018;211(3):564–70.
33. Kanasaki S, Furukawa A, Fumoto K, Hamanaka Y, Ota S, Hirose T, Inoue A, Shirakawa T, Hung Nguyen LD, Tulyeubai S. Acute mesenteric ischemia: multidetector CT findings and endovascular management. Radiographics. 2018;38(3):945–61.
34. Furukawa A, Kanasaki S, Kono N, Wakamiya M, Tanaka T, Takahashi M, Murata K. CT Diagnosis of acute mesenteric ischemia from various causes. Am J Roentgenol. 2009;192(2):408–16.
35. Nuzzo A, Maggiori L, Ronot M, Becq A, Plessier A, Gault N, Joly F, Castier Y, Vilgrain V, Paugam C, Panis Y, Bouhnik Y, Cazals-Hatem D, Corcos O. Predictive factors of intestinal necrosis in acute mesenteric ischemia: prospective study from an intestinal stroke center. Am J Gastroenterol. 2017;112(4):597–605.
36. Schieda N, Fasih N, Shabana W. Triphasic CT in the diagnosis of acute mesenteric ischaemia. Eur Radiol. 2013;23(7):1891–900.
37. Zeng Y, Yang F, Hu X, Zhu F, Chen W, Lin W. Radiological predictive factors of transmural intestinal necrosis in acute mesenteric ischemia: systematic review and meta-analysis. Eur Radiol. 2023;33(4):2792–9.
38. Calame P, Grillet F, Delabrousse E. Reply to "Small-bowel dilatation is the most consistent feature of transmural intestinal necrosis". Am J Roentgenol. 2020;215(4):W43.
39. Zarrouk M, Salim S, Elf J, Gottsäter A, Acosta S. Testing for thrombophilia in mesenteric venous thrombosis—retrospective original study and systematic review. Best Pract Res Clin Gastroenterol. 2017;31(1):39–48.
40. Bagnacci G, Guerrini S, Gentili F, Sordi A, Mazzei FG, Pozzessere C, Guazzi G, Mura G, Savelli V, D'Amico S, Calomino N, Volterrani L, Mazzei MA. Non-occlusive mesenteric ischemia (NOMI) and prognostic signs at CT: reperfusion or not reperfusion that is the question. Abd Imag. 2022;47(5):1603–13.
41. Hauenstein K, Li Y. Radiological diagnosis of portal/mesenteric vein occlusion. Visc Med. 2014;30(6):382–7.
42. Alzubaidi S, Patel I, Saini A, Knuttinen G, Naidu S, Kriegshuaser S, Albadawi H, Oklu R. Current concepts in portal vein thrombosis: etiology, clinical presentation and management. Abdom Radiol (NY). 2019;44(10):3453–62.
43. Michaely HJ, Dietrich O, Nael K, Weckbach S, Reiser MF, Schoenberg SO. MRA of abdominal vessels: technical advances. Eur Radiol. 2006;16(8):1637–50.
44. Zachariah SK, Fenn M, Jacob K, Arthungal SA, Zachariah SA. 'Management of acute abdomen in pregnancy: current perspectives. Int J Wom Health. 2019;11:119–34.
45. Kougias P, Lau D, El Sayed HF, Zhou W, Huynh TT, Lin PH. Determinants of mortality and treatment outcome following surgical interventions for acute mesenteric ischemia. J Vasc Surg. 2007;46(3):467–74.
46. Gnanapandithan K, Feuerstadt P. Mesenteric ischemia. Curr Gastroenterol Rep. 2020;22(4):17.
47. Schoots IG, Levi MM, Reekers JA, Lameris JS, van Gulik TM. Thrombolytic therapy for acute superior mesenteric artery occlusion. J Vasc Interv Radiol. 2005;16(3):317–29.
48. Darwood R, Berridge DC, Kessel DO, Robertson I, Forster R, Berridge DC. Surgery versus thrombolysis for initial management of acute limb ischaemia. Cochrane Datab Syst Rev. 2018;2018(8):CD002784.
49. Tilsed JV, Casamassima A, Kurihara H, Mariani D, Martinez I, Pereira J, Ponchietti L, Shamiyeh A, Al-Ayoubi F, Barco LA, Ceolin M, D'Almeida AJ, Hilario S, Olavarria AL, Ozmen MM, Pinheiro LF, Poeze van Bokhoven M, Triantos G, Fuentes FT, Sierra SU, Soreide K, Yanar H. ESTES guidelines: acute mesenteric ischaemia. Eur J Trauma Emerg Surg. 2016;42(2):253–70.
50. Acosta S, Björck M. Modern treatment of acute mesenteric ischaemia. Br J Surg. 2014;101(1):e100–8.

51. Winzer R, Fedders D, Backes M, Ittermann T, Gründling M, Mensel B, Held H, Kromrey M, Weitz J, Hoffmann R, Bülow R, Kühn J. Local intra-arterial vasodilator infusion in non-occlusive mesenteric ischemia significantly increases survival rate. Cardiovasc Interv Radiol. 2020;43(8):1148–55.
52. Di Minno MND, Milone F, Milone M, Iaccarino V, Venetucci P, Lupoli R, Sosa Fernandez LM, Di Minno G. Endovascular thrombolysis in acute mesenteric vein thrombosis: a 3-year follow-up with the rate of short and long-term sequaelae in 32 patients. Thromb Res. 2010;126(4):295–8.
53. Yoshitomi T, Nagasaki Y. Self-assembling antioxidants for ischemia-reperfusion injuries. Antioxid Redox Signal. 2022;36(1–3):70–80.
54. Garzelli L, Nuzzo A, Hamon A, Ben Abdallah I, Gregory J, Raynaud L, Paulatto L, Dioguardi Burgio M, Castier Y, Panis Y, Vilgrain V, Corcos O, Ronot M. Reperfusion injury on computed tomography following endovascular revascularization of acute mesenteric ischemia: prevalence, risk factors, and patient outcome. Insights Imag. 2022;13(1):194.
55. Roussel A, Castier Y, Nuzzo A, Pellenc Q, Sibert A, Panis Y, Bouhnik Yoram M, Corcos O. Revascularization of acute mesenteric ischemia after creation of a dedicated multidisciplinary center. J Vasc Surg. 2015;62(5):1251–6.
56. Hayashi K, Hayashi K, Narita M, Tsunoda A, Kusanagi H. Still time to perform intestinal revascularization in patients with acute mesenteric ischemia with peritonitis: an analysis of bowel viability in resections. SAGE Open Med. 2020;8:2050312120923227.

Chapter 27
Options on Conservative Treatment in Acute Surgical Emergencies

Leandro Stoll Coelho, Vinicius Rocha-Santos, and Joel Faintuch

Introduction

Along surgical history, decreasing tissue damage through less invasive techniques was always on the scope of the surgeons. Approaches never dreamed before like laparoscopic surgery, image guided percutaneous procedures, angioembolizations to treat aneurisms and hemorrhage, and the cutting-edge technology of robotic assisted surgery remarkably contributed to lessen tissue damage and consequently the immune and metabolic response to trauma, with the same safety and efficacy as conventional open surgeries. The Hippocratic motto *primum non nocere* worked like a moral compass. It probably played a major role on the mental drive of surgeons committed to good medical practice, pushing toward the use of minimally invasive techniques, in order to keep risks and complications at bay.

Can we go further and take one more step into non-invasiveness? Is there any more room for conservative treatment within contexts in which surgery would be first choice? High-definition imaging devices like CT scan, MRI, advanced ultrasound, and PET scan, complemented by cutting-edge PET/MRI, laser-CT scan, laser ultrasound, and

Reproduced from Acute Care Surgery in Geriatric Patients , Petrone P (ed), Springer, 2024, as granted by Springer Bookpermissions on March 31, 2023

L. S. Coelho
Regional Hospital of Registro, Sao Paulo and Regional Hospital Dr. Leopoldo Bevilacqua, Pariquera-Acu, Sao Paulo, Brazil

V. Rocha-Santos
Liver Transplantation Unit, Gastroenterology Division, University of Sao Paulo, Sao Paulo, Brazil
e-mail: vinicius.rocha@hc.fm.usp.br

J. Faintuch (✉)
Department of Gastroenterology, Sao Paulo University Medical School, Sao Paulo, Brazil
e-mail: j.faintuch@hc.fm.usp.br

© The Author(s), under exclusive license to Springer Nature Switzerland AG 2024

J. Faintuch, S. Faintuch (eds.), *Recent Strategies in High Risk Surgery*,
https://doi.org/10.1007/978-3-031-56270-9_27

Table 27.1 Conservative pathways for traditional surgical emergencies

Intensive monitoring (invasive and noninvasive)
Hemodynamic, respiratory, gastrointestinal, neurological
Clinical management
Fluid replenishment, shock management, coagulation factors, antibiotics, antacids, hormones
Interventional radiology
Drainage, embolization, stenting, clot removal
Local bleeding control
Abdominal or thoracic packing, fibrin glue, and hemostatic patches
Endoscopic maneuvers
Blood vessel sclerosis, stricture dilatation, obstruction stenting, collection drainage, visceral by-pass, fistula occluders, and sponges
Hyperbaric oxygen therapy
Refractory anaerobic infections, ischemic lesions and grafts, necrotic wounds
Other options (benign and cancerous lesions)
Radiofrequency ablation
Laser hemostasis
Cryotherapy

endoscopic ultrasound, are making it possible to access body structures with unparalleled precision and reliability, allowing the surgeon to feel more confident with periodic surveillance only. They enabled multiple conservative changes in the handling of traumatic and nontraumatic disorders of gastrointestinal, biliopancreatic, and colorectal viscera. In such circumstances the otherwise uncontested immediate surgical indication gave place to less invasive or completely conservative options (Table 27.1).

Gastroduodenal Problems

Complications of peptic ulcers such as perforation, bleeding, or obstruction have become much less common after the advent of H2 receptor antagonists and notably proton pump inhibitors, associated with wider employment of endoscopy and breath tests which increased *Helicobacter pylori* diagnosis and treatment. Medical and endoscopic treatment is nowadays, by far, the best option of treatment for peptic disease, even in the face of complications such as partial obstruction and limited hemorrhage.

Perforated Peptic Ulcer

One should admit that acute abdomen caused by ulcer perforation, although infrequent still carries serious morbidity, mainly in those with associated health conditions including the elderly patients. Surgical repair is the best option in most cases; however in selected patients conservative management is possible.

According to some sources, in 1870 Redwood reported a patient successfully treated without surgical intervention. It is true that at those early times surgical mortality was so prohibitive that not operating, although fraught with obvious danger, seemed rather natural. Yet even in the first half of the twentieth century with a number of advances in anesthesia, blood and fluid replacement, and antibacterial sulfonamide drugs, Wangensteen defended nonsurgical treatment after spontaneous healing of a perforated ulcer. Taylor first reported a series of 28 patients receiving non-operative management in 1946 naming it the Taylor method, which consisted of nasogastric aspiration, antibiotic therapy, and intravenous fluid replacement. More recently *Helicobacter Pylori* eradication was added to that therapeutic protocol [1].

The Taylor rationale is based on gastric decompression and continuous external drainage which promotes healing. Of course nutritional support was the weak point, in case a prolonged fasting period was required, as modern enteral and parenteral nutrition were not available in the 1940s. Nevertheless Edward Crisp in 1843 had already noticed that inflammatory adhesions and adjacent tissues often blocked perforated ulcers after just a few days, thus preventing fluids spreading into peritoneal cavity. A much more recent French prospective study published by Songne et al. demonstrated a 50% success rate of conservative treatment in a series of 82 consecutive patients.

Clinical Phases of Acute Perforated Ulcer

Phase 1: Chemical peritonitis caused by gastric acid. The leaked fluids have relatively scarce bacteria.

Phase 2: Occurs 6–12 h after the perforation. Pain diminishes somewhat probably due to dilution of the irritating gastric contents by the peritoneal exudates.

Phase 3: Peritoneal infection. Occurs after 12–24 h, whereas bacterial growth and sepsis are the main features [2].

Eligibility to Non-operative Treatment

The candidate should be within the first 12 h after symptom onset, a period in which the abdomen is still sterile or minimal bacterial contamination is present, abdominal pain is limited to the upper abdomen, and hemodynamic variables are stable. Oral food and fluids should be discontinued and a decompressive gastric tube must be used to prevent additional gastric content leak. Intravenous fluids, antibiotics, and injectable proton pump inhibitors must be started. Close surveillance comprising vital signs, physical examination, and pain evaluation at least every 6 h is of vital importance.

Upon signs of hemodynamic instability, worsening of pain suggestive of generalized peritonitis, or any other clinical deterioration, the patient should be taken to the operating room to be surgically treated, preferentially by the laparoscopic approach. Special attention must be given to frail or elderly individuals in whom proportionally minor cardiac, circulatory, or metabolic imbalances could be life-threatening. In principle those admitted with signs of shock, tachycardia, hypotension, generalized peritonitis, fever, or history of onset of symptoms longer than 12 h should not undergo conservative treatment.

Endoscopic Closure of the Perforation

Over-the-scope-clips (OTSC) are a recent attempt to close the ulcer through an endoscopic approach. It is minimally invasive and takes little time (around 10 min) [3]. The peritoneal cavity is supposed not to be infected, otherwise, surgical treatment is the best option. Further prospective randomized studies must be conducted as current evidence is limited.

Acute Appendicitis

With a lifetime risk ranging from 7% to 8%, acute appendicitis is the most common surgical emergency and the most frequent cause of surgical acute abdomen worldwide. McBurney was the first to describe appendectomy in 1894 and the classical abdominal incision bears his name. The laparoscopic approach is related to less wound infections, less postoperative morbidity, shorter hospital stays, and better quality of life, being recommended by the Society of American Gastrointestinal and Endoscopic Surgeons (SAGES) and the European Association for Endoscopic Surgery (EAES) as the gold standard. Mortality of appendectomy is lower than in the past however not negligible, around 0.5%.

Non-operative Handling

Harrington in 1953 and Coldrey in 1959 were among the first to advocate non-operative treatment. Coldrey reported 471 patients treated with antibiotics suffering low mortality (0.2%) and low recurrence rate (14%). Such success notwithstanding, very few followed his lead.

The advantages of conservative treatment would be no wound infection, adhesions, and incisional hernias. Anesthesia-associated risks would also be excluded which could play a positive role on comorbid patients. Furthermore, it presumes shorter hospital stays, lower costs, and shorter absences from work. Failure of antibiotic therapy should not be overlooked, exposing the patient to complicated appendicitis including perforation, fecal peritonitis, and sepsis leading to greater morbidity and mortality. Moreover without removal of the diseased organ, the lifetime risk of appendicitis would remain. Another risk for prolonged use of antibiotics during acute appendicitis would be bacterial resistance.

In the meta-analysis conducted by Prechal, 63% of the non-operated patients were successfully treated within the first year of follow-up. In the surgical (control) group, the success rate was 96%. In the patients who needed secondary appendectomy for failure of antibiotic treatment, the complications were statistically the same as from primary appendectomy. There was no difference in the duration of hospital stay, and absence of work was significantly shorter in the antibiotic group. Surgery provided definitive cure however the conservative did not expose the patients to increased risk.

Long-term effects of nonsurgical antibiotic therapy need to be further studied. The incidence of cancer in uncomplicated appendicitis is very low; however, it still has to be taken into account as it can play a role in prognosis. Given the higher rate of failure of conservative treatment and of recurrence [2], the indication for conservative treatment in this setting should be tailored according to the patient's needs and expectations.

Colonoscopy Perforation

Colonoscopy is a widely performed procedure throughout the world, with over 15 million yearly interventions just in the USA. Although safe and with minimal associated morbidity the technique is not risk-free. Iatrogenic colon perforation (ICP) is probably the most dreaded complication for patients undergoing diagnostic screening or therapy. Reported frequencies are 0.019–0.8% and 0.1–3.0% for diagnostic and therapeutic colonoscopy, respectively. This complication can lead to prolonged hospital stay, emergency surgery with or without a stoma, and sepsis. Mortality range is 5–7% and up to one-third of those requiring operation get a stoma.

Therapeutic colonoscopies have a higher probability of perforation both because they may deal with an already diseased organ, and on account of occasionally complex manipulations. Other aspects contributing to colon perforation include pneumatic dilatation of strictures in Crohn's disease, advanced age (over 75 years), endoscopic mucosal and submucosal dissection for colorectal neoplasia, multiple comorbidities, and female gender.

Up to 60% of ICPs are promptly detected by the endoscopist [4], such as when an intraperitoneal structure appears on the screen during endoscopic examination. Abdominal pain (up to 95% of the cases) and deranged laboratory and radiologic tests demand urgent awareness and should be actively investigated in suspicious circumstances. Such encompass distention, rebound tenderness, fever, diffuse peritonitis, tachycardia, rectal bleeding, along with elevated white blood cell count and C-reactive protein and pneumoperitoneum. If suspicion of perforation persists, computed tomography scan should be done as it can detect not only free air, but also free fluid. Double contrast tomographic colonic imaging (intravenous and rectal) sometimes demonstrates sealed perforations, which may be eligible for non-operative treatment [5].

Signs of sepsis or diffuse peritonitis, immunosuppressed individuals, large perforations (such as those easily identified by the endoscopist during the primary examination), or those related to cancer almost invariably demand immediate surgery.

Conservative Treatment

Localized pain, free air but no free fluids in the abdominal cavity, hemodynamic stability, and absence of fever are usually associated with good prognosis without operation. Intravenous fluids and nutrients, bowel rest, and broad-spectrum antibiotics are mandatory along with close clinical and laboratory surveillance. If the pneumoperitoneum impairs respiration it should be percutaneously needle- or catheter-drained, a maneuver that could help closing the perforation [5]. Initial improvement does not rule out the need for subsequent surgery, therefore the patient should be monitored for several days in the hospital. This means a longer total hospital stay than when primary operation is conducted [4].

Endoluminal Repair

Endoscopic treatment is a minimally invasive and effective alternative. Ideally the damage should be recognized during the procedure and bowel preparation should be adequate. Clip closures are reported since 1997, sealing and healing perforations without surgery [4]. Devices such as through-the-scope (TTS) clips and over-the-scope clips (OTSC) are highly successful in closing ICP . Perforations larger than 1 cm are better treated with such modality which includes more tissue within the clips.

Through-the-scope clips are used primarily for hemostasis; however, they are able to seal full thickness perforations as well. Yet because of the smaller size only submucosa and mucosa tend to be reached. Nevertheless with small defects success rates as encouraging as of 84% have been demonstrated.

If OTSC is the option, a more difficult advance of the colonoscope mounted with the OTSC system could occur in the right colon; however, not in more distal parts of the large bowel. Such barrier notwithstanding, given the overall high success rates in treating ICP, the OTSC system might become the standard approach for this lesion in the near future.

Endoscopic Band Closure

Band-ligation technique was also reported as a method of closing small perforations when the use of an endoscopic clip is difficult. Surrounding tissue and the perforation site are sucked into the banding cap and the band is deployed as usual.

Post-endoscopy management of an ICP should include broad-spectrum antibiotics and bowel rest. A close surveillance is important to prevent clinical deterioration, and surgery must be carried out if severe abdominal pain, peritonitis, or sepsis ensues.

Acute Diverticulitis

Diverticulosis of the sigmoid colon is common in the elderly, affecting approximately 33% of persons older than 60 years of which up to 15% will proceed with an episode of diverticulitis [6]. According to some groups acute diverticulitis is increasing more swiftly than the expected aging of the population, as much as 26% between 1998 and 2005. Complicated diverticulitis can include abscess, fistula, stricture, and partially blocked or free perforation. For a long time treatment of acute diverticulitis with extraluminal air has been emergent resection with or without colostomy, which is associated with high morbidity and mortality (40–44% and 4–24%, respectively). Fortunately recurrence rates are lower compared to younger patients, those free from recurrence representing 83% of those>67 years of age [7].

Non-operative Treatment

Acute left colon diverticulitis (ALCD) is associated with abscess in 20% of the cases. For small collections recommendation is broad-spectrum antibiotic therapy with close clinical monitoring. This approach has a failure rate of 19% if the median size is 4 cm. Larger abscesses are best handled by percutaneous drainage associated with antibiotics, which still carries a failure rate of 21% for abscesses with a median size of 6.1 cm. Surgery should be avoided in stable, younger patients, becoming more urgent in the elderly whenever refractory to the conservative approach, as it is associated with higher mortality [7].

In circumstances of distant free intraperitoneal air and no intraperitoneal fluid, non-operative management is still a possibility if hemodynamic stability and no signs of sepsis are confirmed. The failure rate ranges from 10 to 43%, and experience with the elderly is limited [7]. With just about 2 cm of air in the absence of peritonitis or fluid effusions, 86% success rate and no mortality have been observed. If pericolic air only is detected, as much as 99% healing could be possible.

Trauma—Spleen

The spleen is involved in around 32% of the events of major abdominal trauma. Over the last 40 years, splenic injuries evolved from a mainly surgical to a fundamentally non-operative management (NOM) aiming at spleen conservation in hemodynamically stable patients, thus preventing long-term risks of splenectomy [8] which include immunological impairment and lifelong threat of severe infectious diseases. Moreover, NOM avoids anesthesia, operation, and complication costs and success rate can be as high as 97%, especially with lower injury grades. NOM is also associated with a shorter hospitalization period, thus has become the gold standard for blunt spleen trauma in hemodynamically stable patients, in the absence of peritonitis or associated injuries requiring laparotomy [9].

Conservative and Minimally Invasive Treatment

It includes clinical and hemodynamic observation with or without angiography and embolization. For planning NOM, contrast-enhanced CT scan is crucial in grading lesions with sensitivity and specificity around 96–100% [9]. NOM should only be attempted in centers capable of precise diagnosis of the severity of spleen and other injuries and around-the-clock management including close observation, with intensive care and surgery team easily available.

NOM is classically indicated for minor and moderate spleen lesions, as scored according to the World Society of Emergency Surgery/WSES or the American Association for the Surgery of Trauma/AAST (WSES I, AAST-II/WSES II, AAST III). If a positive blush or early aneurism is present in CT scan angiography should be considered, as those findings are risk factors for re-bleeding. NOM failure rate ranges from 4% to 15%. Age over 55 years is a risk factor for NOM failure which is associated with a higher mortality and longer hospital stay [9], even though the spleen tends to shrink with aging and thus be less vascularized, within the framework of generalized atrophy of immune tissues in the elderly.

Angioembolization

If moderate lesions (WSES III/AAST IV-V) are selected for NOM angiography/angioembolization (AG/AE) is advised regardless of a CT blush. In AAST injury grades above IV, the failure rate of NOM may reach 54.6% [9]. AG/AE has become a powerful ally for spleen trauma treatment enhancing success up to 86–100%. The earlier AG/AE is performed, the lower are the splenectomy odds. NOM failure in the presence of CT contrast blush ranges between 67% and 82% so AG/AE is mandatory in those cases. Nevertheless AG/AE is not complication-free, encompassing major troubles (3.7–28.5%) such as re-bleeding, splenic infarction, splenic abscess, pseudocyst, and severe puncture-related complications, especially when conducted by non-specialized teams or in not well-equipped units. Minor morbidity occurs in 23% to 61% of the candidates including fever, pleural effusion, and coil migration [9].

Liver Trauma

Because of its large size and location in the upper part of the abdomen, the liver is one of the most affected organs by abdominal trauma, both penetrating and blunt, and its rich vascular nature makes it a source of potentially fatal hemorrhage.

Analogous to spleen injuries, NOM depends on grading of the damage by contrast-enhanced CT scan (gold standard). Hemodynamic stability is mandatory for such option as well as no other abdominal injuries requiring surgical treatment like hollow viscus perforation.

Around 80% of blunt hepatic trauma can be conservatively treated and NOM is similarly the treatment of choice for stable patients with stab and gunshot wounds [10]. This applies to liver injuries graded as minor or moderate (WSES I–II and AAST I, II and III), for which success rate reaches around 80% if all modalities of hepatic trauma are considered. For stab wounds more failures are to be expected (50% need for interventions if anterior lesions and 25% if posterior ones).

Clinical and hemodynamic monitoring follows the lines of splenic injuries. Special attention should be given to gunshot wounds as they carry a higher risk of associated lesions and should be conservatively treated only in specialized trauma centers [11].

Angiography/angioembolization should be employed when a contrast blush or early aneurism is present. If NOM is selected for more severe lesions (WSES III and AAST IV-V), admission to the ICU is advised [10]. Interventional radiology should be readily available as additional vascular damage could be present. Drops in hematocrit levels even in the absence of shock should raise the suspicion of active bleeding and immediate angiography should be considered.

As in other contexts angioembolization is occasionally followed by adverse events nominally bile leak, contained biloma, hepatic necrosis, and hepatic abscess.

Pancreatic Trauma

It occurs in less than 1% of all traumas and up to 11% of abdominal trauma. Blunt injuries are the most frequent ones [12]. Their importance stems from the high risk of complications and death. Given the limited experience in most centers, treatment of moderate and severe pancreatic injury (PI) is still a topic of debate. Lesions graded I or II (without main duct injury) are treated conservatively. Main pancreatic duct (MPD) injury is the most important finding on the CT scan and operation is often the choice, although associated with high morbidity and mortality. Pancreatic injury can be associated with other abdominal lesions rendering conservative treatment less likely, notably after penetrating trauma. Despite the dearth of solid evidence, non-operative management (NOM) is increasing in this field [5].

NOM in moderate and severe PI (grades III, IV, and V) has a success rate of 30% however with a high rate of subsequent pseudocysts, ranging from 65% to 74% [12]. Nevertheless these are mostly benign troubles amenable to minimally invasive interventions, particularly endoscopic drainage. After ERCP pancreatic stent insertion could be a successful strategy for grade III PI.

Main Duct Disruption

There is still not consensus on whether NOM is a legitimate approach for MPD. However, if delayed presentation with a well-walled pseudocyst is detected, MPD might benefit from minimally invasive treatment nominally endoscopic cystogastrostomy. To this aim various models of stents contribute to keep the transmural drainage open till the cyst is reabsorbed.

Pancreatic Necrosis and Abscess

Acute pancreatitis is deemed as the most common cause, after gallbladder colic, of serious upper abdominal pain in clinical practice and although the vast majority of cases are mild and self-limited, up to 10% are associated with extensive pancreatic necrosis, which means high morbidity and prolonged hospital stay. In the relatively recent past it could carry a mortality rate of 30%, and even 70% with associated infection.

Pancreatic necrosis may present as an acute necrotic collection (ANC), usually seen in the first 4 weeks and often extending into surrounding fat and retroperitoneal tissues, or walled-off necrosis (WON) which is a more mature, encapsulated pancreatic mass seen 4 weeks or more after the onset of pancreatitis. In both circumstances infection of the necrotic tissue is possible, eventually encompassing anaerobic bacteria [13].

Early laparotomy, debridement and drainage of infected pancreatic necrosis (IPN) was the established approach during many years, yet burdened by major complications (34–95%) and death (11–39%). Recent experience [14] demonstrates that non-operative treatment of IPN is the best alternative. In a series of 31 patients eight were treated with antibiotics only (25.8%), and the remaining ones were handled by drainage procedures (endoscopic and percutaneous). Surgical necrosectomy was necessary in only four patients (12.9%) because of treatment failure. Total mortality was 3.2% (01 death only).

The PANTER trial challenged open necrosectomy versus a less invasive approach named "step-up", in which minimally invasive procedures can be escalated or re-employed for draining IPN. Such encompassed percutaneous drainage, endoscopic transgastric drainage, and minimally invasive retroperitoneal necrosectomy, generally employed in this sequence.

Percutaneous Drainage

Currently this represents indeed the first line of treatment for IPN achieving 25–60% resolution of infection, with a high level of evidence (1A) [13]. Endoscopic transgastric drainage or necrosectomy and video-assisted retroperitoneal debridement are other alternatives, when required. Open surgery should be employed when those less invasive options fail as this approach relates to less new-onset organ failures, although it is more aggressive and may require more interventions.

In cases of disconnected duct syndrome with walled-off necrosis surgical transgastric necrosectomy may be also feasible, with morbidity and mortality around 38% and 2%, respectively [13].

Nonsurgical Pneumoperitoneum

Spontaneous nonlaparoscopy-related pneumoperitoneum indicates hollow viscus perforation and conventionally demands emergent surgical exploration. However, in 5% to 15% of cases it is not associated to perforation and may be conservatively managed.

Common and Infrequent Conditions

Early post-operative pneumoperitoneum can of course be detected after 60% of open surgeries and 25% of laparoscopic procedures. Around two-thirds of the findings will resolve within 2 days and 97% after 5 days. On CT scan free peritoneal air may be recognized for somewhat longer, in about 50% of the cases after 6 days. A decreasing volume without worrisome clinical or peritoneal signs indicates a benign course.

Peritoneal dialysis can be associated with asymptomatic pneumoperitoneum (10–33% of the patients) [14]. Pneumatosis cystoides intestinalis is a rather rare cause of nonsurgical pneumoperitoneum. This condition is characterized by multiple intramural cysts filled with gas that may eventually rupture leading to pneumoperitoneum. Only in exceptional circumstances will intervention be required.

The lungs and thoracic structures may also be a source of nonsurgical pneumoperitoneum as occasionally occurs during prolonged mechanical ventilation with pneumothorax or pneumomediastinum. Risk factors include high airway pressures, noncompliant lungs, obstructive airway disease, and acute respiratory distress syndrome. Pneumoperitoneum in this setting, in the absence of peritoneal signs, could lead to unnecessary imaging investigation and even laparotomy [14].

Although unusually air may enter the peritoneal cavity from the genital tract through the uterus and uterine tubes. Tubal insufflation during an hysterosalpingogram is an obvious mechanism; however, other local manipulations including sexual intercourse could be possible causes. Spontaneous resolution is the rule [14]. Only in circumstances of significant pain or rebound tenderness, fever, elevated white blood cell count, or other signs of peritoneal inflammation should additional work be provided.

Case Report

As previously alluded to, non-operative treatment of infected pancreatic necrosis is the preferred approach nowadays. Especially when percutaneous or endoscopic catheter drainage of the septic focus is feasible, and material can be collected for bacteriologic profile and targeted antibiotic therapy. More than three decades ago interventional radiology and endoscopy were not as available and effective in this condition as nowadays. Mortality with strictly conservative therapy was prohibitive, therefore nearly all services advocated urgent open drainage. A patient seen by one of the authors [15] was a profoundly religious man admitted to an academic hospital.

The involved microbes could not be identified as initial blood cultures were negative, and minimally invasive access to the focus was not available at that time. However, the individual was clinically septic with fever, high white blood cell count, upper abdominal distention and pain, and gas bubbles were identified during the imaging exploration of the pancreatic area, along with extensive retroperitoneal necrosis. As the case was being prepared for operative handling the patient adamantly refused surgical consent. In his opinion either his faith would save him, or otherwise he would peacefully accept that his time of dying has arrived. As he offered no alternative intravenous nutrients and high doses of antibiotics were prescribed, and the medical team crossed fingers hoping for the best. "After the second week the patient rapidly started to improve, to the point that he could be discharged home without operation" [15]. To the best of our knowledge, it was the first report of full regression with medical management only.

Not surprisingly the article was subsequently criticized, not only on account of lack of bacteriologic confirmation, but because the concept of non-operative recovery after such an ominous infection was unconscionable at that time. Only about a decade later did that pathway start to become mainstream and now of course it's commonplace, provided minimally invasive drainage is also accomplished.

We agree that our first plan had not been medical care either, as in the 1980s and 1990s of last century minimally invasive approaches were mostly a distant horizon, and even well-equipped surgical intensive care units (SICUs) were not easy to come by. Only today can one be confident that a critically ill subject will be well monitored when admitted to a SICU. Should conservative therapy fail and unexpected deterioration occur, the surgeon will still be able to change course and provide the required operation.

References

1. Chung KT, Shelat VG. Perforated peptic ulcer—an update. World J Gastrointest Surg. 2017;9(1):1–12. https://doi.org/10.4240/wjgs.v9.i1.1.
2. Salminen P, Tuominen R, Paajanen H, Rautio T, Nordström P, Aarnio M, Rantanen T, Hurme S, Mecklin JP, Sand J, Virtanen J, Jartti A, Grönroos JM. Five-year follow-up of antibiotic therapy for uncomplicated acute appendicitis in the APPAC randomized clinical trial. JAMA. 2018;320(12):1259–65. https://doi.org/10.1001/jama.2018.13201. Erratum in: JAMA 2018 Oct 23;320(16):1711. PMID: 30264120; PMCID: PMC6233612
3. Wei JJ, Xie XP, Lian TT, Yang ZY, Pan YF, Lin ZL, Zheng GW, Zhuang ZH. Over-the-scope-clip applications for perforated peptic ulcer. Surg Endosc. 2019;33(12):4122–7. https://doi.org/10.1007/s00464-019-06717-x.
4. de'Angelis N, Di Saverio S, Chiara O, et al. WSES guidelines for the management of iatrogenic colonoscopy perforation. World J Emerg Surg. 2017;2018(13):5. https://doi.org/10.1186/s13017-018-0162-9.
5. Koganti SB, Kongara R, Boddepalli S, Mohammad NS, Thumma V, Nagari B, Sastry RA. Predictors of successful non-operative management of grade III & IV blunt pancreatic trauma. Ann Med Surg (Lond). 2016;10:103–9. https://doi.org/10.1016/j.amsu.2016.08.003.
6. Khan A, Hawkins AT. Challenging surgical dogma: controversies in diverticulitis. Surg Clin North Am. 2021;101(6):967–80. https://doi.org/10.1016/j.suc.2021.05.024.
7. Fugazzola P, Ceresoli M, Coccolini F, Gabrielli F, Puzziello A, Monzani F, Amato B, Sganga G, Sartelli M, Menichetti F, Puglisi GA, Tartaglia D, Carcoforo P, Avenia N, Kluger Y, Paolillo C, Zago M, Leppäniemi A, Tomasoni M, Cobianchi L, Dal Mas F, Improta M, Moore EE, Peitzman AB, Sugrue M, Agnoletti V, Fraga GP, Weber DG, Damaskos D, Abu-Zidan FM, Wani I, Kirkpatrick AW, Pikoulis M, Pararas N, Tan E, Broek RT, Maier RV, Davies RJ, Kashuk J, Shelat VG, Mefire AC, Augustin G, Magnone S, Poiasina E, De Simone B, Chiarugi M, Biffl W, Baiocchi GL, Catena F, Ansaloni L. The WSES/SICG/ACOI/SICUT/AcEMC/SIFIPAC guidelines for diagnosis and treatment of acute left colonic diverticulitis in the elderly. World J Emerg Surg. 2022;17(1):5. https://doi.org/10.1186/s13017-022-00408-0.
8. Cinquantini F, Simonini E, Di Saverio S, Cecchelli C, Kwan SH, Ponti F, Coniglio C, Tugnoli G, Torricelli P. Non-surgical management of blunt splenic trauma: a comparative analysis of non-operative management and splenic artery embolization-experience from a european trauma center. Cardiovasc Intervent Radiol. 2018;41(9):1324–32. https://doi.org/10.1007/s00270-018-1953-9.
9. Coccolini F, Montori G, Catena F, Kluger Y, Biffl W, Moore EE, Reva V, Bing C, Bala M, Fugazzola P, Bahouth H, Marzi I, Velmahos G, Ivatury R, Soreide K, Horer T, Ten Broek R, Pereira BM, Fraga GP, Inaba K, Kashuk J, Parry N, Masiakos PT, Mylonas KS, Kirkpatrick A, Abu-Zidan F, Gomes CA, Benatti SV, Naidoo N, Salvetti F, Maccatrozzo S, Agnoletti V, Gamberini E, Solaini L, Costanzo A, Celotti A, Tomasoni M, Khokha V, Arvieux C, Napolitano

L, Handolin L, Pisano M, Magnone S, Spain DA, de Moya M, Davis KA, De Angelis N, Leppaniemi A, Ferrada P, Latifi R, Navarro DC, Otomo Y, Coimbra R, Maier RV, Moore F, Rizoli S, Sakakushev B, Galante JM, Chiara O, Cimbanassi S, Mefire AC, Weber D, Ceresoli M, Peitzman AB, Wehlie L, Sartelli M, Di Saverio S, Ansaloni L. Splenic trauma: WSES classification and guidelines for adult and pediatric patients. World J Emerg Surg. 2017;12:40. https://doi.org/10.1186/s13017-017-0151-4.
10. Pillai AS, Kumar G, Pillai AK. Hepatic trauma interventions. Semin Intervent Radiol. 2021;38(1):96–104. https://doi.org/10.1055/s-0041-1724014.
11. Coccolini F, Coimbra R, Ordonez C, Kluger Y, Vega F, Moore EE, Biffl W, Peitzman A, Horer T, Abu-Zidan FM, Sartelli M, Fraga GP, Cicuttin E, Ansaloni L, Parra MW, Millán M, DeAngelis N, Inaba K, Velmahos G, Maier R, Khokha V, Sakakushev B, Augustin G, di Saverio S, Pikoulis E, Chirica M, Reva V, Leppaniemi A, Manchev V, Chiarugi M, Damaskos D, Weber D, Parry N, Demetrashvili Z, Civil I, Napolitano L, Corbella D, Catena F, WSES Expert Panel. Liver trauma: WSES 2020 guidelines. World J Emerg Surg. 2020;15(1):24. https://doi.org/10.1186/s13017-020-00302-7.
12. Coccolini F, Kobayashi L, Kluger Y, et al. Duodeno-pancreatic and extrahepatic biliary tree trauma: WSES-AAST guidelines. World J Emerg Surg. 2019;14:56. https://doi.org/10.1186/s13017-019-0278-6.
13. Leppäniemi A, Tolonen M, Tarasconi A, Segovia-Lohse H, Gamberini E, Kirkpatrick AW, Ball CG, Parry N, Sartelli M, Wolbrink D, van Goor H, Baiocchi G, Ansaloni L, Biffl W, Coccolini F, Di Saverio S, Kluger Y, Moore E, Catena F. 2019 WSES guidelines for the management of severe acute pancreatitis. World J Emerg Surg. 2019;14:27. https://doi.org/10.1186/s13017-019-0247-0.
14. Mularski RA, Sippel JM, Osborne ML. Pneumoperitoneum: a review of nonsurgical causes. Crit Care Med. 2000;28(7):2638–44. https://doi.org/10.1097/00003246-200007000-00078.
15. Faintuch J, Meniconi MT, Speranzini MB, Pinotti HW, Smolentsov H. Clinical regression of infected pancreatic necrosis: case report. Int J Pancreatol. 1991;8(4):379–86. https://doi.org/10.1007/BF02952729.

Part VII
Bedside and Adjunct Procedures

Chapter 28
Percutaneous Ultrasound-Guided Gastrostomy Placement

Samuel B. Fordyce, Rooshi K. Parikh, and Stephen P. Reis

Introduction

Surgical techniques for gastrostomy tubes were first developed in the 1800s, with most of the test subjects perishing due to infection prior to the advent of antibiotics. Fast forward to 1969, two surgeons, Dr. Jeffery Ponsky and Dr. Michael Gauderer, devised and performed the first percutaneous endoscopic gastrostomy tube placement [1]. Other minimally invasive techniques, such as fluoroscopic and ultrasound-guided techniques, were subsequently developed. Today, approximately 250,000 gastrostomy tubes are placed annually in the United States alone [2]. With our ever-aging population and medical capabilities allowing patients to live longer lives, gastrostomy tubes are becoming a vital part of the treatment algorithm, particularly for critically ill patients. The most recently developed technique, ultrasound-guided gastrostomy tube placement, has become a widely adopted technique that holds specific advantages. Apart from surgical approaches for gastrostomy tube placement, open or laparoscopic routes, minimally invasive techniques (endoscopic, fluoroscopic, and ultrasound) are widely preferred, secondary to their low complication risk and lack of general anesthesia; however, they still require special equipment, trained practitioners, and dedicated endoscopic/fluoroscopic suites.

On the other hand, percutaneous ultrasound-guided gastrostomy tube placement has been shown to be effective and safe as a bedside option, using readily available

S. B. Fordyce (✉) · S. P. Reis
Department of Interventional Radiology, Columbia University Irving Medical Center, New York, NY, USA
e-mail: saf9141@nyp.org; sr3321@cumc.columbia.edu

R. K. Parikh
City University of New York School of Medicine, New York, NY, USA
e-mail: rparikh000@citymail.cuny.edu

© The Author(s), under exclusive license to Springer Nature Switzerland AG 2024
J. Faintuch, S. Faintuch (eds.), *Recent Strategies in High Risk Surgery*,
https://doi.org/10.1007/978-3-031-56270-9_28

technology, thereby reducing complications and inconveniences such as transportation of patients [2]. Depending on the specific patient and medical reasoning behind placing a gastrostomy tube, all of the techniques mentioned below have their advantages and disadvantages.

Indications

The main indication for gastrostomy tube placement is the need for supplemental nutrition secondary to insufficient oral intake, contraindication to oral intake through the mouth or gastric decompression; however, there are nuances that need to be carefully considered prior to gastrostomy tube placement [3]. Assuming patients have acceptable baseline nutritional status, they can tolerate up to 10 days of partial fasting prior to significant protein catabolism [3]. On the other hand, patients with chronic illnesses that previously inhibited their oral intake abilities may require the initiation of nutritional support sooner.

Enteral feedings options are most commonly split between nasoenteric and gastroenteric techniques. Typically, nasoenteric options, namely nasogastric tubes, are reserved for short-term enteric supplementation of acutely ill patients, such as immediately postoperatively. Nasogastric tubes have their advantages: they are easily placed and are fairly low risk. As mentioned above, acutely ill patients or patients expected to make a full recovery can benefit from short-term enteral supplementation and gastric decompression without the need for an invasive procedure; however, there are several disadvantages. Nasoenteric alternatives can be associated with skin irritation, gastroesophageal reflux, bleeding, and ulceration, especially with use greater than 2 weeks [3, 4]. Gastrostomy tube placement forgoes many of these complications; however, the procedure itself is more invasive and can lead to complications. One cited reason for gastrostomy tube placement over nasoenteric techniques is the possible reduction of aspiration risk [5, 6].

Patients at a moderate to high risk of malnourishment requiring nutritional support greater than 30 days should consider placement of a gastrostomy tube [3, 7]. A wide variety of conditions/diagnosis are referred for gastrostomy tube placement (Table 28.1); it is important to carefully assess an individual patient's needs, including preferences, diagnosis, goals, and life expectancy. Quality of life should remain a priority.

Table 28.1 Referral diagnosis for gastrostomy tube placement

Neurological disorders	Malignancy	Congenital and neonatal	Miscellaneous
Congenital or acquired neurological disorders interfering with ability to ingest food	Head and neck, esophagus, upper abdomen, brain	Cystic fibrosis, low birth weight, congenital heart disorders	Trauma including traumatic brain injury, burns especially involving face, dysphagia, other digestive aberrations, palliative care

Aspiration Pneumonia

Aspiration pneumonia is the most commonly cited cause of mortality in patients with nasogastric or gastrostomy tubes [6, 8, 9]. Originally, one of the main presumed advantages of gastrostomy over nasogastric tubes was decreased events of aspiration pneumonia. Purely from an anatomical and technical perspective, this assumption makes sense. Nasogastric tubes extend from the patient's nares, through the gastroesophageal sphincter and into the stomach. This keeps the gastroesophageal sphincter partially open, thereby increasing the likelihood of aspiration, especially in chronically ill patients with impaired normal functions. Gastrostomy tubes forgo the need to keep the gastroesophageal sphincter open, which prevents aspiration. Contrary to anatomical logic, past studies and meta-analyses have been unable to elicit statistically significant differences for incidences of aspiration pneumonia between nasoenteric and gastroenteric techniques [10]. On the other hand, dysphagia secondary to stroke, gastrostomy tube placement reduced the risk of aspiration by almost five times, compared to nasogastric tube placement [11]. Regardless of such results, it is well known that both increase the risk compared to patients without either, and it should be considered in the decision-making process [12].

Dementia

Most experts agree that the incidence and prevalence of dementia will proportionally increase with a continuously aging population [13]. A majority of these patients, more than 90%, have dysphagia or other oral intake problems, leading to the placement of long-term enteral feeding options, like gastrostomy tubes, which are considered a prognostic indicator of mortality within a 6-month time period [14]. Patients with dementia who undergo a gastrostomy tube placement have a mortality rate of up to 54% after 1 month and 90% after 1 year [15]. For these reasons, quality of life and improvement in mortality should be of paramount importance [8].

Periprocedural Care and Patient Preparation

Pre-Procedural Care

It's important to conduct a comprehensive physical exam prior to any gastrostomy procedure to ensure certain modalities are not precluded. The oropharynx needs to be evaluated for anatomical variants, congenital anomalies, and facial fractures, which would increase the risk for an endoscopic approach [16]. The endoscopic route with partially obstructing head and neck malignancies is contraindicated and infeasible. Certain conditions may increase procedural complexity, for example, obesity, ascites, and neurological disorders. Any prior imaging and/or obtaining

Table 28.2 Comparison of the advantages and disadvantages of the various gastrostomy tube placement techniques

Technique	PUG	PRG	PEG
Advantages	– Performed at bedside – Shorter ICU and hospital length of stay – Cost savings – No radiation exposure	– Shorter procedure length – Better visualization of gastric insufflation – No cross-contamination of oral flora	– Shorter procedure time – Possible at bedside – No radiation exposure
Disadvantages	– Longer procedure length – Inadequate gastropexy with larger patients	– Radiation exposure – Requirement of a fluoroscopy suite	– Inadequate transillumination in obese patients – No direct visualization of intercepting bowel or liver – Risk of gastrostomy tract tumor seeding

further imaging is advised if you suspect or know of altered anatomy from prior surgery [16, 17]. The delineation of hepatic and colonic anatomy can be a priority as well. Certain patients may warrant pre-procedural ultrasound to delineate the liver edge in order to ensure it isn't accidentally punctured (Table 28.2).

Typically, patients are required to be nothing by mouth (NPO) or nothing per nasogastric tube for 6–8 h prior to the procedure, mainly due to aspiration risk secondary to anesthesia, whether that is moderate or general anesthesia. Additionally, most policies require patients to ingest oral contrast (Barium) 12–24 h prior to the procedure to elucidate colonic anatomy, particularly the transverse colon. Alternatively, patients may be given pre-procedural rectal contrast instead of oral contrast to ensure the transverse colon is clear of the potential needle path.

Antibiotic Prophylaxis

As a "clean-contaminated" procedure, antibiotic prophylaxis has long been standard of practice, as it reduces periprocedural infections, particularly peristomal infections [18]. The guidelines dictating appropriate antibiotic prophylaxis are varied and technique specific. According to the Society of Interventional Radiology (SIR), Standards of Practice Committee (SPC), and American Society for Gastrointestinal Endoscopy (ASGE), 1 g of cefazolin is recommended for the "pull" fluoroscopic and endoscopic-guided techniques, since traversing the oropharynx or nasopharynx is thought to seed bacteria within the stomach and skin tunnel. Special considerations should be considered for patients with head and neck cancer with potential bacterial overgrowth from an obstructing malignancy. Per SIR guidelines, second generation cephalosporins should be used for prophylaxis followed by an oral course of a first generation of cephalosporins [18] (Table 28.3). There is conflicting data concerning antibiotic prophylaxis for "push" techniques and an absence of SIR guidelines [18, 23, 24].

Ultrasound-Guided Placement

Even though there is no consensus, the technique requires traversal of the mouth, increasing the potential of bacterial seeding and the likelihood of periprocedural infections [24]. Therefore antibiotic prophylaxis should be a consideration.

Management of Anticoagulation

According to the SPC, gastrostomy tube placement is considered a "high bleeding risk" procedure, with greater than 1.5% rate of major bleeding [25, 26]. Prothrombin time (PR)/ international normalized ratio (INR) and platelets should be routinely checked and corrected if less than 1.5 and 50,000, respectively [25] (Table 28.3). Per ASGE, warfarin and clopidogrel should be stopped at least 5 and 7 days prior to the procedure, respectively [19]. Patients requiring interim anticoagulation can be given aspirin or low molecular weight heparin; however, they should be held the day of the procedure. Similar guidelines are prescribed by SIR; however, they suggest withholding clopidogrel for 5 days instead of 7 [19].

Anti-Platelet Therapies

These are becoming a widely prescribed class of drugs in patients with cardiovascular disease and strokes. Requiring patients to stop taking these vital drugs prior to percutaneous or radiologically placed gastrostomy tubes is no longer routine practice, with retrospective analysis showing no increased risk of bleeding complications while taking single or dual anti-platelet therapy [27]. As most of the societal guidelines are 5–10 years old, they don't reflect the most up-to-date practices. Regardless of societal guidelines, pre-procedural laboratory values should be confirmed prior to placement.

Table 28.3 Societal guidelines and practices for gastrostomy tube placement

American Gastroenterology Association (AGA) and others	2011 [19]	jvir.org/article/S1051-0443(11)00850-5/fulltext#secd29348500e1435
American Society of Parental and Enteral Nutrition and others	2013 [20]	saxinstitute.org.au/wp-content/uploads/Gastrostomy-guidelines-a-rapid-review.pdf
Cardiovascular and Interventional Radiological Society of Europe (CIRSE)	2016 [21]	pubmed.ncbi.nlm.nih.gov/27184363/
Society of Interventional Radiology—Updated Review	2020 [22]	jvir.org/article/S1051-0443(21)00326-2/fulltext

Post-Procedural Care

Immediately after gastrostomy tube placement, it is important to assess for acute (within 24 h) complications, like bleeding, aspiration perforation, pneumoperitoneum, and developing peritonitis [16]. Typically, providers will begin with a slow infusion of sterile water on the day of insertion followed by the initiation of trickle feeds to be advanced as tolerated by the patient. Historically, providers have waited 24 h prior to the initiation of feeds through the newly placed gastrostomy tubes. Multiple past and ongoing retrospective and prospective trials have shown the safety and feasibility of early feeding, 4 h after the placement of an uncomplicated gastrostomy tube [28]; however, these are primarily focused on endoscopic approaches. Even though extrapolations have been made to transabdominal techniques, like ultrasound and fluoroscopic-guided techniques, there is limited clinical research supporting the current practices. Additionally, no formal guidelines exist for optimal post-procedural feeding time.

Gastronomy Placement Options

Ultrasound-Guided Gastrostomy

Ultrasound has been previously used in tandem with traditional percutaneous endoscopically guided (PEG) and percutaneous radiologic guided (PRG) procedures to enhance visualization and/or reduce radiation exposure/dose [29, 30]. Ultrasound has also been proven useful at the bedside to replace damaged or dislodged gastrostomy tubes through the pre-existing stoma [31]. While there are older reports of a retrograde percutaneous ultrasound-guided (PUG) procedure in both adult and pediatric populations [30, 32, 33], anterograde PUG is a recently established technique with a wide array of applications.

Contraindications

Any electronic implants, such as a pacemaker, may interfere and/or be disrupted using strong magnets [34]. Suboptimal stomach position such as high under the ribs require fluoroscopic visualization using insufflation [2, 24]. A pre-procedure ultrasound measurement spanning from anterior gastric wall to skin greater than 4.5 cm may make needle puncture difficult or infeasible [24, 35]. Additionally, inability to pass two enteric tubes into the patient secondary to nasopharyngeal or oropharyngeal obstruction is a contraindication [24].

Procedure

The oral cavity and oropharynx should be anesthetized with topical spray and the patient should be moderately sedated. If not already present, a nasogastric tube should then be inserted for insufflation of the stomach. Prior to the procedure, it is important to establish known landmarks, most importantly the stomach and the left hepatic lobe. First, the Point-of-care Ultrasound Magnetically Aligned Gastrostomy kit (PUMA-G System; CoapTech, Baltimore MD, USA) orogastric tube (OGT) should be inserted through the mouth and into the stomach. The PUMA-G orogastric tube contains an inflatable balloon with an internal magnetic component to allow for temporary gastropexy of the stomach.

Next, the PUMA-G external handheld magnet should be placed over the epigastrium to attract the internal magnet and the anterior gastric wall toward the abdominal surface, in order to achieve a temporary magnetic gastropexy. Optionally, a gauss meter can be used to locate the internal magnet to ensure appropriate coaptation and plan optimal needle entry. Following coaptation of the internal and external magnets, the orogastric balloon should be inflated with 20–30 ml of saline. Methylene blue can be added to the saline to act as a visual cue for needle entry into the balloon. Using ultrasound, the orogastric balloon should be placed in the field of view. Prior to needle puncture, it's important to ensure the proposed needle track does not traverse interposed loops of bowel, particularly the transverse colon, or the left lobe of the liver. If necessary, the external magnet can be utilized to move the balloon to a more suitable location.

Local anesthetic should be injected into the skin and along the proposed gastrostomy tract. Under direct ultrasound guidance, an 18-gauge needle should be advanced through the anterior abdominal wall and into the fluid-filled orogastric balloon. To avoid tenting of the gastric wall, the needle should be advanced with a short jab into the stomach lumen rather than slowly pushed in. Aspiration of colored sterile saline ensures correct placement of the needle inside the orogastric balloon within the stomach. The PUMA-G pigtail guidewire should be passed through the needle into the orogastric balloon and the orogastric balloon should be deflated to entrap the guidewire. At this point, the orogastric tube and trapped guidewire should be pulled back through the mouth leaving the guidewire running continuously from the mouth through the newly made gastrostomy and out of the anterior abdominal wall (Figs. 28.1 and 28.2).

The guidewire should be cut from the orogastric balloon, and a 20-French gastrostomy tube should be pushed over the guidewire through a small dermatotomy into the stomach. Once the gastrostomy tube is in correct position, the guidewire should be removed. If desired, contrast can be injected through the gastrostomy tube and a portable X-ray image can be used to confirm correct placement [2, 24, 35, 36].

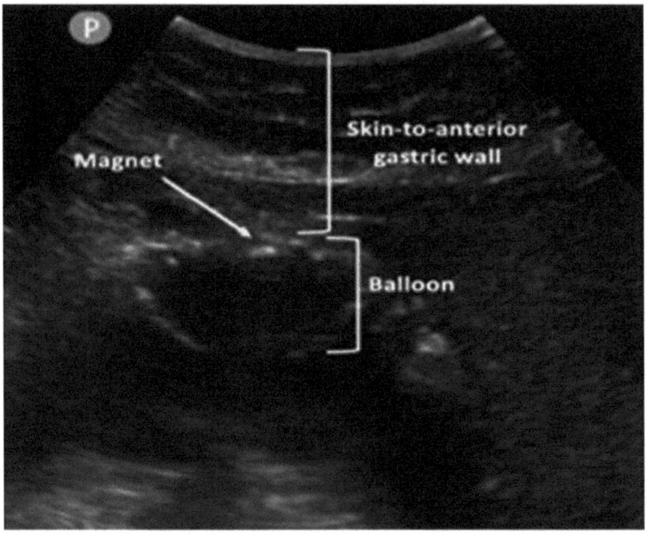

Fig. 28.1 Transverse ultrasound image depicting the OGT ballon with the stomach. Permission of usage granted by CoapTech, Baltimore MD 21230

Advantages

The biggest advantage of PUG placement is the ability to perform this procedure at the bedside without the constraint of an available endoscopic tower or fluoroscopy suite. This allows for earlier gastrostomy tube placement in the intensive care unit (ICU), and in the case of seriously ill candidates in general. PUG is performed on average of 4 days earlier than PEG or PRG [34]. PUG is associated with shorter lengths of hospital stay; approximately 5 less days in the ICU and 10 less days in the hospital [34]. PUG is also associated with cost saving of over $25,000 per patient [34]. Concomitant percutaneous dilatation tracheostomy can be successfully performed along with PUG [37]. Additionally, PUG eliminates radiation dose/exposure to the patient and real-time ultrasound visualization can prevent injury to surrounding organs/tissue.

Disadvantages

PUG has a longer procedure time, around 40–50 min, whereas PEG and PRG procedures last 30–40 min [2, 36, 38]; however, procedure time diminishes with experience. Magnetic gastropexy and subsequent ultrasound visualization is difficult in larger, morbidly obese patients and necessitates fluoroscopic visualization using gastric insufflation. Ultrasound visualization is also a challenge with difficult anatomy including a higher set stomach.

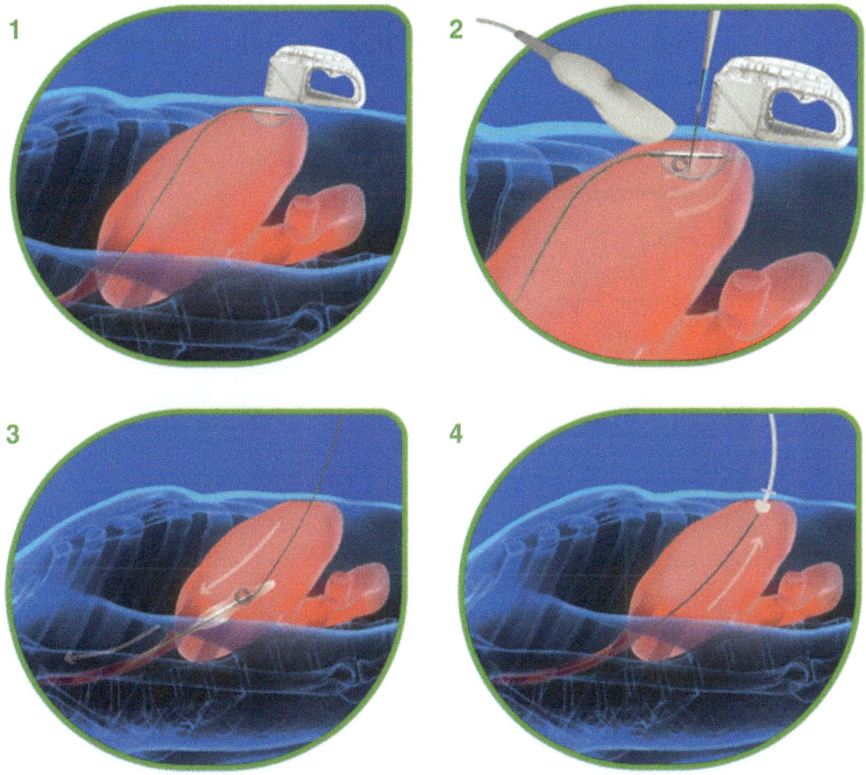

Fig. 28.2 Outlining the four major steps for gastrostomy tube placement using the PUMA-G system. Permission of usage granted by CoapTech, Baltimore MD 21230
Image 1: The PUMA-G: The orogastric route is employed to position the catheter in the stomach. An external magnet is applied on the abdominal wall to attract the balloon, thus simultaneously carrying forward the anterior gastric wall and creating a temporary gastropexy
Image 2: Using ultrasound, the upper abdominal anatomy is reviewed and a tract for needle and guidewire insertion is selected
Image 3: The pigtail guidewire is ensnared by the balloon catheter and both are removed together through the mouth
Image 4: A small abdominal skin incision is made, and the gastrostomy tube is introduced into the stomach by means of the existing guidewire

Complications

Access/stomal site infection is the most reported complication of PUG. Mild aspiration, abdominal wall abscess, and bleeding are also noted [2, 38]. Overall, complications from PUG overlap with complications seen in all other gastrostomy tube placement procedures. Aspiration, bleeding, and ulceration are known to occur in about 1% of all gastrostomy tube placements [16]. Injury to surrounding structures including colon and liver can be avoided by proper pre-procedure visualization.

Finally, in patients with head and neck cancer, transoral gastrostomy has a risk of tumor seeding within the tract and thus a transabdominal approached is preferred [16].

Endoscopic Gastrostomy Tube Placement

The first feasible and readily available alternative to surgically placed gastrostomy tubes was an endoscopic approach developed by two surgeons, Dr. Jeffery Ponsky and Dr. Michael Gauderer, in 1969 [1]. With the advent of advanced endoscopic equipment, it became possible to transilluminate the stomach and "directly" visualize the stomach for a percutaneous approach. Over the years, a variety of different techniques have become available, including the "pull," "push over a wire," and "introducer" techniques [16].

Contraindications

Prior abdominal surgery, more specifically a partial or total gastrectomy, and the potential of interposed organs or anatomical variation are the most significant technique-specific contraindications [3]. Additionally, obstructive oropharyngeal processes, like head and neck malignancies, oropharyngeal stenosis, Zenkers diverticulum or facial fractures, prevent proper passage of the endoscope and are considered contraindications [39]. Other absolute contraindications that are shared among all the non-surgical gastrostomy tube placement techniques are severe ascites, peritonitis, peritoneal carcinomatosis, and coagulation derangement. Compared to radiologically placed gastrostomy tubes, a patient's weight is not considered a contraindication.

Procedure

All methods start with an upper endoscopy to transilluminate the stomach so that a suitable percutaneous entry track can be chosen. Using a catheter and needle, an incision is made in the anterior abdominal wall followed by a small gastrostomy. For the "pull" technique, a string with a metal wire loop is advanced through the needle and snared using the endoscope. Once the string is snared, the endoscope is removed along with the string through the patient's mouth creating a continuous track from the patient's mouth through the stomach and out the newly made gastrostomy. The gastrostomy tube is attached to the wire loop and pulled through the mouth and esophagus into the stomach and out of the anterior abdominal wall and secured in place. For the "push over a wire" technique, the general steps are similar; however, instead of using a piece of string to pull the gastrostomy tube, a wire is used as a track to push a gastrostomy tube from the patients mouth into position in the newly made gastrostomy [16]. The "pull" and "push over a wire" techniques are similar and only differ in the final step of physically placing the gastrostomy tube within the stomach [16].

The "introducer" technique avoids oropharyngeal contamination of the gastrostomy tube prior to placement. This could avoid seeding of bacteria and cancer cells for certain patient populations, such as those with head and neck malignancies. Like the "pull" and "push over wire" techniques, an endoscope is used to transilluminate the stomach, enabling the placement of a needle/trocar system into the stomach. A wire is placed into the stomach and ensnared using the endoscope to secure the newly made gastrostomy. T-bar fasteners, more frequently used in the fluoroscopic-guided gastrostomy techniques, are used to provide preliminary gastropexy of the stomach to the anterior abdominal wall. Once the tract is serially dilated to the appropriate size, the gastrostomy tube can be passed over the wire and secured in place.

Advantages

The biggest advantage of PEG compared to PRG placement techniques is direct visualization of the stomach and needle tract. Compared to the PRG techniques, PEG gives the practitioner the ability to confirm the needle is intraluminal within the stomach, but also that an appropriate location has been chosen for the gastrostomy tube tract.

Disadvantages

The most significant disadvantage of an endoscopic approach is the specialized equipment, including the endoscope and the endoscopic tower, along with the need for a specialized practitioner trained in the use of an endoscope.

Complications

Similar general complications could occur such as bleeding, aspiration pneumonia, and internal organ injury, with the likelihood of any of them being very low. For example, reported major bleeding events range from 0.2% to 2.5% [40]. Overall, complication rates of PEG compared to PRG are comparable at 0–8% and 1.4–5.6%, respectively [39]. Minor differences are seen in a subset of categories. For example, PEG has increased rates of minor post-procedural infections (8–15%) [41]. Tumor seeding is considered a rare complication exclusive to "pull" techniques in circumstances such as esophageal cancer [42].

Fluoroscopic-Guided Gastrostomy Placement

Originally devised in 1981 with the advancement of real-time imaging modalities, PRG tube placement is generally considered to be the gold standard non-surgical technique [43]. Compared to the other gastrostomy tube techniques, PRG is considered the least invasive with the lowest complication rate [43].

Contraindications

Like the ultrasound-guided technique, the most significant contraindication to PRG is an unsafe needle tract, for example, secondary to interposed bowel loops. Additionally, portal hypertension and the presence of varices increase the risk of the procedure, particularly in a non-surgical setting where there are limited opportunities to control potential bleeding [44]. Other similarly important contraindications are inability for patients to tolerate insufflation, anatomical variance specifically with positioning of the stomach, and prior surgical history with possible adhesions and anatomical distortions, leading to a hostile intrabdominal environment preventing safe needle passage or appropriate gastropexy. There are a handful of relative contraindications that don't necessarily preclude patients from receiving gastrostomy tubes but require additional consideration and planning. For example, ascites, altered oropharyngeal anatomy, and obesity [16].

Procedure

Techniques can similarly be divided into the "push" and "pull" type techniques. The initial step for both requires an indwelling nasogastric tube to insufflate the stomach with air, approximately 500–1000 ml. The "pull" technique was originally adopted from endoscopic procedures, gaining access to the stomach via an internal-external approach. Firstly, an 18G needle is used to puncture the stomach and verified with the aspiration of the injected air, or administration of contrast to elucidate the rugal folds. Ideally, the stomach is punctured centrally, in the lower one-third, to avoid the gastroepiploic arteries [43]. Once correct positioning is confirmed, the needle is exchanged over a wire and the placement of a sheath, usually 5-Fr, creates a definitive entry point for the rest of the procedure. Depending the patient's anatomy and procedure difficulty, a catheter and wire are advanced into the esophagus and out of the patients oropharynx [43]. If there is difficulty in gaining access to the patient's esophagus or advancing the catheter/wire, an option is to use a loop snare, advance it anterograde through the oropharynx and esophagus, and snare the wire within the stomach. Depending on institutional policy and the practitioner's comfort, the hydrophilic wire is exchanged for a stiffer wire, attached to the external end of the gastrostomy tube, and pulled from the patient's mouth out of the newly made gastrostomy [43].

Compared to "pull" technique, the "push" technique inserts the gastrostomy tube without the need to traverse the patient's esophagus and oropharynx [43]. Exactly like the "pull" technique, access to the stomach is gained through a 17G needle; however, it is preloaded with an anchor. The anchors are specialized T-bar fasteners (Cope Gastrointestinal Suture Anchor Set; Cook, Bloomington IN, USA) [43]. Depending on institutional and provider practices, a minimum of three fasteners are placed with an optional fourth. By suturing the fasteners tight, a gastropexy is formed. Once secure, the gastric wall is punctured and a gastrostomy tube is pushed into the stomach after appropriate serial dilation of the tract using a peel away sheath [43].

Advantages

Of all the non-surgical gastrostomy tube techniques, PRG has the highest success rate, close to 100% [44]. It is also deemed the least invasive. Risk of tumor cell seeding is eliminated, bypassing postsurgical or obstructed nasopharynx/oropharynx, and surrounding structures are identified in real time during the procedure [45].

Disadvantages

Ionizing radiation occurs and specialized equipment is mandatory. Comparable to endoscopic techniques, a specialized practitioner with the appropriate expertise and skill is required.

Complications

Reportedly PRG has the lowest rate, in the range of 0–6%, compared to up to 9.4% and 19.9% for endoscopic and surgical approaches, respectively [39, 46].

References

1. Strong AT, Ponsky JL. Following the light: a history of the percutaneous endoscopic gastrostomy tube. 2017.
2. Reis SP, et al. Percutaneous ultrasound guided gastrostomy tube placement: a prospective cohort trial. J Intensive Care Med. 2022;37:641–6.
3. Rahnemai-Azar AA, Rahnemaiazar AA, Naghshizadian R, Kurtz A, Farkas DT. Percutaneous endoscopic gastrostomy: indications, technique, complications and management. World J Gastroenterol. 2014;20:7739–51.
4. Mekhail TM, et al. Enteral nutrition during the treatment of head and neck carcinoma: is a percutaneous endoscopic gastrostomy tube preferable to a nasogastric tube? Cancer. 2001;91:1785–90.

5. Long-term use of percutaneous endoscopic gastrostomies: a survey of duration of use and level of maintenance. Internet. J Gastroenterol. 2006;4:4.
6. Preventing aspiration pneumonia in older people: do we have the 'know-how'? HKMJ https://www.hkmj.org/abstracts/v20n5/421.htm; 2015.
7. Vudayagiri L, Hoilat GJ, Gemma R. Percutaneous endoscopic gastrostomy tube. In: StatPearls. StatPearls Publishing; 2022.
8. Parrish, C. R., Plonk Jr., W. M. Nutrition issues in gastroenterology, series #29.
9. Vergis EN, Brennen C, Wagener M, Muder RR. Pneumonia in long-term care: a prospective case-control study of risk factors and impact on survival. Arch Intern Med. 2001;161:2378–81.
10. Gomes CA Jr, et al. Percutaneous endoscopic gastrostomy versus nasogastric tube feeding for adults with swallowing disturbances. Cochrane Database Syst Rev. 2015;2015:CD008096.
11. Ikenaga Y, Kusunoki T, Yamaguchi H. Percutaneous endoscopic gastrostomy reduces aspiration pneumonia rate in stroke patients with enteral feeding in convalescent rehabilitation wards. Prog Rehabil Med. 2021;6:20210031.
12. Lin T-H, Yang C-W, Chang W-K. Evaluation of oropharyngeal dysphagia in older patients for risk stratification of pneumonia. Front Immunol. 2022;12
13. Nichols E, et al. Estimation of the global prevalence of dementia in 2019 and forecasted prevalence in 2050: an analysis for the global burden of disease study 2019. Lancet Public Health. 2022;7:e105–25.
14. Mitchell SL, et al. The clinical course of advanced dementia. N Engl J Med. 2009;361:1529–38.
15. Sanders DS, et al. Survival analysis in percutaneous endoscopic gastrostomy feeding: a worse outcome in patients with dementia. Am J Gastroenterol. 2000;95:1472–5.
16. Rajan A, Wangrattanapranee P, Kessler J, Kidambi TD, Tabibian JH. Gastrostomy tubes: fundamentals, periprocedural considerations, and best practices. World J Gastrointest Surg. 2022;14:286–303.
17. Boeykens K, Duysburgh I. Prevention and management of major complications in percutaneous endoscopic gastrostomy. BMJ Open Gastroenterol. 2021;8:e000628.
18. Venkatesan AM, et al. Practice guideline for adult antibiotic prophylaxis during vascular and interventional radiology procedures. J Vasc Interv Radiol. 2010;21:1611–30.
19. Itkin M, et al. Multidisciplinary practical guidelines for gastrointestinal access for enteral nutrition and decompression from the Society of Interventional Radiology and American Gastroenterological Association (AGA) institute, with endorsement by Canadian interventional radiological association (CIRA) and cardiovascular and interventional radiological Society of Europe (CIRSE). J Vasc Interv Radiol. 2011;22:1089–106.
20. Collins K, Gaffney L, Tan J, Roberts S, Nyulasi I. Gastrostomy guidelines: a rapid review.
21. Sutcliffe J, et al. CIRSE standards of practice guidelines on gastrostomy. Cardiovasc Intervent Radiol. 2016;39:973–87.
22. Crowley JJ, Cahill AM. Society of interventional radiology guidelines and statements division 2020 year-end document review. J Vasc Interv Radiol. 2021;32(918):e1–918.e4.
23. Khashab MA, et al. Antibiotic prophylaxis for GI endoscopy. Gastrointest Endosc. 2015;81:81–9.
24. Accorsi F, et al. Percutaneous ultrasound gastrostomy (PUG): first prospective clinical trial. Abdom Radiol. 2021;46:5377–85.
25. Patel IJ, et al. Society of Interventional Radiology Consensus Guidelines for the Periprocedural Management of Thrombotic and Bleeding Risk in patients undergoing percutaneous image-guided interventions—part II: recommendations: endorsed by the Canadian Association for Interventional Radiology and the cardiovascular and interventional radiological Society of Europe. J Vasc Interv Radiol. 2019;30:1168–84.
26. Baron TH, Kamath PS, McBane RD. Management of antithrombotic therapy in patients undergoing invasive procedures. N Engl J Med. 2013;368:2113–24.

27. Tramel R, Sandow T, April D, Ramalingam V. Safety and feasibility of percutaneous gastrostomy placement in patients on antiplatelet therapy. Ochsner J. 2021;21:158–62.
28. Bechtold ML, et al. Early versus delayed feeding after placement of a percutaneous endoscopic gastrostomy: a meta-analysis. Am J Gastroenterol. 2008;103:2919–24.
29. Chaves DM, et al. EUS-guided percutaneous endoscopic gastrostomy for enteral feeding tube placement. Gastrointest Endosc. 2008;68:1168–72.
30. Shukla PA, et al. Safety and feasibility of ultrasound-guided gastric access for percutaneous transabdominal gastrostomy tube placement. Gastroenterol Res. 2019;12:115–9.
31. Wu TS, Leech SJ, Rosenberg M, Huggins C, Papa L. Ultrasound can accurately guide gastrostomy tube replacement and confirm proper tube placement at the bedside. J Emerg Med. 2009;36:280–4.
32. Bleck JS, et al. Percutaneous sonographic gastrostomy: method, indications, and problems. Am J Gastroenterol. 1998;93:941–5.
33. Church JT, Speck KE, Jarboe MD. Ultrasound-guided gastrostomy tube placement: a case series. J Pediatr Surg. 2017;52:1210–4.
34. Marshall JD, et al. Length of stay and hospital cost reductions after implementing bedside percutaneous ultrasound gastrostomy (PUG) in a critical care unit. J Intensive Care Med. 2022;37:1667–72.
35. Olivieri PP, Abdulmahdi M, Heavner JJ. Bedside percutaneous ultrasound gastrostomy tube placement by critical care physicians. J Clin Ultrasound. 2021;49:28–32.
36. Cool DW, Chung J, Wiseman D, Kribs S, Mujoomdar A. Percutaneous ultrasound gastrostomy: first-in-human experience with the PUMA-G system. J Vasc Interv Radiol. 2020;31:808–11.
37. Olivieri P, Heavner J, Abdulmahdi M. Concomitant percutaneous dilatation tracheostomy and percutaneous ultrasound gastrostomy: methods to ensure safe practice standards during the COVID-19 pandemic. Chest. 2020;158:A2470.
38. Accorsi F, et al. Percutaneous ultrasound gastrostomy (PUG): first prospective clinical trial. Abdom Radiol N Y. 2021;46:5377–85.
39. Yuan Y, Zhao Y, Xie T, Hu Y. Percutaneous endoscopic gastrostomy versus percutaneous radiological gastrostomy for swallowing disturbances. Cochrane Database Syst Rev. 2016;2016:CD009198.
40. González-González JA, et al. Bleeding complications during percutaneous endoscopic gastrostomy treated with hemoclips. Med Univ. 2009;11:270–2.
41. Strijbos D, et al. Percutaneous endoscopic versus radiologic gastrostomy for enteral feeding: a retrospective analysis on outcomes and complications. Endosc Int Open. 2019;7:E1487–95.
42. Sinclair JJ, Scolapio JS, Stark ME, Hinder RA. Metastasis of head and neck carcinoma to the site of percutaneous endoscopic gastrostomy: case report and literature review. JPEN J Parenter Enteral Nutr. 2001;25:282–5.
43. Karthikumar B, et al. Percutaneous gastrostomy placement by intervention radiology: techniques and outcome. Indian J Radiol Imaging. 2018;28:225–31.
44. Shin JH, Park A-W. Updates on percutaneous radiologic gastrostomy/gastrojejunostomy and jejunostomy. Gut Liver. 2010;4:S25–31.
45. Partovi S, Li X, Moon E, Thompson D. Image guided percutaneous gastrostomy catheter placement: how we do it safely and efficiently. World J Gastroenterol. 2020;26:383–92.
46. Wollman B, D'Agostino HB, Walus-Wigle JR, Easter DW, Beale A. Radiologic, endoscopic, and surgical gastrostomy: an institutional evaluation and meta-analysis of the literature. Radiology. 1995;197:699–704.

Chapter 29
Optimal Pharmacotherapy Strategies for Enhanced Postoperative Recovery in High-Risk Surgeries

Richard Parrish and Rachelle Findley

Introduction: General Principles of Perioperative Pharmacotherapy Optimization

Numerous Enhanced Recovery After Surgery (ERAS®) protocols have incorporated evidence-based pharmacotherapy recommendations that aid in minimizing the frequency and severity of postoperative complications (POCs) [1, 2]. A recent report from an ERAS® Center of Excellence validated guideline-informed pharmacotherapies to minimize the incidence of surgical site infection (SSI) and venous thromboembolism (VTE), with lower lengths of stay in hospital (LOSH) and readmission rates in colorectal and gynecologic oncology patients [3] (Fig. 29.1). Decisions to continue or withhold medications in the preoperative phase help to avoid adverse events; however, these require clear and consistent communication with and participation from patients and caregivers to achieve optimum benefit [4, 5].

R. Parrish (✉)
Department of Biomedical Sciences, School of Medicine, Mercer University, Columbus, GA, USA

R. Findley
Faculty of Medicine, Dalhousie University, Halifax, NS, Canada
e-mail: rachelle.findley@nshealth.ca

© The Author(s), under exclusive license to Springer Nature Switzerland AG 2024

J. Faintuch, S. Faintuch (eds.), *Recent Strategies in High Risk Surgery*,
https://doi.org/10.1007/978-3-031-56270-9_29

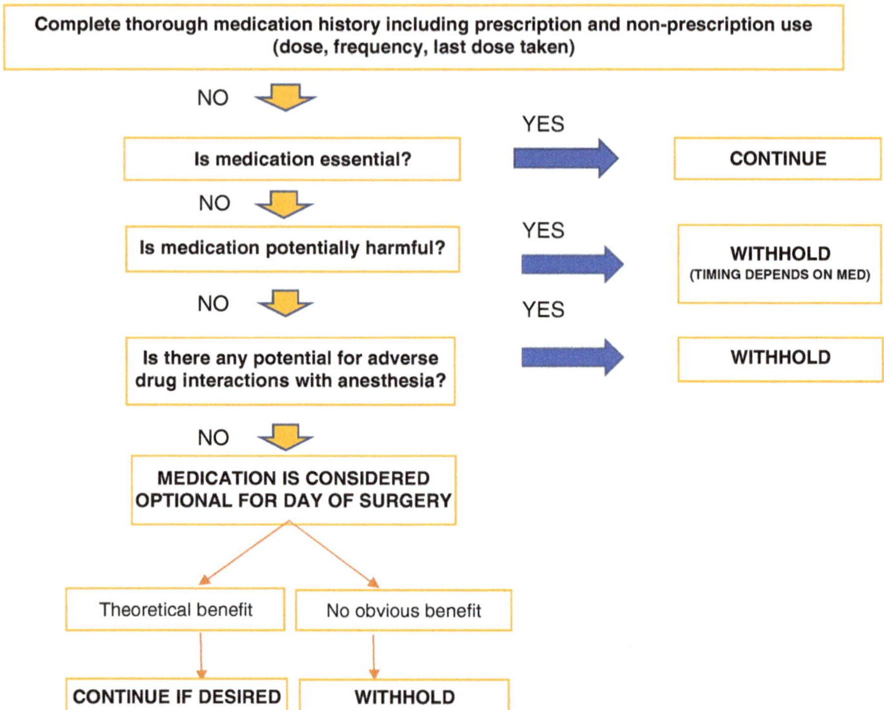

Fig. 29.1 Preoperative medication management decision-making algorithm (continue or withhold) (Cohn, 2021 with permission)

Preoperative Review of Medications

Cardiovascular

Concern in this area is related to medication controlling blood pressure and pulse rate, coagulation, and plaque stabilization [3, 6, 7]. Angiotensin converting enzyme inhibitor (ACEI) and angiotensin receptor blocker (ARB) continuation before non-cardiac surgery may provoke hypotension, but withholding them has no appreciable impact on acute kidney injury (AKI), major adverse cardiac event (MACE), death, or LOSH, suggesting that stopping 24 h preoperatively may be best [6, 7]. AKI is becoming a focus for hospitals in the United States through the Patient Safety Indicator (PSI-10). The PSI-10 is reported across healthcare institutions and is a quality metric for third party payers [8].

For hydroxymethylglutaryl-coenzyme A reductase inhibitors (HMG-CoA inhibitors or "statins"), perioperative initiation is reasonable for patients with vascular procedures and continuation in those already prescribed statins. Perioperative use is important for primary and secondary prevention of plaque rupture [7]. Beta-blockers should not be started in patients undergoing non-cardiac or low risk procedures and may need to be given intravenously in patients having cardiac surgery due to potential gastrointestinal malabsorption [7]. Centrally acting alpha-2 adrenergic agonists (clonidine, dexmedetomidine) are associated with increased hypotension and bradycardia; however, the drug class may lower anesthetic requirements [7].

Anti-Diabetic

Prolonged preoperative fasting should be avoided by providing complex carbohydrate liquids [9]. With the exception of sodium-glucose cotransporter-2 (SGLT2) inhibitors, diabetes medications should be given at the same dose on the day before surgery and withheld on postoperative day zero (POD0) [9, 10] (Table 29.1).

Table 29.1 Preoperative medication management in patients with diabetes (adapted from [9, 10, 58])

Medication	Day before surgery	Day of surgery	Restart
Metformin, DPP4I	Same preoperative doses	Continue at usual dose	Only withhold metformin if glomerular filtration rate < mL/min/1.73 m^2
Sulfonylureas	Same preoperative doses	Withhold	Restart with eating and drinking well
SGLT2I (canagliflozin, dapagliflozin, empagliflozin)	Stop three days before surgery (ertugliflozin—Stop four days before surgery)	Withhold	Restart with eating and drinking well
Injectable non-insulins (GLP-1, GIP)	Same preoperative doses	Continue at usual dose	Continue even if NPO
Glargine, detemir, NPH (long-acting basal insulin)	Same bedtime dose	Half normal morning dose	Continue even if NPO
Combination of long and short acting (mixed insulin; 75/25, 70/30)	Same bedtime dose	Based on fasting blood glucose: If > 200 mg/dL: Half normal dose; If < 200 mg/dL: None	Continue even if NPO

DPP4 Dipeptidil peptidase 4 inhibitors, *SGLT2I* sodium glucose cotransporter 2 inhibitors, *NPO* nothing per os, *GLP-1* glucagon like peptide 1 receptor agonist, *GIP* gastric inhibitory peptide receptor agonist, *NPH* neutral protamine Hagedorn (insulin)

A blood glucose range of between 140 and 180 mg/dL (7.8—10 mmol/L) should be maintained and reassessed every 2 h [10]. Blood glucose can be managed in the operating room with rapid acting insulin, and usually a regular insulin infusion is used in patients with expected temperature and hemodynamic changes, inotrope use, and longer procedure times, as well as in diabetics and those that will miss more than a meal [10].

Anticoagulants and Antiplatelets

While discontinuing aspirin is not associated with inferior outcomes, initiating or resuming aspirin doesn't improve outcomes. In contrast, in myocardial infarction after non-cardiac surgery (MINS), direct oral anticoagulant dabigatran lowered vascular complication risk without significant bleeding. Outcomes for postoperative atrial fibrillation (AFib) are comparable to nonsurgical nonvalvular AFib, and anticoagulation lowers stroke and death risk. Fewer patients are anticoagulated postoperatively [6]. Antiplatelet medications should be stopped prior to neuraxial anesthesia (4–8 h for eptifibatide, 1–2 days for abciximab, and 7 days for clopidogrel); however, aspirin in dual antiplatelet therapy (DAPT) patients should be continued for secondary prevention [7]. Recommendations for anticoagulation with vitamin K antagonists (VKAs), direct oral anticoagulants (DOACs), low molecular weight heparins (LMWHs), aspirin, and $P2Y_{12}$ inhibitors are presented in Figs. 29.2, 29.3, and 29.4 [11–13].

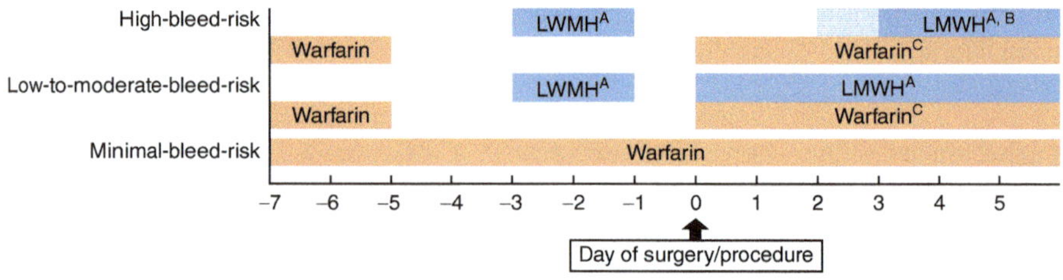

Fig. 29.2 Perioperative management of warfarin (vitamin K antagonists/VKAs) (Douketis et al., 2022 with permission)

[a]Bridging suggested for high thrombotic risk populations with full-dose, subcutaneous LMWH (enoxaparin, dalteparin, or tinzaparin), with the last dose given in the morning of the day before the procedure (POD-1); [b]Low-dose LMWH can be used for first 24–72 h post-procedure, with full-dose LMWH resumed 2–3 days post-procedure; [c]VKAs can be resumed on the evening of the procedure (POD0) for most patients, or the day after procedure (POD1) at the patient's usual maintenance dose; *LMWH* low-molecular-weight heparin, *LMWH* low molecular weight heparin, *VKA* vitamin K antagonist

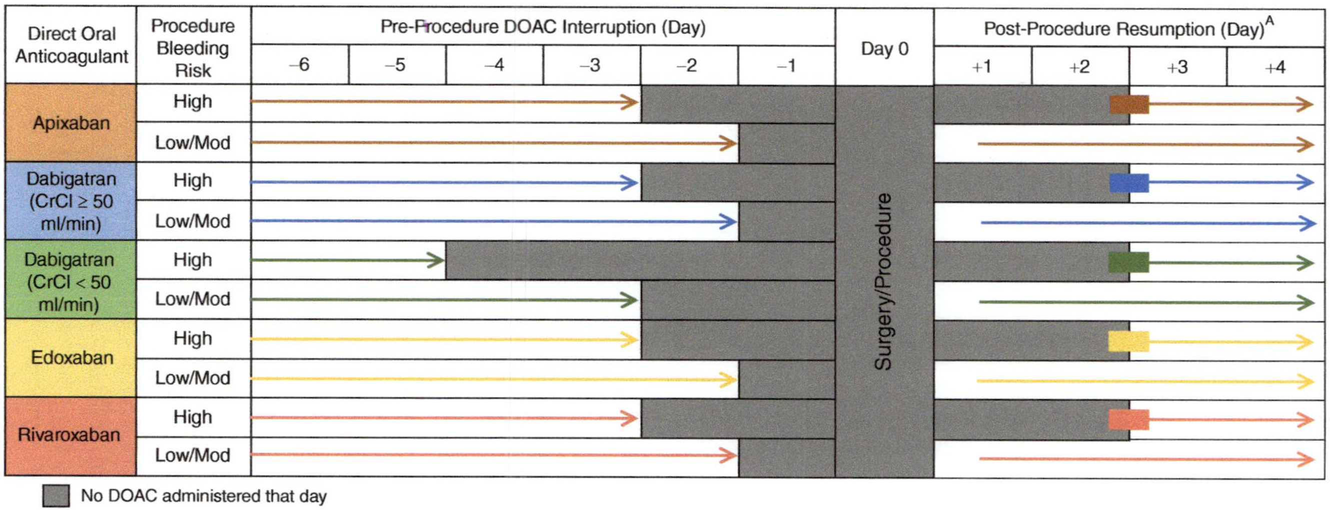

Fig. 29.3 Perioperative management of direct oral anticoagulants (Douketis et al., 2022 with permission)

[a]DOAC can be resumed approximately 24 h after low/moderate-bleed-risk procedures, and 48–72 h after high-bleed-risk procedures. In selected patients at high risk for venous thromboembolism, low-dose anticoagulants can be given for the first 48–72 h post-procedure; *DOAC* direct oral anticoagulants, *CrCl* creatinine clearance

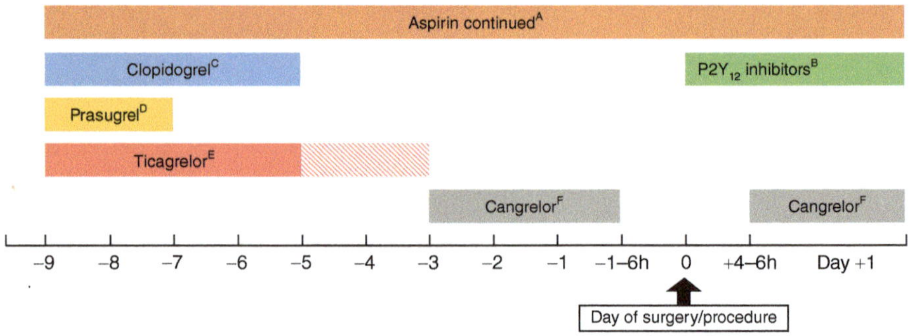

Fig. 29.4 Perioperative management of antiplatelet drugs (Douketis et al. 2022 with permission) [a]Based on surgery/procedure bleed risk assessment; [b]$P2Y_{12}$ inhibitors can be resumed within 24 h post-procedure at a maintenance dose; [c]For ticagrelor, 3–5 days interruption; [d]For clopidogrel, 5 days interruption; [e]For prasugrel, 7–10 days interruption; [f]Routine use not suggested$P2Y_{12}$: Platelet $P2Y_{12}$ receptor inhibitors (antiplatelet agents), such as clopidogrel/ ticagrelor/prasugrel

Neuropsychiatric

Depression, antidepressants, and perioperative anesthetic/analgesic medications interact and may precipitate hypotension, cardiac arrhythmias, and persistent post-operative cognitive dysfunction and pain [14]. Stress-induced proinflammatory cytokines from surgical procedures, such as IL-1, may adversely affect neuronal plasticity and combined with growth factor inhibition, reduce neurogenesis, and magnify depressive symptomatology [14]. Stress also activates the hypothalamus-pituitary-adrenal axis, leading to increased cortisol, growth hormone, and catecholamine release [14, 15]. Patients should continue most antidepressants, anxiolytics, and mood-stabilizing agents (carbamazepine, lamotrigine, oxcarbazepine, and valproate, but not lithium) preoperatively and on POD0 to avoid discontinuation syndrome (dizziness, lethargy, anxiety, confusion, sleep disorders, tremor, delirium, and headache) [14, 15]. Amphetamine and amphetamine-like agents (methylphenidate, atomoxetine) for adult attention deficit hyperactivity should be withheld on POD0; however, guanfacine should be continued [15]. Lithium should be stopped on POD-3 for major procedures, and concomitant ketorolac should be avoided due to precipitous increases in lithium serum levels [14, 15].

Perioperative lidocaine has been shown to reduce tricyclic antidepressant (TCA) cardiotoxicity; however, due to catecholamine depletion, patients may become hypotensive, and fluid boluses with vasopressors may be necessary [14]. Selective serotonin reuptake inhibitors (SSRI) may increase bleeding risk in patients co-administered non-steroidal anti-inflammatories (NSAIDs), such as ibuprofen, ketorolac, and celecoxib [14]. Synthetic opioids and related molecules such as dextromethorphan, meperidine, and tramadol should be avoided in patients on monoamine oxidase inhibitors (MAOI) [14]. Seizure activity should be closely monitored in patients on bupropion, a monocyclic antidepressant structurally similar to amphetamines [14, 15].

Serotonin syndrome (altered mental status, tremor, clonus, hypertonia, and diaphoresis) triggered by SSRIs, TCAs, MAOIs, amphetamines, serotonin norepinephrine inhibitors (SNRIs), and St. John's Wort may be exacerbated from use of common perioperative medications including 5HT2 and 3 inhibitors (granisetron, ondansetron, palonosetron), fentanyl, meperidine, methadone, and metoclopramide [14]. Rare, serious adverse events with analeptics, neuroleptics, volatile anesthetics, and depolarizing neuromuscular blocking agents (NMBs) include neuroleptic malignant syndrome (antipsychotics and dopamine antagonists) and malignant hyperthermia (anesthetics, NMBs) [14, 15].

Corticosteroids and Immunomodulators

Roughly 3% of the perioperative population receive preoperative chronic glucocorticoids which are linked to a three-fold increase (2.9–5%) in surgical site infection (SSI), a 3.4-times increase in wound dehiscence, and a four-fold increase (1.6–6%) in death [16–18]. Dexamethasone and other corticosteroids are often administered to prevent postoperative nausea and vomiting (PONV), airway edema, and stridor. Lower doses (4–5 mg) and more frequent monitoring (every 1 h for 4 h) are suggested for diabetic patients [8]. While withholding glucocorticoids may reduce complications, endogenous steroid production in chronically prescribed patients is often suppressed and discontinuation could precipitate adrenal crisis, which is especially concerning in transplant patients. Return of adrenal function is confirmed with preoperative serum cortisol levels or insulin tolerance and cosyntropin stimulation testing [18].

Reducing steroid dosing to a minimum level is performed on a case-by-case basis [18]. Patients with a history of hypopituitarism should be evaluated accordingly and may require a pre-operative dose of hydrocortisone 100–200 mg prior to surgery. Inhaled steroids should be continued [19]. Purine analogues and methotrexate can be continued; however, all monoclonal antibody and TNF-alpha blockers should be withheld for at least one dosing interval. Tofacitinib and other Janus kinase inhibitors should be withheld beginning POD-7 and ozanimod and other sphingosine-1-phosphate receptor modulators, 60 days prior to procedure [19].

Opioids and Adjunctive Agents

Patients receiving opioids within 90 days of surgery have significantly higher complication rates, especially pain and infection: SSI, urinary tract infection [UTI], and sepsis, with higher healthcare resource utilization (LOSH and hospital costs) [20]. Patients weaned from preoperative use have similar outcomes to opioid-naïve patients [20]. Opioid agonists, mixed agonist-antagonists, calcitonin-gene related peptide (CGRP), antispasmodics (baclofen and tizanidine), and acetaminophen should be continued through the perioperative period while serotonin receptor agonists ("triptans"), opioid antagonists (alvimopan, naltrexone [hold 3–4 days], naloxegol), ergotamine derivatives, butalbital, and centrally acting muscle relaxants should not be given on POD0 morning [21].

Hormones, Bone Medications, Urologicals, and Modulators

Continue all androgenics, antidiuretic hormone, aromatase inhibitors, bromocriptine, cabergoline, calcitonin, cinacalcet, corticosteroids, denosumab, growth hormone, estrogens, progestins, selective estrogen receptor modulators, somatostatin analogues, 5-alpha reductase inhibitors, alpha-1 adrenergic antagonists, antineoplastic urologics, and thyroid preparations [9]. Withhold all bisphosphonates, anticholinergic bladder agents, and PDE5 inhibitors (withhold beginning POD-3 unless used for pulmonary hypertension) on POD0 [19]. Endogenous sex hormone levels are not associated with the same VTE risk as exogenous hormone replacement [22], although elevated levels of estradiol and sex-hormone-binding globulin and free androgen index in polycystic ovarian syndrome may increase risk, especially with hormonal contraception [23].

Since the most likely time for experiencing VTE on estrogen-containing oral contraception (eOCPs) is within 3 months from initiation, whether to discontinue eOCPs throughout the perioperative period is based on patient history and the potential downside risk of a pregnancy in the preoperative period [24]. Of note, sugammadex and aprepitant use may reduce the effectiveness of eOCPs. Patients should be advised to use other non-hormonal contraception for at least 7 days (sugammadex) and 28 days (aprepitant) [25, 26].

Herbals, Vitamins, and Supplements

Chondroitin, ephedra (Ma-Huang), fish oil, garlic, ginseng, glucosamine, kava, milk thistle, saw palmetto, St. John's Wort, valerian, and vitamin E (tocopherol) should be withheld at least till POD-14 while there is no specific recommendation for flaxseed, coenzyme Q10, and green tea [27]. In general, any dietary supplement should be withheld (Table 29.2) between 2 and 3 weeks preoperatively [28].

Table 29.2 Medications that should be withheld preoperatively

Medication or supplement	Preoperative hold
ACEI (captopril, lisinopril, ramipril) or ARB (azilsartan, candesartan, irbesartan, losartan, olmesartan, valsartan, telmisartan)	POD-1 and POD0
Amphetamines, methylphenidate, atomoxetine	POD0
Anticholinergic bladder agents (bethanechol, mirabegron)	POD-1 and POD0 (especially in elderly)
Bisphosphonates (alendronate, risedronate, ibandronate)	POD-3 and POD0
Butalbital	POD0
Centrally acting muscle relaxants (carisoprodol, cyclobenzaprine, metaxalone, methocarbamol, orphenadrine)	POD0
Ergotamine derivatives	POD0
Lithium	POD-3 and POD0
Monoclonal antibody (ustekinumab, natalizumab, vedolizumab)	One dosing interval (usually POD-14 to -28)
Monoamine oxidase inhibitors (phenelzine, tranylcypromine, isocarboxazid, selegiline)	POD-14 with psychiatric consult
Naltrexone	POD-3 or -4
Sphingosine-1-phosphate receptor modulators (ozanimod, fingolimod, siponimod)	POD-60
PDE5 inhibitors (sildenafil, tadalafil, vardenafil)	POD-3 (continue for pulmonary hypertension)
Oral supplements (chondroitin, ephedra [ma-Huang], fish oil, garlic, ginseng, glucosamine, kava, milk thistle, saw palmetto, St. John's wort, valerian, vitamin E [tocopherol])	POD-14-21
TNF-α blockers (adalimumab, infliximab, and biosimilars)	One dosing interval (usually POD-14 to -28)
Janus kinase inhibitors (tofacitinib, baricitinib, ruxolitinib, upadacitinib, fedratinib, abrocitinib, ruxolitinib)	POD-7

ACEI angiotensin converting enzyme inhibitors, *ARB* angiotensin receptor blockers, *PDE5* phosphodiesterase 5 inhibitors

Minimizing Risk from Common Comorbidities

Coexisting Infection

Preoperative sepsis has been identified as an independent predictor of postoperative mortality [29]. Those with sepsis are more likely to require an emergent operation which further increases the perioperative mortality risk [29]. UTI at the time of surgery is also associated with increased risk of infectious and non-infectious complications [30]. Despite the risks of POCs, there are no strong data to support treating asymptomatic bacteriuria. Therefore, it is not recommended to screen for asymptomatic bacteriuria but to treat only if symptomatic [31]. Preoperative respiratory infections, such as pneumonia or COVID-19, have been identified as risk factors for increased postoperative mortality and complications such as prolonged ventilation or need for reintubation [32–34]. It is recommended that surgery be delayed, if possible, until any respiratory infection is treated.

Tobacco Use

Tobacco use is associated with increased risk of POCs including wound healing concerns, infection, pulmonary complications, and prolonged LOSH [35–37]. Historic observations suggested there was increased sputum production and change in cough if smoking stopped within a few weeks of surgery. This has not been substantiated and a meta-analysis demonstrated that there is no increased risk of POCs if smoking cessation occurs within 8 weeks of an operation [35].

While increased complications with smoking cessation have not been shown, a reduction in POCs has also not been definitively shown if there is a short interval between cessation and surgery [37]. Behavioral support and nicotine replacement therapy may improve short-term smoking cessation complaints and should be offered to help minimize discomfort [38]. For motivated patients wishing long-term cessation, there is evidence of benefit for intensive intervention started at least 4 weeks prior to surgery. These patients may have fewer complications overall, with a potentially significant reduction in wound complications [38].

Ethanol Use

Alcohol use is common among patients and national guidelines substantially vary on recommended daily maximum intake. High alcohol intake, or "risky drinking," can be tentatively defined as more than three alcoholic units per day or 21 per week. Indeed, the World Health Organization states that no level of alcohol consumption is safe for health. One unit equals 12 g of ethanol in Italy, Sweden, and some other parts of Europe, or one small glass of wine, with a worldwide range of 8–20 g/unit [39]. While alcohol use can cause disorders of the liver, pancreas, and nervous system, it may also impact other physiologic systems that increase the risk for perioperative complications. Alcohol intake greater than three units per day can compromise the immune response, increase the risk of cardiac insufficiency and arrhythmias, and alter blood clotting time [39].

Available data suggests that short and long-term interventions can decrease alcohol use in the perioperative period, but data are lacking on whether there is a corresponding reduction in complication rates [39]. Preoperative alcohol screening is encouraged to prevent POCs from alcohol withdrawal syndrome, nominally *delirium tremens* which can impact LOSH as well as mortality [40].

Nutritional Status

At least 30% of hospitalized patients undergoing major surgery are malnourished [41, 42]. Malnutrition is an independent predictor of POCs including increased LOSH in both the oncologic and non-oncologic patient group [41, 43, 44]. Large data available from the National Surgical Quality Improvement Program (NSQIP) identifies malnutrition as a modifiable risk factor for reducing postoperative mortality and morbidity [42, 43]. The impacts of malnutrition are broad, including impaired immune function, changes in digestion and absorption, muscle weakness leading to respiratory complications, and wound healing troubles [45].

Defining malnutrition can be challenging. Measurement of serum albumin can be applied to preoperative patients; however, it can be impacted by stress, infection, and organ dysfunction separate from malnutrition [46]. Albumin levels lower than 3 g/dL are associated with significantly higher rates of POCs and 30-day mortality [43]. Other studies suggest that an even higher threshold for hypoalbuminemia should be considered, with a cutoff of 4 g/dL [41]. Body mass index (BMI) may also be a surrogate marker for malnutrition as those with a BMI less than 18.5 kg/m^2, or less than 20 kg/m^2 if older than 65, have higher rates of POCs [42]. A more formal assessment of nutrition status such as the Perioperative Nutrition Screen (PONS) integrates BMI, recent unintentional weight loss, dietary intake, and serum albumin, and vitamin D levels to provide a risk score. It is recommended that those at high risk for malnutrition see a registered dietician for preoperative nutritional optimization [42].

Nutritional support in malnourished patients should ideally begin preoperatively and continue postoperatively [44, 46]. Enteral nutrition is the preferred method for improving nutrition. Optimizing protein intake can reduce complication rates when started at least 5–7 days prior to major surgery [44, 46]. Use of parenteral nutrition is not recommended as there may be increased risk of POCs and infection. This should only be considered in those with an absolute contraindication to enteral feeding [44, 46].

Anemia

Anemia affects at least one-third of preoperative patients [47–49]. Iron deficiency anemia is the most common cause of anemia preoperatively [47, 49]. Preoperative anemia is associated with higher rates of postoperative mortality and morbidity including SSI, cardiac events, and LOSH [47, 49].

Mainstay of treatment is iron supplementation, and red blood cell transfusion should be avoided. Iron can be supplemented either orally or parenterally [47, 49]. Oral iron supplementation must be started 1 or 2 months in advance of surgery whereas parenteral iron should be given at least 2 weeks preoperatively [49, 50]. The use of recombinant erythropoietin (EPO) to stimulate hematopoiesis in bone marrow has come in and out of favor since it became available [45, 47, 48]. Meta-analysis of available studies suggest that EPO in combination with iron supplementation does reduce the risk of transfusion perioperatively [47, 46]. Increased risk of thromboembolism with recombinant EPO products was a concern, but newer research suggests that those risks may be higher in prolonged use of EPO, while short term use immediately preoperatively may not have the same risk [47]. Given this, recombinant EPO can be considered along with iron supplementation in well-selected patients requiring correction of preoperative anemia and to support blood conservation management strategies [50].

High-Risk, Non-cardiovascular Surgeries

High-risk surgeries are defined as procedures with possible significant effect on hemodynamics and blood loss. These procedures include colorectal surgery with bowel resection; kidney transplant; major joint replacement (shoulder, knee, and hip); open radical prostatectomy or cystectomy; and major oncologic general, gynecologic, or head and neck surgery.

Common Postoperative Complications

Nausea and Vomiting

Postoperative nausea and vomiting (PONV) are common complications of surgery and optimal management is sometimes complex [51]. Risk factors include female gender, a history of PONV or motion sickness, nonsmokers, and young age. The choice of anesthetic during surgery can impact these rates. Avoidance of opioids has been shown to reduce PONV and options include opioid-free total intravenous anesthesia (TIVA), regional anesthesia, multimodal analgesia, beta-blockers, and administration of alpha-agonists [51]. Nitrous oxide is a likely risk factor for PONV, but it appears to be related to exposure time as use less than an hour has a significantly lower risk of PONV compared to longer exposures [51].

Preoperative prophylactic acetaminophen significantly decreases opioid use and reduce rates of PONV. Intravenous use is best studied, but oral prophylaxis reduces opioid use and is less expensive [51]. Alpha-2 adrenergic receptor agonist dexmetomidine administration prior to skin incision also reduces opioid use and PONV [51]. Use of neuraxial anesthesia, such as epidural anesthesia and transversus abdominus plane (TAP) blocks are other interesting alternatives [51].

Pharmacologic prophylaxis is recommended and newer guidelines suggest multimodal prophylaxis in those with one or more risk factors. Serotonin 5-HT3 receptor antagonists can be combined with dexamethasone, aprepitant, haloperidol, or betahistine. Non-5HT3 receptor antagonist containing combinations are also described [51].

In those exhibiting PONV despite prophylaxis, using a pharmacologic agent from a different class is recommended as repeated dose of the former options within 6 h has not been shown to provide additional benefit [51]. In those who did not receive prophylaxis, 5-HT3 receptor antagonists are the first-line therapy for treating PONV. Nonpharmacologic therapies such as aromatherapy with isopropyl alcohol or peppermint oil, ginger, and PC6 acupressure may all reduce PONV [51, 52].

Postoperative Ileus (Delayed Gastric Emptying)

Early feeding and early mobilization significantly reduce the rate of postoperative ileus and are core components of ERAS® pathways [53, 54]. Epidural analgesia is also associated with a reduction in ileus compared to systemic analgesia, but may not benefit LOSH [53]. Selective use of nasogastric tube drainage is recommended along with early removal [54]. A variety of pharmacologic and nonpharmacologic approaches has been trialed in the prevention of ileus, without consistent outcomes [55, 56].

The peripherally acting mu-opioid receptor antagonist, alvimopan, significantly reduces the time to bowel recovery. Side-effects include hypokalemia and insomnia [57]. Methylnaltrexone and ghrelin receptor agonists do not reliably reduce the risk of ileus [57]. Data on serotonin receptor agonists as prophylaxis are more limited but mosapride may reduce the time to bowel recovery, whereas metoclopramide does not appear to reliably reduce ileus [57].

Glycemic and Electrolyte Imbalances

Perioperative glycemic control is recommended by most major societies as a strategy to reduce infections complications, lower mortality, and shorten LOSH [58]. This applies to both diabetic and non-diabetic patients. Attention should be paid to which agents are most likely to cause hypoglycemia in patients who are nil per os (NPO), as this is a potentially serious side-effect of anti-diabetic drugs. These higher risk agents, such as short-acting insulin, SGLT-2 inhibitors, meglitinides, and sulfonylureas, should be held until patients are eating well [58]. Other agents can be continued throughout the perioperative period with attention paid to a dose reduction for long-acting insulins [58]. In North America, it is common practice to withhold metformin perioperatively; however, this agent does not cause hypoglycemia and the risk of lactic acidosis is extremely low. Given this, it should only be held if the patient's eGFR is less than 30 mL/min/1.73 m^2 [58]. In patients with blood glucose levels above 180 mg/dL (10 mmol/L), intervention with basal bolus insulin therapy reduces POCs in comparison with traditional sliding-scale insulin regimens [58, 59].

Major electrolyte disturbances can occur in the postoperative period. Patients at higher risk include those with AKI, malnourished patients experiencing refeeding syndrome, patients with a malignancy, and those in the intensive care unit.

Disturbances in sodium levels are typically related to imbalances in total body water with correction being achieved after assessment for total body water excess or deficit. Treatment of hyperkalemia requires removal of additional potassium supplementation in fluids and binding or shifting potassium to facilitate removal. If there are no ECG changes and the patient has a functional bowel, then an oral agent such as sodium polystyrene (Kayexalate) can be used. If more urgent shifting is required, this can be achieved with insulin with accompanying glucose. If ECG changes are present, a parenteral dose of calcium is required for myocardial stabilization.

In the event of hypokalemia, this is replaced orally if the patient is asymptomatic and tolerating enteral nutrition, with the parenteral route used for symptomatic patients, those who cannot tolerate oral supplementation, or those with critically low values. Muild hypophosphatemia and hypomagnesemia are replaced with oral supplementation. Parenteral supplementation is indicated if the refeeding syndrome is suspected, or in those not tolerating enteral nutrition. Magnesium should be infused over a prolonged period, ideally 24 h at up to 1 g/h, to maximize absorption and minimize renal excretion [60].

Acute Kidney Injury

Acute kidney injury (AKI) occurs with an increase in serum creatinine by 50% or greater within 7 days, of greater than or equal to 0.3 mg/dL (26.5 mmol/L) within 48 h, or oliguria in face of adequate fluid intake [61]. Postoperative AKI is associated with increased mortality and LOSH, as well as subsequent chronic kidney disease [61]. The mechanism leading to kidney injury is often multifactorial and can include perfusion related injuries, nephrotoxic medications, urologic obstruction, and vasoconstriction [61]. Nephrotoxic medications may play a role in up to 30% of AKI [61].

NSAIDs may contribute to postoperative AKI, and routine prescription of 0.9% saline is associated with more postoperative AKI compared to balanced crystalloids in those at high risk [62]. Hypotension and prolonged hyperglycemia are both recognized mechanisms [62]. If AKI is recognized, it is key to remove nephrotoxic medications and treat the underlying causes. Initial expansion of the intravascular volume is recommended with balanced crystalloids as opposed to colloids such as albumin. Diuretics can be initially tested provided hydration is maintained (euvolemia), and may be required if there is evidence of volume overload [62].

Urinary Retention

The incidence of postoperative urinary retention varies from 5% to 70% [63]. Risk factors include age over 50, male gender, major abdominal or pelvic surgery, neurologic complications (such as diabetic neuropathy, stroke, multiple sclerosis), prolonged surgery duration, medications, and receiving excess perioperative intravenous fluids [63]. Urinary retention has been precipitated by medications such as anticholinergics, opioids, anesthetics, alpha-adrenergic agonists, calcium channel blockers, detrusor relaxants, and benzodiazepines. Their prescription should be carefully analyzed in those with prostate hypertrophy or previous history of urinary retention [63, 64].

Standard of care management of urinary retention is bladder catheterization, whether this be intermittent or indwelling [63]. Prophylactic alpha-adrenergic blockers such as tamsulosin may attenuate urinary retention in both men and women; however, results are inconsistent [63, 65, 66].

Venous Thromboembolism (VTE)

VTE includes deep vein thrombosis and pulmonary embolism. These are common complications, occurring at rates of 15–38% and just under 1%, respectively, in those undergoing major general or gynecology surgery who do not receive prophylaxis [67, 68]. Appropriate thromboprophylaxis can reduce the rate of VTE by 30–65% with low risk of complications [67]. Studies indicate that despite recommendations 40–60% of patients don't receive appropriate prophylaxis [67].

Conventional guidelines with injectable drugs recommend thromboprophylaxis for all major general, gynecologic, and open urology operations with either low molecular weight heparin/ LMWH, low-dose unfractionated heparin (UFH), or subcutaneous fondaparinux [68]. In gynecologic oncology surgery VTE is decreased by just over 40% with either LMWH or low-dose UFH [67]. Giving aspirin alone is not deemed sufficient in any patient group [68]. Direct oral anticoagulants/DOAC for extended prophylaxis appear to provide a safe alternative to injectable medications and may be more acceptable to patients [69]. The recommended length of postoperative prophylaxis varies widely among surgical groups, procedure type, and patient factors such as malignancy.

Blood Pressure Management

While blood pressure targets for ambulatory patients are clearly defined and well-researched, optimum blood pressure targets in the perioperative setting are less clear [70]. Intraoperative hypotension in non-cardiac surgery is associated with increased morbidity including cardiac and renal dysfunction, delirium, and postoperative mortality [70]. Intraoperative hypertension is not reliably associated with POCs [70]. Based on the available evidence for those undergoing non-cardiac surgery, identifying the patient's baseline blood pressure, and maintaining intraoperative blood pressure within a range of up to 10% variance is suggested [70].

Postoperative Hypotension/Hypertension

A systolic blood pressure of less than 90 mmHg has been found to increase the risk of myocardial injury, stroke, and mortality [71]. This threshold may be higher in someone with preoperative hypertension and avoiding a drop in blood pressure by more than 30% of the patient's baseline is suggested [71]. While many patients have a natural drop in their blood pressure by 10–20% while sleeping, some do not. Therefore, it is important to not ignore prolonged periods of hypotension unless the patient has been demonstrated to have lower blood pressures out of hospital [71].

Postoperative hypertension (systolic pressure greater than 180 mmHg) is associated with increased risk of heart attack, arrhythmia, pulmonary complications, stroke, and bleeding [71]. Curiously there is no demonstrated benefit from lowering blood pressure substantially below 180 mmHg postoperatively [71].

Cardiologic Medications

Continuing already prescribed beta-blockers postoperatively decreases short and long-term mortality. Conversely, holding a beta-blocker has been shown to increase mortality in those undergoing vascular surgery. A beta-blocker should be held postoperatively if a patient develops a third-degree heart block and the dose titrated or held in the setting of hypotension or severe bradycardia [71]. Angiotensin-converting enzyme inhibitors/ACEI and angiotensin receptor blockers/ARB should be restarted within 48 h of surgery unless the patient has an elevation in creatinine levels or low blood pressure. Failure to restart these agents is associated with an increase in 30-day mortality, especially in those under age 60 [71]. Calcium channel blockers/CCBs may reduce cardiac ischemia and arrhythmia in the perioperative period but guidance on reintroduction of these agents is limited by lack of evidence [71]. Similarly, evidence is limited on management of diuretics [71].

Atrial Fibrillation

Atrial fibrillation (AFib) occurs in up to 10% of patients undergoing non-cardiac surgery and the vast majority will revert to sinus rhythm prior to discharge [72]. Despite this, perioperative AFib is associated with an increased risk of early and late stroke (62% higher odds of early, 37% higher odds of late) and mortality (37–44% higher odds), particularly in those undergoing non-cardiac surgery [72]. In the POISE trial evaluating prophylactic metoprolol in the perioperative period, there were fewer new AFib events however significantly higher rates of mortality and stroke [71, 72]. Therefore this practice is not encouraged. In contrast meta-analyses with cardiac surgery cohorts identified risk reduction with such drugs as amiodarone, landiolol, and colchicine.

Patients experiencing AFib in the perioperative period should be managed similar to those in the ambulatory setting. An assessment for predisposing factors preceding the AFib event is key, along with an evaluation on the need for ongoing anticoagulation [73]. According to Canadian guidelines, beta-blockers or nondihydropyridine calcium channel blockers (verapamil, diltiazem) should be considered as first-line therapy for rate control in those with normal cardiac ejection fraction. Cardioversion should be considered for any patients deemed to be vitally unstable [73].

Shock and Hemorrhage

In patients with postoperative shock, 30-day mortality rate is as high as 26%, and independent factors associated with short-term prognosis are the severity of clinical status at ICU admission, worsening organ dysfunction during the first 3 days of ICU admission, and intraoperative coagulation disturbances [74]. The first 3 days of ICU admission are important for overall survival [74]. Long-term mortality (>6 months) is also associated with worsening early organ dysfunction, especially hepatic dysfunction, and intraoperative coagulation disturbances, and the impact of comorbidities [74]. The evolving concept of perioperative goal-directed fluid (hemodynamic) therapy (GDFT) currently includes the use of fluids and/or vasopressors to reach and maintain hemodynamic endpoints (systolic pressure > 90 mmHg, mean arterial pressure 60–65 mmHg) and minimize postoperative circulatory complications [75, 76].

Perioperative GDFT to optimize fluid status and hemodynamics, with the appropriate use of fluids as well as the use of earlier/preemptive inotropes and vasopressors has been adopted in some centers, however not in others [75]. Vasopressor selection (dopamine, norepinephrine, epinephrine, phenylephrine, vasopressin) should be based on rectifying underlying physiologic deficits. Practically speaking, which agent is chosen initially does not seem as important as reaching and maintaining hemodynamic goals. A supraphysiologic goal for cardiac output has not been beneficial and may cause morbidity [75]. A second medication with a different mechanism of action should be added when maximum doses of the initial agent are inadequate [75].

Myocardial Infarction in Non-cardiac Surgeries

Cardiogenic shock (CS) is a feared complication of acute myocardial infarction (AMI), and the mortality rate of patients with CS as a result of AMI is around 40–50%, within any setting [76]. Progression from AMI to CS can develop within hours after severe AMI, as a result of left ventricular systolic and diastolic dysfunction (most common), acute mitral regurgitation, ventricular septal rupture, isolated right ventricular failure, tamponade or cardiac rupture [76]. While guidance for optimal pharmacologic therapy in patients with CS after AMI is scarce, guidelines recommend avoiding renin-angiotensin-aldosterone system inhibitors and beta-blockers until shock resolves [76].

Surgical Site Infection

After implementing an ERAS® protocol for colorectal surgeries, a 2.5-fold decrease in SSI rate has been announced even if compliance with other individual bundle items is below 50%. However, compliance with preoperative antibiotic administration alone is associated with improved outcomes [77]. Alternative non-cephalosporin regimens, especially ertapenem, may be as effective as cephalosporin-based regimens for preventing 30-day SSI; however, recent evidence suggests that alternative regimens may lead to worse outcomes [78].

Evidence of at least moderate certainty indicates reduced SSI risk when IV antibiotics are administered prior to cesarean incision, breast cancer surgery, and hernia repair. Iodine-impregnated adhesive drapes are not recommended, and there is probably no difference in SSI risk when antibiotics are stopped the day of surgery compared to longer duration during colorectal surgery [79]. Optimization of stroke volume and cardiac output is defended by some, so that circulation to the surgical wound area is not compromised [80].

GDFT seems to reduce SSI in cardiac, gastrointestinal, and other non-cardiac surgeries, but not in vascular or orthopedic procedures [80]. Respiratory and urinary system infectious complications were also less frequent, however not sepsis or septic shock [80]. Visceral surgery patients with reported penicillin allergy can be treated with a cephalosporin or ertapenem; however, true cephalosporin allergy requires alternative therapy with gentamicin and clindamycin or metronidazole [81]. Oral antibiotic gut sterilization has very rare indications nowadays, and even for laparoscopic bowel and rectal procedures it is sometimes questioned [55].

Pain Management

As many as 55% of patients have POCs that are related to higher pain levels [82]. Diabetes is an independent predictor of postoperative pain, and about 30% of diabetics experience neuropathic pain [80]. Younger patients experience more pain intensity and this could be explained by reduced renal clearance of opioids in the elderly [82]. See Table 29.3 for a suggested multimodal protocol which reduced the frequency and severity of postoperative pain by 50% in colorectal surgery [82]. Minimally invasive surgery (MIS) is deemed less painful than open surgery, however outcomes are inconsistent, for instance when anterior rectal resection and abdominal perineal rectal excision modalities are compared [82].

IV lidocaine, although beneficial in select cases, is currently not considered the standard of care for acute pain management due to the primarily observational data supporting its safe and effective use, with scarce prospective protocols [83]. Compared with sufentanil, hydromorphone may significantly reduce postoperative pain, with no significant difference in sedation and patient-controlled analgesia requests. In addition, the incidence of PONV and somnolence with hydromorphone could be lower [84].

Table 29.3 Pharmacotherapy recommendations for preventing common postoperative complications (expanded from Parrish et al. [1])

Postoperative complication	Recommendations (consider alternatives for shortages)
Nausea and vomiting	Preoperative complex carbohydrate loading Aprepitant 1–3 h prior for ≥2 risk factors Female patients: Other non-hormonal contraception for at least 28 days postoperatively Scopolamine patch (skin behind ear for 72 h); reduce patch for children and elderly; Intraoperative dexamethasone 8–10 mg IV (half-life 36–54 h); half dose in diabetes; Postoperative (48 h): $5HT_3I$ (ondansetron, granisetron, polonosetron); dopamine (D_2) antagonists (metoclopramide, droperidol, prochlorperazine); Histamine-1 antagonists (diphenhydramine, dimenhydrinate, trimethobenzamide);
Ileus	Alvimopan 12 mg oral if taking opioids; <15 doses due to increased risk of MI; stop upon passing flatus Naloxegol 12.5–25 mg oral Naldemedine 0.2 mg oral
Glycemic and electrolyte imbalances	Previous short-acting insulin, SGLT-2 inhibitors, meglitinides, and sulfonylureas should be held until eating well Other oral agents/long-acting insulin continued at a lower dose Basal bolus insulin therapy (BBIT) for hyperglycemia
Acute kidney injury/AKI	GDFT: Enough fluids to minimize risk of renal injury Hold NSAIDs and other nephrotoxic agents Initial bolus balanced crystalloids if AKI suspected
Urinary retention	GDFT review (dehydration?); minimization of opioids Catheterization if in doubt
Venous thromboembolism	LMWHs or DOACs (>12 h after neuraxial anesthesia) Avoid rivaroxaban/dabigatran for elderly (bleeding risk) Continue 28 days in cancer/other high-risk cases
High blood pressure	ACEI/ARBs re-initiated within 48 h unless hypotensive Hold antihypertensives: Systolic < 90 mmHg or 30% below patient's baseline
Atrial fibrillation	Beta-blockers: Continue if on pre-operatively; Beta-blockers/calcium channel blocker: Initiated if stable Unstable: Consider cardioversion
Delirium	Avoid benzodiazepines/gabapentinoids Avoid fluid fasting; clear liquids until 1–2 h preoperatively Pharmacotherapy elimination (non-essentials) Multimodal opioid-sparing analgesia: Acetaminophen, COX-2 NSAIDs (celecoxib, meloxicam); review opioids (chronic pain);
Shock and hemorrhage	Consider GDFT for raising mean arterial pressure (MAP) Norepinephrine in non-cardiogenic shock if fluid bolus inadequate Add arginine vasopressin, milrinone if MAP still low
Non-CS acute myocardial infarction	Consider LMWH for anticoagulation Avoid renin-angiotensin-aldosterone inhibitors (ACEI, ARB, spironolactone) and beta-blockers until shock resolves

(continued)

Table 29.3 (continued)

Postoperative complication	Recommendations (consider alternatives for shortages)
Fever	Consider blood culture, chest X-ray, empiric antibiotics after 24 h, trauma or shock; eventually tests for viruses, fungi, and parasites
Surgical site infection (one pre-op IV dose <120 min; rarely more prolonged use;	Surviving site infection /SSI bundle: Antibiotic prophylaxis, normothermia, glucose control, appropriate hair removal, oral antibiotic bowel preparation (laparoscopic colon and rectum operations only), preoperative bathing with chlorhexidine, standardized dressing removal/wound care, wound closure protocol; **clean (high-risk)/clean-contaminated procedure SSI risk:1– 8%**; Adults—Cefazolin 2 g (3 g > 120 kg) or cefuroxime 1.5 g; vancomycin (15 mg/kg) if MRSA colonized Children—Cefazolin (or cefuroxime) 50 mg/kg up to adult dose **Contaminated procedure/ anaerobes (SSI risk: 20–25%)** Adults—Cefazolin + metronidazole 500 mg piggyback/ PB Children—Cefazolin plus metronidazole 7.5 mg/kg IV Alternatives—Cefoxitin or cefotetan 2 grams IV or ertapenem 1 gram IV Cephalosporins/ertapenem: Diluted 20 mL, 3–5 min; metronidazole 5 mg/mL PB, 20–60 min Penicillin allergic: Cephalosporin or ertapenem; Cephalosporin allergic: Gentamicin 1.5 mg/kg + metronidazole IVPB 500 mg or clindamycin 600–900 mg IVPB (60 min infusion) Children—Gentamicin + metronidazole as above or clindamycin 10 mg/kg IVPB
Pain management	Multimodal (acetaminophen, NSAIDs, muscle relaxants, neuropathic pain adjuvants) to prevent opioid need Post-discharge opioid exposure (daily MME < 50) 7 days visceral, 15 days musculoskeletal/ neurosurgical procedures Epidural analgesia: Up to 3 days especially open colonic surgery Diabetes (30% neuropathic pain):Gabapentin, duloxetine, venlafaxine Patient-controlled analgesia/PCA: Consider hydromorphone, not sufentanil; transabdominal pain block and wound infiltration preferred over PCA (if repeated IV opioids required)

Considering the current North American opioid epidemic, minimal or no opioid exposure (daily morphine milligram equivalents [MME] < 50) is advised for opioid-naïve patients and limiting duration to 7 days and up to 15 days for those undergoing highly painful musculoskeletal and neurosurgical procedures [81, 85]. Example protocol: acetaminophen 4 g daily given during the whole postoperative period (unless hypertransaminasemic) with or without NSAIDs (anastomotic leakage risk is controversial). Combine with pre-induction thoracic epidural analgesia (TEA with bupivacaine 1 mg/mL, fentanyl 2 μg/mL, and epinephrine 2 μg/mL at a rate of 3–12 mL/h) until POD2 (POD4 in open rectal resection). Continue with long-acting opioids orally twice a day and short-acting opioids orally as needed.

Treatment regimens that include testing for several single nucleotide polymorphisms related to opioids, such as CYP2D6, OPRM1, and ABCB1, may improve therapeutic response and diminish chances of addiction [86].

Delirium

Postoperative delirium occurs in almost two-thirds of patients over age 60, and multiple risk factors have been identified including polypharmacy, use of physical restraints, and indwelling urinary catheters. In particular, gabapentin use in multimorbid older patients has been associated with greater risk of delirium requiring antipsychotic use and conducting to pneumonia [87]. Patients with cognitive impairments, having emergent procedures, or hip surgeries are at greater risk. Management includes eliminating reversible causes and orientation procedures. Routine prescription of antipsychotics and benzodiazepines is not supported by current literature and may exacerbate delirium. Polypharmacy reduction based on the Beers Criteria (potentially inappropriate medications) such as avoiding metoclopramide, benzodiazepines, and anticholinergics could be helpful [88].

Fever

Postoperative fever is defined as an internal (oral) body temperature over 100.4 °F or 38 °C and is related to the release of endogenous cytokines, especially IL-1 [5, 89]. It can be divided into immediate, acute, subacute, and delayed, according to the corresponding period [5]. Immediate fever occurs within hours and typically is caused by administration of blood products, antibiotics, a pre-existing infection, and, rarely, inhalation anesthetics. Often self-limiting with resolution within 2 or 3 days, blood cultures, chest radiograms, or empiric antibiotics are not routinely demanded. Acute postoperative fever (within POD7) is often caused by infections with bacteria from resident skin or bowel flora. For subacute fever occurring 1–4 weeks postoperatively, surgical incision contamination as well as medication reactions (beta-lactam and sulfonamide antibiotics, histamine-2 antagonists, and heparins) should be investigated, and the possibility of *Clostridioides difficile* colitis should be addressed. In patients with cancer, the onset of prolonged fever has been associated with white blood cell counts less than 1000/mm^3 and use of steroids or immunosuppressants, and perioperative oral management is recommended to avoid oral mucositis, dental infections, and fever of unknown origin [90]. Delayed fever, occurring more than 4 weeks postoperatively, is often caused by coagulase-negative Staphylococci leading to a potential subacute bacterial endocarditis. Viral, fungal, and parasitic etiologies need to be ruled out [5].

Very High-Risk Surgeries

Very high-risk surgeries according to some groups, are those with major impact on hemodynamics, fluid shifts, and blood loss. Others adopt the threshold of >10% mortality risk, encompassing also lesser operations in multimorbid, decompensated patients. These procedures typically include certain modalities of aortic, cardiac, or lung operations, extensive oncologic interventions, along with complex transplant procedures (heart, lung, liver).

Amiodarone can continue if initiated 5–6 days ahead of cardiac surgery [7]. Diuretics are associated with AKI, promote hypotension, and have no recognized benefit in heart failure patients undergoing cardiac surgery [7].

Those with liver cirrhosis are known to be at higher risk of infection, including multidrug resistant organisms, and active infection is a contraindication to liver transplantation. Treatment for infection is required prior to transplantation, and surgery need not be delayed as evidence suggests that perioperative complications and mortality rates are not higher even if infection was diagnosed within 1 month of surgery [91].

General Pharmacotherapy Recommendations

Table 29.3 summarizes the most useful approaches for management and prevention of common surgical complications, and Fig. 29.5 provides a timeline pointing out their respective incidence.

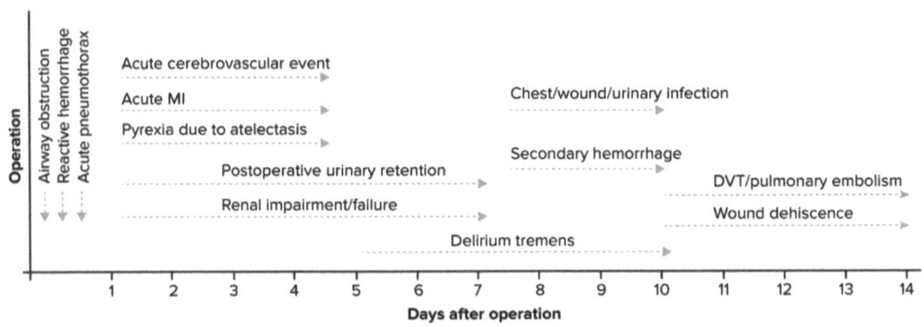

Fig. 29.5 Timeline of common postoperative complications

Acknowledgments The authors are very grateful for the review and insights of Gregg Nelson, MD, PhD, FRCSC, Gourang Patel, PharmD, FCCP, FCCM, BCPS, BCCCP, and Mitchell Kredentser, BA, MA, JD.

References

1. Parrish RH 2nd, Bodenstab HM, Carneal D, et al. Positive patient postoperative outcomes with pharmacotherapy: a narrative review including perioperative-specialty pharmacist interviews. J Clin Med. 2022;11(19):5628.
2. Ljungqvist O, Scott M, Fearon KC. Enhanced recovery after surgery: a review. JAMA Surg. 2017;152(3):292–8.
3. Parrish RH 2nd, Findley R, Elias KM, et al. Pharmacotherapeutic prophylaxis and postoperative outcomes within an enhanced recovery after surgery (ERAS®) program: a randomized retrospective cohort study. Ann Med Surg (Lond). 2021;73:103178.
4. Cohn SL, editor. Decision making in perioperative medicine: clinical pearls. McGraw-Hill; 2021.
5. Stephenson C, Mohabbat A, Raslau D, Gilman E, Wight E, Kashiwagi D. Management of common postoperative complications. Mayo Clin Proc. 2020;95(11)
6. Cohn SL, Grant PJ, Slawski B. Update in perioperative cardiovascular medicine. Cleve Clin J Med. 2019;2019, 86(10)
7. Lomivorotov VV, Efremov SM, Abubakirov MN, Belletti A, Karaskov AM. Perioperative management of cardiovascular medications. J Cardiothorac Vasc Anesth. 2018;32(5)
8. Agency for Healthcare Quality, Department of Health and Human Services, Patient Safety Indicator 10 (PSI 10), Postoperative Acute Kidney Injury Requiring Dialysis Rate, AHRQ Quality Indicators™. Available from: qualityindicators.ahrq.gov; Accessed June 19, 2023;
9. Galway U, Chahar P, Schmidt MT, et al. Perioperative challenges in management of diabetic patients undergoing non-cardiac surgery. World J Diabetes. 2021;12(8)
10. Pfeifer KJ, Selzer A, Mendez CE, et al. Preoperative management of endocrine, hormonal, and urologic medications: Society for Perioperative Assessment and Quality Improvement (SPAQI) consensus statement. Mayo Clin Proc. 2021;96(6)
11. Douketis JD, Spyropoulos AC, Murad MH, et al. Perioperative management of antithrombotic therapy. Available from: journal.chestnet.org/article/S0012-3692(22)01359-9/fulltext; Accessed June 19, 2023.
12. Farge D, Bounameaux H, Brenner B, et al. International clinical practice guidelines including guidance for direct oral anticoagulants in the treatment and prophylaxis of venous thromboembolism in patients with cancer. Lancet Oncol. 2016;17(10):e452–66.
13. Hornor MA, Duane TM, Ehlers AP, et al. American College of Surgeons' guidelines for the perioperative management of antithrombotic medication. J Am Coll Surg. 2018;227(5):521–36.
14. Aroke EN, Robinson AN, Wilbanks BA. Perioperative considerations for patients with major depressive disorder undergoing surgery. J Perianesth Nurs. 2020;35(2)
15. Oprea AD, Keshock MC, O'Glasser AY, et al. Preoperative management of medications for psychiatric diseases: society for perioperative assessment and quality improvement consensus statement. Mayo Clin Proc. 2022;97(2)
16. Garapati A. Adverse effect of preoperative steroid use on surgical outcomes. Surg Sci. 2020;11(12)

17. Ismael H, Horst M, Farooq M, Jordon J, Patton JH, Rubinfeld IS. Adverse effects of preoperative steroid use on surgical outcomes. Am J Surg. 2011;201(3)
18. Ranson WA, White SJW, Cheung ZB, et al. The effects of chronic preoperative steroid therapy on perioperative complications following elective posterior lumbar fusion. Global. Spine J. 2018;8(8)
19. Pfeifer KJ, Selzer A, Whinney CM, et al. Preoperative management of gastrointestinal and pulmonary medications: Society for Perioperative Assessment and Quality Improvement (SPAQI) consensus statement. Mayo Clin Proc. 2021;96(12)
20. Hassinger TE, Krebs ED, Turrentine FE, et al. Preoperative opioid use is associated with increased risk of postoperative complications within a colorectal-enhanced recovery protocol. Surg Endosc. 2021;35(5):2067–74.
21. O'Rourke MJ, Keshock MC, Boxhorn CE, et al. Preoperative management of opioid and non-opioid analgesics: Society for Perioperative Assessment and Quality Improvement (SPAQI) consensus statement. Mayo Clin Proc. 2021;96(5)
22. Holmegard HN, Nordestgaard BG, Schnohr P, Tybjærg-Hansen A, Benn M. Endogenous sex hormones and risk of venous thromboembolism in women and men. J Thromb Haemo. 2014;12(3)
23. Scheres LJJ, van Hylckama VA, Ballieux BEPB, et al. Endogenous sex hormones and risk of venous thromboembolism in young women. J Thromb Haemo. 2019;17(8)
24. Lidegaard O, Lokkegaard E, Svendsen AL, Agger C. Hormonal contraception and risk of venous thromboembolism: national follow-up study. BMJ. 2009;339:b2890–0.
25. Merck and Company, Prescribing Information, Bridion® (sugammadex). Available from: merck.com/product/usa/pi_circulars/b/bridion/bridion_pi.pdf; Accessed June 19, 2023.
26. Merck and Company, Prescribing Information, Emend® (aprepitant). Available from: merck.com/product/usa/pi_circulars/e/emend_iv/emend_iv_lowedta_pi.pdf; Accessed June 19, 2023.
27. King AR, Russett FS, Generali JA, Grauer DW. Evaluation and implications of natural product use in preoperative patients: a retrospective review. BMC Complement Altern Med. 2009;9
28. Kaye AD, Kucera I, Sabar R. Perioperative anesthesia clinical considerations of alternative medicines. Anesthesiol Clin North Am. 2004;22(1):125–39.
29. Vaid S, Bell T, Grim R, Ahuja V. Predicting risk of death in general surgery patients on the basis of preoperative variables using American College of Surgeons National Surgical Quality Improvement Program Data. Perm J. 2012;16(4):10–7.
30. Pokrzywa CJ, Papageorge CM, Kennedy GD. Preoperative urinary tract infection increases postoperative morbidity. J Surg Res. 2016;205(1):213–20.
31. Nicolle LE, Gupta K, Bradley SF, et al. Clinical practice guideline for the management of asymptomatic bacteriuria: 2019 update by the infectious diseases. Society of America; 2019. Available from: idsociety.org/practice-guideline/asymptomatic-bacteriuria/ Accessed June 19, 2023
32. Arozullah AM, Daley J, Henderson WG, Khuri SF. Multifactorial risk index for predicting postoperative respiratory failure in men after major noncardiac surgery. Ann Surg. 2000;232(2):242–53.
33. Jamali S, Dagher M, Bilani N, et al. The effect of preoperative pneumonia on postsurgical mortality and morbidity: a NSQIP analysis. World J Surg. 2018;42(9):2763–72.
34. COVIDSurg Collaborative. Mortality and pulmonary complications in emergency general surgery patients with COVID-19: a large international multicenter study. J Trauma Acute Care Surg. 2022;93(1):59–65.
35. Myers K, Hajek P, Hinds C, McRobbie H. Stopping smoking shortly before surgery and postoperative complications. Arch Intern Med. 2011;171(11)
36. Quan H, Ouyang L, Zhou H, Ouyang Y, Xiao H. The effect of preoperative smoking cessation and smoking dose on postoperative complications following radical gastrectomy for gastric cancer: a retrospective study of 2469 patients. World J Surg Oncol. 2019;17(1):61.

37. Lauridsen SV, Thomsen T, Jensen JB, et al. Effect of a smoking and alcohol cessation intervention initiated shortly before radical cystectomy—the STOP-OP study: a randomised clinical trial. Eur Urol Focus. 2022;8(6):1650–8.
38. Thomsen T, Villebro N, Møller AM. Interventions for preoperative smoking cessation. Cochr Data Syst Rev. 2014;2014(3):CD002294.
39. Egholm JW, Pedersen B, Møller AM, Adami J, Juhl CB, Tønnesen H. Perioperative alcohol cessation intervention for postoperative complications. Cochr Data Syst Rev. 2018;2018(11)
40. Ungur AL, Neumann T, Borchers F, Spies C. Perioperative management of alcohol withdrawal syndrome. Visc Med. 2020;36(3):160–6.
41. Nishiyama VKG, Albertini SM, de Moraes CMZG, de Godoy MF, Natinho JG. Malnutrition and clinical outcomes in surgical patient with colorectal disease. Arq Gastroenterol. 2018;55(4):397–402.
42. Williams DGA, Molinger J, Wischmeyer PE. The malnourished surgery patient. Curr Opin Anaesthesiol. 2019;32(3):405–11.
43. Uppal S, Al-Niaimi A, Rice LW, et al. Preoperative hypoalbuminemia is an independent predictor of poor perioperative outcomes in women undergoing open surgery for gynecologic malignancies. Gynecol Oncol. 2013;131(2):416–22.
44. Martínez-Ortega AJ, Piñar-Gutiérrez A, Serrano-Aguayo P, et al. Perioperative nutritional support: a review of current literature. Nutrients. 2022;14(8):1601.
45. Souza TT, Sturion CJ, Faintuch J. Is the skeleton still in the hospital closet? A review of hospital malnutrition emphasizing health economic aspects. Clin Nutr. 2015;34(6):1088–92.
46. McClave SA, Kozar R, Martindale RG, et al. Summary points and consensus recommendations from the north American surgical nutrition summit. JPEN. 2013;37(Suppl. 5):99S–105S.
47. Ali SME, Hafeez MH, Nisar O, Fatima S, Ghous H, Rehman M. Role of preoperative erythropoietin in the optimization of preoperative anemia among surgical patients—a systematic review and meta-analysis. Hematol Transfus Cell Ther. 2022;44(1):76–84.
48. Kaufner L, von Heymann C, Henkelmann A, et al. Erythropoietin plus iron versus control treatment including placebo or iron for preoperative anaemic adults undergoing non-cardiac surgery. Cochr Data Syst Rev. 2020;2020(8)
49. Ng O, Keeler BD, Mishra A, et al. Iron therapy for preoperative anaemia. Cochr Data Syst Rev. 2019;2019(12)
50. Corwin HL, Shander A, Speiss B, et al. Management of perioperative iron deficiency in cardiac surgery: a modified RAND Delphi study. Ann Thorac Surg. 2022;113(1):316–23.
51. Gan TJ, Belani KG, Bergese S, et al. Fourth consensus guidelines for the management of postoperative nausea and vomiting. Anesth Analg. 2020;131(2):411–48.
52. Maghami M, Afazel MR, Azizi-Fini I, Maghami M. The effect of aromatherapy with peppermint essential oil on nausea and vomiting after cardiac surgery: a randomized clinical trial. Complement Ther Clin Pract. 2020;40:101199.
53. Ashcroft J, Singh AA, Ramachandran B, et al. Reducing ileus after colorectal surgery: a network meta-analysis of therapeutic interventions. Clin Nutr. 2021;40(7):4772–82.
54. Sindell S, Causey MW, Bradley T, Poss M, Moonka R, Thirlby R. Expediting return of bowel function after colorectal surgery. Am J Surg. 2012;203(5):644–8.
55. Gustafsson UO, Scott MJ, Hubner M, et al. Guidelines for perioperative care in elective colorectal surgery: enhanced recovery after surgery (ERAS®) society recommendations: 2018. World J Surg. 2019;43(3):659–95.
56. Gkegkes ID, Minis EE, Iavazzo C. Effect of caffeine intake on postoperative ileus: a systematic review and meta-analysis. Dig Surg. 2020;37(1):22–31.
57. Drake TM, Ward AE. Pharmacological management to prevent ileus in major abdominal surgery: a systematic review and meta-analysis. J Gastrointest Surg. 2016;20(6):1253–64.
58. Ruzycki SM, Harrison TG, Enns E, McKeen J, Helmle K, Cameron A. Quality gaps in screening and monitoring for postoperative hyperglycemia in a Canadian hospital: a retrospective cohort study. BMJ Open Diabetes Res Care. 2021;9(1):e002445.

59. American Diabetes Association Professional Practice Committee. 17. Diabetes advocacy: standards of medical care in diabetes—2022. Diabetes Care. 2022;45(Suppl. 1):S254–5.
60. Sabbatini G, Caccioppola A, Lusardi AC, Pozzi T, Bianco C, Baio S, Chiumello D. Electrolytes, albumin and acid base equilibrium during laparoscopic surgery. Minerva Anestesiol. 2021;87(12):1300–8.
61. Ostermann M, Bellomo R, Burdmann EA, et al. Controversies in acute kidney injury: conclusions from a kidney disease: improving global outcomes (KDIGO) conference. Kidney Int. 2020;98(2):294–309.
62. Prowle JR, Forni LG, Bell M, et al. Postoperative acute kidney injury in adult non-cardiac surgery: joint consensus report of the acute disease quality initiative and PeriOperative quality initiative. Nat Rev Nephrol. 2021;17(9):605–18.
63. Baldini G, Bagry H, Aprikian A, Carli F, Warner DS, Warner MA. Postoperative urinary retention. Anesthesiology. 2009;110(5):1139–57.
64. Verhamme KMC, Sturkenboom MCJM, Stricker BHC, Bosch R. Drug-induced urinary retention. Drug Saf. 2008;31(5):373–88.
65. Ghuman A, Dawidek MT, Athwal MS, et al. Prophylactic tamsulosin and urinary retention rates following elective colorectal surgery: a retrospective cohort study. Int J Color Dis. 2022;37(1):209–14.
66. Chapman GC, Sheyn D, Slopnick EA, et al. Tamsulosin vs placebo to prevent postoperative urinary retention following female pelvic reconstructive surgery: a multicenter randomized controlled trial. Am J Obstet Gynecol. 2021;225(3):274.e1–274.e11.
67. Bisch S, Findley R, Ince C, Nardell M, Nelson G. Efficacy of pre-operative pharmacologic thromboprophylaxis on incidence of venous thromboembolism following major gynecologic and gynecologic oncology surgery: a systematic review and meta-analysis. Int J Gynecol Cancer. 2021;31(2):257–64.
68. Key NS, Khorana AA, Kuderer NM, et al. Venous thromboembolism prophylaxis and treatment in patients with cancer: ASCO Clinical Practice Guideline Update. Clin Oncol. 2020;38(5):496–520.
69. Spénard E, Geerts W, Lin Y, et al. Apixaban for extended postoperative thromboprophylaxis in gynecologic oncology patients undergoing laparotomy. Gynecol Oncol. 2023;172:9–14.
70. Meng L, Yu W, Wang T, Zhang L, Heerdt PM, Gelb AW. Blood pressure targets in perioperative care. Hypertension. 2018;72(4):806–17.
71. McEvoy MD, Gupta R, Koepke EJ, et al. Perioperative quality initiative consensus statement on postoperative blood pressure, risk and outcomes for elective surgery. Br J Anaesth. 2019;122(5):575–86.
72. Lin MH, Kamel H, Singer DE, Wu YL, Lee M, Ovbiagele B. Perioperative/postoperative atrial fibrillation and risk of subsequent stroke and/or mortality. Stroke. 2019;50(6):1364–71.
73. Andrade JG, Aguilar M, Atzema C, et al. The 2020 Canadian cardiovascular society/Canadian Heart Rhythm Society Comprehensive guidelines for the management of atrial fibrillation. Can J Card. 2020;36(12):1847–948.
74. Hamon A, Mokart D, Pouliquen C, et al. Intraoperative hemorrhagic shock in cancer surgical patients: short and long-term mortality and associated factors. Shock. 2020;54(5)
75. Morozowich ST, Ramakrishna H. Pharmacologic agents for acute hemodynamic instability: recent advances in the management of perioperative shock—a systematic review. Ann Card Anaesth. 2015;18(4)
76. Cormican DS, Sonny A, Crowley J, et al. Acute myocardial infarction complicated by cardiogenic shock: analysis of the position statement from the European Society of Cardiology Acute Cardiovascular Care Association, with perioperative implications. J Cardiothorac Vasc Anesth. 2021;35(10)
77. Albert H, Bataller W, Masroor N, et al. Infection prevention and enhanced recovery after surgery: a partnership for implementation of an evidence-based bundle to reduce colorectal surgical site infections. Am J Infect Control. 2019;47(6):718–9.

78. Bowder AN, Yen CF, Bebell LM, Fernandes AR. Intravenous cephalosporin versus non-cephalosporin-based prophylaxis to prevent surgical site infections in colorectal surgery patients: a systematic review and meta-analysis. Ann Med Surg (Lond). 2021;67:102401.
79. Liu Z, Dumville JC, Norman G, et al. Intraoperative interventions for preventing surgical site infection. Cochr Data Syst Rev. 2018;2018(2)
80. Zhao X, Zhang L, Brackett A, Dai F, Xu J, Meng L. Hemodynamic management and surgical site infection: network meta-analysis of randomized controlled trials. J Clin Anesth. 2020;67:110021.
81. Nelson G, Fotopoulou C, Taylor J, Glaser G, Bakkum-Gamez J, Meyer LA, Stone R, Mena G, Elias KM, Altman AD, Bisch SP, Ramirez PT, Dowdy SC. Enhanced recovery after surgery (ERAS®) society guidelines for gynecologic oncology: addressing implementation challenges. Gynecol Oncol. 2023;173:58–67.
82. Scully RE, Schoenfeld AJ, Jiang W, Lipsitz S, Chaudhary MA, Learn PA, Koehlmoos T, Haider AH, Nguyen LL. Defining optimal length of opioid pain medication prescription after common surgical procedures. JAMA Surg. 2018;153(1):37–43.
83. Sachtleben EP, Rooney K, Haddad H, Lassiegne VL, Boudreaux M, Cornett EM, Kaye AD. The role of pharmacogenomics in postoperative pain management. Methods Mol Biol. 2022;2547:505–26.
84. Park CM, Inouye SK, Marcantonio ER, Metzger E, Bateman BT, Lie JJ, Lee SB, Levin R, Kim DH. Perioperative gabapentin use and in-hospital adverse clinical events among older adults after major surgery. JAMA Intern Med. 2022;182(11):1117–27.
85. Lindberg M, Franklin O, Svensson J, Franklin KA. Postoperative pain after colorectal surgery. Int J Color Dis. 2020;35(7):1265–72.
86. Masic D, Liang E, Long C, Sterk EJ, Barbas B, Rech MA. Intravenous lidocaine for acute pain: a systematic review. Pharmacotherapy. 2018;38(12):1250–9.
87. Nie ZB, Li ZH, Lu B, Guo YY, Zhang R. Hydromorphone vs sufentanil in patient-controlled analgesia for postoperative pain management: a meta-analysis. Medicine. 2022;101(3):E28615.
88. Burfeind KG, Navales AAT, Togioka BM, Schenning K. Prevention of postoperative delirium through the avoidance of potentially inappropriate medications in a geriatric surgical patient. BMJ Case Rep. 2021;14(4)
89. Dinarello CA. The history of fever, leukocytic pyrogen and interleukin-1. Temperature. 2015;2(1):8–16.
90. Yamada SI, Soutome S, Hasegawa T, et al. A multicenter retrospective investigation on the efficacy of perioperative oral management in cancer patients. Medicine. 2020;99(10)
91. Ruzzenente A, Bagante F, Bertuzzo F, et al. A novel nomogram to predict the prognosis of patients undergoing liver resection for neuroendocrine liver metastasis: an analysis of the Italian neuroendocrine liver metastasis database. J Gastrointest Surg. 2017;21(1):41–8.

Chapter 30
Blood Component Alternatives During Acute Hemorrhage

Lydia Buzzard and Martin Schreiber

Transfusion in Acute Hemorrhage

Approximately 40% of the 13 million units of blood transfused in the United States each year are used in emergency resuscitation. The principles of resuscitating a patient in hemorrhagic shock are governed by damage control resuscitation (DCR) principles [1] . DCR is designed to normalize physiology by restoring intravascular volume and oxygen carrying capacity while normalizing coagulation with the components that have been lost. This is best done with fresh whole blood or the closest equivalent including either liquid cold-stored whole blood or RBCs (Red blood cells), plasma, and platelets given in a 1:1:1 ratio [2, 3].

Indications for Transfusion

Anemia occurs with red cell mass (below 24 mL/kg in females and 26 mL/kg in males). Anemia causes an increase in cardiac output at a hemoglobin (Hb) level of <7 g/dL. Oxygen extraction increases to assure O_2 uptake by the tissues. Normal humans can survive an 80% loss of red cell mass if they are normovolemic and

L. Buzzard (✉)
Oregon Health and Science University, Portland, OR, USA

University of Wisconsin-Madison School of Medicine and Public Health, Madison, WI, USA
e-mail: lbuzzard@wisc.edu

M. Schreiber
Oregon Health and Science University, Portland, OR, USA
e-mail: schreibm@ohsu.edu

© The Author(s), under exclusive license to Springer Nature Switzerland AG 2024

J. Faintuch, S. Faintuch (eds.), *Recent Strategies in High Risk Surgery*,
https://doi.org/10.1007/978-3-031-56270-9_30

normothermic. The threshold for O_2 delivery to maintain adequate tissue oxygenation is at a hematocrit of 10% and a Hb level of 3 g/dL when breathing 100% O_2 with a normal metabolic rate.

Volume-dependent markers, including hematocrit and Hb, are poor indicators of anemia because they are affected by the ratio of RBC mass to plasma volume. Early in hemorrhagic shock, loss of whole blood causes proportional decreases of RBC mass and plasma volume reflected by a relatively small reduction in hematocrit and Hb. Even after hemorrhage control is achieved, Hb continues to drop as the increase in intravascular volume is usually dominated by an increase in plasma volume from equilibration and crystalloid resuscitation.

Blood Products

Fresh Whole Blood (FWB)

Humans are O_2-dependent organisms, and O_2 depletion causes major damage within minutes. Thus, in the exsanguinating patient, RBCs are transfused to improve O_2 transport, although older blood does not carry oxygen as well. Evidence from military studies has suggested the advantage of fresh whole blood in resuscitation and survival of the exsanguinating patient [4]. The rationale is that FWB has more functions than simply transporting O_2 and provides:

- Oncotic pressure and protection from endothelial and glycocalyx damage (from plasma).
- Near 100% clotting factor and platelet function.
- Temperature homeostasis (from warm circulating fluid).
- FWB is stored at close to 37 °C for up to 8 h and offers RBCs, plasma, and platelets in natural proportions.

A 500 mL unit of FWB has:

- A hematocrit of 38–50%.
- 50,000–400,000/mm^3 fully functional platelets.
- 100% activity of clotting factors diluted only by anti-coagulant.
- Excellent oxygen carrying ability.

Fresh RBCs exhibit better rheological properties than stored blood. The safe use of FWB requires the availability of healthy, pre-screened donors and is generally not available in civilian settings. Because the safety of FWB cannot be guaranteed, it is not FDA-approved for use in the United States. FWB can be stored warm for 8 h. After 8 h it is still considered fresh when stored at 4 °C for 48 h. After 48 h, it is considered cold-stored whole blood which can be stored for 21 days in CPD (Citrate phosphate dextrose) solution and 35 days in CPDA-1 (Citrate phosphate dextrose adenine) solution. Some blood suppliers leukoreduce whole blood which decreases platelet count and function [5]. Liquid cold-stored whole blood can be fully tested for TTD (Transfusion trasmitted diseases) and is FDA-approved, but compared to FWB, it does not have equivalent positive effects on coagulation due to decreases in coagulation factors, platelets and platelet function which worsen as the time of storage increases.

Whole blood can be safely transfused as type-specific or as low anti-A, anti-B titer O whole blood (LTOWB). The utilization of LTOWB may be associated with a lower rate of major transfusions reactions due to the avoidance of clerical errors in matching blood types as low titer type-O whole blood is a universal donor.

Packed Red Blood Cells

Previous hemorrhage management involved resuscitation with excessive amounts of crystalloids and transfusion of RBCs in high ratios compared to other components which diluted native clotting factors, causing hypocoagulation [6]. Crystalloid resuscitation aggravates coagulopathy initiated from the moment of injury due to:

- Loss of warm blood and replacement with cooler fluid, decreasing body temperature.
- Resuscitation with acidic solutions that are high in chloride, resulting in acidosis.
- Dilution of coagulation factors.
- Raising blood pressure in the absence of improved coagulation capacity, displacing established clots.

Biochemical reactions within the body require specific, narrow temperature and pH ranges to proceed. Even without a loss of clotting factors, the coagulation cascade is inhibited when tissue pH is below 7.2 and temperature is below 34 °C. This combination of events is known as trauma-induced coagulopathy (TIC) [6, 7]. TIC occurs endogenously within moments of injury and is mediated through the protein C pathway. Endothelial damage resulting in third-spacing and glycocalyx damage are directly proportional to the volume of crystalloid infused. These processes can be mitigated by transfusion of plasma. Fibrinolysis, fibrinogen dysfunction, platelet dysfunction are also exacerbated by crystalloid resuscitation; these derangements can be mitigated by FWB transfusion.

Component Therapy

Platelets

Platelets are the most problematic component of DCR. Platelets are typically stored at room temperature with agitation for up to 5 days. Their short half-life is due to risk of bacterial contamination. There is evidence that cold-stored platelets have greater hemostatic efficacy and can be stored up to 21 days [8]. Cold platelets are approved for use in the United States for up to 3 days. An exception can be obtained from the FDA to store cold platelets up to 21 days when standard platelets are not available. Cold platelets used by the US military are stored up to 21 days in battlefield settings.

Platelets can be distributed as single donor platelets, equivalent to the number of platelets present in a single unit of whole blood, or as apheresis platelets, a unit of which is equivalent to the number of platelets in 6 units of whole blood. Platelets in the United States are typically suspended in plasma.

Plasma

Plasma utilized in DCR comes in three forms: liquid, thawed, or fresh frozen plasma (FFP). Liquid plasma has never been frozen and thus has superior factor function, as the freeze thaw cycle diminishes clotting factor function. Liquid plasma can be stored for up to 26 days with minimal factor degradation and is immediately available for transfusion.

Fresh Frozen Plasma

FFP is less logistically feasible in DCR because thawing units may take up to 30 min. This can be partially mitigated by thawing units for future use. Thawed FFP can be stored for up to 5 days with minimal factor degradation, but this practice results in increased waste.

Type AB plasma is the universal donor, but Type A plasma is also frequently used.

Cryoprecipitate

Cryoprecipitate contains fibrinogen, von Willebrand factor/factor VIII complex, and fibrin stabilizing factor XIII. Cryoprecipitate may not be required in all cases of acute hemorrhage. One unit (250 mL) of FFP contains 0.5 g of fibrinogen; 1 unit of cryoprecipitate contains 0.25 g fibrinogen, but in 10 mL (rather than 250 mL). Therefore, if a rapid increase in the amount of fibrinogen is required, cryoprecipitate is a useful adjunct.

The CRYOSTAT-1 feasibility study suggested that early cryoprecipitate therapy maintained acceptable blood fibrinogen levels during active bleeding, with a signal for reduced mortality in the treatment arm of the study [9]. The results of the CRYOSTAT-2 trial are pending. A two-year retrospective trauma quality improvement project review of trauma patients receiving four or more units of RBCs showed an association between cryoprecipitate use and improved survival [10].

Fibrinogen Concentrate

The use of fibrinogen concentrate has been reported in trauma patients. The RETIC trial was a single-center, open-label randomized trial comparing initial treatment with 15 mL/kg of FFP or 50 mg/kg of fibrinogen concentrate based on ROTEM (Rotational thromboelastometry) parameters. The trial showed that a single dose of fibrinogen concentrate was more likely to restore normal coagulation in severely injured trauma patients based on ROTEM and resulted in a lower bleeding score [11].

Effects of Transfusing Blood and Blood Products

Stored pRBCs (for a maximum of 42 days) develop defects proportional to the duration of storage, especially in severely ill cases and massive volumes.

Metabolic Effects

- There is a storage-related decrease in ATP (Adenosine triphosphate) which precedes red blood cell membrane deformability and its survival during storage.
- Degradation of 2,3-diphosphoglycerate (2,3-DPG), which affects the affinity of Hb for O_2, occurs after 7–10 days in storage. After 7 days of storage, the O_2-transporting ability of Hb drops by two-thirds. Adenine added to pRBCs may restore levels of 2,3-DPG in vivo after transfusion.
- Increased ammonia release occurs due to release of intracellular protein after disruption of the red cell membrane during storage.
- Blood products are stored in citrate which chelates calcium, a critical component of nearly every reaction of coagulation.

Hyperkalaemia

Despite potassium concentration of >40 mmol/L, short-term potassium elevation often does not need correction.

Coagulation Abnormalities

Conventional coagulation assays either focus on one artificial aspect of clotting (PT/INR and APTT) or report concentrations, as in the case of fibrinogen or platelets, which may not correlate with function. Increasingly, the transfusion of blood components is guided by viscoelastic hemostatic assays (VHA) such as thromboelastography/ thromboelastometry (TEG or ROTEM), which are functional tests of whole blood clotting and provide results within minutes, guiding adjunctive therapies given in addition to empiric DCR.

Other Risks of Transfusion

Transfusion-Transmitted Infections

- Hepatitis A, B, C, and D.
- Human immunodeficiency virus "window period".
- Cytomegalovirus.
- Atypical mononucleosis and a swinging temperature that can be present for 7–10 days post-transfusion.
- Malaria.
- Brucellosis.
- Yersinia.
- Syphilis.

Hemolytic Transfusion Reactions

- Incompatibility: ABO, rhesus (type the blood), and 26 other surface antigens (screen for these).
- To very cold blood, overheated blood or pressurized blood.
- Immediate generalized reaction (plasma).

Immunological Complications

- Major incompatibility reaction (usually caused by "wrong blood" due to administrative errors).
- Graft-versus-host disease which is rare but frequently fatal.
- Transfusion related acute lung injury (TRALI).
- Immunomodulation: Elevations of the ratio of suppressor-to-helper T cells could trigger infection.

Factors Implicated in Hemostatic Failure

- Hypothermia: Blood is stored at 4 °C, but body temperature is 37 °C, so the body needs to provide energy to heat each unit of blood to body temperature.
- Acidosis (from citrate and lactate).

- Dilution, depletion, and decreased production of red cells and platelets.
- Diffuse intravascular coagulation: There is a consumption of clotting factors and platelets within the circulation, which are trapped in the microvascular thrombi created due to fibrin deposition.
  - Extrinsic: Tissue thromboplastins, for example in blunt trauma, surgery, and burns.
  - Intrinsic: Endothelial injury, endotoxin, hypothermia, hypoxia, acidosis, and platelet activation.
- Fibrinolysis.
- Consumption of red cells and platelets.
- Protein C activation.
- Hypocalcemia.

Despite the extensive list quoted above, there is limited evidence regarding the complications of pRBC transfusion, although it could precipitate:

- Wound and systemic infection.
- Organ failures and SIRS.
- Prolonged hospitalization with more severe morbidity and less survival.
- TRALI and ARDS (acute respiratory distress syndrome).
- DVT (deep venous thrombosis).

Leukocyte depletion might contribute to attenuate general and infectious events in this population.

Adjuncts to Enhance Clotting

Adjuncts to enhance clotting as part of the resuscitation of the acutely hemorrhaging patient include:

Prothrombin Complex Concentrate

Prothrombin Complex Concentrate (PCC) is produced by combining plasma from thousands of patients and isolating the complex of vitamin K dependent factors as well as anti-coagulants Protein C and S, anti-thrombin III, and heparin. Despite containing anti-coagulant factors, PCC is overall pro-coagulant. PCC undergoes multiple viral inactivation steps, and anti-HLA antibodies are reduced. PCC can be rapidly reconstituted with a small volume, and 3000 IUs increases coagulation factors by 40–80%. PCC reverses anti-coagulation effects of coumadin much faster than plasma. It is FDA-approved for coumadin reversal in patients requiring life-saving procedures or with life-threatening bleeds.

The use of PCC in combination with plasma in non-anti-coagulated trauma patients has been associated with improved survival and decreased rates of acute kidney injury and ARDS [12]. Due to its short half-life, PCC is given with Vitamin K. Randomized studies evaluating the efficacy and safety of PCC in hemorrhaging, non-anticoagulated patients are underway.

Tranexamic Acid

Tranexamic acid (TXA) is indicated in hemorrhagic shock patients and in massive transfusion protocol patients.

The CRASH-2 trial showed that TXA use significantly reduced mortality [13]; however, fewer than half the patients required red cell transfusion. Further, in those who were transfused, the two arms utilized the same amount of blood, and the mortality rate in both arms did not correlate with that in other studies. In addition, no injury severity comparisons were included. A study of TXA in the military context showed improved coagulation and survival, especially in patients requiring massive transfusion [14].

The STAAMP trial compared the use of TXA to placebo in trauma patients with either hypotension or tachycardia [15]. Overall, there was no survival benefit in the group that received TXA. Subgroup analysis revealed that patients who received TXA within 1 h of injury and patients with an initial systolic blood pressure < 70 mmHg had improved survival [16]. The TXA in TBI trial, another large randomized trial, revealed that patients with CT proven intracranial hemorrhage who received a one-gram bolus of TXA in the field had increased survival and improved disability rating scores compared to patients who received placebo or one-gram in the field and a one-gram infusion in the hospital [15]. Some regions are now giving a two-gram bolus of TXA in the field for hemorrhagic shock and TBI.

Desmopressin (DDAVP)

Desmopressin, an analog of the vasopressin hormone, potentiates the function of platelets and is indicated only for functional platelet disorders, secondary to platelet inhibitors such as aspirin, clopidogrel, ticagrelor, or prasugrel, renal or hepatic failure, hemophilia-A and von Willebrand's disease.

Monitoring Coagulation Status

This is part of the concept of personalized medicine or goal-directed therapy, giving the patient only what is needed and avoiding unnecessary transfusions.

Viscoelastic Hemostatic Assays (VHA)

VHA technology results in a visual profile, or trace, and variables with a reference value, as shown in Fig. 30.1a, b. The most common modalities are Thromboelastography (TEG) and Rotary Thromboelastomerography (RoTEM) [17, 18] (Fig. 30.2).

Standard TEG® and ROTEM® assays can be accelerated with kaolin activation. The contribution of fibrinogen to clot strength can also be evaluated with either assay. VHAs are portable bedside devices. While completion of the test out to LY30

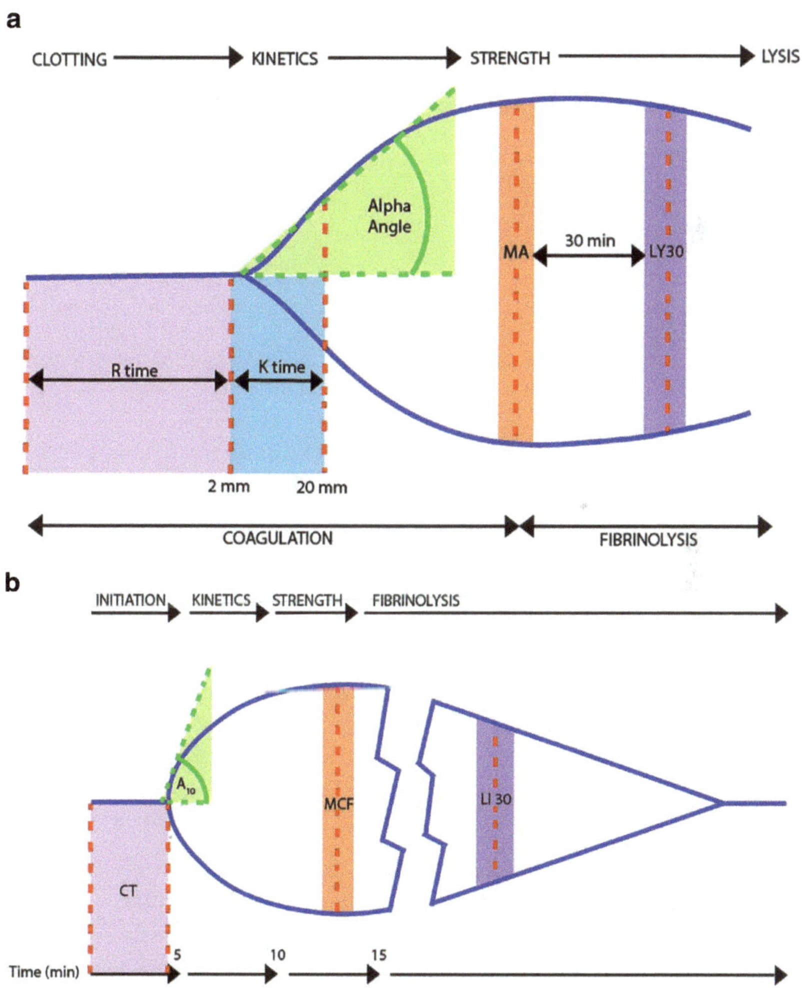

Fig. 30.1 (**a**) Thromboelastogram. *R time* reaction time, *K time* kinetic time, *α (alpha) angle* clot strength, *MA maximum amplitude* maximum clot strength, *Ly30* fibrinolysis after 30 min. (**b**) RoTEM appearance*CT* clotting time, *A10* Amplitude after 10 min, *MCF* maximum clot firmness, *LI30* fibrinolysis after 30 min

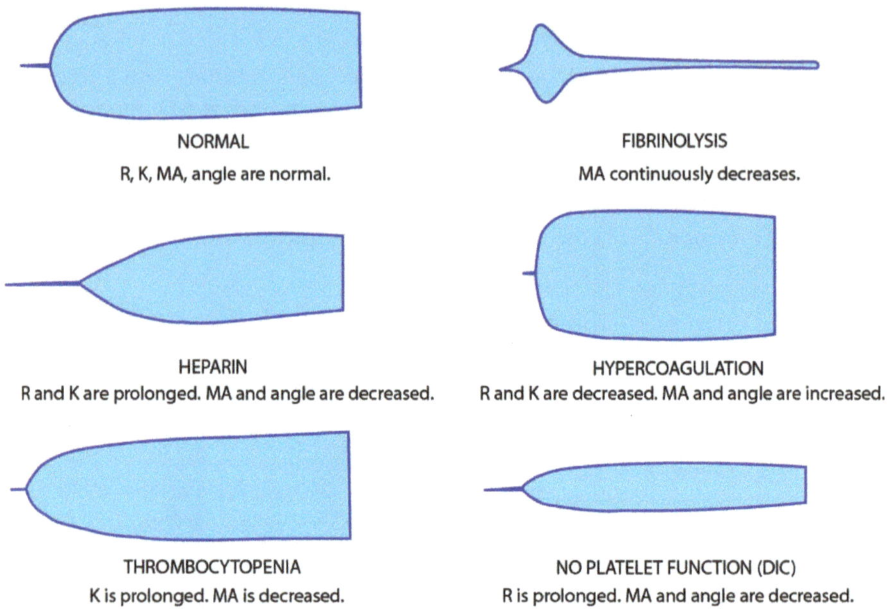

Fig. 30.2 Abnormal appearances of thromboelastography*DIC* disseminated intravascular coagulopathy, *K* kinetic time, *MA* maximum amplitude, *R* reaction time

(thrombolysis after maximum clot strength) can take close to an hour, many results are available within 10 min, in the form of a curve (Fig. 30.1a or b) that can be seen at the bedside in real time. Measured parameters include (Table 30.1):

- R time (reaction time)/clotting time—latency from the time at which the blood is placed in the cup until the clot begins to form.
- The α (alpha) angle—progressive increase in clot strength which is primarily determined by the rate of fibrin crosslinking.
- K time (kinetic time)—window from when R time ends and when the curve reaches 20 mm amplitude.
- MA (maximum amplitude)—maximal clot strength which is primarily determined by platelet function.
- LY30—amount of thrombolysis after 30 min, expressed as percent of the MA.

VHAs allow for goal-directed hemostatic therapy, thereby only treating with what is needed. One of several international validated algorithms is shown in Table 30.1. Furthermore, VHAs elucidate if the bleeding is surgical or coagulopathic/pathological, depends on clotting factor deficiency, or the function of platelets, and whether fibrinolysis is evolving normally. Transfusion of blood components, coagulation factors, and additional medication can be administered rationally, based on VHA results. During a massive transfusion when coagulation status is rapidly changing, VHAs can be used in addition to DCR to determine adjunctive therapies [17, 18].

Table 30.1 Interpretation of the parameters of the TEG and ROTEM

Measurement	TEG parameter (normal range)	ROTEM parameter (normal range)	Abnormalities and corrections
Activity of clotting factors	*R* (3–8 min)	CT_{EXTEM} (38–79 s) CT_{INTEM} (100–240 s)	*R* 10–14 min, ExTEM 80–100 s, InTEM 200–240 s: Give FFP 20 mL/kg *R* > 14 min, ExTEM > 100 s, InTEM > 240 s: Give FFP 30 mL/kg OR prothrombin complex concentrate Difference in R Hep TEG® versus standard TEG® *R* > 2 min (InTEM CT/HepTEM CT > 1.25): give protamine 50–100 mg OR FFP 10–20 mL/kg
Maximum clot strength kinetics	*K* (1–3 mm)		*K* > 4 min: Give cryoprecipitate 5 mL/kg OR fibrinogen concentrate 30 mL/kg OR prothrombin complex concentrate
Clot strength rate of increase	*α* (55–69°)	$A_{10\ EXTEM}$ (43–65 mm)	*α* < 65°: Give cryoprecipitate 5 mL/kg OR fibrinogen concentrate 30 mg/kg OR DDAVP
Maximum clot strength	MA (51–69 mm)	MCF_{EXTEM} (50–72 mm)	MA 45–49 mm and FF_{MA} > 14: Give platelets 5 mL/kg MA < 45 mm and FF_{MA} > 14: Give platelets 10 mL/kg
Clot lysis at 30 min	Ly30 (<4%)	LI30 (94–100%)	LY30 > 3–8% or LI30 < 94%: Give TXA 10 g or 10–20 mg/kg
Fibrinogen activity (level)	FF_{MA} (14–24 mm)	FibTEM MCF (9–16 mm)	FF_{MA} 7–14 mm: Give FFP 20 mL/kg OR cryoprecipitate 3 mL/kg OR FF_{MA} 0–7 mm: Give FFP 30 mL/kg

Thrombelastography (TEG®): Rotational thromboelastometry (ROTEM®): *R* reaction time, *CT* clotting MCF time, *K* K time, *α* Alpha angle, A_{10} Amplitude after 10 min, *MA* maximum amplitude, *MCF* maximum clot firmness, *Ly30* fibrinolysis after 30 min, *LI30* fibrinolysis after 30 min, FF_{MA} functional fibrinogen, *Fib* fibrinogen, *TXA* tranexamic acid, *FFP* fresh frozen plasma, *rFVIIA* recombinant factor VIIa, *DDAVP* desmopressin, *Sec* seconds

Autotransfusion

Autotransfusion eliminates the risk of incompatibility, the risk of disease transmission from donors, and the need for crossmatching [19, 20]. In-line filters minimize microembolization by removing gross particles and macroaggregates [19].

Cell-washing and centrifugation diminishes free Hb reinfusion, however the possibility of infection remains.

Bleeding from the chest seems ideal for immediate autotransfusion as the contents of the thoracic cavity are sterile, in contrast with abdominal bleeding, where visceral injury and contamination may coexist. The simplest effective method is to use the sterile chest drain container. Saline is used to create the fluid valve at the end of a chest drainage tube, to which it is added 1000 IU fractionated heparin. The contents of the bottle may be hung and (using a microfilter to collect microaggregates) immediately reintroduced intravenously. Blood collected from the chest may cause fibrinolysis due to pleural exposure, and coagulopathy due to depletion of coagulation factors.

Within the oncologic setting no adverse outcomes have been observed [20], and even in the presence of contaminated trauma laparotomy, complication rate does not seem to be significantly affected.

Massive Hemorrhage/Massive Transfusion

Definition

The blood volume of a healthy young adult is approximately 70 mL/kg. Massive transfusion has traditionally been defined as administration of 10 units of RBCs or more in 24 h. Patients who die early with severe blood loss may not survive long enough to receive 10 units, and patients with low intensity bleeding may reach 10 units over 24 h without being in hemorrhagic shock. The critical administration threshold (CAT) was described to address these issues and is defined as greater than or equal to three units of RBCs transfused in the first hour [21].

There is danger of death when blood loss is more than 150 mL per minute or 50% of blood volume in 20 min. Acidosis, hypothermia, and hypocalcemia are the most relevant dangers. Bicarbonate use in the treatment of acidosis remains controversial. Use of sodium bicarbonate in the acidotic trauma patient is associated with an increase in mortality [22]. Hypocalcemia caused by citrate is typically associated with massive or rapid transfusions. Calcium gluconate or chloride should be given empirically in all patients undergoing massive transfusion. Core temperature should be monitored and not allowed to drop <34 °C, as blood clotting and survival particularly in trauma subjects could be impaired.

Massive Transfusion Protocol (MTP)

An algorithm of coordinated action incorporating many hospital departments (surgery, blood bank, ICU, anesthesiology), known as a massive transfusion protocol (MTP) is activated upon the arrival of a patient with massive hemorrhage. The MTP provides roles for the personnel, actions to be taken, medications and blood products to be transfused. The goal is increased survival of these patients. The basis of MTPs has been knowledge acquired from modern battlefields. Ideally, MTPs should include:

- Blood (LTOWB or balanced ratios of RBCs, plasma, and platelets) given until bleeding is stopped.
- Early delivery of empiric calcium, with levels followed.

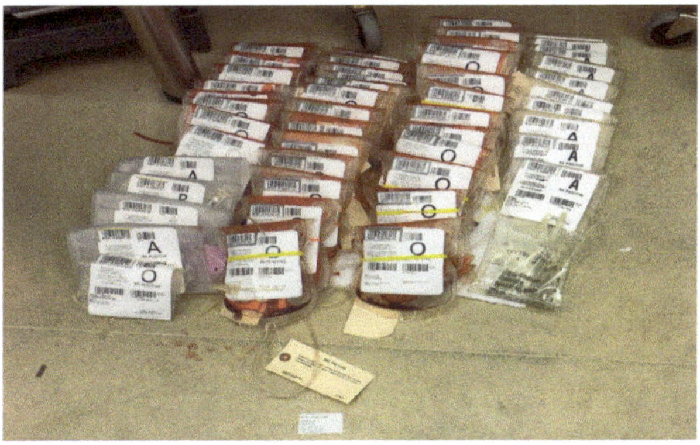

Fig. 30.3 A well-organized blood bank for patients requiring the massive transfusion protocol

- TXA.
- Viscoelastic testing, performed frequently to guide adjunctive therapies.
- A designated organizer to guide resuscitation [23].

Figure 30.3 is an example of a well-organized MTP.

Topical Hemostatic Adjuncts/Tissue Adhesives

Fibrin

Both autologous (Vivostat system; Vivolution A/S Birkeroed, Denmark) and heterologous (Tisseel/Tissucol, Baxter Hyland Immuno, Vienna, Austria) sources have been advocated. The following steps could be useful:

- Before application, tamponade the bleeding surface.
- Compress with a warm pad for a few minutes.
- The pad is taken away, air is sprayed, followed by short bursts of fibrin.

Patches

Tachosil®

TachoSil® (Takeda Nycomed AS, Asker, Norway) is a fixed, widely available, ready-to-use combination of a collagen sponge coated with a dry layer of the human coagulation factors fibrinogen and thrombin, making it easy to employ. It is most suitable for oozing from the raw surfaces of solid organs or to seal air leaks from lung injuries.

HemoPatch®

Similarily HemoPatch® (Baxter Hyland Immuno, Vienna) has recently become available. It triggers natural clotting and is resorbed within 6–8 weeks.

Collagen Fleece

Collagen fleece (e.g., TissoFleece, Baxter, Vienna) as well as FloSeal (Baxter, Vienna) are other options for persistent mild bleeding, alone or in combination with a thin layer of fibrin.

Celox Gauze (Celox Medical, Crewe, UK)

Celox gauze is composed of chitosan and has been shown to have bacteriostatic properties. This product is largely used by the British military.

QuikClot Combat Gauze

QuikClot Combat Gauze is imbedded with kaolin. Kaolin is an inorganic mineral that functions by potently activating factor XII, producing accelerated clotting through the extrinsic clotting cascade. This is the same product that is used to accelerate clot formation in thrombelastography. QuikClot Combat Gauze does not produce an exothermic reaction. It is carried by the US military and is present in Stop the Bleed kits sold commercially in the United States. Both QuikClot and Celox come in the format of packable gauzes that are ideal for bleeding wounds. They are approved for external use only.

Conclusions

The successful management of hemorrhaging patients involves rapid arrest of hemorrhage and damage control resuscitation to replace volume and maintain normal physiology. Both whole blood and blood components have indications depending on hemorrhage severity, risk of coagulopathy, product availability, and other circumstances. Adjunctive therapies that accelerate clotting or prevent fibrinolysis may improve outcomes. The use of thromboelastometry may help guide resuscitation therapy.

References

1. Holcomb JB, Jenkin D, Rhee P, Johannigman J, Mahoney P, et al. Damage control resuscitation: directly addressing early coagulopathy of trauma. J Trauma. 2007;62:307–10.
2. Holcomb JB, Tilley BC, Baraniuk S, Fox EE, Wade CE, Podbielski JM, et al. Transfusion of plasma, platelets, and red blood cells in a 1:1:1 vs a 1:1:2 ratio and mortality in patients with severe trauma: the PROPPR randomized clinical trial. JAMA. 2015;313(5):471–82. https://doi.org/10.1001/jama.2015.12.
3. Holcomb JB, del Junco DJ, Fox EE, Wade CE, Cohen MJ, Schreiber MA, et al. The prospective, observational, multicenter, major trauma transfusion (PROMMTT) study. J Trauma Acute Care Surg. 2013;75(Suppl. 1):S1–2. https://doi.org/10.1097/TA.0b013e3182983876.
4. Nessen SC, Eastridge BJ, Cronk D, Craig RM, Berseus O, et al. Fresh whole blood use by forward surgical teams in Afghanistan is associated with is associated in improved survival compared to component therapy without platelets. Transfusion. 2013;53(Suppl. 1):107S–13S.
5. Remy KE, Yazer MH, Saini A, Mehanovic-Varmaz A, Rogers SR, et al. Effects of platelet-sparing leukocyte reduction and agitation methods on in vitro measures of hemostatic function in cold-stored whole blood. JTACS. 2018;84:S104–14.
6. Hess JR, Brohi K, Dutton RP, Hauser CJ, Holcomb JB, Kluger Y, et al. The coagulopathy of trauma: a review of mechanisms. J Trauma. 2008;65(4):748–54. https://doi.org/10.1097/TA.0b013e3181877a9c.
7. Ishikura H, Kitamura T. Trauma-induced coagulopathy and critical bleeding: the role of plasma and platelet transfusion. J Intensive Care. 2017;5:2. https://doi.org/10.1186/s40560-016-0203-y.
8. Reddoch-Cardenas KM, Bynum JA, Meledeo MA, Nair PM, Wu X, et al. Cold-stored platelets: a product with function optimized for hemorrhage control. Transfus Apher Sci. 2019;58:16–22.
9. Curry N, Rourke C, Davenport R, Beer S, Pankhurst L, et al. Early cryoprecipitate for major hemorrhage in trauma: a randomised controlled feasibility trial. Br J Anaesth. 2015;115:76–83.
10. Ditillo M, Hanna K, Casatanon L, Zeeshan M, Kulvatunyou N, et al. The role of cryoprecipitate in massively transfused patients: results from the trauma quality improvement program database may change your mind. JTACS. 2020;89:336–43.
11. Innerhofer P, Fries D, Mittermayr M, Innerhofer M, von Langen D, et al. Reversal of trauma-induced coagulopathy using first-line coagulation factor concentrates or fresh frozen plasma (RETIC): a single-Centre, parallel-group open-label, randomised trial. Lancet Haematol. 2017;4:e258–71.
12. Zeeshan M, Hamidi M, Feinstein AJ, Gries L, Jehan F, et al. Four-factor prothrombin complex concentrate is associated with improved survival in trauma-related hemorrhage: a nationwide propensity-matched analysis. JTACS. 2019;87:274–81.
13. CRASH-2 Trial Collaborators. Effects of tranexamic acid on death, vascular occlusive events, and blood transfusion in trauma patients with significant hemorrhage (CRASH-2): a randomised, placebo-controlled trial. Lancet. 2010;376:27–32.
14. Morrison JJ, Dubose JJ, Rasmussen TE, Midwinter MJ. Military application of tranexamic acid in trauma emergency resuscitation (MATTERs) study. Arch Surg. 2012;147(2):113–9. https://doi.org/10.1001/archsurg.2011.287.
15. Rowell SE, Meier EN, McKnight B, Kannas D, May S, et al. Effect of out-of-hospital tranexamic acid vs placebo on 6-month functional neurologic outcomes in patients with moderate or severe traumatic brain injury. JAMA. 2020;8:961–74.
16. Guyette FX, Brown JB, Zenati MS, Early-Young BJ, Adams PW, et al. Tranexamic acid during prehospital transport in patients at risk for hemorrhage after injury: a double-blind, placebo-controlled, randomized clinical trial. JAMA Surg. 2020;156:11–20.

17. Stensballe J, Ostrowski SR, Johansson PI. Viscoelastic guidance of resuscitation. Curr Opin Anaesthesiol. 2014;27(2):212–8.
18. TEG/ROTEM. Available from www.surgicalcriticalcare.net/Guidelines. (Accessed online Dec 2018).
19. Hughes LG, Thomas DW, Wareham K, Jones JE, John A, Rees M. Intra-operative blood salvage in abdominal trauma: a review of 5 years' experience. Anaesthesia. 2001;56:217–20.
20. Sutton TL, Pasko J, Kelly G, Maynard E, Connelly C, Orloff S. Enestvedt CK intraoperative autologous transfusion and oncologic outcomes in liver transplantation for hepatocellular carcinoma: a propensity matched analysis. HPB (Oxford). 2022;24(3):379–85.
21. Moradi S, Jahanian-Najafabadi A, Roudkenar MH. Artificial blood substitutes: first steps on the long route to clinical utility. Clin Med Insights Blood Disord. 2016;9:33–41.
22. Wilson RF, Spencer AR, Tyburski JG, Dolman H, Zimmerman LH. Bicarbonate therapy in severely acidotic trauma patients increases mortality. J Trauma Acute Care Surg. 2013;74(1):45–50.
23. Moore EE, Moore HB, Chapman MP, Gonzalez E, Sauia A. Goal-directed hemostatic resuscitation for trauma induced coagulopathy: maintaining homeostasis. J Trauma Acute Care Surg. 2018;84(Suppl. 1):S35–40.

Part VIII
Wound Care

Chapter 31
Skin Wound Complications in High-Risk Surgery

Corey Keenan, Elof Eriksson, and Kristo Nuutila

Introduction

High-risk surgery is accompanied by a high risk of complications in the healing wound. In 1980, Cruse and Foord (1980) published a seminal study on wound complications in over 62,000 patients at the Foothills Hospital in Calgary, Canada. They studied how many different factors contributed to wound complications, and they also introduced methods to reduce their incidence, which to a large extent are still true [1]. There are many recent excellent studies, particularly the ones from the American College of Surgeons (ACS) and other surgical national and international organizations [2, 3]. The Center for Disease Control (CDC) is also continually collecting data and publishing reports on SSI [4].

Lifestyle and Comorbidities

Abnormal healing, leading to chronic wounds and fibrotic scars, is uncommon in healthy patients and is usually associated with various underlying risk factors such as infection, diabetes, malnutrition, ischemia, smoking, old age, cancer, immunosuppression, and obesity [5]. Annually in the United States, 6.5 million patients need treatment for non-healing wounds with an estimated $25 billion USD spent.

C. Keenan
Department of Surgery, William Beaumont Army Medical Center, El Paso, TX, USA

E. Eriksson
Harvard Medical School, Boston, MA, USA

K. Nuutila (✉)
United States Army Institute of Surgical Research, JBSA Fort Sam Houston, TX, USA
e-mail: kristo.j.nuutila.ctr@health.mil

© The Author(s), under exclusive license to Springer Nature Switzerland AG 2024

J. Faintuch, S. Faintuch (eds.), *Recent Strategies in High Risk Surgery*,
https://doi.org/10.1007/978-3-031-56270-9_31

This burden is growing yearly due to the expanding incidence of obesity and diabetes, further increasing the importance to address these complications. Infections are another concern significantly prolonging hospitalization and increasing costs [6]. It has been calculated that a patient who experiences a surgical site infection (SSI) will incur an extra $11,000 USD on average, and an increase in the average hospital length of stay by 9.7 days. All SSIs annually cost the US healthcare system up to $10 billion in spite of being potentially preventable 60% of the time [7, 8].

Wound Healing Process

Superficial (loss of epidermis) and partial-thickness (loss of epidermis and dermis) wounds, not involving abdominal cavities or visceral procedures, heal through re-epithelialization. Keratinocytes migrate from the wound edges and the skin adnexal structures (hair follicles and glands) if they have remained intact, to close the wound. Full-thickness wounds involve all the layers of skin (epidermis, dermis, and hypodermis) and can reach muscle, tendons, bone, and viscera [9]. If untreated, these wounds heal through contraction, granulation tissue formation, and re-epithelialization from the wound edges. Full-thickness wounds are typically managed by surgical intervention including primary or secondary closure, and if necessary also flaps and grafts [10].

Biomolecules, Immune Reactions, and Tissue Repair

Wound healing is a process regulated by different cell types, growth factors, cytokines, and chemokines. It is traditionally divided into four overlapping phases of hemostasis, inflammation, proliferation, and remodeling [11]. Hemostasis, or clotting, is the first phase of the wound healing process and its purpose is to prevent excessive blood loss [12]. Subsequently, in the inflammation phase, the wound bed is cleared from pathogens to prevent infection. This occurs immediately after wounding and lasts for about 2–4 days [13]. The proliferation phase occurs approximately 2–10 days after wounding, and in this phase, the injured tissue is rebuilt by proliferating cells. Remodeling, the last phase, begins around 10–14 days after wounding and can last for up to 2 years following injury. During this phase, granulation tissue matures into scar, tissue tensile strength increases, collagen realigns, all of the processes activated after the injury discontinue, and the cells that are no longer needed undergo apoptosis [14].

Healing Pathology

The wound is usually defined as chronic if it fails to heal within 30 days [15]. Chronic wounds do not follow the steps of normal healing and stay stuck in the inflammation phase. Thus, the healing process is prolonged, incomplete, and uncoordinated, resulting in a poor healing outcome [16, 17]. Chronic healing can also lead to fibrosis when the injured tissue does not regenerate. In fibrosis, prolonged inflammation increases fibroblast to myofibroblast transition that facilitates excessive growth of granulation tissue and wound contraction. This process commonly results in the formation of scar tissue, which is described as either hypertrophic scarring or keloid formation [18, 19].

Factors Influencing Wound Healing

Underlying comorbid conditions such as diabetes, as well as factors related to the patient's lifestyle such as smoking, alcohol consumption, and unhealthy diet, often play a role in the processes of wound inflammation and repair (Fig. 31.1) [20].

Diabetes

Diabetes is an important factor compromising all phases of wound healing. Firstly, hyperglycemia causes peripheral microvascular disease resulting in poor blood flow to the skin. This decreases tissue oxygenation and nutrition delivery, especially to the lower extremities. Hypoxia in the wound tissue causes prolonged inflammation and promotes chronicity of the wounds [21]. Secondly, wounds in diabetic patients are more susceptible to infection. Microvascular disease reduces leukocyte migration

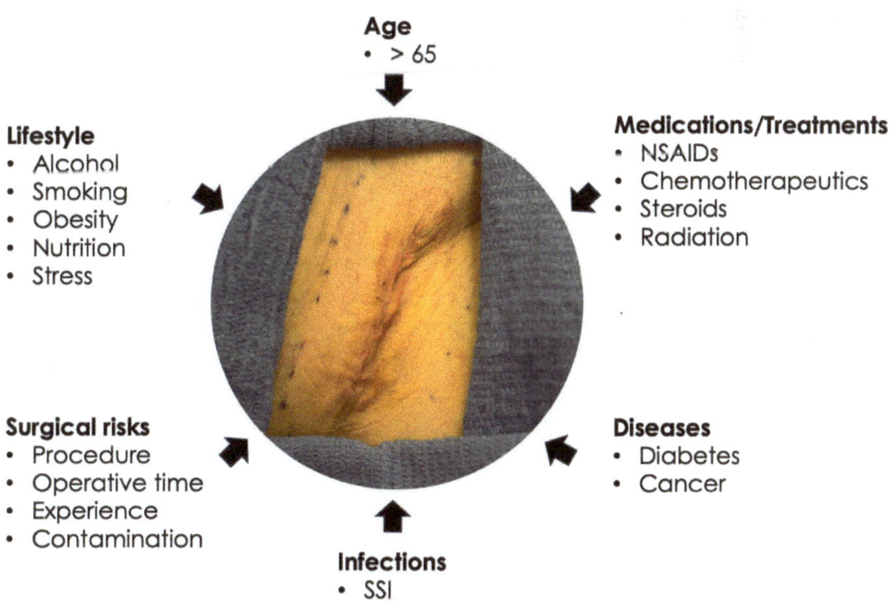

Fig. 31.1 Common risk factors affecting wound healing post-surgery

into the wound, and hyperglycemia further impairs leukocyte function, weakening the immune defense. Additionally, a local hyperglycemic wound environment promotes bacterial growth increasing infection risk [22]. A recent meta-analysis showed that diabetes increased a patient's risk of developing an SSI by 1.5 times [23].

Smoking

Smoking cigarettes and vaping have been associated with prolonged wound healing times, dehiscence, tissue flap necrosis, anastomotic leakage, decreased wound tensile strength, and infection [20]. Cigarette smoke contains numerous toxic compounds like nicotine, carbon monoxide, and hydrogen cyanide impairing wound healing. Nicotine acts as a vasoconstrictor reducing blood flow to the injured area causing hypoxia and limiting supply of nutrients and other important factors to the wound. Carbon monoxide binds to hemoglobin, and thus reduces blood's oxygen content causing hypoxia in the wound tissue that delays healing [24]. Studies have shown that carbon monoxide has a 200–300 greater affinity to bind hemoglobin than oxygen, forming carboxyhemoglobin. Hydrogen cyanide affects tissue oxygenation by binding to mitochondrial cytochrome oxidase which inhibits the oxidative metabolism and oxygen transport at the cellular level. Cessation of smoking has been shown to decrease complications related to wound healing [25].

Alcohol

Alcohol use interferes with both inflammation and proliferation in wound healing. During the inflammation phase, it suppresses the release of pro-inflammatory cytokines, inhibits neutrophil recruitment to the wound site, and reduces phagocytic function of the macrophages [26]. This weakens the ability to fight against pathogens, thus making the wound more prone to infections. Furthermore, it has been shown that acute exposure to alcohol affects the restoration of the connective tissue, which leads to decrease in collagen production and alterations in protease balance at the injured area [20]. In addition, during the proliferation phase, exposure to alcohol impairs wound angiogenesis by up to 60%. The decrease in wound microcirculation causes hypoxia and oxidative stress that further impairs wound healing [27].

Age

Aging affects the metabolic activity of the cells with declined tissue regeneration during wound healing [28]. Immune response is also impaired in the elderly which makes their wounds more vulnerable to infections. In addition, collagen production slows down affecting the tensile strength of the healing wound. This population exhibits increased risk of developing chronic wounds, even in the absence of major comorbidities, since the inflammation phase of wound healing is prolonged and the production of reactive oxygen species (ROS) is increased [29].

Malnutrition

The deficiency of many nutrients such as antioxidants, amino acids (proteins), fatty acids, carbohydrates, and vitamins has been associated with prolonged inflammation, decreased angiogenesis, collagen synthesis, and fibroblast proliferation [30]. Malnutrition has also been linked to reduced wound tensile strength, making the wound more prone to breakdown and increased infection rates. Malnourished patients can develop chronic wounds such as pressure ulcers, and besides global nutritional replenishment could require special nutrients aimed at correcting nutrition deficiencies responsible for the impaired healing [31].

Obesity

There is often increased tension on the wound edges in obese patients that may result in wound dehiscence. Other common complications include seromas along with development of pressure and venous stasis ulcers. Obese people may suffer from vascular compromise that impair oxygen delivery to the wound tissue causing prolonged inflammation and delayed healing [20]. Obesity has also been connected to oxidative stress due to an imbalance of pro- and antioxidants in the cells, that can further cause tissue damage. Sarcopenic obesity, a modality of muscle atrophy eventually associated with protein deficiency, could also impair wound healing. Moreover, obesity is connected to stress and depression that can also be reasons for poor wound healing [32].

Medications

The most well-known drug classes which interfere with wound healing are corticosteroids, non-steroidal anti-inflammatory drugs (NSAIDs), cancer chemotherapeutics, and anticoagulants causing hematomas [20]. During the inflammation phase of wound healing, corticosteroids such as dexamethasone decrease the expression of multiple cytokines, thus suppressing the inflammatory response. In addition, they inhibit macrophage infiltration to the injured area. In the proliferation phase, corticosteroids inhibit fibroblast proliferation and re-epithelialization by down-regulating the expression of growth factors. In the remodeling phase, they mitigate collagen synthesis and decrease tensile strength.

The use of vitamin A to mitigate these wound healing complications is well-known in animal models; however, experience in patients on chronic corticosteroid therapy is limited and results are still debated [33–35]. NSAIDs, such as ibuprofen, negatively affect wound healing by decreasing cell proliferation and tensile strength, thus delaying wound closure and increasing infection risk. Chemotherapeutic drugs, such as cyclophosphamide, inhibit the inflammation phase by blocking cell metabolism, cell division, and angiogenesis. This further delays wound healing and increases the risk of infection [36–38].

Radiation

Radiation therapy used to kill cancer cells and shrink tumors has side effects that impact wound healing. Acutely it upregulates the inflammatory response affecting the cell's ability to produce growth factors and cytokines [39]. Late consequences include skin atrophy, dryness, telangiectasia, dyschromia, dyspigmentation, fibrosis, and ulcer formation. Radiation therapy–related complications occur in approximately 60% of previously radiated surgical patients [40].

Surgical Risk Factors

Emergent surgeries greatly increase the risk of wound complications compared to elective surgeries from 6% to 16%, with half of those cases requiring prolonged hospitalization. They are also at three times higher risk of returning to the operating room [41]. Operative time can also be a factor. Procedures in patients who developed SSIs were only 30 min longer than in patients who did not experience infection [42]. This stresses not only the importance of working expeditiously in the operating room (OR) but also the importance of preoperative planning to reduce dwell time in the OR. Another factor, although debated, is surgeon experience to include case volume and subspecialty training, which could increase technical precision and shorten OR time [2]. Often, the most skilled surgeons have a full schedule, and high-risk operations end up being done by less skilled surgeons. Surgical drains and intraoperative transfusion requirement are also deemed deleterious [43].

Bacterial Contamination

This is one of the most studied mechanisms since the twentieth century. Altemeier (1979) stated that the dose of bacterial contamination multiplied by the virulence and divided by the host resistance ultimately yields the risk of wound contamination [44]. Furthermore, Robson and Heggers in 1969 showed that a microbial load of $>10^5$ CFU/g of tissue is diagnostic of wound infection [45]. Classically the most common pathogen associated with SSI is *Staphylococcus aureus*, comprising approximately 21% of all SSIs [46]. Nevertheless, surgical location plays a large role in the causative pathogen. SSIs that occur in surgery that involves violation into the gastrointestinal tract often involve *E. coli* most commonly at 48% and secondly enterococcus species at 13% [47, 48].

Surgical Site Infections

A patient who experiences an SSI will incur an extra cost of $11,000 on average and an increase in the average hospital length of stay by 9.7 days [7]. Prevention is achieved through a thorough understanding of the different types of SSI that can occur, pre- and postoperative risk stratification, and utilizing mitigation strategies to prevent the occurrence.

Types of SSI

The National Healthcare Safety Network of the CDC publishes updated guidelines each year detailing the classification of surgical site infections [4]. Broadly, there are three main categories: superficial incisional, deep incisional, and organ space infections. Superficial incisional SSIs involve the skin and soft tissue around the incision, occur within 30 days postoperatively, and have localized swelling, pain, tenderness, erythema, or heat present. Superficial incisional infections also must have either purulent drainage, an organism identified on microbiological testing of infection site, or else the surgeon deliberately opens wound to drain. Superficial incisional SSIs can be primary (SIP) or secondary (SIS) based on if the infection is in the primary incision (e.g. midline incision in an open exploratory laparotomy) versus a drain site [4].

Deep Incisional SSIs

They involve deeper soft tissue structures, such as muscle or fascia, and occur either in less than 30 days postoperatively in a category I procedure, or less than 90 days for a category II procedure. Examples of category I procedures include most intra-abdominal and vascular procedures, limb amputations, and transplant operations, whereas category II includes most orthopedic procedures, breast, and cardiac surgery. For a full list of each category, visit the most recent NHSN SSI publication on CDC.gov. To be categorized as a deep incisional SSI, it must also possess purulent drainage, have presence of an abscess, or be deliberately drained by the surgeon with positive identification of an organism on microbiological testing, along with fever, pain, or tenderness in the area. It can be further categorized into deep incisional primary (DIP) or deep incisional secondary (DIS) [4].

Similar to deep incisional, an organ/space SSI must occur within 30 days for category I procedures and 90 days for category II procedures. It must also possess either purulent drainage, positive organism identified on microbiological testing, or an abscess. There are also further criteria at specific sites that are listed on the NHSN publication found on CDC.gov, of which is too lengthy to detail in this chapter [4].

Surgical Wound Classification

Categorizing a patient's wound class preoperatively and having the ability to recategorize it during the procedure will help to mitigate complications in the postoperative period. Table 31.1 outlines the current CDC's surgical wound classification (SWC).

Initially defined in 1964 by the National Research Council, this four-category classification system has been extensively adopted by hospitals and surgeons throughout the world [49]. Nevertheless, it is also criticized because new categories appear all the time and are difficult to classify. Moreover since its creation, the risk of infection of each class has substantially changed. Prevention and treatment strategies continue to advance, whereas this is offset by more high risk and aged patients undergoing procedures. Initially, clean wounds were found to have 1.5% risk of postoperative surgical site infection (SSI), 7.7% risk for clean-contaminated, 15.2% for contaminated, and 40% risk of postoperative SSI in a dirty wound [1]. According to recent ACS-NSQIP data of all surgical specialties, clean cases harbor a risk of

Table 31.1 Surgical wound classification

Class	Cleanliness	Definition	Infection rates %	Examples
Class I	Clean	Uninfected, no inflammation. Does not enter GI, urinary, respiratory, genital tracts	2.5	Lipoma excision, breast surgery, ophthalmic, cosmetic facial procedures
Class II	Clean-contaminated	Controlled entry into GI, urinary, respiratory, genital tracts. No spillage/contamination into surrounding tissues	6.7	Appendectomy/cholecystectomy without gross spillage/perforation. Lung lobectomy.
Class III	Contaminated	Fresh, open wounds with frank spillage/contamination usually from GI tract or abscesses	8.6	Perforated appendectomy. Spillage of bile during cholecystectomy
Class IV	Dirty	Devitalized, necrotic tissue resulting from lack of source control or days of contamination/infection	11.8	Necrotizing fasciitis, chronic wounds, prolonged trauma and perforated viscus

ACS-NSQIP American College of Surgeons-The National Surgical Quality Improvement Program [3, 50]

postoperative SSI around 2.5%, clean-contaminated at 6.7%, contaminated at 8.6% and dirty at 11.8% [3]. In the review of Mioton et al. over 15,000 plastic surgery cases in the NSQIP database, lower rates of developing a postoperative SSI in clean-contaminated, contaminated, and dirty procedures were detected, at 2.8%, 4.9%, and 5.1%, respectively [50].

SSI Scores

The first multivariate index (1970) derived from 58,000 surgical patients predicted the occurrence of SSI with almost twice greater accuracy than the Surgical Wound Classification (Goodman-Kruskal G statistic 0.67 vs 0.36 respectively), using four risk factors that can be assessed at the end of the case. These risk factors are abdominal operation, operation lasting >2 h, contaminated or dirty (class 3 or 4), and having three or more diagnoses which yielded four categories depending on the diagnosis (0–4; 0 = very low risk and 4 = very high risk) [51]. Many more scores can be found in the recent literature, although search for the ideal index still proceeds.

Mitigation Strategies

The treatment of infection starts with prevention through optimization of the patient preoperatively. In high-risk patients, surgery should be avoided or minimized in order to prevent postoperative complications such as SSI. Systemic factors that should be addressed include diabetes, smoking, nutrition, medications, and exogenous steroid use. Local factors that are detrimental to wound healing include decreased tissue perfusion and oxygenation, radiation, neoplasm, bacteremia, and necrotic/devitalized tissue [52].

Optimization of the Patient

A meta-analysis of almost half a million patients who underwent a total joint arthroplasty showed that patients who were malnourished, as proven by serologic lab testing, had significantly higher rates of wound disruption, both superficial and deep incisional SSIs, and organ space SSIs [53, 54]. Strategies for ensuring nutritional support in the perioperative and postoperative periods encompass identifying those at high risk, avoiding prolonged fasting, reestablishing oral or enteral feeding as early as possible after surgery, and mobilizing the patient early after surgery to facilitate muscle function and protein synthesis [55]. Although this number is highly surgeon and patient-dependent, there have been multiple studies showing benefits from cessation of smoking 4 weeks or more before surgery, such as decreased pulmonary complications and surgical wound infections [56, 57]. In women undergoing mastectomy, whether a patient was a light or heavy smoker, this significantly increased their risk of wound infection, flap necrosis, and epidermolysis. Other optimization strategies are controlling the patient's blood glucose perioperatively and attempting to achieve a normal or decreased BMI whenever overweight or obese, if there is enough time [58].

Preoperative Antibiotic Use

The use of preoperative prophylactic antibiotics is continuing to become more routine in almost any procedure carried out in the operating room. Literature shows that optimal timing of preoperative administration is between 30 and 60 min prior to skin incision [59, 60]. Selection is often based on which bacteria may be encountered during that specific surgery in a certain anatomic region (for instance, in abdominal surgery with the possibility of gross spillage, infected joint with hardware, etc.) [61].

Modern Wound Dressings

Appropriate choice of dressing is also a mitigation strategy against SSIs. Dressings can be used to optimize the wound environment to prevent infection and allow for faster and better healing. Besides promoting healing, reducing pain, and protecting the wound against infection, the dressings should be easy to apply and remove. Over the years, novel dressings and advanced wound care solutions have replaced the traditional dry dressings made of gauze, lint, or cotton. Research has extensively demonstrated the importance of moist wound environment. Therefore, modern wound healing dressings are moist, generally derived from natural and synthetic biomaterials, and often incorporated with antimicrobial agents. Moist wound dressings include films, foams, hydrocolloids, hydrogels, and alginate dressings. Other advanced wound care solutions include bioengineered skin products that include biomaterials containing cells and growth factors. The purpose of bioengineered or artificial skin products is to mimic normal skin and promote skin regeneration while protecting the injured area [62–64]. In addition, the use of negative pressure wound therapy (NPWT) systems has been established in the treatment of all kinds of wounds from chronic wounds to surgical incisions. This approach promotes wound healing by enhancing wound bed microcirculation and stimulating granulation tissue formation. It also reduces edema and pathogens by removing excessive wound fluid. The controlled application of negative pressure also promotes wound contraction and facilitates wound closure [65, 66].

Additional Prevention Strategies

Six additional strategies, backed by randomized control trials, have been reported in a large meta-analysis to lower rates of SSIs, summarized in Table 31.2 [67].

Table 31.2 Postoperative infection prevention strategies

Prevention strategy	Infection rate without strategy	Infection rate with strategy
Removal of hair with clipper	4.4% (with razor)	2.5%
Intranasal and skin decolonization using anti-staphylococcal agents	2%	0.8%
Forced-air warming device intraoperatively	13%	4.7%
Glucose control post-operatively (<150)	16% (glucose >150)	9.4%
Incisional negative pressure wound therapy	15% (standard dressing)	9.7%

Adapted from Seidelman et al. [45]

Other Complications

Other common wound healing complications post-surgery include dehiscence, incisional hernia, hematoma, and seroma.

Dehiscence

A wound complication seen more frequently in high-risk surgery is wound dehiscence. This can be classified into superficial and deep dehiscence. Superficial dehiscence involves the wound edges separating, and deep dehiscence involves separation of the underlying fascia. In abdominal surgery, wound dehiscence has been shown to occur in up to 3% of cases and the mortality rate can be up to 40% (46). Additionally, the NIS database shows an added hospital length of almost 10 days and an increase of over $40,000 in excess hospital charges when dehiscence occurs (hcup-us.ahrq.gov). Risk factors for wound dehiscence include diabetes, smoking, poor nutrition, infection, and radiation [68].

For superficial dehiscence, management usually includes washing out the wound, debriding any necrotic tissue, and allowing for the wound to heal by secondary intent. If unacceptable, the scar can be revised at a later time. Importantly, abdominal binders are recommended to prevent the worsening of dehiscence and potential for progression to deep dehiscence, which is a surgical emergency [68]. Dehiscence of fascia in abdominal surgeries can lead to evisceration which must be promptly recognized, kept moist with surgical towels, and taken to the operating room emergently.

One way to mitigate the risks of developing wound dehiscence is to know when to perform a delayed closure. In the setting of heavy contamination, such as colonic perforation, the skin should be left open [69]. Additionally, fascia should not be closed under tension and a continuous running stitch using a monofilament suture, such as polydioxanone (PDS), should be used. It was shown that when a suture to wound length ratio of 4:1 was used, the rate of dehiscence went from 6.6% to 3.8% [70]. This technique, first suggested by Jenkins in 1974, describes using 1 cm bites at 1 cm intervals [71]. In a 2015 randomized control trial, 21% of patients who underwent abdominal closure with large bites (1 cm bites every 1 cm) developed an incisional hernia versus 13% of patients closed with small bites (0.5 cm bites every 0.5 cm) at 1 year follow-up [72]. The rates of adverse events did not differ significantly between groups.

If there is tension on the fascial edges, retention sutures can be placed to decrease the tension. This can be as simple as placing horizontal mattress sutures with non-absorbable material. Using specifically designed closure systems such as the novel adhesive suture retention device is another option [73]. The use of prophylactic retention sutures in an abdominal midline closure in patients at high risk for wound dehiscence was found to decrease rate of dehiscence from 13.5% to 4.1% in a randomized control trial in 2013 [74].

Nevertheless, retention sutures are associated with abdominal compartment syndrome, a condition with not much less mortality than total dehiscence. In this sense, it is useful to measure intra-abdominal pressure. Values in the range of 20 mmHg or higher should be avoided.

Incisional Hernia

It has been found to occur in as many as 15% of abdominal surgeries [75]. Risk factors for developing incisional hernias include high BMI (>25), surgical wound class III or IV, preoperative chemotherapy, need for blood transfusion, old age, and female sex [76]. Presentation can range from a small bulge noticed during Valsalva maneuvers to a large hernia sac unable to be reduced. The dreaded risk of an incisional hernia is an incarcerated and strangulated bowel, which occurs in about 7% of the cases and is a surgical emergency [77].

Managing incisional hernias can be as simple as observation in the case of a small asymptomatic bulge. Yet complex abdominal wall repair can be required in more demanding circumstances. Component separation techniques (CST), although multiple variations exist, can help span fascial gaps up to 20 cm [78]. Loss of domain can occur in large incisional hernias from separation of the fascia, leading to mechanical offloading, disuse atrophy, and muscular fibrosis [79]. Furthermore, the use of mesh applied in an underlay technique in combination with CST has gained traction, both allowing for the ability to close large defects with good outcomes [80]. Mitigating the risk of developing an incisional hernia can be achieved using similar strategies, as mentioned above, for preventing dehiscence: a suture to wound length of 4:1, small bites, and limiting fascial tension during closure.

Hematoma and Seroma

The formation of fluid collections such as hematomas and seromas during wound healing can have detrimental effects on wound healing. The incidence of postoperative hematomas varies widely depending on the type of procedure, yielding proportions of about 6% in laparoscopic cases, 10% in abdominoplasties, and 1% in breast surgery cases [81–83]. Negative healing outcomes include infection, delayed wound healing, increased pressure on overlying skin/incision leading to necrosis or dehiscence, and poor cosmesis. Mechanisms of hematomas and seromas can be multifactorial to include anticoagulation medication encompassing systemic coagulopathy, inadequate hemostasis, shearing forces on tissue, lymphatic disruption, and surgical dead space [84]. Although simple in theory, achieving hemostasis can be challenging in practice due to factors such as unforeseen coagulopathy, retraction of injured vessels, and high abdominal insufflation pressure that temporarily tamponades smaller bleeding vasculature [85].

The surgeon's ability to achieve hemostasis at the conclusion of a case has been improved by novel hemostatic adjuncts such as fibrin sealants, collagen, gelatin, oxidized regenerated cellulose, and cyanoacrylates adhesives [86]. Table 31.3 summarizes common hemostatic agents to be utilized in the operating room, categorized by mechanical, active, flowables, and sealants. Mechanical agents work by acting as a barrier and causing tissue swelling. Active agents promote activity in the coagulation cascade. Flowable agents usually contain either bovine or porcine derived gelatin and allow for the application into hard-to-reach areas. Lastly, fibrin sealants contain fibrinogen or thrombin and help with providing hemostasis [87].

Preventing hematoma or seroma formation should start preoperatively, by ruling out any coagulopathy, and carefully evaluating anti-platelet/anticoagulant medication. Obtaining hemostasis intraoperatively and leaving drains when large defects are created will help decrease postoperative fluid collections. And lastly, evacuating large seroma and hematomas postoperatively will help to decrease wound healing complications [84].

Table 31.3 Common hemostatic adjuncts

Class	Product	Mechanism
Mechanical	Gelfoam (Pfizer)	Absorbable porcine gelatin
	Surgicel (Johnson & Johnson)	Absorbable cellulose hemostat
	Arista (Medafor)	Absorbable polysaccharide hemostat
Active	Evithrom (Johnson & Johnson)	Thrombin
Flowable	Floseal (Baxter healthcare co.)	Bovine gelatin & HPP thrombin
Sealant	Tisseal (Baxter healthcare co.)	PH thrombin and fibrinogen, aprotinin, plasminogen

Adapted from Fagan et al. [87]
HPP human pooled plasma, *PH* pooled human

Recommendations

- It is very important to recognize and record every SSI, by surgical procedure, hospital area, and the name of the surgeon. Regular feedback should be provided to area and surgeon.
- High-risk surgery should be delayed, avoided, or at least minimized whenever feasible.
- The patient's pre-, intra- and postoperative condition should be optimized by frequent evaluations and a multidisciplinary perioperative team.
- Preparation of the surgical site, surgical technique, and postoperative wound management should be standardized in accordance with the most recent validated recommendations.
- Surgical departments should try to establish methods to preoperatively match the high-risk procedures with the more skilled surgeons. There are probably surgeons who should refrain from doing high-risk surgery.

Disclaimer The views expressed in this chapter are those of the author(s) and do not reflect the official policy or position of the U.S. Army Medical Department, Department of the Army, DOD, or the U.S. Government.

References

1. Cruse PJ, Foord R. The epidemiology of wound infection. A 10-year prospective study of 62,939 wounds. Surg Clin North Am. 1980;60(1):27–40.
2. Mahar AL, McLeod RS, Kiss A, Paszat L, Coburn NG. A systematic review of the effect of institution and surgeon factors on surgical outcomes for gastric cancer. J Am Coll Surg. 2012;214(5):860–8.
3. ACS National Surgical Quality Improvement Program. [cited Jun 15, 2023]. Available from: facs.org/quality-programs/data-and-registries/acs-nsqip/; Accessed June 26, 2023.
4. Surgical Site Infection Event (SSI). CDC.gov: 2023 January. Available at cdc.gov/nhsn/pdfs/pscmanual/9pscssicurrent.pdf; Accessed June 26, 2023.
5. Wilkinson HN, Hardman MJ. Wound healing: cellular mechanisms and pathological outcomes. Open Biol. 2020;10(9):200223.
6. Sen CK. Human wounds and its burden: an updated compendium of estimates. Adv Wound Care (New Rochelle). 2019;8(2):39–48.
7. Schweizer ML, Cullen JJ, Perencevich EN, Vaughan Sarrazin MS. Costs associated with surgical site infections in veterans affairs hospitals. JAMA Surg. 2014;149(6):575–81.
8. American College of Surgeons and Surgical Infection Society: Surgical Site Infection Guidelines, 2016 Update Available from : tnpatientsafety.com/pubfiles/mrsa/1.pdf; Accessed June 26, 2023.
9. Beam JW. Management of superficial to partial-thickness wounds. J Athl Train. 2007;42(3):422–4.
10. Rivera AE, Spencer JM. Clinical aspects of full-thickness wound healing. Clin Dermatol. 2007;25(1):39–48.
11. Gurtner GC, Werner S, Barrandon Y, Longaker MT. Wound repair and regeneration. Nature. 2008;453(7193):314–21.
12. Singer AJ, Clark RA. Cutaneous wound healing. N Engl J Med. 1999;341(10):738–46.

13. Almadani YH, Vorstenbosch J, Davison PG, Murphy AM. Wound healing: a comprehensive review. Semin Plast Surg. 2021;35(3):141–4.
14. Kruse CR, Nuutila K, Lee CCY, Kiwanuka E, Singh M, Caterson EJ, et al. The external microenvironment of healing skin wounds. Wound Repair Regen. 2015;23(4):456–64.
15. Järbrink K, Ni G, Sönnergren H, Schmidtchen A, Pang C, Bajpai R, et al. Prevalence and incidence of chronic wounds and related complications: a protocol for a systematic review. Syst Rev. 2016;5(1):152.
16. Eriksson E, Liu PY, Schultz GS, Martins-Green MM, Tanaka R, Weir D, et al. Chronic wounds: treatment consensus. Wound Repair Regen. 2022;30(2):156–71.
17. Han G, Ceilley R. Chronic wound healing: a review of current management and treatments. Adv Ther. 2017;34(3):599–610.
18. Burgess M, Valdera F, Varon D, Kankuri E, Nuutila K. The immune and regenerative response to burn injury. Cells. 2022;11(19):3073.
19. Knowles A, Glass DA. Keloids and hypertrophic scars. Dermatol Clin. 2023;41(3):509–17.
20. Guo S, DiPietro LA. Factors affecting wound healing. J Dent Res. 2010;89(3):219.
21. Spampinato SF, Caruso GI, De Pasquale R, Sortino MA, Merlo S. The treatment of impaired wound healing in diabetes: looking among old drugs. Pharmaceuticals (Basel). 2020;13(4):60.
22. Ackermann PW, Hart DA. Influence of comorbidities: neuropathy, vasculopathy, and diabetes on healing response quality. Adv Wound Care (New Rochelle). 2013;2(8):410–21.
23. Martin ET, Kaye KS, Knott C, Nguyen H, Santarossa M, Evans R, et al. Diabetes and risk of surgical site infection: a systematic review and meta-analysis. Infect Control Hosp Epidemiol. 2016;37(1):88–99.
24. McDaniel JC, Browning KK. Smoking, chronic wound healing, and implications for evidence-based practice. J Wound Ostomy Continence Nurs. 2014;41(5):415–2.
25. Silverstein P. Smoking and wound healing. Am J Med. 1992;93(1A):22S–4S.
26. Curtis BJ, Hlavin S, Brubaker AL, Kovacs EJ, Radek KA. Episodic binge ethanol exposure impairs murine macrophage infiltration and delays wound closure by promoting defects in early innate immune responses. Alcohol Clin Exp Res. 2014;38(5):1347–55.
27. Choudhry MA, Chaudry IH. Alcohol intoxication and post-burn complications. Front Biosci. 2006;11:998–1005.
28. Gosain A, DiPietro LA. Aging and wound healing. World J Surg. 2004;28(3):321–6.
29. Khalid KA, Nawi AFM, Zulkifli N, Barkat MA, Hadi H. Aging and wound healing of the skin: a review of clinical and pathophysiological hallmarks. Life (Basel). 2022;12(12):2142.
30. Barchitta M, Maugeri A, Favara G, Magnano San Lio R, Evola G, Agodi A, et al. Nutrition and wound healing: an overview focusing on the beneficial effects of curcumin. Int J Mol Sci. 2019;20(5):1119.
31. Stechmiller JK. Understanding the role of nutrition and wound healing. Nutr Clin Pract. 2010;25(1):61–8.
32. Pierpont YN, Dinh TP, Salas RE, Johnson EL, Wright TG, Robson MC, et al. Obesity and surgical wound healing: a current review. ISRN Obes. 2014;2014:638936.
33. Corball M, O'Dwyer P, Brady MP. The interaction of vitamin a and corticosteroids on wound healing. Irish J Med Sci. 1985;154(8):306–10.
34. Polcz ME, Barbul A. The role of vitamin a in wound healing. Nutr Clin Pract. 2019;34(5):695–700.
35. Wicke C, Halliday B, Allen D, Roche NS, Scheuenstuhl H, Spencer MM, et al. Effects of steroids and retinoids on wound healing. Arch Surg. 2000;135(11):1265–70.
36. Khalil H, Cullen M, Chambers H, McGrail M. Medications affecting healing: an evidence-based analysis. Int Wound J. 2017;14(6):1340–5.
37. Zhao-Fleming H, Hand A, Zhang K, Polak R, Northcut A, Jacob D, et al. Effect of non-steroidal anti-inflammatory drugs on post-surgical complications against the backdrop of the opioid crisis. Burns Trauma. 2018;6:25.
38. Deptuła M, Zieliński J, Wardowska A, Pikuła M. Wound healing complications in oncological patients: perspectives for cellular therapy. Postepy Dermatol Alergol. 2019;36(2):139–46.

39. Dormand E, Banwell PE, Goodacre TEE. Radiotherapy and wound healing. Int Wound J. 2005;2(2):112–27.
40. Haubner F, Ohmann E, Pohl F, Strutz J, Gassner HG. Wound healing after radiation therapy: review of the literature. Radiat Oncol. 2012;7:162.
41. Sørensen LT, Hemmingsen U, Kallehave F, Wille-Jørgensen P, Kjaergaard J, Møller LN, et al. Risk factors for tissue and wound complications in gastrointestinal surgery. Ann Surg. 2005;241(4):654–8.
42. Cheng H, Chen BP, Soleas IM, Ferko NC, Cameron CG, Hinoul P. Prolonged operative duration increases risk of surgical site infections: a systematic review. Surg Infect. 2017;18(6):722–35.
43. Zabaglo M, Sharman T. Postoperative wound infection. In: StatPearls. Treasure Island, FL: StatPearls Publishing; 2023.
44. Altemeier WA. Principles in the management of traumatic wounds and in infection control. Bull N Y Acad Med. 1979;55(2):123–38.
45. Robson MC, Heggers JP. Bacterial quantification of open wounds. Mil Med. 1969;134(1):19–24.
46. Zarb P, Coignard B, Griskeviciene J, Muller A, Vankerckhoven V, Weist K, et al. The European Centre for Disease Prevention and Control (ECDC) pilot point prevalence survey of healthcare-associated infections and antimicrobial use. Euro Surveill. 2012;17(46):4–19.
47. Alexiou K, Drikos I, Terzopoulou M, Sikalias N, Ioannidis A, Economou N. A prospective randomised trial of isolated pathogens of surgical site infections (SSI). Ann Med Surg. 2017;21:25–9.
48. Hassan RSEE, Osman SOS, Aabdeen MAS, Mohamed WEA, Hassan RSEE, Mohamed SOO. Incidence and root causes of surgical site infections after gastrointestinal surgery at a public teaching hospital in Sudan. Pat Safety Surg. 2020;14(1):45.
49. Hart D, Postlethwait RW, Brown IW Jr, Smith WW, Johnson PA. Postoperative wound infections: a further report on ultraviolet irradiation with comments on the recent (1964) national research council cooperative study report. Ann Surg. 1968;167(5):728–43.
50. Mioton LM, Jordan SW, Hanwright PJ, Bilimoria KY, Kim JY. The relationship between preoperative wound classification and postoperative infection: a multi-institutional analysis of 15,289 patients. Arch Plast Surg. 2013;40(5):522–9.
51. Haley RW, Culver DH, Morgan WM, White JW, Emori TG, Hooton TM. Identifying patients at high risk of surgical wound infection. A simple multivariate index of patient susceptibility and wound contamination. Am J Epidemiol. 1985;121(2):206–15.
52. Myers WT, Leong M, Phillips LG. Optimizing the patient for surgical treatment of the wound. Clin Plast Surg. 2007;34(4):607–20.
53. Zhang D, Zhang X. Effect of serologic malnutrition on postoperative wound infection problems after total joint arthroplasty: a meta-analysis. Int Wound J. 2023;20(2):261–8.
54. Lim SC, Koh AJH. Nutrition and the elderly surgical patients. MOJ Surg. 2017;4(5):114–20.
55. Quan H, Ouyang L, Zhou H, Ouyang Y, Xiao H. The effect of preoperative smoking cessation and smoking dose on postoperative complications following radical gastrectomy for gastric cancer: a retrospective study of 2469 patients. World J Surg Oncol. 2019;17(1):61.
56. Wong J, Lam DP, Abrishami A, Chan MTV, Chung F. Short-term preoperative smoking cessation and postoperative complications: a systematic review and meta-analysis. Can J Anaesth. 2012;59(3):268–79.
57. Sørensen LT, Hørby J, Friis E, Pilsgaard B, Jørgensen T. Smoking as a risk factor for wound healing and infection in breast cancer surgery. Eur J Surg Oncol. 2002;28(8):815–20.
58. Gyssens IC. Preventing postoperative infections: current treatment recommendations. Drugs. 1999;57(2):175–85.
59. Galandiuk S, Polk HC, Jagelman DG, Fazio VW. Re-emphasis of priorities in surgical antibiotic prophylaxis. Surg Gynecol Obstet. 1989;169(3):219–22.
60. Crader MF, Varacallo M. Preoperative antibiotic prophylaxis. In: StatPearls. Treasure Island, FL: StatPearls Publishing; 2023.
61. Kolimi P, Narala S, Nyavanandi D, Youssef AAA, Dudhipala N. Innovative treatment strategies to accelerate wound healing: trajectory and recent advancements. Cells. 2022;11(15):2439.
62. Brumberg V, Astrelina T, Malivanova T, Samoilov A. Modern wound dressings: hydrogel dressings. Biomedicines. 2021;9(9):1235.

63. Nuutila K, Eriksson E. Moist wound healing with commonly available dressings. Adv Wound Care (New Rochelle). 2021;10(12):685–98.
64. Argenta LC, Morykwas MJ. Vacuum-assisted closure: a new method for wound control and treatment: clinical experience. Ann Plast Surg. 1997;38(6):563–76.
65. Anghel EL, Kim PJ. Negative-pressure wound therapy: a comprehensive review of the evidence. Plast Reconstr Surg. 2016;138(Suppl. 3):129S–37S.
66. Shanmugam VK, Fernandez SJ, Evans KK, McNish S, Banerjee AN, Couch KS, et al. Postoperative wound dehiscence: predictors and associations. Wound Repair Regen. 2015;23(2):184–90.
67. Seidelman JL, Mantyh CR, Anderson DJ. Surgical site infection prevention: a review. JAMA. 2023;329(3):244–52.
68. Rosen RD, Manna B. Wound dehiscence. In: StatPearls. Treasure Island, FL: StatPearls Publishing; 2023.
69. Cameron JL, Cameron AM. Current surgical therapy. 14th ed. The Netherlands: Elsevier; 2022.
70. Tolstrup M, Watt SK, Gögenur I. Reduced rate of dehiscence after implementation of a standardized fascial closure technique in patients undergoing emergency laparotomy. Ann Surg. 2017;265(4):821–6.
71. Jenkins TP. The burst abdominal wound: a mechanical approach. Br J Surg. 1976;63(11):873–6.
72. Deerenberg EB, Harlaar JJ, Steyerberg EW, Lont HE, van Doorn HC, Heisterkamp J, et al. Small bites versus large bites for closure of abdominal midline incisions (STITCH): a double-blind, multicentre, randomised controlled trial. Lancet. 2015;386(10000):1254–60.
73. Roybal LL, Blattner CM, Young J, Lear W. A novel adhesive suture retention device for the closure of fragile skin under tension. JAAD Case Rep. 2020;6(2):109–14.
74. Khorgami Z, Shoar S, Laghaie B, Aminian A, Hosseini Araghi N, Soroush A. Prophylactic retention sutures in midline laparotomy in high-risk patients for wound dehiscence: a randomized controlled trial. J Surg Res. 2013;180(2):238–43.
75. Bosanquet DC, Ansell J, Abdelrahman T, Cornish J, Harries R, Stimpson A, et al. Systematic review and meta-regression of factors affecting midline incisional hernia rates: analysis of 14,618 patients. PLoS One. 2015;10(9):e0138745.
76. Itatsu K, Yokoyama Y, Sugawara G, Kubota H, Tojima Y, Kurumiya Y, et al. Incidence of and risk factors for incisional hernia after abdominal surgery. Br J Surg. 2014;101(11):1439–47.
77. Ozbagriacik M, Bas G, Basak F, Sisik A, Acar A, Kudas I, et al. Management of strangulated abdominal wall hernias with mesh; early results. North Clin Istanb. 2015;2(1):26–32.
78. Berrevoet F. Prevention of incisional hernias after open abdomen treatment. Front Surg. 2018;5:11.
79. Parker SG, Halligan S, Blackburn S, AaO P, Archer L, Mallett S, et al. What exactly is meant by "loss of domain" for ventral hernia? Systematic review of definitions. World J Surg. 2019;43(2):396–404.
80. Heller L, Chike-Obi C, Xue AS. Abdominal wall reconstruction with mesh and components separation. Semin Plast Surg. 2012;26(1):29–35.
81. Marcovici I. Significant abdominal wall hematoma from an umbilical port insertion. JSLS: J Soc Laparoend Surg. 2001;5(3):293–5.
82. Stocchero IN. Ultrasound in the diagnosis and management of fluid collection complications following abdominoplasty. Ann Plast Surg. 2004;52(3):331.
83. Kaoutzanis C, Winocour J, Gupta V, Ganesh Kumar N, Sarosiek K, Wormer B, et al. Incidence and risk factors for major hematomas in aesthetic surgery: analysis of 129,007 patients. Aesth Surg J. 2017;37(10):1175–85.
84. Bullocks J, Basu CB, Hsu P, Singer R. Prevention of hematomas and seromas. Semin Plastic Surg. 2006;20(4):233–40.
85. de Rosnay P, Chandiramani M, Usman S, Owen E. Injury of epigastric vessels at laparoscopy: diagnosis and management. Gynecol Surg. 2011;8(3):353–6.
86. Masci E, Santoleri L, Longoni M. Topical hemostatic agents in surgical practice. Transf Apher Sci. 2011;45(3):305–11.
87. Fagan NL, Chau J, Malesker M. Topical hemostats. US Pharm. 2010;35(11):HS2–8.

Chapter 32
Can Negative Pressure Dressings Prevent Wound Infection After Surgery?

Richard J. B. Walker and Paul J. Karanicolas

Abbreviations

CDC	Centers for Disease Control and Prevention
CI	Confidence interval
NNT	Number needed to treat
NPWT	Negative-pressure wound therapy
RCT	Randomized controlled trial
RR	Relative risk
SSI	Surgical site infection
WHO	World Health Organization

Introduction

Surgical site infections (SSIs) harm patients and substantially increase the cost to health systems. Organizations including the World Health Organization (WHO) and Centers for Disease Control and Prevention (CDC) have published guidelines targeted toward reducing the incidence of SSIs with evidence-based recommendations spanning the pre-, intra-, and postoperative periods [1, 2]. Nonetheless, SSIs remain relatively common, with incidence rates up to 25% in some populations [3]. More work needs to be done to reduce the incidence of these morbid and costly complications.

R. J. B. Walker · P. J. Karanicolas (✉)
Division of General Surgery, Department of Surgery, University of Toronto, Toronto, ON, Canada

Institute of Health Policy, Management, and Evaluation, Dalla Lana School of Public Health, University of Toronto, Toronto, ON, Canada

Division of General Surgery, Sunnybrook Health Sciences Centre, Toronto, ON, Canada
e-mail: richard.walker@mail.utoronto.ca; paul.karanicolas@sunnybrook.ca

© The Author(s), under exclusive license to Springer Nature Switzerland AG 2024

J. Faintuch, S. Faintuch (eds.), *Recent Strategies in High Risk Surgery*,
https://doi.org/10.1007/978-3-031-56270-9_32

Negative-pressure wound therapy (NPWT) is a relatively recent wound care advancement that has been studied in a variety of settings including open wounds, pressure ulcers, diabetic foot infections, traumatic wounds, skin grafts, burns, and closed incisions [4]. The approach involves applying a porous dressing to a wound, placing an occlusive material on top of the dressing to create an air-tight seal, and applying suction to the dressing via an external device.

History of Negative-Pressure Wound Therapy

The concept of using negative pressure to promote healing has been explored for centuries; there are reports of the Roman army employing healers to apply direct suction to wounds sustained in battle using their mouths [5]. However, it was not until the 1980s that NPWT was evaluated by the scientific community. Russian investigators found that negative pressure could reduce the bacterial burden in purulent wounds and improve healing [6, 7]. In parallel to this work, others developed a technique to apply negative pressure to enterocutaneous, lymphatic, and urinary fistulas as well as large abdominal wounds [8]. Promising results from these pioneering experiments were followed by the first iterations of the vacuum-assisted closure (V.A.C.) device that is still used today [9].

The initial device comprised of a fenestrated tube embedded into a polyurethane ether foam dressing. Early experiments involved placing the foam within an open wound and covering the foam with an adhesive drape to create a seal. The tubing was then attached to a fluid collection container and a vacuum pump. When a pressure differential of −125 mmHg was applied to the system, the porous structure of the foam allowed for an even distribution of negative forces across the wound. In a study of 300 wounds where this technique was applied, there was a significant reduction in tissue edema and subsequent increase in the formation of granulation tissue [9]. The authors hypothesized that the mechanism for these improvements came from the removal of interstitial fluid, resulting in a decrease in capillary afterload and promoting improved circulation to the wound. However, the authors noted that one patient developed an enteric fistula when the foam was left in direct contact with compromised intestine. Nonetheless, the success of these early experiments resulted in an explosion of interest in NPWT [4].

The use of NPWT for closed surgical incisions was first reported in 2006. Patients with persistently draining hematomas or surgical incisions from high-risk orthopedic procedures were randomized to receive either a NPWT dressing on top of their closed incision or a standard dressing [10]. Patients treated with the NPWT dressing had a significantly reduced duration of drainage. Patients with persistently draining hematomas also demonstrated a significantly reduced rate of SSIs. Up until this point, NPWT had mostly been used for open wounds to promote healing by secondary intent or to facilitate a delayed primary closure. However, with the promise of this new application for NPWT, manufacturers began designing NPWT devices specifically for closed incisions.

There have been additional advancements in NPWT systems since the 1990s. Different foams have been developed with variations in pore size, hydrophilic versus hydrophobic polymers, and ionic silver impregnated into the material for its antimicrobial effects [4]. Other developments have included variable vacuum settings, battery improvements to facilitate portability, and alarm systems to notify providers and patients of air leaks or when a fluid collection canister is full [11, 12]. Despite these advancements, the fundamental concept of applying negative pressure evenly across a wound via a porous dressing has remained relatively constant since the technology's inception.

Mechanism of Action

The process of wound healing is generally divided into four consecutive and overlapping stages: hemostasis, inflammation, proliferation, and remodeling [13]. Hemostasis involves the contraction of vessels and coagulation of blood in the wound to form a scab composed of platelets and a fibrin network. The inflammatory stage typically lasts approximately 72 h and involves the activation and recruitment of immune cells including neutrophils, monocytes, and mast cells to destroy microorganisms and promote vasodilation and further immune cell migration. The proliferative stage can last several weeks and involves the formation of granulation tissue, angiogenesis, and re-epithelialization. Finally, remodeling involves the replacement of type III collagen with mature type I collagen and scar formation [13]. NPWT primarily affects the inflammatory and proliferative stages of wound healing. The specific mechanisms by which NPWT may accelerate wound healing and thereby reduce wound-related complications can be divided into four main categories: macrodeformation, microdeformation, removal of fluid, and stabilization of the wound environment [4]. The subsequent sections will explore these mechanisms in more detail.

Macrodeformation

Macrodeformation refers to wound contraction that occurs with the application of negative pressure (Fig. 32.1) [4]. There is an inherent tension in skin that predisposes wounds to be pulled apart. For open wounds, macrodeformational forces oppose this tension and significantly decrease the wound surface area [14]. As well, wound shrinkage paradoxically creates an increase in pressure at the wound edge, which has been shown to stimulate the release of vasodilatory mediators and promote angiogenesis [15, 16]. For closed incisions, NPWT reduces lateral tensile forces, which may help hold the wound together and theoretically prevent dehiscence. One biomechanical modeling study estimated that the use of NPWT at −80 mmHg reduced the force on individual sutures by 69% [17].

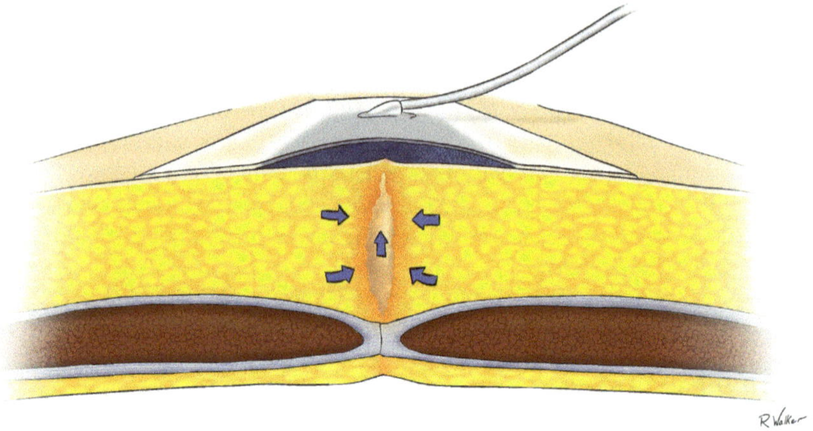

Fig. 32.1 Illustration of negative pressure wound therapy (NPWT) applied to a closed abdominal incision

Microdeformation

Microdeformation refers to the forces on cells at the foam-wound interface as tissue is pulled against the porous structure of the dressing [18, 19]. Cells that are mechanically stretched have been shown to proliferate and differentiate at increased rates [20]. In vitro experiments have found that negative-pressure applied to fibroblasts upregulates genes responsible for the production of growth factors and collagen in addition to inducing cellular proliferation [21]. The extent of these microdeformations can be controlled by adjusting device properties; for example, larger foam pore sizes can cause greater microdeformations and may result in greater tissue growth [22]. However, standard gauzes are still capable of producing microdeformations [18]. While microdeformation appears to be an important mechanism of action for NPWT applied to open wounds, it is less likely to be a significant factor for closed wounds where injured tissues are not in direct contact with the porous dressing.

Fluid Removal

NPWT has been shown to facilitate the removal of edema and excess interstitial fluid from the wound. Evacuating this fluid may decompress small blood vessels and improve perfusion to nearby tissues [4, 23]. Catabolites and inflammatory mediators are also removed along with edema, which may assist in controlling the extent of the inflammatory response [16]. Some investigators have hypothesized that the removal of fluid in the wound bed reduces the bacterial burden; however, one randomized controlled trial (RCT) of 54 patients found no difference in the bacterial load in wounds treated with NPWT compared to conventional moist gauze

[24]. Nonetheless, the removal of excess fluid using NPWT appears to improve wound healing.

Stabilization of the Wound Environment

Lastly, NPWT dressings provide a warm, hydrated environment while also acting as a barrier to external bacterial contamination [4]. A hydrated wound environment has been shown to increase angiogenesis, collagen synthesis, and the breakdown of fibrin and necrotic tissue [25]. While traditional dressings are also capable of creating this environment, it would be remiss to not mention this as a mechanism by which NPWT may improve healing.

Clinical Evidence

The Burden of SSIs

Patients who experience SSIs have an increased risk of ICU admission and death during their hospitalization [26]. Morbidity from these infections can also extend beyond the initial hospitalization; perioperative infections increase a patient's risk of subsequent infections and mortality up to 1 year after the index operation [27]. As well, health-related quality of life at 30 days following a laparotomy is significantly worse in patients who develop SSIs [28]. Oncologic outcomes in patients undergoing surgery for cancer have also been shown to be negatively impacted by perioperative infections. A meta-analysis of 43 studies including 154,981 patients undergoing surgery for colorectal cancer found that infective complications were associated with a significant decrease in overall and cancer specific survival [29].

A causal effect on oncologic outcomes is thought to be through two mechanisms: (1) an increase in cytokines in response to infection and circulating bacterial components that may promote tumor growth, and (2) a deregulated immune response that may weaken the body's ability to fight cancer cells [30].

Resource Utilization and Cost

Healthcare costs for patients who experience an SSI are approximately twice the amount of those who do not have an SSI [31]. In one large population-based study of a variety of surgical patients, the 6891 cases of SSIs accounted for an additional 406,730 hospital days and over 1.6 billion USD in additional costs from the index admission and subsequent readmissions [32]. Given the substantial burden of SSIs on patients and healthcare systems, effective measures to reduce the incidence of SSIs have the potential to be of great impact.

The Benefits of NPWT for Patients with Closed Incisions

There have been many RCTs evaluating the effects of NPWT on closed, non-infected surgical wounds and recent meta-analyses of their results [33, 34]. A Cochrane review published in 2022 provides an up-to-date synthesis of the available experimental evidence for this indication [33]. The review included RCTs that compared NPWT to any other type of wound dressing. Excluded RCTs were those evaluating NPWT for skin grafts (donor or recipient sites), flap closures, and wounds following delayed primary closure. Sixty-two RCTs were eligible, with a total of 13,340 participants undergoing obstetric, orthopedic, vascular, and general surgeries. In most studies, NPWT was applied to wounds for 7 days or less. The review concluded with moderate certainty evidence from 44 of the studies that NPWT results in fewer SSIs than standard dressings (relative risk [RR] 0.73; 95% confidence interval [CI] 0.63–0.85). The certainty of the evidence was downgraded for risk of bias attributed largely to a lack of blinding, which would understandably be difficult for such an intervention.

One subgroup analysis categorized trials by surgical indication, without significant differences. Thirteen RCTs evaluated general surgery procedures and included a total of 1823 patients. Despite the confidence bands crossing 1.0, indicating a questionable result, the effect estimate for this subgroup remained relatively similar (RR 0.78; 95% CI 0.57–1.05). The same was true for cesarean sections (RR 0.78; 95% CI 0.65–0.95) and hepatopancreatobiliary surgeries (RR 0.58; 95% CI 0.23–1.45). The similar direction of the estimates, absence of a statistically significant difference between groups, and conceptual validity of NPWT improving healing regardless of anatomical site suggest that the pooled estimate from all trials are applicable across surgical indications [33].

Deeper Surgical Infections

The CDC defines superficial incisional SSIs as an infection within 30 days following an operation that involves the skin or subcutaneous tissue [35]. Deep incisional SSIs are those occurring within 30 days if there is no synthetic implant (or within 1 year if there is an implant) that involve the deep soft tissues. For abdominal surgeries, these include the fascial and muscle layers. Finally, organ/space SSIs are those that involve organs or spaces other than the incision that were opened or manipulated during surgery. These include intraperitoneal infections, osteomyelitis, septic joints, and intracranial infections. In a subgroup analysis, there was a significant association between NPWT and decreased rates of superficial SSIs (RR 0.70; 95% CI 0.53–0.92; $p = 0.01$) [33]. However, there was not a significant association for deep or organ/space SSIs (RR 0.95; 95% CI 0.76–1.18). This aligns with our understanding of the mechanism of NPWT; it is conceivable that negative pressure applied to the surface of a wound would not have a substantial effect on deeper layers, let alone spaces such as the intraperitoneal cavity.

Degrees of Contamination

The CDC has defined four classes of wounds: clean, clean-contaminated, contaminated, and dirty or infected [36]. Clean wounds are those that are uninfected and where the respiratory, alimentary, genital, or urinary tracts are not entered. A common example would be an inguinal hernia repair. Clean-contaminated wounds are those in which the respiratory, alimentary, genital, or urinary tracts are entered without unusual contamination. This category would include procedures such as a laparoscopic cholecystectomy. Contaminated wounds include accidental wounds, those with major breaks in sterile technique, those with gross spillage from the GI tract, and those where acute, non-purulent inflammation is encountered. A fresh stab wound would be an example of a contaminated wound. Finally, dirty wounds include old traumatic wounds and those involving perforated viscera. An example would be a bowel resection for ischemic colitis complicated by perforation. The classification system provides a coarse framework for thinking about the risk of SSI. The Cochrane review found no evidence for a significant difference in results based on degree of contamination [33]. Therefore, NPWT may still be useful in preventing SSIs in wounds with gross contamination.

Major and Minor Outcomes

The Cochrane review found no clear difference in mortality, wound dehiscence, reoperation, readmission, or seromas in patients treated with NPWT compared to those treated with standard dressings [33]. Another recent meta-analysis with broad inclusion criteria found no difference in length of hospitalization for patients treated with NPWT compared to standard dressings (Table 32.1) [34]. Nonetheless, the potential for NPWT to significantly decrease the rate of superficial SSIs for all types of surgeries and wound classifications is meaningful. The Global Guidelines for the Prevention of Surgical Site Infection published by the WHO in 2018 gave a

Table 32.1 Summary of the Norman et al. and Shirokey et al. meta-analyses comparing NPWT to standard dressings

Outcome	Number of participants (studies)	Effect estimate (95% CI)
SSI	11,403 (44)	RR 0.73 (0.63, 0.85)
Wound dehiscence	8724 (23)	RR 0.97 (0.82, 1.16)
Seroma	5436 (15)	RR 0.82 (0.65, 1.05)
Hematoma	5909 (17)	RR 0.79 (0.48, 1.30)
Mortality	6384 (11)	RR 0.78 (0.47, 1.30)
Reoperation	6272 (18)	RR 1.13 (0.91, 1.41)
Skin blisters	5015 (11)	RR 3.55 (1.43, 8.77)
Length of hospitalization (days)[a]	576 (4)	MD −1.17 (−2.19, −0.16)

NPWT negative pressure wound therapy, *RR* relative risk, *MD* mean difference
[a]Length of hospitalization was derived from the meta-analysis by Shirokey et al. (2020)

conditional recommendation for the use of prophylactic NPWT in adult patients on primarily closed incisions in high-risk wounds, while accounting for resource use [2].

The Evidence for NPWT Treatment Parameters

As of 2023, the leading NPWT systems for closed surgical incisions are the Prevena (3M, Saint Paul, MN, USA) and the PICO 7 (Smith & Nephew, Hull, UK). The Prevena applies 125 mmHg of continuous negative pressure, whereas the PICO 7 applies 80 mmHg of continuous negative pressure. There are no RCTs comparing NPWT devices for closed incisions head-to-head [33]. However, subgroup analyses according to the type of dressing [34] addressed the Prevena (3 M, Saint Paul, MN), the PICO 7 (Smith & Nephew, Hull, UK), the V.A.C. (3 M, Saint Paul, MN, USA), the V.S.D. (Wuhan Medical Science & Technology, Wuhan, China), and dressings constructed from available hospital supplies (i.e., home-made), without differences on SSI rates [34].

For open incisions, a small RCT compared 125 mmHg to 75 mmHg of negative pressure in 40 patients with diabetic food wounds [37]. There was no difference in the proportion of wounds that were ultimately closed surgically or wounds that demonstrated a 50% or greater surface area reduction after 4 weeks. These results may not apply to closed surgical incisions.

Experimental Models

One study compared the Prevena, PICO 7, and Platform Wound Dressing (Medela, Baar, Switzerland) applied to closed incisions in porcine models [38]. There were no significant differences between devices in the amount of granulation tissue at the end of 9 days. Regarding the optimal waveform for NPWT, experiments on porcine models have demonstrated that intermittent suction produces superior tissue granulation compared to continuous suction [23, 39]. However, intermittent suction may cause more pain to patients [39]. Both the Prevena and PICO 7 apply continuous pressure to closed incisions.

Duration

In general, dressing systems for closed incisions are recommended for a maximum of 7 days postoperatively, although some may be applied for longer [11, 12]. In a recent meta-analysis, the duration of therapy ranged from 2 to 14 days; dressings were most often removed between day 5 and 7 [34].

Cost-Effectiveness

Variability in results for cost-effectiveness [33] has likely arisen from several factors, including, but not limited to, how cost has been measured, the costs themselves as these commonly vary between centers and systems, the baseline SSI rate in the patient population as this affects the number needed to treat (NNT), and the observed effect of NPWT on SSIs in that population.

The PICO 7 cost as low as 120 pounds in one UK trial [40]. Conversely, the Prevena cost up to 544 USD in a trial from Pennsylvania [41]. These costs can vary substantially even for the same device; therefore, clinicians interested in the cost-effectiveness of NPWT in their practice may consider familiarizing themselves with the costs at their center.

Measures of cost-effectiveness would ideally consider the healthcare costs averted by preventing SSIs and not just the cost of the NPWT device alone. An RCT of women with a body mass index (BMI) ≥30 undergoing a cesarean section estimated an incremental cost-effectiveness ratio (ICER) of 15,000 USD for each SSI prevented; however, this RCT calculated the ICER based only on the device cost and the number needed to treat (NNT) to prevent one SSI [41]. Additional dressings, wound care, prolonged hospitalization, follow-up appointments, and any subsequent complications or procedures should be considered as well. Another RCT from Australia of obese women undergoing a cesarean section included hospital and outpatient care into their cost calculation, and estimated an ICER of 1347 Australian dollars (AUD) for each SSI prevented [42]. Yet another trial of obese women undergoing a cesarean section found NPWT to be cost-saving when considering inpatient and outpatient costs [43]. This trial estimated that NPWT would be cost-saving up to a device cost of 192 USD for their population.

Markov Microsimulation Models

These can be used to study the cost-effectiveness of interventions while accounting for many potential disease states, their probabilities of occurring, and their associated costs. Advantages of simulation studies include the ability to apply results from a variety of high-quality sources (including RCTs and meta-analyses) and to consider the impact of rare events. With elective open right hemicolectomy used as the base case [44], the cost of several potential consequences of superficial and deep SSIs were considered. These consequences included emergency room (ER) presentation, readmission, the need for home care, dehiscence with reoperation, or hernia as a result of SSI. The authors found that prophylactic NPWT resulted in a cost-saving of USD $17.07 per patient and 0.09 quality adjusted life years gained [44].

High Baseline Risk of SSI

The Cochrane review estimated an absolute risk reduction of 31 fewer SSIs per 1000 people with NPWT [33]. This was based on a baseline risk of SSIs with standard dressings of 11.7% and equates to an NNT of 32.3 to prevent one SSI. Operations with higher risks of SSIs would require a lower NNT to prevent on SSI and therefore have improved cost-effectiveness. A prospective international cohort study of 12,539 patients from 343 hospitals and 66 countries undergoing elective or emergency gastrointestinal surgeries found 30-day SSI rates of 9.5%, 22.5%, and 25.0% for clean-contaminated, contaminated, and dirty procedures, respectively [3]. If we take the baseline SSI risk of 25.0% for dirty procedures and assume an RR of 0.73 with NPWT compared to standard dressings, NPWT would result in 68 fewer SSIs per 1000 people. This equates to an NNT of 14.7.

The Markov microsimulation study likewise performed subgroup analyses to examine the effect of NPWT on patients at an elevated risk of SSI [44]. Cost-savings increased to US$85.83, $92.33, and $188.50 for patients who are smokers, diabetic, or obese. Table 32.2 lists the NNT for several common general surgery procedures using reported average SSI risks and the RR for NPWT from the Cochrane review [33, 45, 46].

The Cochrane review probable advantages of NPWT for cesarean sections in obese women, however not for fracture surgery or for deep SSIs [33].

The Risks

Based on low-certainty evidence from 11 trials (5015 participants), patients treated with NPWT may be more likely to develop skin blisters compared to those treated with standard dressings (RR 3.55; 95% CI 1.43–8.77) [33]. No clear difference in incisional pain compared to those with standard dressings was detected; however, the ability to pool estimates was limited by differing outcome definitions. With regard to hematoma, the review was uncertain based on pooled results from 17 trials (RR 0.79; 95% CI 0.48–1.30). Product manuals for the Prevena and PICO 7 advise

Table 32.2 Hypothetical number needed to treat with NPWT to prevent one SSI for a variety of abdominal procedures

Procedure	Average risk of SSI[a]	NNT[b]
Laparoscopic cholecystectomy	1.1%	336.7
Appendectomy for perforated appendicitis	4.7%	78.8
Anterior resection	11.5%	32.2
Repair of perforated small bowel	12.5%	29.6
Pancreaticoduodenectomy	27.9%	13.3

NNT number needed to treat, *SSI* surgical site infection, *NPWT* negative pressure wound therapy
[a]Average SSI risk was derived from the American College of Surgeons NSQIP Surgical Risk Calculator [45], except for pancreaticoduodenectomy, where the risk was derived from Javed et al. [46]
[b]NNT calculated assuming a RR of 0.73 [33]

caution when using the device for patients at an elevated risk of bleeding [11, 12]. The user manual for the PICO 7 also warns users that the dressing should not be placed in contact with exposed vessels due to a risk of erosion [12]. Finally, as with most dressings, there is a risk of allergic reaction to the dressing materials and adhesives. Of note, the Prevena foam is impregnated with silver, which may also cause skin reactions in patients with sensitivities and allergies to the metal.

Contraindications

NPWT devices are relatively straightforward to use; however, there are some practical considerations worth noting. Please note that this information should not be used in lieu of a product manual.

Contraindications for all types of NPWT include malignant wounds, untreated osteomyelitis, fistulae, and exposed organs or blood vessels [4, 11].

Malignant Wounds

There are concerns that NPWT may promote tumor growth and expedite metastases by the same mechanisms that it promotes wound healing [47]. However, there have been case reports of patients having good responses to NPWT for abdominal wounds with gross tumor involvement in the palliative context [47, 48]. In these reports, NPWT decreased odor and exudate, reduced the frequency of potentially painful dressing changes, and, in one case, facilitated a delayed primary closure [47, 48]. The PICO 7 user manual acknowledges the device may still be used in the palliative setting for patients with malignancy in the wound bed [12].

Osteomyelitis

NPWT does not substitute for antibiotics and conventional treatments. In one retrospective study of patients with post-sternotomy osteomyelitis, NPWT had no added benefit over antimicrobial therapy alone [49].

Non-enteric or Unexplored Fistulas

NPWT may increase the volume of fluid passing through a fistula, thereby delaying its closure [4, 12]. However, if the primary goal for a patient's fistula is to keep the surrounding skin clean, NPWT may be helpful. There have been reports of using

NPWT in patients with enteroatmospheric fistulas to keep the wound clean, enhance granulation tissue formation, and reduce local inflammation [50, 51]. Nonetheless, NPWT should be cautioned in wounds with fistulas, and wound care experts or experienced providers should be consulted if it is being considered in this setting.

Exposed Organs or Blood Vessels

The concern here is erosion [4]. One study followed patients in whom a V.A.C. was used to manage an open abdomen after laparotomy. The device was applied with a fenestrated layer between the bowel and foam, and negative pressure was applied at −125 mmHg. A total of 6/29 patients (20%) developed intestinal fistulas at a median of 20 days from the start of therapy [52]. This contraindication is not a concern for closed incisions.

References

1. Berríos-Torres SI, Umscheid CA, Bratzler DW, et al. Centers for Disease Control and Prevention guideline for the prevention of surgical site infection, 2017. JAMA Surg. 2017;152:784–91.
2. WHO. Global guidelines for the prevention of surgical site infection. 2nd ed. World Health Organization; 2018. Available at: iris.who.int/handle/10665/250680. Accessed September 22, 2023
3. GlobalSurg Collaborative. Surgical site infection after gastrointestinal surgery in high-income, middle-income, and low-income countries: a prospective, international, multicentre cohort study. Lancet Infect Dis. 2018;18:516–25.
4. Huang C, Leavitt T, Bayer LR, Orgill DP. Effect of negative pressure wound therapy on wound healing. Curr Probl Surg. 2014;51:301–31.
5. Miller C. The history of negative pressure wound therapy (NPWT): from "lip service" to the modern vacuum system. J Am Coll Clin Wound Spec. 2012;4:61–2.
6. Davydov IA, Larichev AB, Smirnov AP, Flegontov VB. Vacuum therapy of acute suppurative diseases of soft tissues and suppurative wounds. Vestn Khir Im I I Grek. 1988;141:43–6. (Article in Russian), 48
7. Kostiuchenok BM, Kolker II, Karlov VA, et al. Vacuum treatment in the surgical management of suppurative wounds. Vestn Khir Im I I Grek. 1986;137:18–21. (Article in Russian)
8. Chariker ME, Gerstle TL, Morrison CS. An algorithmic approach to the use of gauze-based negative-pressure wound therapy as a bridge to closure in pediatric extremity trauma. Plast Reconstr Surg. 2009;123:1510–20.
9. Argenta LC, Morykwas MJ. Vacuum-assisted closure: a new method for wound control and treatment: clinical experience. Ann Plast Surg. 1997;38:563–76. discussion 577
10. Stannard JP, Robinson JT, Anderson ER, et al. Negative pressure wound therapy to treat hematomas and surgical incisions following high-energy trauma. J Trauma. 2006;60:1301–6.
11. KCI. Prevena 125 therapy unit with Prevena 45 ml Canister and accessories: instructions for use; 2019. Available at: acelity.com/-/media/Project/Acelity/Acelity-Base-Sites/shared/PDF/420236a-gde-prevena-125-150ml-canister-clinician-denovo-web.pdf. Accessed September 22, 2023.
12. Smith & Nephew. PICO 7: Single use negative pressure wound therapy system user manual; 2020. Available at: possiblewithpico.com/sites/default/files/picoImages/documents/

IFUs/35053_PICO%2014%20Patient%20and%20caregiver_US.pdf. Accessed September 22, 2023.
13. Alhajj M, Goyal A. Physiology, granulation tissue. In: StatPearls. Treasure Island, FL: StatPearls Publishing; 2023.
14. Borgquist O, Ingemansson R, Malmsjö M. The influence of low and high pressure levels during negative-pressure wound therapy on wound contraction and fluid evacuation. Plast Reconstr Surg. 2011;127:551–9.
15. Kairinos N, Solomons M, Hudson DA. The paradox of negative pressure wound therapy—in vitro studies. J Plast Reconstr Aesthet Surg. 2010;63:174–9.
16. Lancerotto L, Bayer LR, Orgill DP. Mechanisms of action of microdeformational wound therapy. Semin Cell Dev Biol. 2012;23:987–92.
17. Loveluck J, Copeland T, Hill J, et al. Biomechanical modeling of the forces applied to closed incisions during single-use negative pressure wound therapy. Eplasty. 2016;16:e20.
18. Borgquist O, Gustafsson L, Ingemansson R, Malmsjö M. Micro- and macromechanical effects on the wound bed of negative pressure wound therapy using gauze and foam. Ann Plast Surg. 2010;64:789–93.
19. Saxena V, Hwang C-W, Huang S, et al. Vacuum-assisted closure: microdeformations of wounds and cell proliferation. Plast Reconstr Surg. 2004;114:1086–96. discussion 1097–1098
20. Ingber DE. Mechanical control of tissue growth: function follows form. Proc Natl Acad Sci U S A. 2005;102:11571–2.
21. Lu F, Ogawa R, Nguyen DT, et al. Microdeformation of three-dimensional cultured fibroblasts induces gene expression and morphological changes. Ann Plast Surg. 2011;66:296–300.
22. Heit YI, Dastouri P, Helm DL, et al. Foam pore size is a critical interface parameter of suction-based wound healing devices. Plast Reconstr Surg. 2012;129:589–97.
23. Morykwas MJ, Argenta LC, Shelton-Brown EI, McGuirt W. Vacuum-assisted closure: a new method for wound control and treatment: animal studies and basic foundation. Ann Plast Surg. 1997;38:553–62.
24. Mouës CM, Vos MC, van den Bemd G-JCM, et al. Bacterial load in relation to vacuum-assisted closure wound therapy: a prospective randomized trial. Wound Repair Regen. 2004;12:11–7.
25. Junker JPE, Kamel RA, Caterson EJ, Eriksson E. Clinical impact upon wound healing and inflammation in moist, wet, and dry environments. Adv Wound Care (New Rochelle). 2013;2:348–56.
26. Kirkland KB, Briggs JP, Trivette SL, et al. The impact of surgical-site infections in the 1990s: attributable mortality, excess length of hospitalization, and extra costs. Infect Control Hosp Epidemiol. 1999;20:725–30.
27. O'Brien WJ, Gupta K, Itani KMF. Association of postoperative infection with risk of long-term infection and mortality. JAMA Surg. 2020;155:61–8.
28. Pinkney TD, Calvert M, Bartlett DC, et al. Impact of wound edge protection devices on surgical site infection after laparotomy: multicentre randomised controlled trial (ROSSINI trial). BMJ. 2013;347:f4305.
29. Lawler J, Choynowski M, Bailey K, et al. Meta-analysis of the impact of postoperative infective complications on oncological outcomes in colorectal cancer surgery. BJS Open. 2020;4:737–47.
30. Tsujimoto H, Ichikura T, Ono S, et al. Impact of postoperative infection on long-term survival after potentially curative resection for gastric cancer. Ann Surg Oncol. 2009;16:311–8.
31. Broex ECJ, van Asselt ADI, Bruggeman CA, van Tiel FH. Surgical site infections: how high are the costs? J Hosp Infect. 2009;72:193–201.
32. de Lissovoy G, Fraeman K, Hutchins V, et al. Surgical site infection: incidence and impact on hospital utilization and treatment costs. Am J Infect Control. 2009;37:387–97.
33. Norman G, Shi C, Goh EL, et al. Negative pressure wound therapy for surgical wounds healing by primary closure. Cochrane Database Syst Rev. 2022;4:CD009261.
34. Shiroky J, Lillie E, Muaddi H, et al. The impact of negative pressure wound therapy for closed surgical incisions on surgical site infection: a systematic review and meta-analysis. Surgery. 2020;167:1001–9.

35. Horan TC, Gaynes RP, Martone WJ, et al. CDC definitions of nosocomial surgical site infections, 1992: a modification of CDC definitions of surgical wound infections. Infect Control Hosp Epidemiol. 1992;13:606–8.
36. Garner JS. Guideline for prevention of surgical wound infections, 1985: supersedes guideline for prevention of surgical wound infections published in 1982. Am J Infect Control. 1986;14:71–80.
37. Lavery LA, La Fontaine J, Thakral G, et al. Randomized clinical trial to compare negative-pressure wound therapy approaches with low and high pressure, silicone-coated dressing, and polyurethane foam dressing. Plast Reconstr Surg. 2014;133:722–6.
38. Nuutila K, Broomhead M, Proppe K, Eriksson E. Study comparing platform wound dressing, a negative-pressure device without a filler, with three conventional negative-pressure wound therapy systems in the treatment of excisional and incisional wounds. Plast Reconstr Surg. 2021;147:76–86.
39. Malmsjö M, Gustafsson L, Lindstedt S, et al. The effects of variable, intermittent, and continuous negative pressure wound therapy, using foam or gauze, on wound contraction, granulation tissue formation, and ingrowth into the wound filler. Eplasty. 2012;12:e5.
40. Nherera LM, Trueman P, Karlakki SL. Cost-effectiveness analysis of single-use negative pressure wound therapy dressings (sNPWT) to reduce surgical site complications (SSC) in routine primary hip and knee replacements. Wound Repair Regen. 2017;25:474–82.
41. Ruhstaller K, Downes KL, Chandrasekaran S, et al. Prophylactic wound vacuum therapy after cesarean section to prevent wound complications in the obese population: a randomized controlled trial (the ProVac study). Am J Perinatol. 2017;34:1125–30.
42. Heard C, Chaboyer W, Anderson V, et al. Cost-effectiveness analysis alongside a pilot study of prophylactic negative pressure wound therapy. J Tissue Viability. 2017;26:79–84.
43. Hyldig N, Joergensen JS, Wu C, et al. Cost-effectiveness of incisional negative pressure wound therapy compared with standard care after caesarean section in obese women: a trial-based economic evaluation. BJOG. 2019;126:619–27.
44. Cheung DC, Muaddi H, de Almeida JR, et al. Cost-effectiveness analysis of negative pressure wound therapy to prevent surgical site infection after elective colorectal surgery. Dis Colon Rectum. 2022;65:767–76.
45. Bilimoria KY, Liu Y, Paruch JL, et al. Development and evaluation of the universal ACS NSQIP surgical risk calculator: a decision aid and informed consent tool for patients and surgeons. J Am Coll Surg. 2013;217:833–42.
46. Javed AA, Teinor J, Wright M, et al. Negative pressure wound therapy for surgical-site infections: a randomized trial. Ann Surg. 2019;269:1034–40.
47. Cai SS, Gowda AU, Alexander RH, et al. Use of negative pressure wound therapy on malignant wounds—a case report and review of literature. Int Wound J. 2017;14:661–5.
48. Riot S, de Bonnecaze G, Garrido I, et al. Is the use of negative pressure wound therapy for a malignant wound legitimate in a palliative context? "The concept of NPWT ad vitam": a case series. Palliat Med. 2015;29:470–3.
49. Tocco MP, Ballardini M, Masala M, Perozzi A. Post-sternotomy chronic osteomyelitis: is sternal resection always necessary? Eur J Cardiothorac Surg. 2013;43:715–21.
50. Bobkiewicz A, Walczak D, Smoliński S, et al. Management of enteroatmospheric fistula with negative pressure wound therapy in open abdomen treatment: a multicentre observational study. Int Wound J. 2017;14:255–64.
51. Gunn LA, Follmar KE, Wong MS, et al. Management of enterocutaneous fistulas using negative-pressure dressings. Ann Plast Surg. 2006;57:621–5.
52. Rao M, Burke D, Finan PJ, Sagar PM. The use of vacuum-assisted closure of abdominal wounds: a word of caution. Color Dis. 2007;9:266–8.

Part IX
Innovative Approaches

Chapter 33
Practical Implementation of Extracorporeal Membrane Oxygenation in the Critically Ill Surgical Patient

Taylor N. Ziegler and Shaun L. Thompson

Abbreviations

BMI	Body mass index
CaO_2	Arterial oxygen content
CO	Cardiac output
CPR	Cardiopulmonary resuscitation
DO_2	Oxygen delivery
DTI	Direct thrombin inhibitor
ECLS	Extracorporeal life support
ECMO	Extracorporeal membrane oxygenation
EF	Ejection fraction
HIT	Heparin-induced thrombocytopenia
ICU	Intensive care unit
INR	International normalized ratio
LDH	Lactate dehydrogenase
LV	Left ventricle
LVOT	Left ventricular outflow tract
MAP	Mean arterial pressure
PEEP	Positive end expiratory pressure
RPM	Rotations per minute
RRT	Renal replacement therapy
RV	Right ventricle
SvO_2	Venous oxygen saturation
TAPSE	Tricuspid annular plane systolic excursion
TIVA	Total intravenous anesthesia
UFH	Unfractionated heparin
VA-ECMO	Veno-arterial extracorporeal membrane oxygenation

T. N. Ziegler · S. L. Thompson (✉)
Department of Anesthesiology, University of Nebraska Medical Center, Omaha, NE, USA
e-mail: taylor.ziegler@unmc.edu; slthomps@unmc.edu

© The Author(s), under exclusive license to Springer Nature Switzerland AG 2024

J. Faintuch, S. Faintuch (eds.), *Recent Strategies in High Risk Surgery*,
https://doi.org/10.1007/978-3-031-56270-9_33

VILI	Ventilator-induced lung injury
VO_2	Volume oxygen (extraction)
VTI	Velocity time integral
VV-ECMO	Veno-venous extracorporeal membrane oxygenation

Introduction

Extracorporeal membrane oxygenation (ECMO), also known as extracorporeal life support (ECLS), is a mechanical device which supports cardiopulmonary physiology in patients with refractory circulatory or respiratory failure, until functional recovery occurs, or a more durable device and/or transplantation are provided.

The most common indications are cardiogenic shock from acute myocardial infarction, decompensated heart failure, and acute respiratory distress syndrome (ARDS). Extracorporeal cardiopulmonary resuscitation (CPR) when conventional CPR fails to restore circulation, massive pulmonary embolus, status asthmaticus, anaphylactic shock, pulmonary hemorrhage, septic shock, malignant arrhythmias, fulminant myocarditis, severe hypothermia, and trauma could also require such assistance.

Morbidity and in-Hospital Mortality

These events can exhibit rates of as much as 80% and 50–60%, respectively [1, 2]. Therefore, the providing physician should give careful consideration to patient selection and the associated risks and benefits. Is the patient's underlying pathology potentially reversible (unless ECMO support is used as a bridge to transplantation)? An irreversible pathology with no plan for successful decannulation is the absolute contraindication [3]. Relative contraindications include pre-terminal or terminal cases of malignancy, detrimental neurologic injury, extremes of age and BMI, severe liver disease, contraindications to anticoagulation, immunosuppression, and overall futility in patient prognosis [3]. Age over 60 years is associated with an increased risk of in-hospital mortality [2].

Physiology

The ultimate function of ECMO is to improve oxygen delivery and perfusion to tissue. Oxygen consumption (VO_2) in adults is ~3–5 mL/kg/min. For homeostasis to be maintained, a ratio of oxygen delivery (DO_2) to oxygen consumption (DO_2/VO_2), where DO_2 = CO (cardiac output) $\times$ CaO_2 (arterial oxygen content), must be at least

2:1 to prevent anaerobic metabolism. In a healthy adult at rest, the DO_2/VO_2 will be close to 5:1. The venous oxygen saturation (SvO_2) reflects the DO_2/VO_2 ratio and will be 50% and 80% at 2:1 and 5:1, respectively. CaO_2 is determined by 1) oxygen carried by red blood cells and 2) oxygen dissolved within the plasma calculated as CaO_2 = [Hgb (g/dL) × oxygen saturation (SpO_2) × 1.34 (cc/g)] + [PaO_2 (mmHg) × 0.003 (cc/dL/mmHg)].

During illness, metabolic rate and oxygen consumption significantly increases which is often met by more substantial cardiac output of up to 50%. In cardiogenic shock or severe respiratory failure, homeostasis is not able to be maintained. When ECMO is in use, DO_2 can be calculated as: (native cardiac output × CaO_2 of native lung) + (ECMO flow in L/min × CaO_2 of membrane lung).

Veno-Venous (VV-ECMO) vs. Veno-Arterial (VA-ECMO)

VV-ECMO delivers blood from the patient's venous circulation to the ECMO circuit for oxygenation/ventilation and is delivered back to the patient's venous circulation. Therefore, it is capable of supporting only respiratory physiology. VA-ECMO assists both respiratory and circulatory physiology. If circulatory support is not required, VV-ECMO is preferable due to less complications associated with venous cannulation versus arterial cannulation, and the lack of higher afterload resulting in more heart effort [4]. As a disease process progresses, reconfiguration could be necessary. Hybrid models have been used more frequently in recent years: V-AV, VV-AV, VV-A.

VV-ECMO

It may be considered during respiratory failure when conventional therapies are insufficient and expected mortality is greater than 50% defined by arterial partial pressure of oxygen (PaO_2)/inspired oxygen concentration (FiO_2) < 150 on FiO_2 > 90% and/or Murray Score 2–3 (see Fig. 33.1). VV-ECMO is *indicated* when mortality is greater than 80% defined as PaO_2/FiO_2 < 100 on FiO_2 > 90% and/or Murray Score 3–4 despite optimal care for 7 h or more. The RESP score can also be utilized to predict in-hospital mortality for VV-ECMO (see Fig. 33.2) [5, 6]. A relative contraindication for VV-ECMO is patients who have received mechanical ventilation for more than 7 days with plateau pressure > 30 cm H_2O and FiO_2 > 90%, as irreversible pulmonary damage has likely occurred [3]. The therapy could be envisaged as well during severe air leak syndromes, intubation requirement for patient awaiting lung transplantation, primary lung graft dysfunction after transplant, refractory hypercapnia with pH < 7.25 on optimal mechanical ventilation with pressure limitations (plateau pressure > 30), and adjunct in management during tracheobronchial or lung surgery [3]. (Table 33.1).

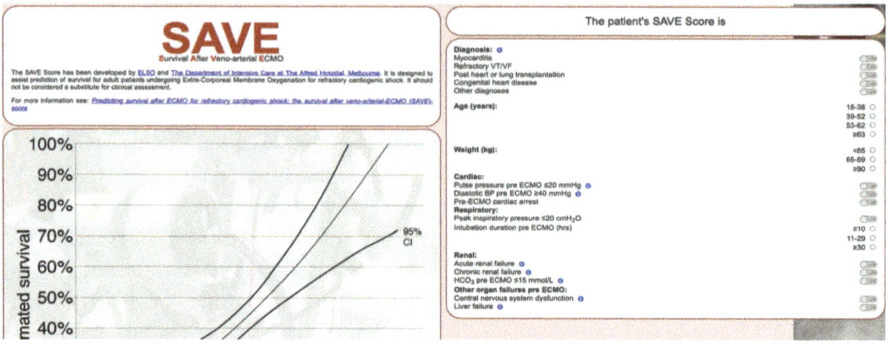

Fig. 33.1 SAVE score used to predict potential outcomes for patients needing VA ECMO. Accessed at elso.org/savescore/index.html

Transport: **Before Leaving**

- ☐ Full O_2 tank
- ☐ Tubing clamp available

After Returned

- ☐ Wall power/O_2/med. air returned to wall supply
- ☐ O_2 returned to flow meter (from O_2 tank)
- ☐ Water turned on/run

Fig. 33.2 Checklist for transport of ECMO patients at UNMC. Courtesy of Jordanna Knott

Table 33.1 Murray Score stratifies severity of acute lung injury and can be utilized for ECMO patient selection [7]

Murray score	0	1	2	3	4
Consolidation on CXR	None	1 quadrant	2 quadrants	3 quadrants	4 quadrants
PaO_2/FiO_2	>300	225–299	175–224	100–174	<100
PEEP (cm H_2O)	<5	6–8	9–11	12–14	>15
Compliance (mL/cm H_2O) Vt/(PIP-PEEP)	>80	60–79	40–59	20–39	<19

VA-ECMO

It should ideally be employed within 6 h of identifying cardiogenic shock that is refractory to conventional therapies. The SAVE score can be used to predict in-hospital survival for VA-ECMO patients in the setting of cardiogenic shock but does not apply to the post-cardiotomy setting. Some functional and structural cardiovascular conditions are considered relative contraindications for VA-ECMO including severe aortic regurgitation, acute aortic dissection, and severe vascular disease of the aorta and peripheral arteries. Compared to VV-ECMO, a disadvantage of VA-ECMO is the significant increase in left ventricle (LV) afterload and distension leading to poor LV function and ischemia. Prompt treatment should be employed in such circumstances. Options include pharmacological agents (e.g. diuretics, vasodilators, inotropes), reducing ECMO flows, LV assist device, intraaortic balloon pump, or catheter-based LV venting [8]. If poor ejection through the aortic valve impairs regular opening, life-threatening thrombosis of the left ventricle or aorta may occur. Further, pulmonary edema is common when LV pressures are increased.

Extracorporeal Circuit

The basic ECMO circuit consists of a pump, oxygenator, and cannulas. The functional capacity of each component must be considered when deciding on the type of circuit to utilize and should be capable of fully supporting the patient. (Partial support is permissible if ECMO is being utilized only for CO_2 removal such as in an asthma exacerbation.)

Pump

A centrifugal pump, however also axial rotary, modified roller, and peristaltic pumps are available. The rotations per minute (RPM) are set/adjusted for centrifugal pumps which determine the L/min of blood flow. Suction (inlet) pressure should not exceed −300 mmHg; otherwise, the tubing could shake or "chatter" leading to hemolysis or even worse, cavitation of air within the circuit could lead to air embolus. Drainage (outlet) pressure should not exceed +400 mmHg. ECMO pumps should have a battery back-up and hand crank in case of emergency power failure.

Oxygenator

The oxygenator (or "membrane lung") is where gas exchange occurs and is determined by the membrane surface area. The flow describes the rate at which desaturated blood can be fully saturated per minute, or maximal O_2 delivery. If the blood flow required for total support of oxygen delivery in a patient exceeds an oxygenator's rated flow, an additional oxygenator can be used in parallel. A gas blender attached to the oxygenator mixes air and oxygen allowing for adjustment of fraction of delivered oxygen ($F_D O_2$). Increasing $F_D O_2$ will increase PaO_2. A flowmeter regulates the gas flow ("sweep flow") in L/min to the membrane. In most circumstances, the sweep gas will be 100% oxygen with a rate equal to the blood flow rate (1:1). Increasing the sweep flow increases CO_2 clearance because CO_2 diffuses approximately ten times more efficiently than oxygen. However, increasing the sweep flow does not significantly affect oxygenation.

Heat Exchanger

An external water bath heats the circulating blood to warm (or cool) the patient, toward the desired temperature.

Console

Parameters are displayed such as the blood flow, pump speed, pre- and post-membrane lung pressure, oxyhemoglobin saturations, hematocrit, and temperature.

Cannulas

They are named in relation to the ECMO circuit and not the patient. The inflow ("drainage") cannula carries deoxygenated blood from the patient to the ECMO circuit, and the outflow ("return") one does the opposite. Surface heparin coating or other polymer coatings are often present to decrease blood surface interaction. The cannula should support approximately 3 $L/m^2/min$ (60 mL/kg/min) in the adult patient [4]. The resistance of blood flow is proportional to the length and inversely proportional to the radius of the cannula tubing (Poiseuille's Law). A large one could precipitate distal ischemic injuries or direct injuries to vessels [9].

Cannulation

The Seldinger technique or surgical cut-down are alternatives. Ultrasound guidance and visualization of the guidewire within the targeted vessel is highly recommended for confirmation of placement. Further, utilization of echocardiogram and/or fluoroscopic assessment is critical for confirmation of correct positioning. Chest and abdominal films can subsequently be used to evaluate location of cannulas if troubleshooting is needed.

Veno-arterial ECMO can be centrally placed, with the drainage cannula positioned within the right atrium and the return cannula within the ascending or descending thoracic aorta. Given the invasive nature, central cannulation is commonly performed post-cardiotomy or sternotomy. However, it could be considered if peripheral vasculature is too small or diseased.

Peripheral Cannulation

The inflow cannula is inserted into the femoral or internal jugular vein with the cannula tip in the distal inferior or superior vena cava, respectively. The outflow cannula is inserted into the common femoral artery, subclavian artery, or axillary artery.

Veno-Venous ECMO

A dual-lumen single cannula (DLSC) or two single-lumen cannulas can be employed. DLSCs are designed to be inserted into the internal jugular vein with drainage ports to rest in the IVC and SVC with the infusion port projected towards the tricuspid valve. It offers the potential for increased patient mobility. Two single-lumen cannulas are often placed in femoral-femoral, femoral-internal jugular or internal jugular-femoral configuration. The two cannulas should have at least 8–10 cm between the tips in order to prevent significant recirculation of oxygenated blood back through the circuit [4].

Management of the ECMO Patient

Monitoring and Vascular Access

In order to maintain adequate tissue perfusion and oxygenation, non-invasive monitors including continuous pulse oximetry, electrocardiography, blood pressure, and temperature are available. Additionally, near-infrared spectroscopy can be used to evaluate limb and cerebral perfusion. Invasive monitors include intra-arterial blood pressure monitoring, pulmonary arterial catheter, and indwelling urinary catheter for urine output and color. Pulse oximetry and/or an invasive radial arterial blood pressure monitor should be located on the right upper extremity to detect differential oxygenation and surrogate for oxygenation in the proximal aortic arch. An invasive blood pressure monitor will also allow you to assess native cardiac contractility based on pulse pressure. Central venous access is highly recommended. Routine lab monitoring to assess end organ function and perfusion should be drawn at least daily if stable including metabolic panel, liver function panel, lactate, and mixed venous blood saturation. Point of care echocardiography is an invaluable tool to help guide management of ECMO [8].

Hemodynamics

In general, a goal MAP of at least 65 mmHg is recommended. If there is evidence of ongoing end organ ischemia, higher values are advised. Contrarily, if mixed venous blood saturation remains greater than 70%, it may be reasonable to allow lower MAPs. As VV-ECMO does not support circulatory physiology, vasopressor support is needed via pharmacological agents if the patient's own physiology is unable to maintain adequate tissue perfusion. During VA-ECMO, hemodynamics is based on blood flow (i.e. pump flow plus native cardiac function) and vascular/circuit resistance. If mixed venous saturation is less than 70% and/or MAPs are below goal, increasing the pump flow is indicated until perfusion is sufficient. This may require additional volume, whether blood products or crystalloids, to achieve increased flows [10]. During initiation of ECMO, significant vasoplegia may develop due to inflammatory response to the circuit, which may require high vasopressor support.

VA-ECMO: Cardiac Output and "Pulsatility"

If the pulse pressure on the arterial waveform becomes narrow or even flat, this could be a sign the left ventricle is not able to eject. This can lead to stasis of blood within the left ventricle and eventually thrombus formation which is a catastrophic complication that needs to be avoided at all costs. Increased vasopressor support to increase contractility can be implemented. As VA-ECMO increases afterload significantly, high VA-ECMO flows can paradoxically limit left ventricular output so a reduction in flows could help improve pulse pressure and allow cardiac ejection as well. Unfortunately, in patients with severe heart failure needing ECMO support, reductions in flow are typically not well tolerated.

Fluid Management

The initial goal of volume status and fluid management is to provide enough volume to achieve adequate blood flows through the circuit as this determines oxygen delivery. However, excessive fluid administration should be avoided. A positive fluid balance on day 3 of ECMO has been shown in some studies to be associated with increased mortality [11]. There is strong evidence to support a negative fluid balance in patients until dry weight is reached if hemodynamics tolerate it once initial stabilization on ECMO is achieved [11].

Mechanical Ventilation and Hypoxemia

Patients with respiratory failure who require ECMO support for oxygenation should receive lung protective ventilation strategies to limit ventilator-induced lung injury (VILI). As ventilation and oxygenation improves with initiation of ECMO support, ventilator settings should be continued to wean. Further needs for escalation in ventilation or oxygenation should be employed via the ECMO circuit as able, not by increasing ventilator settings. Recommended ventilation settings are inspiratory pressure less than 25 cm H_2O, positive end expiratory pressure/PEEP > 10 to prevent atelectasis, tidal volumes 4–8 mL/kg of IBW, respiratory rate of 4–15 breaths/min, and FiO_2 as low as possible [3, 12]. A select population of patients may even be able to tolerate extubation; however, this should be approached with great caution.

Hypoxemia still frequently occurs while on ECMO despite the oxygenation support of the circuit. Because delivery of oxygen while on ECMO is determined by circuit flow, increasing flows will often improve hypoxemia by increasing oxygen delivery/consumption ratio (DO_2/VO_2). Thorough evaluation of the circuit and cannulas should be performed as well, to ensure the problem is not mechanical, along with evaluation for factors that may be increasing oxygen consumption (e.g. fever, sepsis, agitation, shivering, high metabolic state) [3]. Two concepts specific to ECMO must also be included in the differential diagnosis of hypoxemia—"differential oxygenation" and "recirculation".

Differential Oxygenation

Also known as Harlequin Syndrome or North-South Syndrome, it occurs when the lower body is being perfused by oxygen-rich blood from the VA-ECMO circuit but portions of the upper body (i.e. coronaries, right arm and brain) are perfused with hypoxemic blood as the LV recovers function, leading to hypoxic insult of the brain or heart. Identification of differential oxygenation can be made with pulse oximetry or blood gas analysis from the right upper extremity. Improving native lung function or adding an additional return cannula to the jugular vein (VAV ECMO) may help to improve detrimental effects [8].

Recirculation

During VV-ECMO oxygenated blood from the return cannula can be sucked into the drainage cannula without reaching systemic circulation. This most commonly occurs in femoral-jugular cannula configuration. Detection of recirculation can be made by a bright red color of blood within the drainage cannula, increased venous saturation, and/or paradoxical decrease in systemic saturation despite increasing ECMO flows [3]. Canula tips should be repositioned in such circumstance.

Anticoagulation and Monitoring

Systemic therapeutic anticoagulation is indicated in most clinical scenarios where ECMO is employed. However, it can pose a great challenge for the provider in the setting of unbalanced coagulation homeostasis inherent to critically ill patients and the inflammatory response related to foreign material of the ECMO circuit. Patients are at very high risk for both bleeding and clotting, approximately 37% and 42% respectively. Approximately 20% of patients will experience both complications [13]. No specific protocol or anticoagulation strategy has been proven ideal by large, randomized control trials to date.

Retrospective studies demonstrate that it is feasible to utilize VV-ECMO with low-dose heparin or without therapeutic systemic anticoagulation, with no increase in thrombosis risk and further benefit of less bleeding and decreased transfusion requirements [14–16]. Few studies have investigated safety and feasibility of not employing therapeutic anticoagulation in VA-ECMO, though the limited data available did report no increase in thrombotic complications [17]. It therefore remains an investigational routine.

Conventional Heparin

Unfractionated heparin (UFH) is the most adopted therapeutic anticoagulation on ECMO [15]. Advantages of UFH include being inexpensive, easy to monitor with lab tests, and with a convenient antidote for rapid reversal (i.e. protamine). Disadvantages encompass resistance and/or variable patient dose response due to plasma protein binding and the rare, but devastating risk of heparin-induced thrombocytopenia (HIT), which is estimated to occur in 0.2–5% of adult patients [18].

Direct Thrombin Inhibitors (DTI)

DTIs such as bivalirudin and argatroban are endowed with more predictable dose response, do not rely on activity of antithrombin or bind plasma proteins, are short-acting, and can be used in HIT. Reversal agents are very expensive and not available in all markets (although short half-life makes this less of a concern), the drugs are intrinsically more costly, and lack lab monitoring tests. In the case of severe bleeding secondary to DTI use, recombinant factor VIIa has been used [18].

Several laboratory tests are available to monitor anticoagulation, but often have discordant results. Many experts suggest using anti-Xa assays to monitor UFH anticoagulation. However, aPTT is often used in many institutes as well and is the test of choice for DTI anticoagulation. Expert consensus suggests achieving anti-Xa level of 0.3–0.5 U/mL with UFH or aPTT of 50–70 s (or 2–2.5 times above normal) as strong evidence is still lacking in safety of low-dose anticoagulation strategies. It is important for the provider to be aware of how patient characteristics (e.g. hyperbilirubinemia, hemolysis, leukocytosis, liver failure, renal failure) can alter these laboratory tests and the need for anticoagulation dose adjustment [15].

As cytopenias, hemolysis, and other disturbances in the coagulation cascade are common in ECMO patients, laboratory tests should be monitored frequently and include complete blood count, platelet count, fibrinogen, plasma-free hemoglobin, lactate dehydrogenase/LDH, antithrombin activity, international normalized ratio/INR, and thromboelastography/thromboelastometry.

Maintenance of ECMO Circuit

Routine inspection of circuit components for visible blood clots should be performed frequently. Areas with the lowest flows or highest resistance are most likely to form clots first. Pressures within the circuit (i.e. pump inlet pressure, pre- and post-membrane pressures, delta pressure) should be monitored for changes and trends. Increasing negative pressures of the pump inlet may indicate increased resistance within the pump (e.g. thrombosis), hypovolemia, or drainage cannula malposition/kinking. Increasing positive pressures of the pre-membrane may indicate oxygenator thrombosis, increased patient afterload, or return cannula malposition/kinking.

Increased post-membrane pressures may also indicate elevated patient afterload or return cannula malposition/kinking. Increases in delta pressure (i.e. pre-membrane minus post-membrane pressure) indicates obstruction inside the oxygenator. Once the cause of pressure changes is identified, prompt action should be taken to mitigate the issue and may require exchange of failing pumps or oxygenators. An additional parameter is the post-oxygenator pO_2. Results should exceed 300 mmHg when the gas flow FiO_2 is 100% [19].

Complications

Overall incidence is upwards of 80% in some reports. Mechanical complications occur because of device insertion failure or malfunction. Examples include circuit failure, cannula displacement, inappropriate size or positioning of cannula, and mechanical obstruction of blood flow. Routine inspection and maintenance of the circuit and assessment of cannula sites and position should be employed.

Medical complications are numerous and have the potential to be devastating, such as bleeding, thrombosis, embolic events, distal limb ischemia, vascular injury, coagulopathy, renal failure, neurologic events, fluid overload, and infection.

Distal Limb Ischemia

It occurs more often with larger cannula size and femoral artery cannula placement. The risk of ischemia can be decreased from approximately 25–10% by placing a distal perfusion catheter into the superficial femoral artery. This is highly recommended for all femoral arterial cannulas [8]. Near-infrared spectroscopy can be used to monitor the tissue saturation in the extremities to assure there is no ongoing ischemia. Saturations should be above 50% but ideally above 60% with less than 20% difference between extremities. Cannula placement in the upper limb tends to lead to hyperperfusion and swelling more often than ischemia.

Acute Kidney Injury and Fluid Overload

These are common occurrences and are associated with increased mortality. Renal replacement therapy (RRT) is often employed early in those who respond poorly to diuretics. In-line RRT or hemofilter with the ECMO circuit can both be effective and are a good alternative to placing additional access for dialysis in the anticoagulated, critically ill patient [11].

Prophylactic Antibiotics

They are not routine prescribed; however, signs and symptoms of infection should be closely monitored. Unlike removing a central venous access that becomes infected, removing ECMO cannulas is not always possible and generally not needed. The clinician should also be aware of the increased volume of distribution associated with the ECMO circuit, potentially altering the pharmacokinetics and pharmacodynamics of antibiotics (and other medications).

Perioperative Considerations

Besides needing care in the operating room for removal of ECMO, many patients will require other non-cardiac procedures while they are on ECMO support. Several of these procedures become necessary because of complications from ECMO, including source control for bleeding, fasciotomy for compartment syndrome due to limb ischemia, and exploratory laparotomy for mesenteric ischemia.

Transport of the ECMO Patient

Movement of the ECMO patient from the ICU to the operating room is no small feat and takes significant time, effort, and teamwork to do safely. Providers involved typically are anesthesiologists, operating room nurses, surgeons, and perfusionists. Making certain ECMO flows are maintained and interventions can be quickly applied in the event of emergencies are top priorities for safe transport. Having a checklist of supplies to carry and assigning duties to each team member helping with transport of the patient helps to mitigate disaster. The most vital supplies to have for transport are adequate oxygen supply for the membrane lung, tubing clamps in the event of accidental decannulation, and medications and fluids for resuscitation should a complication occur.

Mechanical Ventilation

Similar ventilator settings should be utilized in the operating room as in the ICU. Severe respiratory failure may be present and continuation of the mechanical ventilation strategy used in the ICU is important to continue lung rest while in the operating room. Use of lung protective settings with tidal volume of <6 mL/kg IBW in order to keep plateau pressures under 25 cm H_2O, driving pressure less than 10 cm H_2O, and mechanical power under 12 J/min is recommended.

Metabolic Homeostasis

Arterial pH of 7.35–7.45, $PaCO_2$ of 40, and PaO_2 of 60–80 mmHg are relevant [10]. According to the extracorporeal life support organization/ELSO, optimization of the ECMO circuit to achieve these goals should occur prior to changes on the ventilator, to reduce risk of further lung damage that may be caused by increasing mechanical ventilator settings.

Hypoxemia can occur despite being on VA- or VV-ECMO and troubleshooting in the operating room can be difficult. Many times, increasing flows on either VV- or VA-ECMO can help to remedy hypoxemia, but evaluation of the circuit and the patient must be done to ensure no other issues are ongoing. Increased intrathoracic pressure can lead to decreased venous drainage resulting in poor flows and decreased oxygenation. Pneumothorax, hemothorax, or even intraabdominal hypertension are possible. An intraoperative x-ray and/or echocardiography to confirm proper cannula placement may be necessary to ensure enough distance exists between the cannulas to reduce recirculation as previously described. Blood transfusion can also be considered to increase hemoglobin in an attempt to increase oxygen carrying capacity, especially in the setting of intraoperative blood loss. However, there is a relation between blood transfusion and worse outcomes on ECMO, so caution should be applied to this practice [20].

Intraoperative Hemodynamics

Maintenance of blood pressure should follow goals as previously defined while in the ICU, if necessary with the help of vasopressors. Sudden reductions in flow are typically mechanical in nature or related to hypovolemia as discussed above. If this situation arises in the operating room, care should be taken to inspect the cannulas to make sure they have not migrated in any way during transport. The tubing and membrane lung should be inspected as well for thrombus to be sure this is not the reason for decreased flows. Thrombus formation in the membrane lung can also be a reason for hypoxemia and poor flows which may require exchange of the membrane lung. An arterial blood gas measurement from the circuit post-oxygenator can be performed. If the value of the PO_2 is under 200 mmHg, then exchanging the membrane lung should be discussed [20].

Maintenance of Anesthesia

Due to the fact that many patients on ECMO have underlying lung disease, and in the light of the fact that a fraction of blood volume will be bypassed around the lungs, titrating an appropriate depth of anesthesia with volatile anesthetics can be difficult. Because of this, total intravenous anesthesia (TIVA) is recommended [20].

Most agents used for anesthesia and analgesia are lipophilic and highly protein bound which makes them very susceptible to sequestration in the ECMO circuit and membrane lung. Higher doses may be necessary in order to achieve the desired levels of sedation. Table 33.2 shows commonly used intravenous agents and their level of uptake by the ECMO circuit. Propofol, benzodiazepines, and dexmedetomidine have a high uptake in the ECMO circuit with nearly 70–85% decrease in drug level noted after 60 min of infusion [21].

Opioids remain a necessary treatment for patients on ECMO as there is a high level of discomfort relating to the presence of cannulas, mechanical ventilation, and other invasive procedures. As these agents are highly lipophilic, their uptake in the ECMO circuit is quite high as well. Up to 97% of fentanyl is lost to the circuit, while the hydrophilic drug, morphine, has 0% loss [21]. There is also evidence that when hydromorphone is used compared to fentanyl, there is less drug sequestration and outcomes are improved for ECMO patients [21]. In our practice, it is common to start with fentanyl infusions for analgesia; however, if the patient is going to require a longer ECMO run (I.e. >5–7 days), then hydromorphone is used for pain control.

Ketamine is a non-selective N-methyl-D-aspartate receptor inhibitor and has both sedative and analgesic properties. It is lipophilic, similar to other agents, but it has

Table 33.2 Uptake of sedatives and analgesics by ECMO circuit [21]

Sedation/analgesic agent	Uptake percentage by ECMO circuit
Propofol	70–85%
Dexmedetomidine	67–93%
Fentanyl	97%
Hydromorphone	24%
Ketamine	10–30%
Midazolam	>50%

lower protein binding which may make it a better option when trying to avoid sequestration in the circuit [21]. Many reports have noted the need for rapid uptitration of ketamine to achieve sedation levels. Because of this, the recommended dosing is a bolus of 1.0–4.5 mg/kg followed by an infusion at 0.05 mg/kg/h [21, 22].

Weaning and Decannulation from ECMO

Recovery of native lung function is a crucial variable. This can be noted in improved chest x-rays, decreased mechanical ventilation needs, decreased fraction of inspired oxygen, decreased amounts of PEEP, and finally, decreased support from the VV-ECMO circuit itself. Many times, improvements on the arterial blood gas will be noted and will continue to hold steady as flows and sweep gas settings are decreased on the VV-ECMO circuit. Once patients are able to be stabilized with minimal flow (around 2 L/min) and minimal sweep gas flow (1 L/min), they are likely ready to be decannulated from VV-ECMO. Removal of VV-ECMO is typically performed at the bedside with purse string sutures placed around the site of cannulation followed by the cannulas being removed with sutures cinched down. Pressure can be applied as needed to achieve hemostasis. It is important to note that any time flows on ECMO are reduced to lower than 3 L/min; it is paramount that systemic anticoagulation is on board and the patient is at therapeutic levels, to reduce the chances of catastrophic thrombus formation in the circuit.

Weaning from VA-ECMO

This can be more challenging and can lead to very poor outcomes if performed too quickly. Typically, patients will exhibit improvements in pulse pressure, decreased needs for vasopressors and inotropes, decreased sweep gas flows, and normalization of other organ dysfunction if present. If these findings are confirmed, then evaluation with echocardiography can be helpful in determining if the patient will potentially tolerate removal of VA-ECMO. A "turndown" study can be performed with real-time echocardiography to evaluate cardiac function as ECMO support is reduced in a stepwise fashion. As the ECMO support is reduced, cardiac chamber and function parameters such as left ventricular chamber diameter in systole and diastole, right ventricular chamber diameter in systole and diastole, right ventricular tricuspid annular plane excursion (TAPSE), systolic left ventricular outflow tract velocity time integral ($LVOT_{VTI}$), and estimated ejection fraction (EF) can be assessed to determine viability of ECMO removal.

Parameters suggestive of successful separation are an EF of >20%, $LVOT_{VTI} > 12$ cm per contraction, and right ventricular TAPSE of >10 mm [20]. It is important to note that patients who need high amounts of vasoactive or inotropic support do not tolerate being removed from ECMO well and typically have a high mortality rate [20, 22].

References

1. Extracorporeal Life Support Organization (ELSO). Registry report on extracorporeal life support, International Summary; 2022.
2. Rajsic S, Treml B, Jadzic D, et al. Extracorporeal membrane oxygenation for cardiogenic shock: a meta-analysis of mortality and complications. Ann Intensive Care. 2022;12:93.
3. Tonna JE, et al. Management of adult patients supported with Venovenous extracorporeal membrane oxygenation (VV ECMO): guideline from the extracorporeal life support organization (ELSO). ASAIO J. 2021;67(6):601–10.
4. Sorokin V, et al. Choosing the appropriate configuration and cannulation strategies for extracorporeal membrane oxygenation: the potential dynamic process of organ support and importance of hybrid modes. Eur J Heart Fail. 2017;19(Suppl. 2):75–83.
5. Thalanany MM, et al. Methods of data collection and analysis for the economic evaluation alongside a national, multi-centre trial in the UK: conventional ventilation or ECMO for Severe Adult Respiratory Failure (CESAR). BMC Health Serv Res. 2008;8:1–2.
6. Schmidt M, et al. Predicting survival after extracorporeal membrane oxygenation for severe acute respiratory failure. The respiratory extracorporeal membrane oxygenation survival prediction (RESP) score. Am J Respir Crit Care Med. 2014;189(11):1374–82.
7. Murray JF, et al. An expanded definition of the adult respiratory distress syndrome. Am Rev Respir Dis. 1988;138(3):720–3.
8. Lorusso R, et al. ELSO interim guidelines for venoarterial extracorporeal membrane oxygenation in adult cardiac patients. ASAIO J. 2021;67(8):827–44.
9. Kim J, et al. Impact of cannula size on clinical outcomes in peripheral venoarterial extracorporeal membrane oxygenation. ASAIO J. 2019;65(6):573–9.
10. Brogan T, et al. Extracorporeal life support: the ELSO red book. 5th ed. Ann Arbor, MI: ELSO; 2017.
11. Bridges BC, et al. Extracorporeal life support organization guidelines for fluid overload, acute kidney injury, and electrolyte management. ASAIO J. 2022;68(5):611–8.
12. Peek GJ, et al. Efficacy and economic assessment of conventional ventilatory support versus extracorporeal membrane oxygenation for severe adult respiratory failure (CESAR): a multicentre randomised controlled trial. Lancet. 2009;374(9698):1351–63.
13. Nunez JI, et al. Bleeding and thrombotic events in adults supported with venovenous extracorporeal membrane oxygenation: an ELSO registry analysis. Intensive Care Med. 2022;48(2):213–24.
14. Kurihara C, et al. Feasibility of venovenous extracorporeal membrane oxygenation without systemic anticoagulation. Ann Thorac Surg. 2020;110(4):1209–15.
15. Helms J, et al. Anticoagulation in adult patients supported with extracorporeal membrane oxygenation: guidance from the scientific and standardization committees on perioperative and critical care Haemostasis and thrombosis of the international society on thrombosis and Haemostasis. J Thromb Haemost. 2023;21(2):373–96.
16. Krueger K, et al. Venovenous extracorporeal membrane oxygenation with prophylactic subcutaneous anticoagulation only: an observational study in more than 60 patients. Artif Organs. 2017;41(2):186–92.
17. Wood KL, et al. Venoarterial-extracorporeal membrane oxygenation without routine systemic anticoagulation decreases adverse events. Ann Thorac Surg. 2020;109(5):1458–66.
18. McMichael ABV, et al. 2021 ELSO adult and pediatric anticoagulation guidelines. ASAIO J. 2022;68(3):303–10.
19. Gajkowski EF, et al. ELSO guidelines for adult and pediatric extracorporeal membrane oxygenation circuits. ASAIO J. 2022;68(2):133–52.
20. Mazzeffi MA, et al. Intraoperative management of adult patients on extracorporeal membrane oxygenation: an expert consensus statement from the society of cardiovascular anesthesiologists: Part II, Intraoperative management and troubleshooting. J Cardiothorac Vasc Anesth. 2021;35(12):3513–27.

21. Patel JS, et al. A narrative review of the impact of extracorporeal membrane oxygenation on the pharmacokinetics and pharmacodynamics of critical care therapies. Ann Pharmacother. 2023;57(6):706–26.
22. Pappalardo F, et al. Timing and strategy for weaning from venoarterial ECMO are complex issues. J Cardiothorac Vasc Anesth. 2015;29(4):906–11.

Chapter 34
Improving the Selection of Patients for High-Risk Surgery: The Ethical Use of Artificial Intelligence

Russell Seth Martins and Charles E. Binkley

Introduction to Patient Selection

The Ethics of Patient-Centered Care

It is vital for the objective assessment of operability to be appraised within a framework of fundamental ethical considerations: To what extent does surgery benefit the patient? What are the risks or harms that an operation may entail, and how do potential risks compare with potential benefits? Do the anticipated outcomes of surgery align with the patient's personal values and goals of care? This last concern is one that is of increasing relevance, as patient-reported measures continue to grow in importance alongside traditional clinical outcomes. Patient autonomy has long been touted as one of the ethical keystones of medicine. Yet, the decision to operate, based on careful weightage of pros and cons, has historically fallen upon the surgeon (i.e., surgeon autonomy). While surgeons unquestionably have their patients' best interests at heart, their judgment regarding the overall appropriateness of an operation is made against the backdrop of their own personal experience, values, and cognitive biases, and is rooted in paternalism. It is thus essential that the decision to operate or not is made with consideration of the patient's own interpretation of the risks and benefits of surgery, while considering how the patient themself defines benefit and burden. The responsibility of comprehensively apprising patients

R. S. Martins
Division of Thoracic Surgery, Department of Surgery, JFK University Medical Center, Hackensack Meridian Health, Edison, NJ, USA
e-mail: russellseth.martins@hmhn.org

C. E. Binkley (✉)
Hackensack Meridian Health, Edison, NJ, USA

Department of Surgery, Hackensack Meridian School of Medicine, Nutley, NJ, USA
e-mail: charles.binkley@hmsom.edu

© The Author(s), under exclusive license to Springer Nature Switzerland AG 2024

J. Faintuch, S. Faintuch (eds.), *Recent Strategies in High Risk Surgery*, https://doi.org/10.1007/978-3-031-56270-9_34

of their objective risk profiles lies with the surgical care team. The patient must then be allowed to evaluate the balance of absolute benefit and absolute risk through the lens of their own personal values, so as to arrive at a decision of whether to proceed with an operation or not. Patient values may be broadly understood as the unique lens through which individual patients interpret clinical information [1] and may be a function of each patient's unique beliefs, life experiences, and sociocultural backgrounds. This is important for several reasons. First, being thoroughly informed about their risk profile empowers patients with knowledge which may make them less anxious about the operation they are due to undergo [2]. Moreover, patients, especially those at high risk for adverse postoperative outcomes, generally underestimate the magnitude of risks they face [2]. Patients who are well-informed of their risk profile may even express the desire to postpone surgery and participate in prehabilitation programs to decrease perioperative risks [2].

This emphasizes the importance of incorporating the patient's perspective and values into the patient selection process, making surgery-related decision-making a collaboration between the surgeon and the patient. Patients may be better informed and empowered in the decision-making dynamic by use of decision aids, which are tools that help patients understand a range of management options. Decision aids increase patients' active participation in the decision-making process by increasing their knowledge of various options and the risks and benefits associated with them, managing expectations, reducing decisional uncertainty, and lowering surgeon-patient decisional conflict.

Of note, whereas patient autonomy is deeply entrenched as one of the guiding principles in medicine in the Western world, this is not necessarily the case in other cultures [3]. In fact, the imposition of the principle of autonomy in medical practices in non-Western cultures has been described as a form of ethical imperialism [3]. Active involvement in high-stakes decision-making may also be a source of anxiety for patients [4], and these feelings of anxiety may reciprocally affect the quality of decision-making by the patient [5]. Thus, some patients may still prefer to have their surgeon, or another family member make the decision for them. Instead of seeing this as contrasting with patient-centered care, it should be viewed as empowering patients with the ability to decide how their surgical decisions are made and by whom.

Managing Surgeon-Patient Conflicts

Ultimately, decision aids can help to align patients' values with eventual therapeutic choices. However, ethical conundrums may arise when there is decisional conflict between the surgeon and patient even after the patient fully understands their options. Specifically, a patient may refuse an operation that the surgeon has judged to be more beneficial than risky, or a patient may request an operation that the surgeon has judged to be more risky than beneficial. Each scenario requires the application of different ethical considerations. In the first instance, the surgeon may choose to evaluate whether the patient has medical decision-making capacity and ascertain that the decision is voluntary. If the patient is judged to have medical decision-making capacity, it is important for the surgeon to better understand the patient's reasons for informed refusal. Is fear interfering with the decision-making process and can the patient's fears be addressed? Is the patient making unspoken assumptions about the operation and post-operative recovery? Part of the surgeon's responsibility is to explore the patient's reasons for refusal and try to address them without being coercive.

When patients request an operation that a surgeon may deem to either not be beneficial or prohibitively risky, the surgeon must seek to confirm that their risk and benefit assessment of the patient is objective and not influenced by cognitive or other biases. In particular, it is important for surgeons to avoid making decisions about what quality of life is acceptable or unacceptable to their patients [6]. It may also help to seek a second opinion to validate their recommendation and to offer the patient another assessment. In both cases, the surgeon must also explore the patient's reasoning behind their decision and address any concerns they may have. While doing so, it is of utmost importance that the surgeon respects the patient's autonomy, and that the decision-making discussion is free from elements of coercion.

Improving on Surgeon Judgment

Appropriate patient selection for surgery is critical to achieving desired outcomes. The decision to operate is founded on a synthesis of relevant clinical information, which mainly includes factors related to the medical condition (e.g., severity, acuity, and prognosis) and patient characteristics (e.g., age, comorbid conditions, and frailty) [7]. Over the centuries, the tools used by surgeons to assess operability have gradually grown in sophistication and objectivity. At one end of the spectrum is the personal clinical judgment of the operating surgeon, which is biased by the surgeon's own preferences and experience. At the other end of the spectrum are surgical risk calculators, such as the American College of Surgeons (ACS) National Surgical Quality Improvement Program (NSQIP) Surgical Risk Calculator [8], which leverage clinical data from large national databases to provide risk estimates with a higher degree of certainty. The use of automated, standardized, and validated risk assessment tools leads to demonstrable improvements in the quality of surgical care and postoperative clinical outcomes [9].

Even the best surgical risk calculators currently in use have their limitations. Given the improving trends in surgical outcomes brought about by the evolution of surgical technology and standards of care, traditional surgical risk calculators may become outdated and require newer iterations with increasing frequency [10]. The input data required to produce a risk assessment may be time-consuming and infeasible to acquire [11, 12]. Additionally, the clinical variables considered by risk calculators are generally those that are reported in large databases, many of which lack granularity. The static cutoff values employed by risk calculators, as well as the inflexible statistical regression models used in calculator design, are a poor representation of the complex pathophysiological processes and associations for an individual patient [13–16]. Moreover, most calculators do not take into account variables beyond the patient and their condition, despite many such indirect factors being recorded in large databases and having shown to have a significant impact on perioperative outcomes. These include surgeon characteristics (experience, volume, etc.) [17], hospital characteristics (infrastructural and human resources, institutional pathways [18], quality accreditations etc.), and hospital volume [19]. What is intriguing is that even if these additional variables were to be included in mainstream risk calculators, a considerable amount of variability in outcomes may remain unexplained [18]. The presence of these "blind spots" highlights that there is still considerable room for improvement in patient selection methods, especially in a data-rich world where unprecedented volumes of highly granular data may be acquired for an individual patient.

Artificial Intelligence in Patient Selection

Understanding Artificial Intelligence: A Surgical Primer

As the field of artificial intelligence (AI) continues to advance, its applications in healthcare are becoming increasingly widespread. AI technology has the potential to offer much more sophisticated, robust, holistic, efficient, and accurate data synthesis, analysis, and predictions compared to traditional statistical methods. These superior capabilities may be of particular benefit in surgical patient selection and clinical decision support systems (CDSS), where AI could perform a more comprehensive assessment to provide more customized and patient-specific decisions. Thus, as AI assumes an integral role in patient-centered surgical healthcare delivery, surgeons must aim to become broadly familiar with AI systems and approaches that are commonly used in AI CDSS.

Machine Learning (ML) is a subfield of AI that focuses on developing models that enable computers to adapt processing when exposed to new data, without specific programming to do so (simulating "learning from experience") [20–22]. This learning may be "unsupervised" or "supervised". In unsupervised learning, the AI model adapts its processing based on hidden, underlying patterns within the data without any explicitly provided instructions or data labeling. It may be leveraged to perform exploratory analysis using large datasets with many variables, or multiple datasets, with the intent to identify important associations that are not immediately apparent. On the other hand, supervised learning is leveraged for predictive modeling, whereby an algorithm is initially trained on labeled data and can then apply its "experience" to new, unlabeled data. A third category of learning, termed "reinforcement learning", allows the ML algorithm to learn from its own successes and failures by receiving external feedback or validation of its outputs. ML-based predictive modeling has been consistently shown to outperform conventional statistical models [23–25], with further improvements in accuracy made possible by using ensemble ML (i.e., multiple algorithms working together) to consolidate data from multiple sources.

Artificial neural networks (AAN) are used in ML and are designed to simulate the human brain by finding complex, interrelated relationships between data. An AAN comprises many computational units ("neurons") that each receive input data, perform operations, and forward output to the next "neuron". Thus, data is processed through a layer of algorithms that create specific output patterns that can be applied to decision-making [26]. Deep learning is a subtype of AANs that consists of many layers that are able to explore deeper, hidden layers of relationships between the input and output data [27]. Convolutional neural networks are another class of AAN that process and analyze grid-like structured data, such images or time series data. AANs have shown to outperform traditional risk calculators [28] and have demonstrated predictive accuracy in excess of 95% [29].

Computer vision is a branch of AI that focuses on enabling algorithms (ML and AAN, among others) to gain a high-level understanding of visual data [30], such as digital images, videos, and multidimensional data from medical imaging [31]. This affords object and scene recognition that has important implications in healthcare, such as computer-aided diagnosis from medical imaging and image-guided surgical interventions [32–34]. In addition, it also allows rich visual data to be incorporated into risk prediction models and CDSS [35, 36], which is currently not possible using existing large databases that do not include granular imaging-related data. Intraoperative imaging, in particular, has the potential to yield unprecedented amounts of unexplored surgical data that can be factored into decision-making algorithms in ways that have not been possible previously.

Natural language processing (NLP) focuses on enabling algorithms to understand human language and can be applied for the analysis of free-text content in electronic medical records and other narrative medical documentation. NLP models incorporate an understanding of semantics and syntax in their processing [37], allowing greater flexibility in the input text it can analyze. The applications of NLP include not only data recognition for the purpose of historical complication detection, coding, and billing [38], but has also been used to develop predictive models for the occurrence of future complications. For example, in an NLP model predicting postoperative anastomotic leak after colorectal resections, the algorithm was able to consider not only clinical variables but also surgeon-perceived difficulty of operation and patient-reported mood and feelings (e.g., feelings of irritation and tiredness). The model was able to achieve a sensitivity of 100% in prediction of anastomotic leaks [39].

The Application of Artificial Intelligence to Surgical Patient Selection

With improvements in AI technology and the ability to utilize vast amounts of granular clinical information, AI-guided patient selection for surgery may be just around the corner and has the potential to revolutionize clinical practice. Already, systems currently in use can analyze computed tomography (CT) scans of patients with cancer and suggest optimized, tailored radiotherapy aimed at minimized locoregional radiation injury [40]. In fact, the superiority of AI-based selection systems over surgeons' personal decision-making process is becoming evident even with modern AI technology. A deep learning algorithm trained using supervised ML was able to use preoperative CT images to predict the complexity of hernia operations with significantly greater accuracy than a panel of experienced surgeons [41]. Similarly, an ML algorithm using electronic health records data was able to outperform physicians with regard to making accurate preoperative risk assessments [42]. Furthermore, augmentation of physicians' decision-making process with input from the ML algorithm also significantly improved the ability to predict postoperative adverse events [42]. Apart from this, AI is also being successfully applied in breast cancer risk calculation, prognostication, and clinical decision support [43–45], management planning [46], and genomics-based precision medicine [47, 48].

The Potential for Benefit and for Harm When Using Artificial Intelligence to Improve Patient Selection for High-Risk Surgery

Patient selection for high-risk surgery may involve several complex, high-stakes decisions. Traditionally, the onus of decision-making lies largely with the surgeon. However, the judgment of surgeons is not infallible and existing patient selection tools are far from perfect. There are many sources of bias that may originate at the level of the individual surgeon, each with the capacity to significantly impact decision-making [49]. Even risk tolerance thresholds, which differ widely across surgeons, can lead to differences in recommendations for or against an operation [50]. Thus, it is no surprise that errors in judgment are among the most common causes of preventable harm experienced by surgical patients [51]. Apart from the direct consequences borne by the patient, medical errors also leave long-lasting negative impacts on the surgeon who shoulders responsibility for the lapse in judgment leading to the error. These effects may include feelings of guilt or shame, loss of confidence, and even loss of reputation, all of which may lead to more serious mental health issues such as depression, substance abuse and burnout [52]. AI-based patient selection tools can help alleviate the burden of decision-making related to surgery and eliminate surgeon-level biases. Thus, the surgeon acts less in the role of decision-maker and serves more as an intermediary who communicates the AI-provided risk assessment to the patient and offers a recommendation if solicited. As a consequence, surgeons would also be alleviated of the burden of having to make accurate clinical predictions based on limited information and would perceive less responsibility for unfavorable outcomes. This may lead to significantly less psychological distress for surgeons with regard to their decision-making.

AI-based patient selection tools may also act as an equalizer for the balance of decision-making power between the surgeon and the patient and may allow for a more pragmatic approach to the incorporation of patient values in decision-making. In fact, some of the paternalism underlying the surgeon-patient decision-making dynamic may be attributable to surgeons believing they "know better" than surgical risk calculators (due to their broader appreciation of factors beyond those considered by the calculator) and "know more" than patients (due to their deeper appreciation of clinical benefits and risks accompanying management options). AI-based systems have the potential to level this playing field by performing highly sophisticated syntheses of a greater volume and broader scope of data to provide highly accurate outputs for patient risk profiles. These attributes lend themselves to increasing patient understanding regarding management options and allowing patients to be more accurately informed and empowered participants in the surgery-related decision-making processes. As a result of this increased involvement in their healthcare decisions, patients may experience more satisfaction with their surgical care, better quality of life, and possibly even better clinical outcomes [53]. As mentioned earlier, AI systems may also redefine the role of the surgeon in the decision-making process from "predictor" and "assessor" to "counselor" and "guide". This shift may also reduce possible conflicts of interest that may arise when a surgeon engages with their patient to make a management-related decision based on their own risk predictions. By allowing AI to offer its most accurate risk assessment and prediction, surgeons can foster patient-centered care by engaging in a more transparent and shared decision-making process.

The Ethical Concerns When Using Artificial Intelligence for Patient Selection

There are several issues that warrant consideration in light of the potential shift in the surgeon-patient decision-making dynamic. Although AI holds great promise for improving patient selection for high-risk surgery, there are several ethical concerns that should be addressed before these systems are deployed for patient care. Even if the concern cannot be completely resolved, ethically justifiable options should be considered and acted upon.

Explainability

Because AI systems find patterns in data in order to make predictions, it is not currently possible to understand the specific associations used to make a prediction for an individual patient. Thus, it is not possible to explain to patients the system's "reason" for recommending whether a patient should or should not undergo surgery. This is a significant concern since it limits the patient's ability to fully participate in shared decision-making and the process of informed consent. It is also problematic for surgeons to speculate as to why the system made the prediction that it did. Such speculation can reinforce the surgeon's potentially erroneous logic which the surgeon could apply to other patients, resulting in harm if their logic was wrong.

Transparency

Unlike other members of the operative team who play a role in the patient's care, such as the surgeon and anesthesiologist, the AI system can remain hidden from the patient. Patients may never know that their surgeon collaborated with a third party, an AI system, in deciding whether or not to offer an operation to a patient. Part of showing respect for the patient is being transparent and fully informing them, not only about the decision itself, but also how the surgeon made the decision. Whether there was agreement or disagreement between the surgeon's decision and the AI system's prediction, patients may find it beneficial to know that an AI system made a personalized prediction, even if that prediction cannot be explained. A related concern is whether or not patients should consent to have the AI system make a prediction in the first place. Informed consent discussions are a moral, ethical, and legal cornerstone of surgery, as they lay a foundation of trust and confidence in the physician-patient relationship throughout the continuum of surgical care. A contrary perspective to requiring that patients give consent for their surgeon to collaborate with an AI system is that it is the prerogative of the surgeon whether or not to consult with the system in order to make a clinical decision. In turn, the surgeon's duty is to inform the patient of the collaboration in the context of shared decision-making.

Privacy and Confidentiality

In order to receive a prediction, AI systems must be given access to information from the patient's electronic medical record (EMR). Moreover, this information, along with the patient's outcome, may be used as part of the AI system's ongoing learning. One of the key strengths of an AI-based risk assessment system is its capacity to make incremental algorithmic course-corrections with each new datapoint fed into it. There are two concerns here. One is that patient data is being given to the system in exchange for a prediction. This implies that as a condition for receiving potentially beneficial information, patients must contribute their personal health information. Second, apart from HIPAA (Health Insurance Portability and Accountability Act) exceptions, patients generally have a right to determine how their private health information is used and with whom it is shared [54, 55]. It is crucial that patients' rights, especially those of privacy and data security, be prioritized while these dilemmas are addressed [56]. While over 100 countries worldwide have data protection laws in place, only a few address issues related to AI [56]. One such regulatory body with preliminary AI-related data protection standards in place is the Ibero-American Data Protection Network, which consists of over 20 institutions in Central and South America and the Caribbean [57].

Benefit and Harm

It is important that AI clinical decision-making systems are proven to be more beneficial and/or less harmful than the current manner in which clinical decisions are made before they are deployed. For AI systems used to make surgical predictions, it would be important to demonstrate, at minimum, that a surgeon collaborating with the AI system to determine a patient's candidacy for surgery results in improved patient outcomes and decreased patient harm than a surgeon making the determination alone. One challenge is that surgeons may have varying skills and tolerance for risk. Surgeons may be more or less skillful at patient selection, and surgeons may be more or less risk averse in the patients they select. The infrastructure of the health system, the volume of complex cases performed, and the availability of specialty services such as critical care and interventional radiology may also play a role in surgical decision-making. Prospectively establishing a system's overall clinical benefit will require evaluation across multiple sites and surgeons, with additional validation needed for each individual surgeon using the system.

Bias

Several deficiencies exist in the current large data sources that could be potentially used to train AI models. These include inaccuracies in the collection, recording, and labeling of data, and lack of representativeness in patient populations. There are also concerns that AI may perpetuate historical biases that have faced minority groups and are ingrained into existing databases that may be used to train AI models [58, 59]. As a result, decision-making based on AI may also reflect these biases. Subsequent outcomes based on these decisions may be used to further train the AI model, thus reinforcing biases in a self-fulfilling prediction loop [60].

Conflicts of Interest

AI systems used for surgical patient selection may have encoded values other than what is in the best interest of the patient, such as the interests of the surgeon or hospital. Systems may be trained not only to maximize benefit and to minimize harm, but to also increase profit and reduce costs. The system may have set the threshold for harm so as to minimize the risk of prolonged ICU stays, even if the system predicted an overall benefit for the patient. It is possible for systems to both prioritize the patient's benefit and also increase revenue and reduce costs. The ethically relevant point is that the primary interest should always be the patient's benefit.

Patient Values

AI systems used for surgical selection will assume a desired outcome, such as survival, functional status, or relief of suffering, and make a prediction based on achieving that outcome. Some patients may not value that outcome, or there may be limits to what the patient finds acceptable in order to achieve that outcome. One way of incorporating patient values into AI systems is to use the prediction as the starting point for a model of physician-patient communication in which the surgeon predicts the likely outcome, and the patient applies their values to the process of shared decision-making [61].

Surgeon Autonomy

It is unclear how AI-based systems will impact surgeon autonomy. Decisional conflict may arise when AI-based systems provide a risk assessment that a surgeon does not agree with [62]. Matters may become even more complicated if a patient desires to undergo an operation based on an AI-based risk assessment that the surgeon does not agree with. It is likely that the AI system has considered a great many more variables than the surgeon has, and its decision is less likely to be affected by personal biases compared to the surgeon's. While currently a surgeon's clinical impression may be considered superior to the risk assessment provided by a standardized risk calculator, this may not be the case when patient selection systems are AI-based and become increasingly sophisticated.

If AI-based clinical decision systems are proven to be superior to the assessment of an individual surgeon, several important dilemmas may arise. To begin with, surgeons may feel some degree of distrust and resentment toward the AI-based system as it may undermine their training and experience. Surgeons may come to feel more like an assistant to the AI system. In addition, it is also possible that surgeons suffer economic losses as AI increasingly replaces aspects of their job related to patient assessment and decision-making. Surgeons may also experience feelings of loss of ownership over their patients, which may lead to a more transactional and dehumanized healthcare experience [56]. Additionally, surgeons may also experience moral distress if there is external pressure from payers, medical groups, and health systems to accept the AI system's prediction even against their own judgment. This may lead to over-reliance on AI-driven decisions and automation complacency, whereby surgeons make less of an effort to perform an independent risk assessment, as well as automation bias, whereby surgeons do not question potential errors in an AI-derived risk assessment. It may also tarnish the learning process for trainees and junior surgeons as they get less practice learning how to assess patients' suitability for surgery. Lastly, the new normal in the decision-making dynamic could have the potential to equilibrate as a futuristic form of paternalism, i.e., one where the "AI knows best" [63]. This concern has been voiced by the Office of the United Nations High Commissioner for Human Rights in 2020 [56].

Accountability for Surgeon-AI Collaborations

It is also important to consider the new landscapes of accountability and legal liability that will arise as the surgery-related decision-making process becomes increasingly reliant on AI-based systems. In the frameworks existing today, surgeons are considered to be at the helm of the decision-making dynamic and are thus held responsible for any harm that occurs to a patient. In many instances, the surgeon may also be liable for medical malpractice and may potentially face serious legal consequences. However, as AI systems become more sophisticated and assume the predominant role in patient selection for surgery, the burden of accountability may shift away from the surgeon. The shifting dynamic of equalization of decision-making roles for the surgeon and patient may thus be mirrored by a trend toward shared accountability. In fact, as use of AI-based clinical decision systems becomes the standard of care, surgeons may be more prone to liability and malpractice issues if they choose to go against the AI-recommended course of action [64, 65].

These considerations also prompt a realization that advancements in AI clinical decision systems must be paralleled by advancements in regulatory frameworks. The intersection between AI and medical ethics is a nascent field, and it will be crucial to have appropriate expertise represented in formal ethics guidelines and on ethics boards, both for clinical and research applications [66]. Existing ethics frameworks related to AI in healthcare are limited and fragmented [67]. The United Nations Educational, Scientific and Cultural Organization (UNESCO), the World Commission on the Ethics of Scientific Knowledge and Technology, and the International Bioethics Committee only briefly discuss important elements of a governance framework for AI in healthcare [68–70]. Similarly, there are few medicolegal precedents related to the use of AI in medicine, and the legal system will undoubtedly face challenges while navigating this new territory. The French Government, in the latest version of its national bioethics law endorsed in 2019, emphasizes key principles for consideration in AI-related medicolegal issues. These include standards that underline the continued need for human supervision and human warranty of AI systems, as well as data safety and security in big data initiatives. Lastly, even the education systems for medicine, healthcare management, ethics, and law should seek to include a degree of AI competency, as it may play an integral role in their day-to-day professional operations. Lastly, it will be important to install regulatory frameworks for quality assurance of AI-based clinical decision systems.

Training and Validating the Performance of Artificial Intelligence Systems

However, as the applications of AI in patient selection continues to grow, it is important to remain cognizant of the risk of system malfunction, and to mitigate the harm that may result if the system begins to fail. To begin with, any AI-based output is only as good as the data that it uses as input. The lack of granularity in existing big data repositories that AI can be trained on could lead to poor real-world clinical applicability of outputs. In addition, given that most registries lack meaningful long-term data, training AI on these datasets runs the risk of ingraining a focus on achieving short-term outcomes within the algorithm. AI-based patient selection models that are trained on large national databases will also require local validation by hospitals to ensure the most context-specific output. This can help account for variables such as the surgeons' operative experience, institutional resources, and local outcomes. In addition, many important variables are not routinely reported in national databases but may be more feasible to source at the institutional level. These include patient-reported outcome variables such as health-related quality of life and psychological well-being, functional status, and satisfaction with care. These outcomes represent rich data that can be leveraged by AI approaches such as NLP to allow for their incorporation, through patients' electronic medical records, into clinical decision-making.

AI can also help tap into the vast amount of patient biometric data that can be sourced from personal devices, such as smartphones and smartwatches, and potentially use this information in risk assessment. However, while exploring the use of these systems using active learning AI systems, it is vital that ethical boundaries be clearly defined with regard to patient privacy. A certain degree of supervision is important to maintain direction over an AI model's use of data and ensure that its output continues to be in line with ethical standards. This could entail periodic reviews of the data utilized by the model, assessing model performance, and evaluating impact on patient outcomes to detect biases or unintended risk factor selection. Moreover, it is paramount that safeguards be in place to protect against data breaches, misuse, or other hacking, as the consequences of such misdemeanors in a healthcare setting could be serious.

Lastly, the "black box" nature of many AI algorithms significantly limits their verifiability and explainability, which may hinder their adoption in clinical practice. This matter of explainability is further compounded by differences in expertise and understanding across involved stakeholders (i.e., data scientists or ML engineers, healthcare professionals, patients etc.). A lack of explainability also has the potential to complicate issues when AI-based decisions contradict those made by experienced clinicians. This may lead to skepticism from healthcare professionals and could ultimately manifest as hesitation in adopting AI-based patient selection tools into routine clinical practice.

Future Directions for Artificial Intelligence in Surgery

The applications of AI in patient selection for surgery holds immense promise and potential for improving healthcare delivery and outcomes. However, to ensure harmony in this future landscape, it is imperative that stakeholders seek to actively explore, engage, and address critical issues that arise. Medical and surgical education and training programs must adapt to embrace the growing intersection between AI and medicine. This may include incorporating AI concepts and related ethics frameworks within the formal curriculum and promoting interdisciplinary educational collaborations. Hospitals must also recognize their responsibility to invest in robust infrastructure, information management systems, and cybersecurity expertise to ensure the efficient and safe use of AI within their institution. Moreover, hospitals must also seek to promote an organizational culture that facilitates trust and collaboration between clinicians, AI experts, and hospital management. In addition, hospitals should also strive to educate patients regarding the role that AI can play in their management and help them manage their concerns and expectations regarding AI's capabilities, limitations, and potential risks. These discussions can be made simpler by achieving greater explainability for AI models, and AI experts and data scientists must continue to recognize the importance of explainability and strive toward developing more explainable AI.

It is also key that health systems develop regulatory frameworks which guide the responsible use of AI technology and regularly monitor performance outcomes of AI systems within the hospital setting. This prospective performance assessment of the real-world clinical utility of AI-based patient-selection systems can generate important data to support its utilization as the standard of care in patient management. However, it is equally important that appropriate ethical and medicolegal structures be established to ensure the proper implementation and oversight of AI in a clinical setting. In fact, the composition of institutional ethics committees should include individuals with expertise in AI. Clear guidelines, rules, and regulations, undergirded by ethical considerations, are essential for the safe, successful, and equitable use of AI. These include being able to deal with issues of liability and accountability, ensuring patient data privacy and protection, and attention to the ethical concerns for transparency, explainability, and the clinical benefit of AI models. In addition, the involvement of private AI companies in the use of AI in the healthcare setting must be navigated with due caution to ensure regulatory oversight, data security and privacy, and avoidance of financial conflicts of interest.

Lastly, it is also important to understand the implications of AI-based healthcare as it relates beyond the immediate clinical setting. As the uptake of AI continues to grow globally, existing surgical healthcare disparities between high- and low-resource settings may be exacerbated. While the utilization of AI can improve surgical healthcare delivery in high-resource settings, low-resource settings may encounter major challenges in adopting AI due to limited technological infrastructure. However, with proper collaborations and partnerships across the global surgical network, AI can actually be leveraged to transform surgical healthcare in low-resource settings by providing diagnostic support, decision-making expertise, and remote intraoperative consultation. Again, careful attention must be given to the ethical implications and equitable implementation of AI systems. Balancing the benefits of AI-based patient selection with the preservation of ethical principles, and equitable access to the technology, will be crucial in harnessing the full potential of AI to enhance surgical healthcare for the well-being of patients around the world.

References

1. Lockwood S. "Evidence of me" in evidence based medicine? BMJ. 2004;329(7473):1033–5.
2. Raymond BL, Wanderer JP, Hawkins AT, Geiger TM, Ehrenfeld JM, Stokes JW, et al. Use of the American College of Surgeons national surgical quality improvement program surgical risk calculator during preoperative risk discussion: the patient perspective. Anesth Analg. 2019;128(4):643–50.
3. Thompson GA, Segura J, Cruz D, Arnita C, Whiffen LH. Cultural differences in patients' preferences for paternalism: comparing Mexican and American patients' preferences for and experiences with physician paternalism and patient autonomy. Int J Environ Res Public Health. 2022;19(17):10663.
4. Margalith I, Shapiro A. Anxiety and patient participation in clinical decision-making: the case of patients with ureteral calculi. Social Sci Med. 1997;45(3):419–27.
5. LeVasseur N, Li H, Cheung W, Myers P, Mckevitt E, Warburton R, et al. Effects of high anxiety scores on surgical and overall treatment plan in patients with breast cancer treated with neoadjuvant therapy. Oncologist. 2020;25(3):212–7.
6. Binkley CE, Reynolds JM, Shuman A. From the eyeball test to the algorithm—quality of life, disability status, and clinical decision making in surgery. N Engl J Med. 2022;387(14):1325–8.
7. Gunaratnam C, Bernstein M. Factors affecting surgical decision-making—a qualitative study. Rambam Maimonides Med J. 2018;9(1):e0003.
8. Bilimoria KY, Liu Y, Paruch JL, Zhou L, Kmiecik TE, Ko CY, et al. Development and evaluation of the universal ACS NSQIP surgical risk calculator: a decision aid and informed consent tool for patients and surgeons. J Am College Surg. 2013;217(5):833–42.
9. Kuy S, Romero RAL. Decreasing 30-day surgical mortality in a VA medical center utilizing the ACS NSQIP surgical risk calculator. J Surg Res. 2017;215:28–33.
10. Imam N, Sudah SY, Manzi JE, Sirch F, Nicholson AD, Denard PJ, et al. Perioperative risk stratification tools for shoulder arthroplasty: a systematic review. J Should Elbow Surg. 2023;32(6):e293–304.
11. Leeds IL, Rosenblum AJ, Wise PE, Watkins AC, Goldblatt MI, Haut ER, et al. Eye of the beholder: risk calculators and barriers to adoption in surgical trainees. Surgery. 2018;164(5):1117–23.
12. Légaré F, Ratté S, Gravel K, Graham ID. Barriers and facilitators to implementing shared decision-making in clinical practice: update of a systematic review of health professionals' perceptions. Patient Educ Counseling. 2008;73(3):526–35. Epub 2008/08/30
13. Loftus TJ, Brakenridge SC, Croft CA, Smith RS, Efron PA, Moore FA, et al. Neural network prediction of severe lower intestinal bleeding and the need for surgical intervention. J Surg Res. 2017;212:42–7.
14. Singh PP, Zeng IS, Srinivasa S, Lemanu DP, Connolly AB, Hill AG. Systematic review and meta-analysis of use of serum C-reactive protein levels to predict anastomotic leak after colorectal surgery. Br J Surg. 2014;101(4):339–46.

15. Kim S, Kim W, Park RW. A comparison of intensive care unit mortality prediction models through the use of data mining techniques. Healthc Inform Res. 2011;17(4):232–43. Epub 2012/01/20
16. Dybowski R, Weller P, Chang R, Gant V. Prediction of outcome in critically ill patients using artificial neural network synthesised by genetic algorithm. Lancet (London, England). 1996;347(9009):1146–50.
17. Billingsley KG, Morris AM, Dominitz JA, Matthews B, Dobie S, Barlow W, et al. Surgeon and hospital characteristics as predictors of major adverse outcomes following colon cancer surgery: understanding the volume-outcome relationship. Arch Surg (Chicago, IL: 1960). 2007;142(1):23–31. discussion 2; Epub 2007/01/17
18. Martins RS, Chang YH, Etzioni D, Stucky CC, Cronin P, Wasif N. Understanding variation in in-hospital mortality after major surgery in the United States. Ann Surg. 2023. Epub 2023/03/31;278:865.
19. Birkmeyer JD, Siewers AE, Finlayson EV, Stukel TA, Lucas FL, Batista I, et al. Hospital volume and surgical mortality in the United States. N Engl J Med. 2002;346(15):1128–37.
20. Bishop CM, Nasrabadi NM. Pattern recognition and machine learning. Springer; 2006.
21. Mitchell TM. Does machine learning really work? AI Mag. 1997;18(3):11.
22. Mintz Y, Brodie R. Introduction to artificial intelligence in medicine. Minim Invasive Ther Allied Technol. 2019;28(2):73–81.
23. Soguero-Ruiz C, Fei WM, Jenssen R, Augestad KM, Álvarez JL, Jiménez IM, et al. Data-driven temporal prediction of surgical site infection. AMIA Annual Symp Proc AMIA Symp. 2015;2015:1164–73.
24. Wang PS, Walker A, Tsuang M, Orav EJ, Levin R, Avorn J. Strategies for improving comorbidity measures based on Medicare and Medicaid claims data. J Clin Epidemiol. 2000;53(6):571–8.
25. Bergquist SL, Brooks GA, Keating NL, Landrum MB, Rose S. Classifying lung cancer severity with ensemble machine learning in health care claims data. Proc Mach Learn Res. 2017;68:25–38. Epub 2017/08/01
26. Deo RC. Machine learning in medicine. Circulation. 2015;132(20):1920–30.
27. Hinton GE, Osindero S, Teh Y-W. A fast learning algorithm for deep belief nets. Neural Comput. 2006;18(7):1527–54.
28. Mofidi R, Duff MD, Madhavan KK, Garden OJ, Parks RW. Identification of severe acute pancreatitis using an artificial neural network. Surgery. 2007;141(1):59–66.
29. Monsalve-Torra A, Ruiz-Fernandez D, Marin-Alonso O, Soriano-Payá A, Camacho-Mackenzie J, Carreño-Jaimes M. Using machine learning methods for predicting inhospital mortality in patients undergoing open repair of abdominal aortic aneurysm. J Biomed Inform. 2016;62:195–201. Epub 2016/07/11
30. Hashimoto DA, Rosman G, Witkowski ER, Stafford C, Navarette-Welton AJ, Rattner DW, et al. Computer vision analysis of intraoperative video: automated recognition of operative steps in laparoscopic sleeve gastrectomy. Ann Surg. 2019;270(3):270.
31. Huang T. Computer vision: evolution and promise. 1996.
32. Kenngott HG, Wagner M, Nickel F, Wekerle AL, Preukschas A, Apitz M, et al. Computer-assisted abdominal surgery: new technologies. Langenbeck's Arch Surg. 2015;400(3):273–81. Epub 2015/02/24
33. Szeliski R. Computer vision: algorithms and applications. Springer Nature; 2022.
34. Volkov M, Hashimoto DA, Rosman G, Meireles OR, Rus D. Machine learning and coresets for automated real-time video segmentation of laparoscopic and robot-assisted surgery. In: 2017 IEEE international conference on robotics and automation (ICRA). IEEE; 2017.
35. Bonrath EM, Gordon LE, Grantcharov TP. Characterising 'near miss' events in complex laparoscopic surgery through video analysis. BMJ Qual Safety. 2015;24(8):516–21.
36. Natarajan P, Frenzel JC, Smaltz DH. Demystifying big data and machine learning for healthcare. CRC Press; 2017.
37. Nadkarni PM, Ohno-Machado L, Chapman WW. Natural language processing: an introduction. J Am Med Inform Assoc. 2011;18(5):544–51.

38. Murff HJ, FitzHenry F, Matheny ME, Gentry N, Kotter KL, Crimin K, et al. Automated identification of postoperative complications within an electronic medical record using natural language processing. JAMA. 2011;306(8):848–55. Epub 2011/08/25
39. Soguero-Ruiz C, Hindberg K, Rojo-Alvarez JL, Skrovseth SO, Godtliebsen F, Mortensen K, et al. Support vector feature selection for early detection of anastomosis leakage from bag-of-words in electronic health records. IEEE J Biomed Health Inform. 2016;20(5):1404–15.
40. Thompson RF, Valdes G, Fuller CD, Carpenter CM, Morin O, Aneja S, et al. Artificial intelligence in radiation oncology: a specialty-wide disruptive transformation? Radiother Oncol. 2018;129(3):421–6.
41. Elhage SA, Deerenberg EB, Ayuso SA, Murphy KJ, Shao JM, Kercher KW, et al. Development and validation of image-based deep learning models to predict surgical complexity and complications in abdominal wall reconstruction. JAMA Surg. 2021;156(10):933–40.
42. Brennan M, Puri S, Ozrazgat-Baslanti T, Feng Z, Ruppert M, Hashemighouchani H, et al. Comparing clinical judgment with the MySurgeryRisk algorithm for preoperative risk assessment: a pilot usability study. Surgery. 2019;165(5):1035–45. Epub 2019/02/23
43. Jiang X, Wells A, Brufsky A, Neapolitan R. A clinical decision support system learned from data to personalize treatment recommendations towards preventing breast cancer metastasis. PLoS One. 2019;14(3):e0213292.
44. Somashekhar SP, Sepúlveda MJ, Puglielli S, Norden AD, Shortliffe EH, Rohit Kumar C, et al. Watson for oncology and breast cancer treatment recommendations: agreement with an expert multidisciplinary tumor board. Ann Oncol. 2018;29(2):418–23.
45. Nindrea RD, Aryandono T, Lazuardi L, Dwiprahasto I. Diagnostic accuracy of different machine learning algorithms for breast cancer risk calculation: a meta-analysis. Asian Pacific J Cancer Prev. 2018;19(7):1747–52. Epub 2018/07/28
46. Sherbet GV, Woo WL, Dlay S. Application of artificial intelligence-based technology in cancer management: a commentary on the deployment of artificial neural networks. Anticancer Res. 2018;38(12):6607–13.
47. Low S-K, Zembutsu H, Nakamura Y. Breast cancer: the translation of big genomic data to cancer precision medicine. Cancer Sci. 2018;109(3):497–506.
48. Xu J, Yang P, Xue S, Sharma B, Sanchez-Martin M, Wang F, et al. Translating cancer genomics into precision medicine with artificial intelligence: applications, challenges and future perspectives. Human Genet. 2019;138(2):109–24.
49. Loftus TJ, Tighe PJ, Filiberto AC, Efron PA, Brakenridge SC, Mohr AM, et al. Artificial intelligence and surgical decision-making. JAMA Surg. 2020;155(2):148–58.
50. Sacks GD, Dawes AJ, Tsugawa Y, Brook RH, Russell MM, Ko CY, et al. The association between risk aversion of surgeons and their clinical decision-making. J Surg Res. 2021;268:232–43.
51. Healey MA, Shackford SR, Osler TM, Rogers FB, Burns E. Complications in surgical patients. Arch Surg (Chicago, IL: 1960). 2002;137(5):611–7. discussion 7–8; Epub 2002/05/02
52. Helo S, Moulton CE. Complications: acknowledging, managing, and coping with human error. Transl Androl Urol. 2017;6(4):773–82. Epub 2017/09/15
53. Vahdat S, Hamzehgardeshi L, Hessam S, Hamzehgardeshi Z. Patient involvement in health care decision making: a review. Iran Red Crescent Med J. 2014;16(1):e12454. Epub 2014/04/11
54. Price WN 2nd, Cohen IG. Privacy in the age of medical big data. Nat Med. 2019;25(1):37–43.
55. Murdoch B. Privacy and artificial intelligence: challenges for protecting health information in a new era. BMC Med Ethics. 2021;22(1):122. Epub 2021/09/17
56. World Health Organization. Ethics and governance of artificial intelligence for health: WHO guidance. 2021.
57. Red Iberoamericana de Protecci6n de datos. General recommendations for the processing of personal data in artificial intelligence (2019); 2019.
58. Obermeyer Z, Powers B, Vogeli C, Mullainathan S. Dissecting racial bias in an algorithm used to manage the health of populations. Science (New York, NY). 2019;366(6464):447–53. Epub 2019/10/28

59. Dastin J. Amazon scraps secret AI recruiting tool that showed bias against women. Ethics of data and analytics. Auerbach Publications; 2018. p. 296–9.
60. Binkley CE, Kemp DS, Scully BB. Should we rely on AI to help avoid bias in patient selection for major surgery? AMA J Ethics. 2022;24(8):773–80.
61. Emanuel EJ, Emanuel LL. Four models of the physician-patient relationship. JAMA. 1992;267(16):2221–6. Epub 1992/04/22
62. Binkley CE, Green BP. Does intraoperative artificial intelligence decision support pose ethical issues? JAMA Surg. 2021. Epub 2021/06/17;156:809.
63. McDougall RJ. Computer knows best? The need for value-flexibility in medical AI. J Med Ethics. 2019;45(3):156–60. Epub 2018/11/24
64. Froomkin AM, Kerr I, Pineau J. When AIs outperform doctors: confronting the challenges of a tort-induced over-reliance on machine learning. Ariz L Rev. 2019;61:33.
65. Price WN 2nd, Gerke S, Cohen IG. Potential liability for physicians using artificial intelligence. JAMA. 2019;322(18):1765–6.
66. Blackman R. Ethical machines: your concise guide to totally unbiased, transparent, and respectful AI. 2022.
67. Jobin A, Ienca M, Vayena E. The global landscape of AI ethics guidelines. Nat Mach Intell. 2019;1(9):389–99.
68. UNESCO International Bioethics Committee. Report of the IBC on big data and health. Paris; 2017.
69. COMEST U. Report of COMEST on Robotics Ethics. World Commission on the Ethics of Scientific Knowledge and Technology (COMEST) Online: https://unesdoc.unesco.org/ark:/48223/pf0000253952.
70. Board UE. Preliminary study on the technical and legal aspects relating to the desirability of a standard-setting instrument on the ethics of artificial intelligence: 206 EX/42. Paris; 2019.

Chapter 35
Artificial Intelligence Surgery: How Autonomous Actions and Surgiomics Can Decrease Risk in High-Risk Surgery

Nouredin Messaoudi and Andrew A. Gumbs

Abbreviations

AI	Artificial Intelligence
AICD	Automatic Implantable Cardioverter Defibrillator
AIS	Artificial Intelligence Surgery
AR	Augmented Reality
ASA	American Society of Anesthesiologists
CV	Computer Vision
DL	Deep Learning
MDTB	Multi-Disciplinary Tumor Boards
MIS	Minimally Invasive Surgery
ML	Machine Learning
NLP	Natural Language Processing
NOTES	Natural Orifice Transluminal Endoscopic Surgery
RAS	Robotic-Assisted Surgery

Introduction

High-risk surgery refers to surgical procedures that carry a significant probability of adverse events or complications due to various factors. These surgeries are typically complex, involving intricate techniques, extensive tissue manipulation, or critical

N. Messaoudi
Department of Hepato-Pancreato-Biliary Surgery, Vrije Universiteit Brussel (VUB), Universitair Ziekenhuis Brussel (UZ Brussel) and Europe Hospitals, Brussels, Belgium

A. A. Gumbs (✉)
Department of Surgery, American Hospital of Tbilisi, Tbilisi, Georgia

Department of General-, Visceral-, Vascular and Transplantation Surgery, University of Magdeburg, Magdeburg, Germany

© The Author(s), under exclusive license to Springer Nature Switzerland AG 2024
J. Faintuch, S. Faintuch (eds.), *Recent Strategies in High Risk Surgery*,
https://doi.org/10.1007/978-3-031-56270-9_35

anatomical structures. Patients undergoing high-risk surgery often have underlying medical conditions, advanced age, or other risk factors that increase their susceptibility to complications. The potential risks associated with high-risk surgery include excessive bleeding, infection, organ failure, prolonged recovery, and mortality. Due to the inherent complexities and increased risks involved, high-risk surgeries require planning, expertise, and advanced resources to ensure optimal patient outcomes and minimize complications. Two emerging tools that are possible because of advances in Artificial Intelligence (AI) (Fig. 35.1), autonomous actions and Surgiomics, have the potential to decrease risk in high-risk surgery.

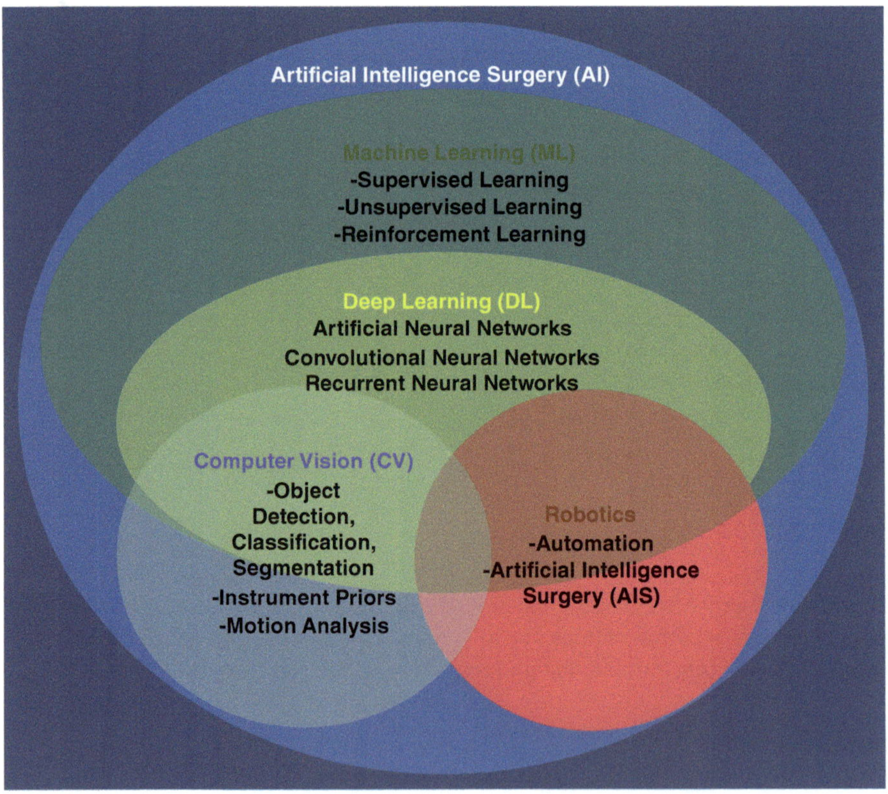

Fig. 35.1 Artificial Intelligence (AI), whose four pillars include: (1) Machine Learning (ML), Deep Learning (DL), Computer Vision (CV), and Natural Language Processing (NLP). (Gumbs AA, Alexander F, Karcz K, Chouillard E, Croner R, Coles-Black J, de Simone B, Gagner M, Gayet B, Grasso V, Illanes A, Ishizawa T, Milone L, Ozmen MM, Piccoli M, Spiedel S, Spolverato G, Sylla P, Vilaccedila J, Abu Hilal M, Swanstrom LL. White paper: definitions of artificial intelligence and autonomous actions in clinical surgery. Art Int Surg 2022; 2:93–100. https://doi.org/10.20517/ais.2022.10)

Artificial Intelligence

AI is a computer system created to perform tasks traditionally requiring human intelligence. One modality is Machine Learning (ML), namely algorithms created that can solve problems that they weren't necessarily designed to solve. Deep Learning (DL) is an architecture of ML that is based on the human neocortex with many decision layers, utilized to permit for more complex solutions. Computer Vision (CV) uses DL architectures of ML to enable a computer to understand visual data and images, a task that is surprisingly difficult to accomplish with surgical video as it often requires the resident or attending surgeon to annotate to teach the computer [1]. Natural Language Processing (NLP) is a technique that has been created to enable computers to interpret spoken messages and the written word.

Autonomous action, commonly mistaken for current robotic surgery or robotic-assisted surgery, implies the use of devices that are not simply automatic, but that also interpret data from sensors and modify actions based on this information [2]. Ultimately, one wonders if the goal of AI should be for robots to perform specific tasks during surgery with no (or minimal) human intervention, or if a future where the surgeon remains in the loop should be sought [3]. While the concept of fully autonomous surgeries is still evolving, certain aspects can already benefit from AI by enhancing surgical precision, dexterity, and visualization.

Surgiomics

Analogously to radiomics, radiogenomics and other categories of precision medicine, it involves the use of advanced analytics, AI-powered predictive modeling, and real-time data analysis to enhance surgical decision-making and patient management. By integrating various sources of patient data such as medical imaging, genetic profile, biopsy results, and patient history, Surgiomics aims to provide surgeons with valuable insights and predictive tools.

High Risk Surgery: Navigating Complexity

High-risk surgeries may involve extensive tissue dissection, major organ manipulation, or complex reconstructions. These procedures often require a higher level of surgical skill, specialized equipment, and advanced perioperative care. Patients undergoing high-risk surgery are often those with underlying health conditions, advanced age, or multiple comorbidities. These factors can increase the risk of complications during and after surgery. The presence of cardiovascular disease, diabetes, or respiratory disorders can impact the patient's physiological reserves and ability to tolerate the surgical stress. Additionally, patients who have previously undergone surgeries or treatments in the same area may have altered anatomy and adhesions, further increasing the complexity and risks associated with subsequent surgeries. Emergency surgeries, performed under urgent or life-threatening circumstances, also tend to be high-risk due to the limited time available for preoperative optimization and planning.

Surgical Risk Score

These assessments consider the patient's medical history, comorbidities, physiological reserves, and other relevant factors to estimate the likelihood of adverse events. Risk prediction models, such as the American Society of Anesthesiologists (ASA) Physical Status Classification System and the Surgical Risk Calculator developed by the American College of Surgeons (NSQIP), assist surgeons in evaluating and communicating the risks associated with a specific procedure to the patient.

However, these classifications do not fully cover the extent of risk related to the surgical interventions and fail at suggesting mitigating strategies to prevent complications. In addition, the management of high-risk surgeries requires a multidisciplinary approach [4]. A specialized team consisting of surgeons, anesthesiologists, nurses, and other healthcare professionals collaborates to optimize patient care and mitigate risks. Preoperative strategies such as optimizing medical conditions, managing medications, and addressing nutritional deficiencies (Prehabilitation), are implemented to minimize the potential risks associated with surgery. Intraoperative monitoring, advanced imaging techniques, and minimally invasive approaches can be utilized to enhance safety and reduce complications during the surgical procedure.

Surgical Technology

Such advancements have significantly contributed to improving outcomes in high-risk surgeries [5]. Surgiomics enables the development of predictive models based on large data analysis that assess patient-specific risks before and after surgery. The integration of these new technologies provides personalized risk assessment and surgical planning, while autonomous actions offer real-time feedback and decision support, resulting in a synergistic approach to risk mitigation in high-risk surgical interventions.

Autonomous Actions

Autonomous Actions: Automation Versus Autonomy

Most people think that a fully functioning autonomous robot must be functioning independently for it to be artificially intelligent. The simplest way to understand this is to compare automatic actions from autonomous ones. During an automatic action, an action is initiated, usually via a button, and the device makes the action occur. Conversely, during an autonomous action, some interpretation of information/data is occurring, and the device or machine is modifying its action based on an interpretation of this information. These 2 different types of actions have also been designated as weak and strong AI, respectively.

Autonomous Actions: What Is "Surgery" Today?

Perhaps the best way for non-interventional doctors to understand this phenomenon is the observation that surgery no longer includes only traditional open or minimally invasive surgery (MIS). MIS itself is divided into endoscopic surgery (i.e. laparoscopic, arthroscopic, thoracoscopic) and robotic-assisted surgery. Robotic-assisted surgery has been divided into console and non-console complete surgical systems, but also into collaborative robotic surgery (corobotic-assisted) and handheld robotic surgery. The reality is that the dominant complete robotic surgical system (da Vinci, Intuitive Surgical, Sunnyvale, CA, USA) is really just a tele-manipulator (i.e. it uses a console to move the robotic arms) not a true robot. The best way to understand this subtly is to understand the 6 levels of surgical autonomy. Notably, the situation is even more complex, because surgery no longer involves these concepts of surgery, but also interventional endoscopy and natural orifice transluminal endoscopic surgery (NOTES), and other interventional disciplines such as interventional radiology, interventional cardiology, and interventional pulmonary.

Autonomous Actions: The Six Levels of Surgical Autonomy

The six levels of surgical autonomy are based on the six levels of autonomously driving cares [6]. Level 0 is when there is an absence of any autonomy and level 1 is when a tele-manipulator is used, but all actions are still controlled by a human. This is the case in current robotic-assisted surgery with complete robotic surgical systems such as the da Vinci (Intuitive Surgical, Sunnyvale, CA, USA) and Versius (CMR, Cambridge, UK) robots. Level 2 is when there is some autonomous action, but under the control of the surgeon, this one corresponds to a gastrointestinal powered stapler with a sensor (Signia, Medtronic, Dublin, Ireland) that will not fire if the tissue is not the appropriate thickness, or will slow down the stapling if the tissue is thick (Fig. 35.2).

Level 3 is when the surgeon has several options to choose from, and great example is the Ligasure device (Valleylab, Boulder, Colorado, USA), which has three buttons and is a vessel sealing device that uses an algorithm that analyzes over 434,000 data points to determine when a vessel is properly sealed and tells the surgeon when it is safe to cut the vessel. Level 4 is when most of the procedure is done by the device autonomously, but the procedure still needs to be performed with the aid of the surgeon and a nice example is an intra-cardiac ablation where the device needs to be placed into the atrium by the interventional cardiologist, but where the device then autonomously detects the area of arrythmia and does the ablation on its own. It is not too hard to then see that an Automatic Implantable Cardioverter Defibrillator (AICD) that can detect a life-threatening arrythmia and give a life-saving therapy all on its own is a perfect example of level 5 autonomy in action.

Autonomous Actions: Surgemes and Dexemes

Although the road to level 5 autonomy may have already arrived in interventional cardiology, any surgeon can tell that this level of autonomy during an open or minimally invasive surgery is much farther off. Nonetheless, when we break down to the steps needed to get there, we can see that we are not as far as we think. A pancreatoduodenectomy, or Whipple procedure in English-speaking countries, involves many steps and multiple phases of reconstruction. A procedure like this can be broken down into surgemes. The Whipple procedure could be divided in to four main

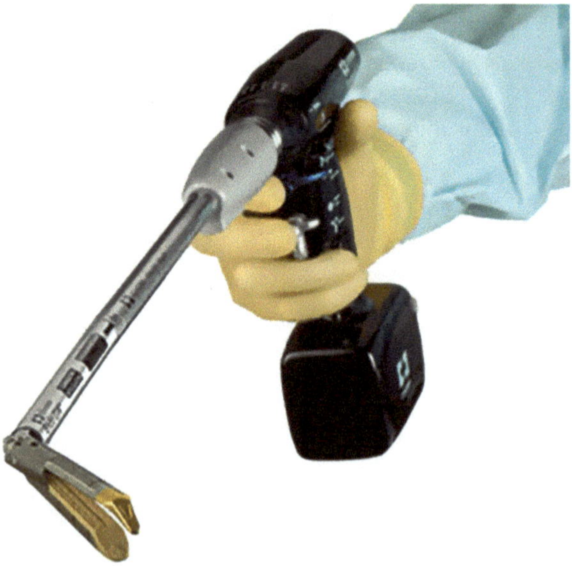

Fig. 35.2 A powered linear gastrointestinal anastomosis (GIA) stapler with a sensor to detect tissue thickness (Signia, Medtronic, Dublin, Ireland). (Gumbs AA, Abu-Hilal M, Tsai TJ, Starker L, Chouillard E, Croner R. Keeping surgeons in the loop: are handheld robotics the best path toward more autonomous actions? (A comparison of complete vs. handheld robotic hepatectomy for colorectal liver metastases). Art Int Surg 2021; 1:38–51. https://doi.org/10.20517/ais.2021.07)

surgemes: (1) the resection of the head of the pancreas duodenum, common bile duct, gastric antrum, and gallbladder if present; (2) the hepatico-jejunostomy; (3) the pancreatico-jejunostomy; and (4) the gastro-jejunostomy. These surgemes can then be separated into their various dexemes. The gastrojejunostomy, the fourth surgeme, could be divided into: (1) identification of the proximal jejunum and placement next to the gastric remnant and stay suture placements; (2) the creation of the enterotomy and gastrotomy; (3) the creation of the linear stapled anastomosis; and (4) closure of the remaining gastro-enterostomy. When we see this, we can see that the third dexeme for the fourth surgeme has already been rendered autonomous, specifically, a powered-stapler with a sensor (Signia, Medtronic, Dublin, Ireland) already exists that can perform a stapled gastrointestinal anastomosis.

Autonomous Actions: Why Artificial Intelligence Surgery Will be Better than Current Robotic-Assisted Surgery

Autonomous actions entail the use of AI-driven robotic systems to perform specific tasks during surgery, referred to as Artificial Intelligence Surgery (RAS), with minimal human intervention. While the concept of fully autonomous surgeries is still evolving, certain aspects of surgery can already benefit from more autonomous actions. Autonomous surgical systems can offer enhanced precision and accuracy compared to traditional surgical techniques. These systems utilize console and handheld robotics with highly precise movements, eliminating the risks associated with human error. By minimizing the margin of error, autonomous actions can reduce complications such as tissue damage, nerve injuries, or inadvertent bleeding during high-risk surgeries. Equipped with sensors and imaging technologies that provide real-time feedback and monitoring, autonomous surgical systems continuously assess the surgical site, vital parameters, and tissue characteristics [7]. This real-time information helps surgeons make informed decisions and take immediate actions to prevent complications. Autonomous actions can adapt to the patient's specific anatomy and physiological characteristics. Through preoperative imaging and intraoperative data analysis, the system can map the patient's anatomy and optimize the surgical approach accordingly. This adaptability reduces the risk of unintended damage to critical structures, supports organ-preservation strategies, improves surgical precision, and minimizes complications associated with anatomical variability [8]. If any abnormalities or potential complications are identified, the autonomous system can take immediate action, such as adjusting instrument pressure, modifying tissue manipulation, thereby facilitating proactive risk mitigation during high-risk surgeries.

Autonomous actions can also contribute to the standardization of surgical techniques across different surgeons and surgical teams. The system can capture and analyze data from previous successful procedures, identify best practices, and create standardized approaches to high-risk surgeries using iterative learning processes.

This standardization reduces variations in surgical techniques and outcomes, leading to improved safety, cost-effective procedures, and decreased complication rates. In addition, AIS can enable minimally invasive techniques, which may carry lower risks compared to open surgeries. By using smaller incisions, robotic instruments, and advanced imaging systems, surgeons can perform high-risk procedures with reduced blood loss, lower infection rates, and faster recovery times. Lastly, autonomous surgical systems may facilitate remote or tele-surgical procedures, where interventions can be performed on patients located at a different site. This can be particularly beneficial in high-risk surgeries, as it allows expert surgeons to provide their expertise and guidance to remote areas or challenging situations where immediate access to specialized care is limited.

Surgiomics

Surgiomics: Big Data Analysis Unveiling Surgical Insights

Surgery remains a high-risk endeavor; however, among surgeons, certain procedures are more high risk than others. Advances in technology help us reduce complications and mortality and surgery has made incredible advances due to enhanced preoperative optimization of patients nutritional and medical status, but also due to improved diagnostic modalities in the intra- and post-operative periods. The reality, however, is that we have arrived at a bottleneck in man's ability to synthesize more data at a rate that can benefit patients. All surgical oncologists know that survival and outcomes data in peer-reviewed articles are already old by the time they are published. This is frankly because surgeons are busy and it takes a long time to shift through patient data, clean it up, analyze it and then write and publish it.

A similar phenomenon can be noted in the actual operating room. The shear amount of information that can be accessible to a surgeon in a modern operating room can be at times hard to process in a timely and effective manner and is probably a cause of the severe burnout that the specialty is currently facing. It is hard to comprehend how augmented reality (AR) and ever-increasing amounts of cancer-specific dyes and intra-operative imaging modalities will be able to be digested by operating surgeons. Although society is apprehensive about many aspects of artificial intelligence, it is hard to imagine a hospital and operating of the future without some form of AI assistance.

The tendency has been for researchers to attach the suffix "-omics" to highlight the fact that large amounts of data are being analyzed. The first technology to use this suffix was "genomics" in the late 1980s. Since then, innumerable other terms have been developed such as proteomics, transcriptomics, radiomics, and pathomics. Radiomics refers to the analysis of vast radiological image repositories to ascertain information that cannot be gleaned from the naked eye but needs complex computing to flush out. Similarly, pathomics is the analysis of entire histopathological images. The term Surgiomics is becoming more utilized, but its exact definition is still being realized. At first glance, surgiomics could simply be the analysis of vast quantities of video recordings of procedures with various types of imaging enhancement such as cancer specific dyes. However, to perform surgery, the surgeon must incorporate an understanding of radiographic, histopathologic and if available genomic data to best determine if, how and when to operate.

Overall, Surgiomics involves the comprehensive analysis of patient-specific data, including clinical records, imaging studies, genetic profiles, histopathologic findings, and real-time intraoperative data. It aims to generate actionable insights that aid in risk assessment, surgical planning, and personalized interventions. Surgiomics can play an important role in preoperative risk assessment by identifying patients who are at higher risk for complications or adverse events before. By analyzing large datasets and applying predictive algorithms, surgeons can gain a better understanding of individual risk factors and make more informed decisions regarding the surgical approach, timing, or adjunctive therapies. Another advantage of Surgiomics is its contribution in intraoperative monitoring in which real-time data analysis of key physiological parameters during surgery can provide surgeons with continuous feedback and early detection of potential complications. By integrating data from various monitoring devices, such as electrocardiography, blood pressure, oxygen saturation, tissue perfusion monitors, or even wearables, Surgiomics can help identify critical events or deviations from normal ranges, allowing for timely intervention. By integrating peri-operative data, appropriate techniques, instruments, and strategies tailored to each patient can be accurately selected, thereby decreasing the risk of adverse events during the procedure. In addition, Surgiomics can provide surgeons with decision support tools that aid in surgical planning, and postoperative care. By combining patient-specific data with evidence-based guidelines and best practices, Surgiomics can assist surgeons in making optimal choices, such as selecting the most appropriate surgical strategy (or even abandon due to futile outcome), adjusting chemotherapy regimens, or predicting patient prognosis.

Surgiomics: Optimizing Autonomous Actions in a Feedback Loop for Ongoing Refinement

Continuous improvement and learning through the analysis of Surgiomics data plays a crucial role in enhancing the quality of high-risk surgeries. By leveraging Surgiomics data, surgeons can identify areas for improvement by analyzing surgical outcomes, trends, and performance metrics. This allows for the identification of patterns and trends specific to high-risk surgeries, leading to the dissemination of best practices for risk mitigation. Moreover, integrating these findings into autonomous systems enables the refinement of autonomous surgical platforms, incorporating Surgiomics insights to optimize performance and patient outcomes [9]. Establishing a feedback loop between Surgiomics, autonomous actions, and surgical teams promotes iterative improvement and refinement based on previous experiences anywhere and anytime. This continuous feedback loop ensures that lessons learned from analyzing Surgiomics data are applied to enhance surgical practices and further optimize the autonomous systems used. Ultimately, continuous improvement and learning driven by Surgiomics analysis foster ongoing refinement, resulting in improved surgical outcomes and patient safety.

Surgiomics: Balancing Innovation and Ethics for Patient Data Safety

Privacy and security concerns surrounding surgical data must be addressed to ensure the confidentiality and integrity of patient information. Ethical considerations and patient consent are paramount, necessitating the ethical use of Surgiomics data and autonomous actions [10]. Informed consent and active patient involvement in decision-making processes are essential to uphold patient autonomy and promote shared decision-making. Additionally, regulatory frameworks need to be established to govern the integration of Surgiomics and autonomous actions, providing guidelines and standards for their implementation (Fig. 35.3). Addressing these challenges and will promote the responsible and effective utilization of Surgiomics and autonomous actions in high-risk surgery, ensuring patient privacy, ethical conduct, and regulatory compliance.

Future Perspectives

The Impact of AI on Surgery and Surgeons

To better understand how AI will affect surgeons, we launched the journal, Artificial Intelligence Surgery (AIS), in 2021 with the first issue getting published in December 2021. This is the first journal dedicated exclusively to AI and Surgery. We consciously called the journal AIS and not AI "in" surgery to differentiate AI "in" the pre-operative and post-operative period from procedures that were being done with an element of AI, specifically, with an element of autonomy in an interventional device.

One of the main impetuses for creating this journal was the realization that we as surgeons do not really understand the fundamentals of robotics [11]. However, at the same time current RAS was rapidly growing in popularity and even being used in the most complex procedures, specifically, the ones with the highest risk [12]. As we have discussed, current RAS systems are simply tele-manipulators and have the lowest level of autonomy. The word "robot" comes from the Slavic for "servant," or

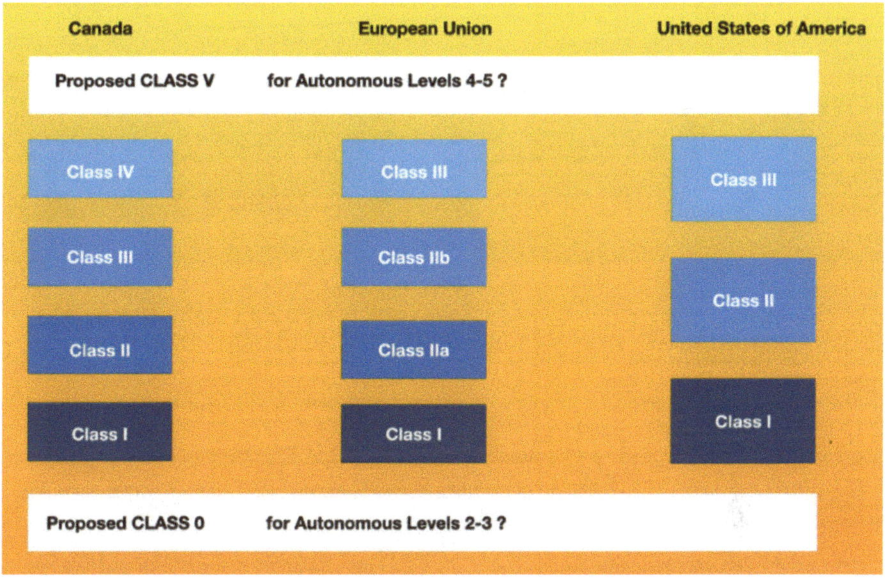

Fig. 35.3 Classes of new devices based on risk in Canada, the European Union, and the United States. It has been proposed that additional levels of risk need to be determined for devices that incorporate Artificial Intelligence (AI). With higher levels for fully autonomous devices, but perhaps lower levels of risk to encourage the development of more "intelligent" devices with sensors that could enhance safety. (Gumbs AA, Gayet B. Why Artificial Intelligence Surgery (AIS) is better than current Robotic-Assisted Surgery (RAS). Art Int Surg 2022; 2:207–12. https://doi.org/10.20517/ais.2022.41)

possibly more accurately "slave." With a tele-manipulator, the servant/slave is the surgeon and not the complete robotic surgical system, as a result, the modern-day usage of "robotic surgery" is no more than an oxymoron. Some authors have attempted to address this by calling it RAS, but the point is clear, without more surgeons having a better understanding of robotics, autonomy, and AI, it will be difficult for us as a group to advance.

Because of the reality that corporations may subconsciously hijack the evolution of RAS, it is becoming ever more paramount that we begin to address, debate, and embrace these new innovations. Newer robotic systems are being developed with haptics, however, because of our natural resting tremor, the haptic feedback creates too much shaking, and this mode has to be turned off (Versius, CMR, Cambridge, U.K.). Some console complete robotic systems have begun to address the fact that having the surgeon unsterile and away from the patient may not be ideal and have created draping mechanisms that enable surgeons go from the console to the bedside while sterile (Dexter, Distalmotion, Épalinges, Switzerland) (Fig. 35.4). Others have done away with the console all together and have the surgeon at the bedside throughout the procedure (Maestro, Moon Surgical, Paris, France) (Fig. 35.5). Lastly, we must also give more consideration to handheld robotics (Figs. 35.6 and 35.7), or so-called collaborative robots (cobots). Whether or not these cheaper

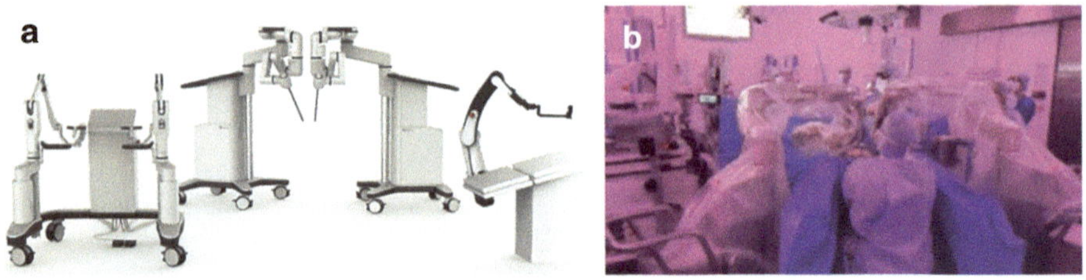

Fig. 35.4 Complete Robotic Surgical system with console that enables the surgeon to remain sterile throughout the entire procedure (Dexter, Distalmotion, Épalinges, Switzerland). (Gumbs AA, Gayet B. Why Artificial Intelligence Surgery (AIS) is better than current Robotic-Assisted Surgery (RAS). Art Int Surg 2022; 2:207–12. https://doi.org/10.20517/ais.2022.41)

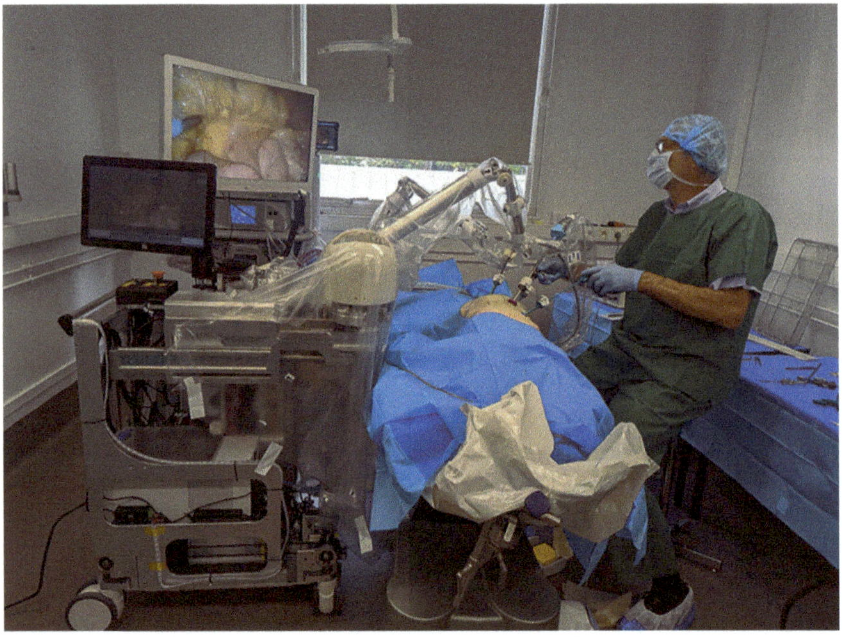

Fig. 35.5 Non-console robotic system with the surgeon at the patient's bedside throughout the surgery (Maestro, Moon Surgical, Paris, France). (Gumbs AA, Gayet B. Why Artificial Intelligence Surgery (AIS) is better than current Robotic-Assisted Surgery (RAS). Art Int Surg 2022; 2:207–12. https://doi.org/10.20517/ais.2022.41)

variants have any advantages to more traditional robotics is unknown, but no one can deny that their affordability may enable more patients to enjoy the benefits or robotic technology.

Perhaps the most eye-opening thing that we need to consider when evaluating the potential for AI to shape the future of surgery is the fact that Intuitive surgical is currently collecting data of instrument priors and movements from every da Vinci procedure done. This massive database could one day lead to level 5 surgical

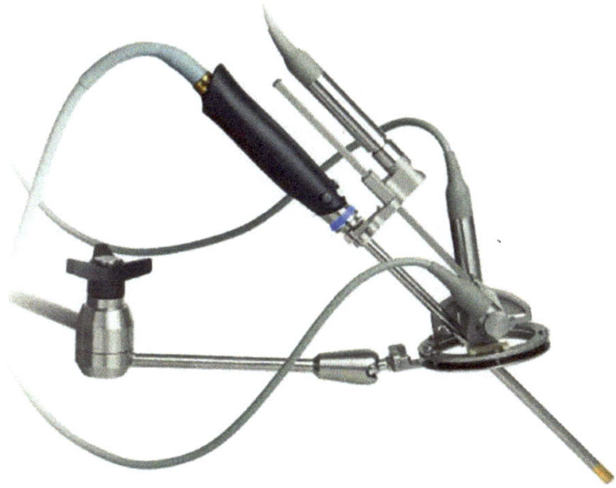

Fig. 35.6 Handheld laparoscope holder that is autoclavable and fits right on the operating room table (VideoendosKopY-ViKY, Endocontrol, Grenoble, France). (Gumbs AA, Abu-Hilal M, Tsai TJ, Starker L, Chouillard E, Croner R. Keeping surgeons in the loop: are handheld robotics the best path toward more autonomous actions? (A comparison of complete vs. handheld robotic hepatectomy for colorectal liver metastases). Art Int Surg 2021; 1:38–51. https://doi.org/10.20517/ais.2021.07)

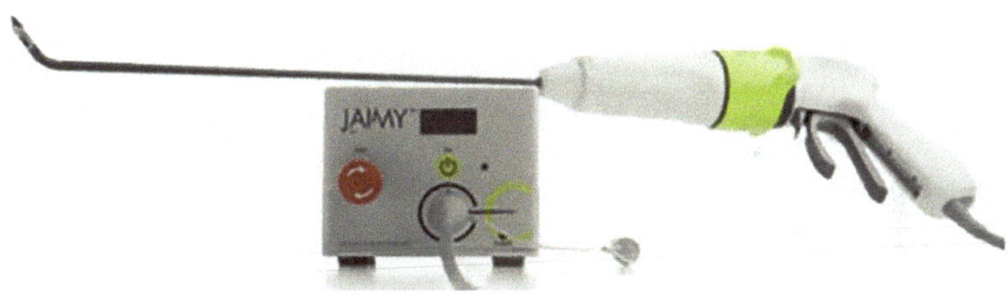

Fig. 35.7 Handheld surgical robotic grasper (Jaimy, Endocontrol, Grenoble, France). (Gumbs AA, Abu-Hilal M, Tsai TJ, Starker L, Chouillard E, Croner R. Keeping surgeons in the loop: are handheld robotics the best path toward more autonomous actions? (A comparison of complete vs. handheld robotic hepatectomy for colorectal liver metastases). Art Int Surg 2021; 1:38–51. https://doi.org/10.20517/ais.2021.07)

autonomy of traditional surgery. Moreover, the STAR robot can now do open and minimally invasive robotic bowel anastomoses that have found to be superior to ones done by humans [13].

Surgiomics Revolutionizing Surgical Oncology

During Multi-Disciplinary Tumor Boards (MDTB) meetings, all the various specialties involved in the care of the cancer patient meet, review the available radiology images, pathology data and any mutational status information to decide timing of neoadjuvant and adjuvant therapies and determine if surgery is indicated. This process has become the standard of care, but it is limited by the fact that only a limited amount of data is actually analyzed. Currently, entire human genomes are not sequenced, because there is no realistic way to get relevant data from this information. Even though the human genome contains approximately 25,000 genes and total genomic sequencing costs only about $1000, most tests of mutational status never look at more than around 500 genes.

To maximize the potential of AI, we have begun an initiative called the AiRGOS, which stands for the Artificial intelligence Radiomics, Genomics, Oncopathologic (Pathomics) and Surgiomics. This multi-centric international project is creating a secure data depository of radiological, histopathological, genomic, and clinical information of patients with pancreatic cancer. We chose pancreatic cancer because it is a primary tumor with generally poor outcomes. Future studies will involve metastatic cancers such as colorectal liver metastases. Deep learning architectures have been utilized to split groups into short- and long-term survivors and once the algorithm is trained, the algorithm can accurately differentiate patients into these categories before treatment is initiated. Osaka University has shown that a single contrast enhanced arterial level image of a hepatocellular cancer is all that is needed to differentiate patients into those that will survive 2 years and those that will not [14].

This blows the lid off of the traditional function of cross-sectional imaging, namely is a tumor resectable or not. We believe that interpreting radiographic images in this way is an example of Surgiomics, because this information impacts whether or not surgery should be offered at all, regardless of whether or not the tumor is resectable. To better understand the difference between Radiomics and Surgiomics in this instance is to consider one of the most popular ways to use radiomics in pancreatic surgery. Multiple radiomic studies have analyzed pancreatic cystic tumors and have been able to identify, which pancreatic cysts will transform into a malignancy and thus should be removed [15].

AiRGOS will attempt to enhance this capability by analyzing all the images of a pancreatic protocol CT scan and not a single image. Furthermore, we hope that combining entire genomic sequencing data, the algorithm will be even more powerful. This approach will be particularly useful for even rarer tumors such as uterine sarcoma, a so-called orphan cancer, where very limited resources have been allocated to identify actionable targets. The combination of entire cross-sectional images with and without contrast, entire genomic sequencing, pathomics with chemotherapy, immunotherapy and radiation therapy regimens should enable us to create a MDTB that can give our patients the best chance at longer-term survival and even cure. The urgency of this project is that we have the data, and we have the technology, we just don't have the funds to remove guessing from cancer therapy. This model could be duplicated in other solid organ cancers, but even in other pathologies such as inflammatory bowel disease, amyloidosis, and sarcoidosis.

Conclusions

The integration of Surgiomics and autonomous actions offers a synergistic approach to decrease risk in high-risk surgeries. Through personalized risk assessment, real-time decision support, precision and adaptability, early detection and intervention, and tele-surgery, Surgiomics and autonomous technologies have the potential to revolutionize high-risk surgical practices. By leveraging these advancements, surgeons can enhance patient safety, improve outcomes, and reduce complications in high-risk surgeries. It's important to note that while these technologies hold promise for reducing risks in high-risk surgeries, they are still evolving fields of study. Extensive research, rigorous testing, and regulatory approvals are necessary to ensure their safety, efficacy, and widespread implementation. Surgeons and healthcare professionals will continue to play a critical role in integrating these technologies into surgical practice while prioritizing patient safety and optimizing outcomes.

References

1. Taher H, Grasso V, Tawfik S, Gumbs A. The challenges of deep learning in artificial intelligence and autonomous actions in surgery: a literature review. Art Int Surg. 2022;2:144–58. https://doi.org/10.20517/ais.2022.11.
2. Gumbs AA, Perretta S, Bernard D, Chouillard E. What is artificial intelligence surgery. Art Int Surg. 2021;1:1–10. https://doi.org/10.20517/ais.2021.01.
3. Gumbs AA, Abu-Hilal M, Tsai T-J, Starker L, Chouillard E, Croner R. Keeping surgeons in the loop: are handheld robotics the best path toward more autonomous actions? (a comparison of complete vs. handheld robotic hepatectomy for colorectal liver metastases). Artif Intell Surg. 2021;
4. Gumbs AA, Lorenz E, Tsai T-J, Starker L, Flanagan J, Benedetti Cacciaguerra A, Yu NJ, Bajul M, Chouillard E, Croner R, et al. Study: international multicentric minimally invasive liver resection for colorectal liver metastases (SIMMILR-CRLM). Cancers. 2022;14:1379. https://doi.org/10.3390/cancers14061379.
5. Gumbs AA, Croner R, Lorenz E, Cacciaguerra AB, Tsai T-J, Starker L, Flanagan J, Yu NJ, Chouillard E, Abu Hilal M. Survival study: international multicentric minimally invasive liver resection for colorectal liver metastases (SIMMILR-2). Cancers. 2022;14:4190. https://doi.org/10.3390/cancers14174190.
6. Gumbs AA, Frigerio I, Spolverato G, Croner R, Illanes A, Chouillard E, Elyan E. Artificial intelligence surgery: how do we get to autonomous actions in surgery? Sensors. 2021;21:5526. https://doi.org/10.3390/s21165526.
7. Gumbs AA, Grasso V, Bourdel N, Croner R, Spolverato G, Frigerio I, Illanes A, Abu Hilal M, Park A, Elyan E. The advances in computer vision that are enabling more autonomous actions in surgery: a systematic review of the literature. Sensors (Basel). 2022;22(13):4918. https://doi.org/10.3390/s22134918.

8. Gumbs AA, Gayet B. Why artificial intelligence surgery (AIS) is better than current robotic-assisted surgery (RAS). Art Int Surg. 2022;2:207–12. https://doi.org/10.20517/ais.2022.41.
9. Gumbs AA, Alexander F, Karcz K, Chouillard E, Croner R, Coles-Black J, de Simone B, Gagner M, Gayet B, Grasso V, Illanes A, Ishizawa T, Milone L, Ozmen MM, Piccoli M, Spiedel S, Spolverato G, Sylla P, Vilaccedila J, Abu Hilal M, Swanstrom LL. White paper: definitions of artificial intelligence and autonomous actions in clinical surgery. Art Int Surg. 2022;2:93–100. https://doi.org/10.20517/ais.2022.10.
10. Capelli G, Verdi D, Frigerio I, Rashidian N, Ficorilli A, Grasso SV, Majidi D, Gumbs AA, Spolverato G. Artificial intelligence surgery editorial board study group on ethics. White paper: ethics and trustworthiness of artificial intelligence in clinical surgery. Art Int Surg. 2023;3:111–22. https://doi.org/10.20517/ais.2023.04.
11. Gumbs AA, De Simone B, Chouillard E. Searching for a better definition of robotic surgery: is it really different from laparoscopy? Mini-invasive Surg. 2020;4:90. https://doi.org/10.20517/2574-1225.2020.110.
12. Gumbs AA, Croner R, Chouillard E. Is robotic pancreatic surgery ready or prime time? Hepatobiliary surgery & nutrition. Hepatobiliary Surg Nutr. 2020;9(5):650–3. https://doi.org/10.21037/hbsn.2019.12.05.
13. Gya Saeidi H, Opfermann JD, Kam M, Wei S, Leonard S, Hsieh MH, Kang JU, Krieger A. Autonomous robotic laparoscopic surgery for intestinal anastomosis. Sci Robot. 2022;7(62):eabj2908. https://doi.org/10.1126/scirobotics.abj2908.
14. Kinoshita M, Ueda D, Matsumoto T, Shinkawa H, Yamamoto A, Shiba M, Okada T, Tani N, Tanaka S, Kimura K, Ohira G, Nishio K, Tauchi J, Kubo S, Ishizawa T. Deep learning model based on contrast-enhanced computed tomography imaging to predict postoperative early recurrence after the curative resection of a solitary hepatocellular carcinoma. Cancers (Basel). 2023;15(7):2140. https://doi.org/10.3390/cancers15072140.
15. Boutros C, Singh V, Ocuin L, Marks JM, Hashimoto DA. Artificial intelligence in hepato-pancreaticobiliary surgery—promises and perils. Art Int Surg. 2022;2:213–23. https://doi.org/10.20517/ais.2022.32.

Chapter 36
Machine Learning and High-Risk Cardiac Surgery Risk Scoring

Michael P. Rogers, Haroon Janjua, Meagan Read, Emily Grimsley, and Paul C. Kuo

Introduction

Patients undergoing high-risk cardiac surgery are a heterogeneous and complex cohort with varying degrees of comorbid conditions and peri-operative surgical risk. These patients may have undergone multiple prior cardiac surgical procedures, necessitate vasoactive medications for maintaining blood pressure, or require mechanical circulatory support for hemodynamic instability and shock. Early identification and risk stratification of patients at risk for adverse outcomes is crucial for pre-operative planning and informed decision making. Ultimate success is contingent on careful patient selection as well as pre-operative optimization and post-operative management. Accordingly, several risk models have been developed to inform physicians and patients and include the Society of Thoracic Surgeons Predicted Risk of Mortality (STS-PROM), European System for Cardiac Operative Risk Evaluation (EuroSCORE) II, the age, creatinine, ejection fraction (ACEF) score, and Society of Thoracic Surgeons–American College of Cardiology Transcatheter Valve Therapy (STS-ACC TVT) score for Transcatheter Aortic Valve Replacement (TAVR), among others [1–5]. These scoring systems employ a combination of patient demographics, clinical variables, and comorbidities to provide estimated risk. However, predictions are often limited in high-risk clinical scenarios where these models have incomplete or limited data from which to estimate. Further, traditional statistical models used in risk scoring often assume linear relationships between clinical variables and outcomes. Surgical risk, however, is a multifactorial phenomenon influenced by complex, nonlinear interactions among variables.

M. P. Rogers (✉) · H. Janjua · M. Read · E. Grimsley · P. C. Kuo
OnetoMAP Analytics, Department of Surgery, University of South Florida Morsani College of Medicine, Tampa, FL, USA
e-mail: mrogers6@usf.edu; hmjanjua@usf.edu; mread@usf.edu; grimsley@usf.edu; paulkuo@usf.edu

© The Author(s), under exclusive license to Springer Nature Switzerland AG 2024

J. Faintuch, S. Faintuch (eds.), *Recent Strategies in High Risk Surgery*,
https://doi.org/10.1007/978-3-031-56270-9_36

Consequently, statistical models may not fully capture these intricate relationships, resulting in suboptimal predictive accuracy. These models may also not encompass all relevant clinical variables, potentially missing crucial risk factors that could impact patient outcomes. These limitations have spurred interest in the application of machine learning (ML) algorithms.

Recent enthusiasm for artificial intelligence and machine learning has burgeoned interest as a potential method to overcome limitations of previous scoring schemes. Machine learning-based models have shown superior predictive ability and the ability to personalize risk stratification, allowing for improved clinical decision making and patient counseling. Further, ML-based models are able to incorporate a broader range of patient-specific data, including genetic and imaging data, and adapt to changes in patient characteristics in real time. In this chapter, we aim to highlight the use of machine learning and artificial intelligence in high-risk cardiac surgery risk scoring and identify future directions as this technology evolves.

Machine Learning Techniques in High-Risk Cardiac Surgery

Machine learning is a subset in the field of artificial intelligence that employs the use of algorithms to learn patterns in data and make predictions based on those patterns. These algorithms can be used to develop predictive models for surgical and procedural intervention, assist in diagnosis, and interpret imaging or pathologic studies. Within cardiac surgery, these tools have shown exceptional performance when compared to traditional statistical techniques for risk prediction and identifying novel variables that may contribute to patient outcome. The potential to progress beyond traditional methods has incited a firestorm of enthusiasm and effort in employing these algorithms to improve clinical risk prediction.

The two main categories of ML algorithms commonly employed in risk scoring include supervised and unsupervised learning. Supervised learning involves the training of models on 'labeled' data (i.e., patient laboratory values), where the outcomes are known, to make new predictions on novel, unlabeled data. Unsupervised learning trains models on unlabeled data, where outcomes are not known, in an effort to identify patterns or clusters in those data. Various techniques within these broad categories may be used for risk prediction with varying results.

Supervised Learning Algorithms

Numerous supervised learning models have been used to quantify cardiac surgical risk. Techniques have included multivariable logistic regression, random forest, support vector machines, decision trees and neural networks, among others. In these approaches, a model is trained using input data and corresponding output labels, allowing the model to 'learn' the underlying patterns and relationships within the data. As these algorithms are trained on 'labeled' data, they depend on robust clinic data from which to train prior to testing and making novel predictions. Each machine learning algorithm has their respective strengths and weaknesses.

Logistic Regression

Logistic regression is a fundamental technique in supervised machine learning and is used widely in various domains for binary classification tasks. This approach is versatile and widely applicable to risk prediction modeling. Rooted in the principles of generalized linear models, this approach extends the linear regression framework to tackle binary classification problems. This model is generally evaluated by the log-odds ratio and likelihood function. The log-odds ratio (i.e., logit function) is a key component of logistic regression and represents the logarithm of the ratio of the probability of the positive class to the probability of the negative class. Mathematically, this is represented as the following:

$$\text{logit}(p) = \log\left(\frac{p}{(1-p)}\right)$$

where p represents the probability of the positive class outcome, and (1—p) represents the probability of the negative class outcome. The log-odds ratio maps the probability values between 0 and 1 onto an entire real number line, allowing for a linear relationship between the predictor variables and the log-odds of the outcome.

Similarly, the likelihood function is a fundamental concept in regression that is the basis of estimating the model parameters. This function quantifies the probability of observing the given set of outcomes in the training data, given the model parameters. In logistic regression, the likelihood function is derived from the assumption that the outcome probabilities follow binomial distribution. Mathematically, this is expressed as the following:

$$L(\Theta) = \pi\left[p^{yi} * (1-p)^{(1-yi)}\right]$$

Here, Θ represents the model parameters, yi represents the observed class labels (0 or 1) for training, and p represents the predicted probability of the positive class outcome. The likelihood function calculates the joint probability of observing the class labels in the training data under the logistic regression model.

The goal of logistic regression is to determine the optimal set of model parameters that maximize the likelihood function. This is accomplished by a process of maximum likelihood estimation. This process finds the values of the model parameters that maximize the likelihood of observing the training data. By maximizing the likelihood function, the negative log-likelihood function is minimized, thereby penalizing the model for incorrect predictions and encouraging the model to converge toward the optimal parameter values that best fit the data. Through iteratively optimizing the log-loss function using optimization algorithms, logistic regression estimates the optimal parameters that define the decision boundary separating the positive and negative class instances in feature space. These estimated parameters can then be used to predict the probabilities of class membership for novel instances.

Practical applications of logistic regression in cardiac surgery or critical care risk scoring include the Parsonnet Score, EuroSCORE, STS-PROM, ACEF, and Acute Physiology and Chronic Health Evaluation (APACHE) scores. These scoring schemes represent some of the most widely used and validated risk calculators. Each model incorporates various factors such as age, comorbidities, nature of the cardiac surgical procedure, and procedural details to provide risk of morbidity and/or mortality. Presently, the most commonly used and validated of these scoring schemes is the STS-PROM.

Evidence supporting the STS-PROM risk calculator is derived from multiple studies that have evaluated its performance and accuracy. The calculator is based on data collected from more than 1500 participating hospitals across the United States, allowing for a robust collection of granular data from which to build a model. Using multivariable logistic regression, the model incorporates various patient-specific factors such as age, sex, comorbidities, and procedural characteristics. This model has been rigorously validated across patient populations and surgical procedures prospectively and has consistently demonstrated accurate risk estimates. Further, discriminative ability and calibration of the scoring system has been excellent. The risk calculator, in concert with clinical judgment, has shown to have practical value as a tool to guide surgical decision making and pre-operative optimization strategies.

Random Forest

Random Forest (RF) is an ensemble learning model that combines multiple decision trees to make predictions. The moniker 'forest' refers to a collection of multiple decision trees. The algorithm uses labeled input features (independent variables) with their associated target labels (dependent variables) to construct multiple decision trees using a method known as bootstrapping. This technique involves randomly selecting subsets of the original dataset to create different training sets for each tree. At each decision point (or node) of a decision tree, a subset of features is considered for splitting the data. Random Forest enhances this process by selecting a random set of features for each tree, thereby reducing correlation among trees. Each tree is then recursively partitioned based on the selected features. This process involves finding the best split point that optimizes a given criterion with the goal of creating a homogenous subset of data at the leaf nodes of the tree. Once all trees are successfully constructed, the Random Forest algorithm can make predictions. For classification, each tree in the forest 'casts a vote' for the class label with the final prediction being determined by majority voting. For regression, Random Forest determines the average or median of the predicted values from all trees as the final prediction. When the algorithm is presented with new data, each decision tree independently classifies or predicts the outcome, with the aggregate result from all trees used to make the final prediction.

Random Forest modeling has been employed in high-risk cardiac surgery risk scoring. Recently, the authors published an automated machine learning approach employing RF modeling to the National Surgical Quality Improvement Program (NSQIP) database for adult patients undergoing coronary artery bypass grafting, open and transcatheter approaches to valve replacement, aortic root replacement, and valvuloplasty with a predicted 30-day post-operative mortality probability of 10% or greater as determined by the NSQIP calculator [6]. While the final model used differed from RF, the results of RF model were nonetheless meaningful.

Random Forest is a powerful machine learning tool with often superb discriminative and predictive ability. However, it can be computationally taxing, especially when encountering a large number of trees or features. Additionally, practical interpretation may be difficult due to the complex nature of the ensemble.

Support Vector Machines

Support Vector Machines (SVM) is another powerful supervised learning model that can be used for classification and regression tasks alike. In particular, it is useful for solving binary classification problems but may also be expanded to deal with multi-class classification problems. The SVM algorithm uses labeled input features and their corresponding target labels to find an optimal 'hyperplane' in the feature space that separates the data points belonging to different classes with the maximum margin. A hyperplane is a decision boundary that divides the feature space into separate regions corresponding to different classes. The margin refers to the distance between the hyperplane and the nearest points from each class. The SVM algorithm attempts to find the hyperplane that maximizes this margin in an effort to generalize well to previously unseen data. The model is then trained through optimization of the hyperplane parameters and then used to predict the class of new data points, assigning a class label accordingly. There are numerous advantages of SVM, including the ability to handle high-dimensional data and efficacy in problems where the number of input values is greater than the number of samples. However, SVM is not without drawbacks, as the algorithm can be computationally complex when using large datasets and fine tuning of the parameters is necessary to optimize the algorithm.

Support vector machines algorithm has been used in predicting the development of acute kidney injury following cardiac surgery, cardiogenic shock following surgical or transcatheter valve replacement, and in mortality risk prediction [7–9]. These methods have shown excellent Area Under the Curve values, however, have not been prospectively validated in these patient populations.

Local Interpretable Model Agnostic Explanations (LIME)

Local Interpretable Model Agnostic Explanations (LIME) is a technique used to provide explanations for individual predictions made by complex machine learning algorithms. As ML algorithms are often considered "black-boxes" with regard to how they make their predictions, LIME offers interpretable insights into the decision-making process at the local level through data perturbation and feature importance sampling. LIME begins by selecting an instance from the dataset and models its behavior locally by generating a "neighborhood" of similar instances around the selected instance. The model then perturbs the features of the instance while keeping the label fixed. LIME is then able to evaluate the importance of each feature by evaluating the model's prediction and the similarity between the model's perturbed instance and measuring the Euclidean distance between the two values. Each feature's degree of importance and weight as it contributes to the model is then determined and allows for insight into model decision making. The explanations given by LIME are specific to the selected instance, or patient, and provide insight to that particular instance. In this way, LIME affords the user an understanding of the relative influence of different features of the prediction.

LIME modeling offers several advantages, including the ability to be applied to any black-box model. By providing insight into the decision process the user is able to understand certain predictions. Additionally, elucidating the degree to which variables contribute to model predictions allows the user to determine which factors to target to decrease mortality. The author's recent analysis of the NSQIP dataset using LIME modeling to analyze mortality prediction in high-risk cardiac surgery provided detailed, patient-specific, prognostication (Fig. 36.1).

Overall, LIME offers a robust and valuable tool for understanding complex black-box machine learning models and provides predictions at the local level, allowing for model transparency and instilling trust in the decision-making process of models.

Unsupervised Learning Algorithms

Unsupervised machine learning approaches can be powerful tools in high-risk cardiac surgery risk scoring by analyzing large amounts of patient data and identifying previously unrealized patterns or patient clusters that may uncover novel associations or factors impacting morbidity and mortality. Unsupervised learning algorithms differ from supervised approaches in that the models have no previous knowledge of labeled data and their outcome, and instead search for similarities between data around which to cluster. Data collection may involve collecting relevant patient data from electronic medical records, including medical history,

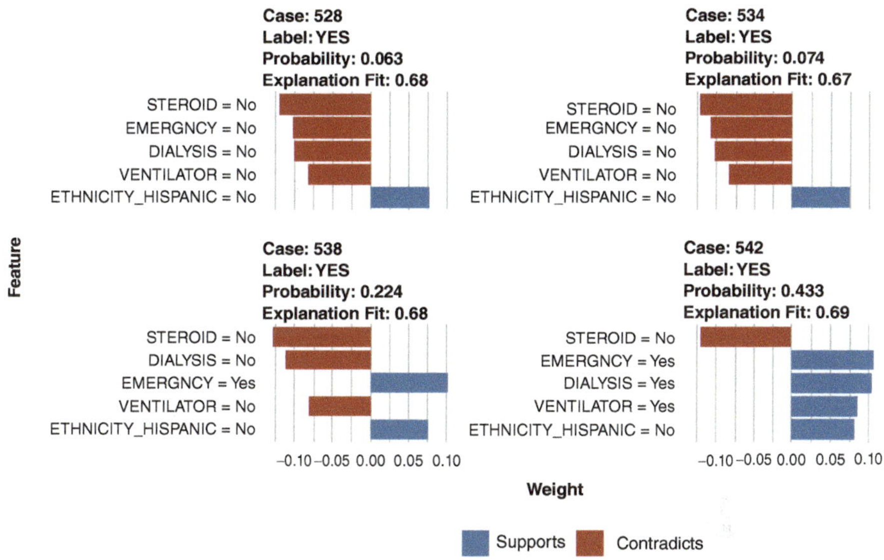

Fig. 36.1 GBM and LIME modeling example with four separate patient cases. Modeling was performed on high-risk cardiac surgical patients and comorbidities analyzed for supporting or contradicting mortality, with probability of mortality and explanation of fit provided for each patient

demographics, diagnostic tests, and other metrics. These data are then preprocessed to ensure compatibility, handle missing values, normalize numerical variables, and encode categorical data. In this technique, features are extracted by identifying key attributes or measurements that may potentially influence cardiac surgical risk. Methods for feature extraction include principal component analysis or independent component analysis to reduce data dimensionality and are beyond the purview of this book chapter. Unsupervised algorithms include *k*-means clustering, hierarchical cluster, or Gaussian mixture models with the goal of grouping similar data based on inherent patterns or structures within the data. The algorithm performance is then evaluated based on traditional metrics and testing, and then may be applied to novel data.

Examples of unsupervised algorithms used in cardiac surgery have included the recognition of epicardial adipose tissue subtypes with distinct atrial fibrosis profiles in patients with persistent atrial fibrillation, unsupervised learning of ECG waveforms to identify bundle branch morphology, and in determining patients at risk for cardiac allograft vasculopathy [10–12].

It should be noted that unsupervised machine learning techniques are unable to provide direct causal relationships or explicitly identify risk factors. Rather, they are a tool to assist in discovering novel patterns or associations within the data, allowing for valuable insights for further investigation and decision support in high-risk cardiac surgery.

References

1. Chalmers J, Pullan M, Fabri B, et al. Validation of EuroSCORE II in a modern cohort of patients undergoing cardiac surgery. Eur J Cardiothorac Surg. 2013;43(4):688–94.
2. Garcia-Valentin A, Mestres CA, Bernabeu E, et al. Validation and quality measurements for EuroSCORE and EuroSCORE II in the Spanish cardiac surgical population: a prospective, multicentre study. Eur J Cardiothorac Surg. 2016;49(2):399–405.
3. Nashef SA, Roques F, Sharples LD, et al. EuroSCORE II. Eur J Cardiothorac Surg. 2012;41(4):734–44. discussion 44–5
4. Ranucci M, Pistuddi V, Scolletta S, de Vincentiis C, Menicanti L. The ACEF II risk score for cardiac surgery: updated but still parsimonious. Eur Heart J. 2018;39(23):2183–9.
5. Rogers MP, Janjua H, DeSantis AJ, Grimsley E, Pietrobon R, Kuo PC. Machine learning refinement of the NSQIP risk calculator: who survives the "hail Mary" case? J Am Coll Surg. 2022;234(4):652–9.
6. Rogers MP, Janjua H, Fishberger G, et al. A machine learning approach to high-risk cardiac surgery risk scoring. J Card Surg. 2022;37(12):4612–20.
7. Tseng PY, Chen YT, Wang CH, et al. Prediction of the development of acute kidney injury following cardiac surgery by machine learning. Crit Care. 2020;24(1):478.
8. Fan Y, Dong J, Wu Y, et al. Development of machine learning models for mortality risk prediction after cardiac surgery. Cardiovasc Diagn Ther. 2022;12(1):12–23.
9. Lawlor MK, Hamid N, Kampaktsis P, et al. Incidence and predictors of cardiogenic shock following surgical or transcatheter tricuspid valve intervention. Catheter Cardiovasc Interv. 2022;99(5):1668–78.
10. Cui C, Qin H, Zhu X, et al. Unsupervised machine learning reveals epicardial adipose tissue subtypes with distinct atrial fibrosis profiles in patients with persistent atrial fibrillation: a prospective 2-center cohort study. Heart Rhythm. 2022;19(12):2033–41.
11. Feeny AK, Rickard J, Trulock KM, et al. Machine learning of 12-lead QRS waveforms to identify cardiac resynchronization therapy patients with differential outcomes. Circ Arrhythm Electrophysiol. 2020;13(7):e008210.
12. Moayedi Y, Teuteberg JJ. Predicting where patients will be, rather than just seeing where they are: establishing trajectories of cardiac allograft vasculopathy. Circulation. 2020;141(24):1968–70.

Chapter 37
Multidimensional Frailty Instruments for Cardiac Surgery

Habib Jabagi, Taleen Haddad, and Louise Y. Sun

Introduction

In the span of the last century, global life expectancy has more than doubled from 29 years in 1900 to 73 years in 2022 [1, 2]. This accomplishment has been attributed to improved nutrition, hygiene [3], and importantly, advances in the medical and surgical management of cardiovascular disease [4], which is the leading cause of death globally [5]. While a remarkable achievement, it has drastically transformed the medical and surgical landscape today, resulting in the average age of patients seeking and undergoing cardiac surgery being significantly older, with increased comorbidities and frailty [6, 7].

Frailty remains a poorly recognized and poorly investigated syndrome in patients undergoing cardiac surgery [8–10] and thus presents complex challenges and unique implications for clinicians working to optimize perioperative outcomes [7, 8, 11]. In this chapter, we will explore the concept of frailty as a whole, its unique impact on patients undergoing cardiac surgery, and the important role of frailty assessments in prognostication and management of this patient population.

H. Jabagi · T. Haddad · L. Y. Sun (✉)
Division of Cardiovascular Surgery, Ichan School of Medicine, Mount Sinai and Division of Cardiothoracic Surgery, Valley Hospital, Ridgewood, NJ, USA

Division of Geriatric Medicine, Queen's University, Kingston, ON, Canada

Division of Cardiothoracic Anesthesiology, Stanford University School of Medicine, Stanford, CA, USA
e-mail: sunl@stanford.edu

© The Author(s), under exclusive license to Springer Nature Switzerland AG 2024

J. Faintuch, S. Faintuch (eds.), *Recent Strategies in High Risk Surgery*,
https://doi.org/10.1007/978-3-031-56270-9_37

Defining Frailty

Often described as a diminished resiliency or marked vulnerability to stress, frailty is a commonly encountered clinical syndrome in older adults, and increases in prevalence with age [11, 12]. It is present in approximately 10–15% of individuals between 65 and 75 years of age, and greater than 50% of those over 80 years of age [13–15]. Frailty is a syndrome comprised of (1) decreased physiological reserve, (2) increased burden of accumulated comorbidities, and (3) declined function across multiple physiologic systems [8, 16].

Although more common in older adults, frailty is not synonymous with aging. Older adults are also a very heterogeneous population with respect to health status [17], with some maintaining excellent physical and cognitive function, while others progressively deteriorate as a result of chronic diseases and/or disabilities [18]. While advanced age is a well-known risk factor for poor health-related outcomes [19], disparities in health status between individuals of the same age can often be explained by frailty. It is well recognized that frailty increases the risk of adverse health outcomes [8], including falls [20], delirium [21], institutionalization [22], incident disability [22], mortality [23], and worse health prognoses [19, 20, 24, 25]. These associated risks and complications likely account for some of the prominent differences between chronological and physiological age [25].

Frailty is also an independent risk factor for poor outcomes after surgery. In patients undergoing major non-cardiac surgery, frailty has been shown to be associated with increased mortality, surgical site infections, prolonged hospitalizations, increased susceptibility to deconditioning and faster functional decline, and higher readmission rates [26–31]. Even minor [32] and ambulatory [33] procedures can pose high risk for frail patients, suggesting an effect that is independent of level of operative stress. Indeed, in a large retrospective study of 432,828 patients undergoing non-cardiac surgical procedures, Shinall et al. [32] demonstrated patients with frailty had a significantly higher risk of postoperative complications and mortality across all levels of operative stress.

Frailty is also associated with higher overall healthcare resource use [34] and expenditure [35]. This has piqued the interest of key stakeholders in the care of older adults, as well as policymakers, and has become a driver for healthcare systems to better understand the patterns and determinants of frailty [16, 36].

Unidimensional Versus Multidimensional Frailty Assessment Scales

Frailty remains an emerging concept in current state-of-the-art medical and surgical practices [24, 37–40]. In the absence of a universally accepted clinical definition [16, 41, 42], a plethora of clinical and administrative frailty assessment tools have been developed [43–45], each with their own strengths, limitations, validity, and applicability [7, 38, 43]. In general, these instruments can be subdivided into two different conceptualizations or approaches to measuring frailty: unidimensional and multidimensional scales [40, 45].

Based on these definitions, early frailty assessments had often focused on singular aspects of frailty, usually the physical domain of functioning, such as mobility, grip strength, or endurance [40, 45, 46]. The advantage of this approach is simplicity of administration in busy clinical settings, allowing for easy workflow integration. However, a major limitation of such tools is that it overlooks other dimensions of frailty, such as cognitive impairment, psychological well-being, and social support [40, 42]. Consequently, this may lead to an incomplete understanding of a patient's overall health status and the potential impact of treatment decisions.

On the other hand, multidimensional frailty scales afford a more holistic and integrative assessment of an individual's frailty status, by including social, psychological, and even environmental domains in addition to physical features [47–51]. While multidimensional assessments provide a broader picture of an individual's health, they can be complex and time-consuming, often requiring additional resources and training. Today, multidimensional assessments for frailty are the preferred approach [45, 49–51].

Numerous studies have analyzed similarities and differences among unidimensional scales [52–55], multidimensional scales [56], as well as drawing comparisons between uni- and multidimensional measures [40, 45, 57, 58]. All conclude that comparisons are difficult as each instrument captures a different group of frail individuals. Consequently, in medicine and surgery, the choice between unidimensional and multidimensional frailty assessment really depends on the specific context and goals of assessment, aiming for a balance between simplicity and thoroughness. Healthcare professionals must carefully weigh the pros and cons of each approach based on the needs of individual patients, ensuring that their assessments align with the patient's overall health status and treatment requirements.

Frailty in Cardiac Surgery

Frailty is prevalent in up to 20% of cardiac surgical patients. Patients presenting for cardiac surgery with pre-existing frailty have a greater than 1.5-fold increase in major adverse cardiac events (MACE) and are less likely to have adequate functional recovery [11, 59, 60]. Frailty in cardiac surgery has also been shown to be associated with increased operative and long-term mortality [8, 9, 61], the need for cardiac resuscitation [27, 62], failure to rescue [61, 63], prolonged hospital and intensive care unit stay [8, 62], postoperative delirium [64], surgical site infections [8], nonhome discharge [61, 63], and readmission [27], all of which contribute to markedly increased healthcare resource utilization and expenditure [7].

Compared to other surgical fields, the prevalence of frailty in cardiac surgery is significantly higher [6, 11]. This higher prevalence can be attributed to several factors unique to the cardiac surgery population, including advanced patient age, the presence of multiple acute and/or chronic illnesses, polypharmacy, and higher rates of physical and cognitive impairment at baseline. Together, these factors make cardiac patients more susceptible to functional decline and adverse outcomes, making frailty a much larger problem in the context of cardiac surgery.

Advanced Patient Age

Age-related risks represent a significant challenge in cardiac surgery, where patients are predominantly older [6]. With the fastest-growing demographic worldwide being those over the age of 65, surgical volume in this field is expected to increase dramatically compared to other surgical fields [6, 65]. In the last decade, the number of elderly patients undergoing cardiac surgery has markedly increased [66, 67], with 70% of procedure-based work derived from those ≥65 years of age in the US [6]. Since advanced age is a known risk factor for frailty [68], cardiac surgeons would be well-served to monitor this clinical syndrome by including it as a routine item in the preoperative risk stratification and assessment process.

Multimorbidity

Improved life expectancy [1, 2] has contributed to a growing geriatric population [69] with an increasing burden of multimorbidity [69–72]. The presence of comorbidities in surgical patients complicates surgical decision-making and patient management, owing to risks of adverse operative outcomes and medical costs [69, 73].

While frailty and multimorbidity are two distinct clinical manifestations of age-related processes, they often coexist in the elderly to adversely affect their clinical course and outcomes [74]. This overlap is especially common in cardiac patients who frequently present with hypertension, diabetes, heart failure, hyperlipidemia, chronic kidney disease, arrhythmias, and respiratory conditions [74–80]. The presence of multimorbidity also contributes to overall frailty status, further compromising stress tolerance and successful recovery in an already high-risk population [74, 79, 81].

Surgical Complexity and Technological Advancements

Coronary artery bypass grafting (CABG), valve replacement/repair, and aortic interventions occasionally require periods of cardiac and/or whole body circulatory arrest. These procedures place significant physiological stress on the body and require intensive care as a part of the initial postoperative recovery, especially in frail and elderly individuals [9, 82, 83].

Furthermore, the challenges posed by frailty in cardiac surgery are amplified by continued technological advancements in the field, which have broadened our capacity to treat elderly and more medically compromised individuals. While this offers life-saving opportunities it also results in a surgical candidate pool of much higher risk.

Given the aging population and increasing prevalence of cardiovascular diseases, the importance of frailty in the context of cardiac surgery is growing. By recognizing its unique challenges in this patient population, clinicians and policy makers are made increasingly aware of how frailty disproportionally affects the surgical success and recovery course of cardiac surgery patients as compared to other surgical fields. Identifying and addressing frailty in the preoperative assessment and perioperative care of cardiac surgery patients are therefore essential for improving outcomes and providing personalized, patient-centered care.

Current State-of-the-Art Cardiac Surgery Risk Assessment

While numerous cardiac surgery risk scores are available [84–88], perioperative risk assessment in cardiac surgery primarily relies on the European System for Cardiac Operation Risk Evaluation II (EuroSCORE II) [89] and the Society of Thoracic Surgeons (STS) Predicted Risk of Mortality (PROM) score [90]. As the two most widely used scoring tools [85, 91], both have demonstrated satisfactory ability in predicting perioperative risk [89–91] and guiding patient selection for cardiac surgery [84]. Notably, both of these risks scores perform poorly in elderly patients [84, 85, 92, 93], as they were not comprehensively designed to assess the complex interaction between comorbidities and biological versus physiological aging [8, 94]. This shortcoming is primarily a result of both tools using chronological age, medical diagnoses, and comorbidities [85, 94], and omitting other relevant factors associated with increased risk, particularly frailty and disability [84, 95].

Despite its prognostic importance [7, 66, 84, 85, 96, 97], instruments that measure frailty are not part of routine cardiac surgery risk stratification and have yet to be included in recognized cardiac surgery risk scores [89, 90]. Risk assessment for most cardiac patients are often confounded by other age-related factors [85, 98]. Specifically, the EuroSCORE tends to overestimate mortality at lower score levels (≤ 6), and underestimate mortality at higher scores (>13) [85, 99]. With respect to other perioperative risks (i.e. morbidity), the EuroSCORE strongly overestimates risk in high-risk patients [100, 101], while the STS PROM score slightly underestimates perioperative risk [102].

Recently, there has been growing interest in integrating factors that describe a patient's physiological age [85] to improve risk assessments in patients undergoing cardiac surgery [16, 26, 83, 84]. Recognizing frailty as a component of preoperative risk assessment not only improves risk stratification, but may also identify potentially modifiable factors that can be optimized preoperatively, improving a patient's likelihood of a successful outcome [7, 8, 66, 83, 103].

Challenges of Assessing Frailty in Cardiac Surgery

With literature primarily consisting of only small series, and based on unidimensional frailty instruments [7, 10, 11, 18], the concept of frailty in cardiac surgery is not well established yet. Consequently, little research is available to guide clinicians on frailty management and patient optimization [11].

The clinical frailty scale (CFS) is a validated tool that can be applied to a variety of different clinical settings, including in the perioperative cardiac surgery setting [7, 11, 104, 105]. This tool assigns a score based on a 9-point scale that provides a way to categorize individuals based on their overall health, functioning, and vulnerability to stressors using visual cues [106] (Fig. 37.1). This score can be used together with other relevant clinical data to assist with prognostication and clinical decision-making in the context of perioperative care. The CFS has been found to be as accurate as other frailty instruments in terms of prognostication, but also has higher feasibility and acceptability measures [11, 94, 105]. Other frailty assessment methods used in cardiac surgery include the following: (A) the frailty (or physical frailty) phenotype [46, 107], which looks at the presence of 5 components (Fig. 37.2); (B) the frailty (or deficit-accumulation) index [108, 109], which considers a set of age-related findings; and (C) the Edmonton Frailty Scale [110] assigns a score from 0–2 for 9 domains to determine degree of frailty.

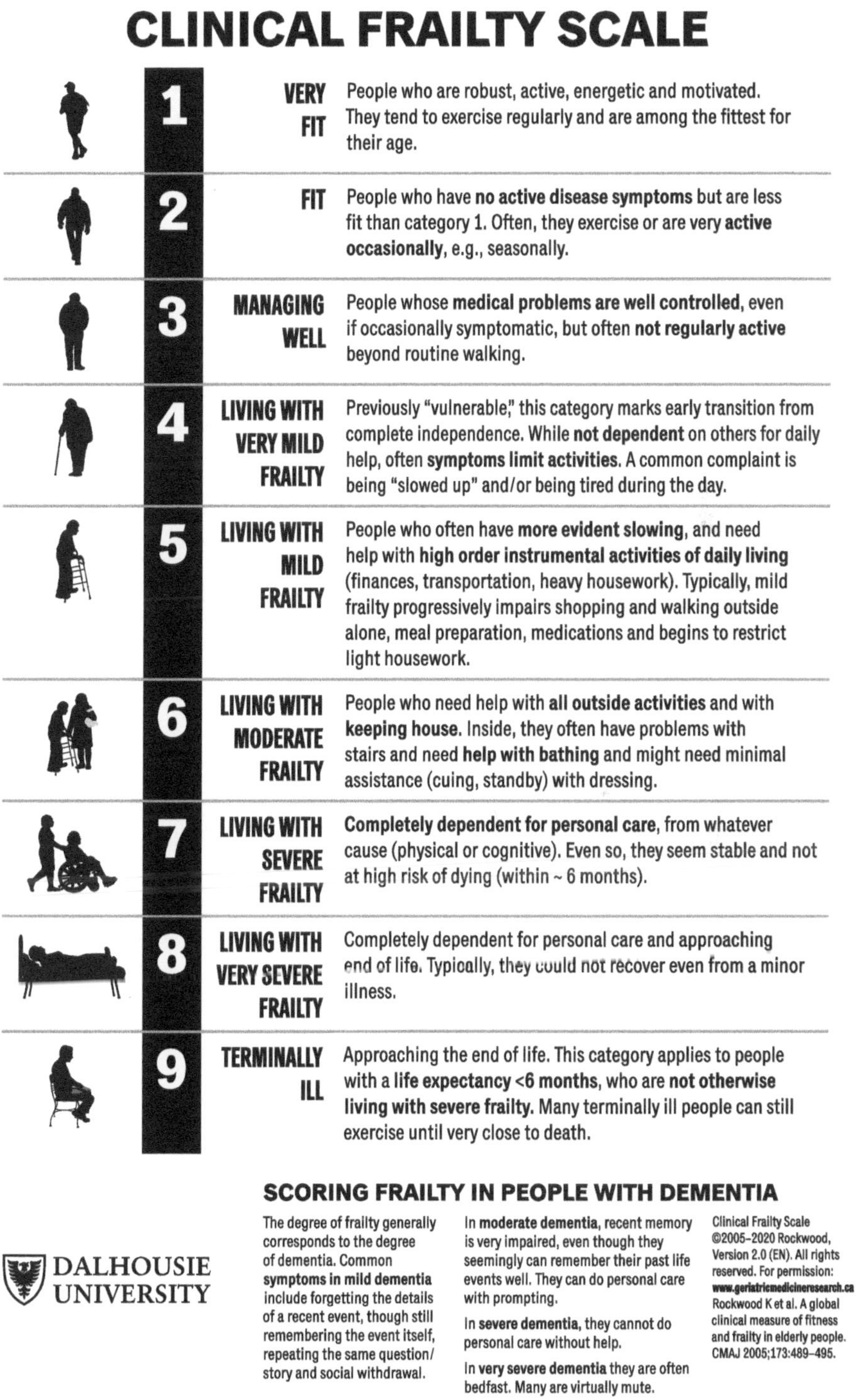
CLINICAL FRAILTY SCALE
1
VERY FIT
People who are robust, active, energetic and motivated. They tend to exercise regularly and are among the fittest for their age.
2
FIT
People who have no active disease symptoms but are less fit than category 1. Often, they exercise or are very active occasionally, e.g., seasonally.
3
MANAGING WELL
People whose medical problems are well controlled, even if occasionally symptomatic, but often not regularly active beyond routine walking.
4
LIVING WITH VERY MILD FRAILTY
Previously "vulnerable," this category marks early transition from complete independence. While not dependent on others for daily help, often symptoms limit activities. A common complaint is being "slowed up" and/or being tired during the day.
5
LIVING WITH MILD FRAILTY
People who often have more evident slowing, and need help with high order instrumental activities of daily living (finances, transportation, heavy housework). Typically, mild frailty progressively impairs shopping and walking outside alone, meal preparation, medications and begins to restrict light housework.
6
LIVING WITH MODERATE FRAILTY
People who need help with all outside activities and with keeping house. Inside, they often have problems with stairs and need help with bathing and might need minimal assistance (cuing, standby) with dressing.
7
LIVING WITH SEVERE FRAILTY
Completely dependent for personal care, from whatever cause (physical or cognitive). Even so, they seem stable and not at high risk of dying (within ~ 6 months).
8
LIVING WITH VERY SEVERE FRAILTY
Completely dependent for personal care and approaching end of life. Typically, they could not recover even from a minor illness.
9
TERMINALLY ILL
Approaching the end of life. This category applies to people with a life expectancy <6 months, who are not otherwise living with severe frailty. Many terminally ill people can still exercise until very close to death.
SCORING FRAILTY IN PEOPLE WITH DEMENTIA
The degree of frailty generally corresponds to the degree of dementia. Common symptoms in mild dementia include forgetting the details of a recent event, though still remembering the event itself, repeating the same question/story and social withdrawal.
In moderate dementia, recent memory is very impaired, even though they seemingly can remember their past life events well. They can do personal care with prompting.
In severe dementia, they cannot do personal care without help.
In very severe dementia they are often bedfast. Many are virtually mute.
Clinical Frailty Scale ©2005–2020 Rockwood, Version 2.0 (EN). All rights reserved. For permission: www.geriatricmedicineresearch.ca
Rockwood K et al. A global clinical measure of fitness and frailty in elderly people. CMAJ 2005;173:489–495.
DALHOUSIE UNIVERSITY

Fig. 37.1 The clinical frailty scale (CFS: version 2.0)
Reproduced with permission from the authors [106]

Frailty Criterion	Definition
Unintentional weight lose	**Meets criteria for weight loss if:** Lost >5% body weight unintentionally in last year, or BMI <18.5kg/m^2 Equipment; scale for body weight; stadiometer for height.
Exhaustion	**Meets criteria for exhaustion if answer:** Felt unusually tired or unusually weak 'all of the time' or 'most of the time' or reported energy level was ≤3, using the following questions. **1.a. "In the past month, on the average, have you been feeling unusually tired during the day?"** Yes □ No □ Refused □ Don't Know □ **1.b. "If yes, have you been feeling unusually tired:"** □ All of the time □ Most of the time □ Some of the time □ Refused / Don't Know **2.a. "In the past month, on the average, have you felt unusually weak?"** Yes □ No □ Refused □ Don't Know □ **2.b. "If yes, have you been feeling weak:"** □ All of the time □ Most of the time □ Some of the time □ Refused / Don't Know **3. "Using the scale below, please rate your usual energy level on a scale from 0 to 10 where 0 is no energy and 10 is the most energy that you have ever had. Please give a number between 0 and 10 that describes your usual energy level while awake in the last month?"** Energy Level: ______
Slowness	**Meets criteria for slow walking speed over 4 meters if:** **Men** ≤0.65m/s for height ≤173 cm (68 inches) ≤0.76m/s for height >173 cm (68 inches) **Women** ≤0.65m/s for height ≤159cm (63 inches) ≤0.76m/s for height >159cm (63 inches) Equipment: 4-meter course, a stopwatch. Participant attempts to walk 4-meter length twice at his or her usual pace. Use average of 2 trials.
Low Activity Level	**Meets criteria for low activity if:** **Men:** <128 kcal of physical expenditure on activity scale per week (6 items[1]) **Women:** <90 kcal of physical expenditure on activity scale per week (6 items[1])
Weekness	**Meets criteria for grip strength weakness if:** **Men** ≤29 kg for BMI ≤24 ≤30 kg for BMI 24.1–26 ≤30 kg for BMI 26.1–28 ≤32 kg for BMI >28 **Women** ≤17 kg for BMI ≤23 ≤17.3 kg for BMI 23.1–26 ≤18 kg for BMI 26.1–29 ≤21 kg for BMI >29 Equipment: (Jamar) hand dynamometer. Participant attempst to squeeze the dynamometer maximally 3 times with the dominant hand. Use maximal score with dominant hand.

[1] Physical activity is based on modified Minnesota Leisure Time Activities Questionnaire, asking about walking (w = 3.5), strenuous household chores (w = 4.5), strenuous outdoor chores (w = 4.5), dancing (w = 5.5), bowling (w = 3.0), and exercise (w = 4.5).
To compute kcals expended per week, use the formula: Kcals (Kilocalories / week) = w * Frequency (sessions per week) * Duration per session (minutes) * Body Weight (kg)/60, where w is the task-specific MET intensity score.

Fig. 37.2 The physical frailty phenotype
Scoring: ≥3/5 criteria met indicates frailty; 1–2/5 indicates pre-or-intermediate frailty; 0/5 indicates non-frail
BMI body mass index, *MET* metabolic equivalent
Reproduced with permission from the authors [46]

Importance of Multidimensional Frailty Instruments

Unidimensional frailty assessments like the frailty phenotype can provide a quick snapshot of a patient's physical capabilities [40, 46], helping surgeons determine their readiness for a procedure. For instance, assessing a patient's ability to perform daily activities like walking and climbing stairs can give insight into their recovery potential. However, relying solely on this information might neglect other factors that could influence surgical outcomes, such as cognitive function or social support [47, 104, 111]. By incorporating multiple domains, multidimensional frailty instruments provide a more comprehensive assessment of a patient's frailty status, aiding surgeons in making better informed surgical decisions and more personalized postoperative care plans [7, 10].

Choosing Which Tool to Use

While agreement exists that frailty measurements in surgery should be operationalized using a multidimensional approach [7, 11, 45, 112], each scale predicts best certain outcomes and exhibits weaknesses regarding others, suffering from some degree of outcome-dependence [7, 109, 117] (Figs. 37.3 and 37.4).

Characteristic	PACE, No. (%) (n = 20 387)	No PACE, No. (%) (n = 68 069)	HR (95% CI)	P value
ACG	4621 (22.7)	10 314 (15.2)	1.66 (1.60-1.71)	<.001
HFRS				
Score per 0.1 unit, mean (SD)	4.7 (5.1)	2.8 (3.8)	1.10 (1.09-1.10)	<.001
0.1-2.0	4162 (20.4)	17 604 (25.9)	1.29 (1.23-1.34)	<.001
2.1-5.0	5340 (26.2)	16 496 (24.2)	1.81 (1.74-1.89)	<.001
≥5.1	6960 (34.1)	12 533 (18.4)	3.30 (3.17-3.43)	<.001
PFI				
Score per 0.1 unit, mean (SD)	0.16 (0.09)	0.12 (0.08)	1.75 (1.73-1.78)	<.001
0.05-0.10	4317 (21.2)	20 367 (29.9)	1.76 (1.65-1.87)	<.001
0.11-0.20	8252 (40.5)	24 859 (36.5)	2.79 (2.63-2.96)	<.001
0.21-0.44	6497 (31.9)	12 362 (18.2)	4.84 (4.55-5.14)	<.001
0.45-1.00	48 (0.2)	52 (0.1)	10.39 (7.79-13.86)	<.001

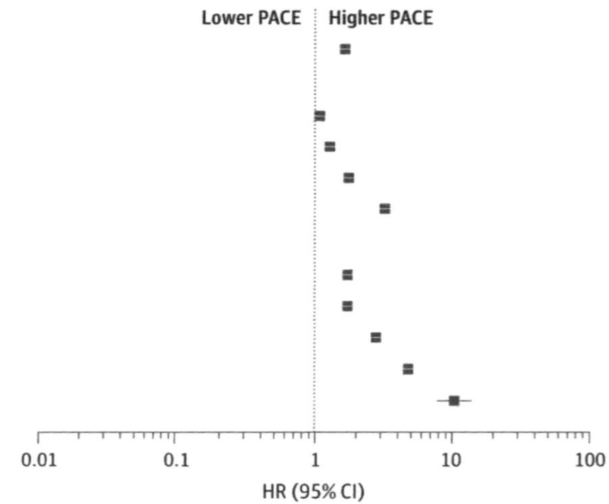

Fig. 37.3 Unadjusted cumulative incidence and hazard ratios of patient-defined adverse cardiovascular and noncardiovascular events for each frailty instrument
Patients meeting ACG criteria (HR, 1.66) and those with higher HFRS (HR, 1.10) and PFI scores (HR, 1.75) had higher rates of PACE. A p-value of <0.05 was considered statistically significant
ACG Johns Hopkins Adjusted Clinical Groups, *CI* confidence intervals, *HFRS* hospital frailty risk score, *HR* hazard ratios, *PACE* patient-defined adverse cardiovascular and noncardiovascular events, *PFI* preoperative frailty index, *SD* standard deviation
Reproduced with permission from the authors [7]

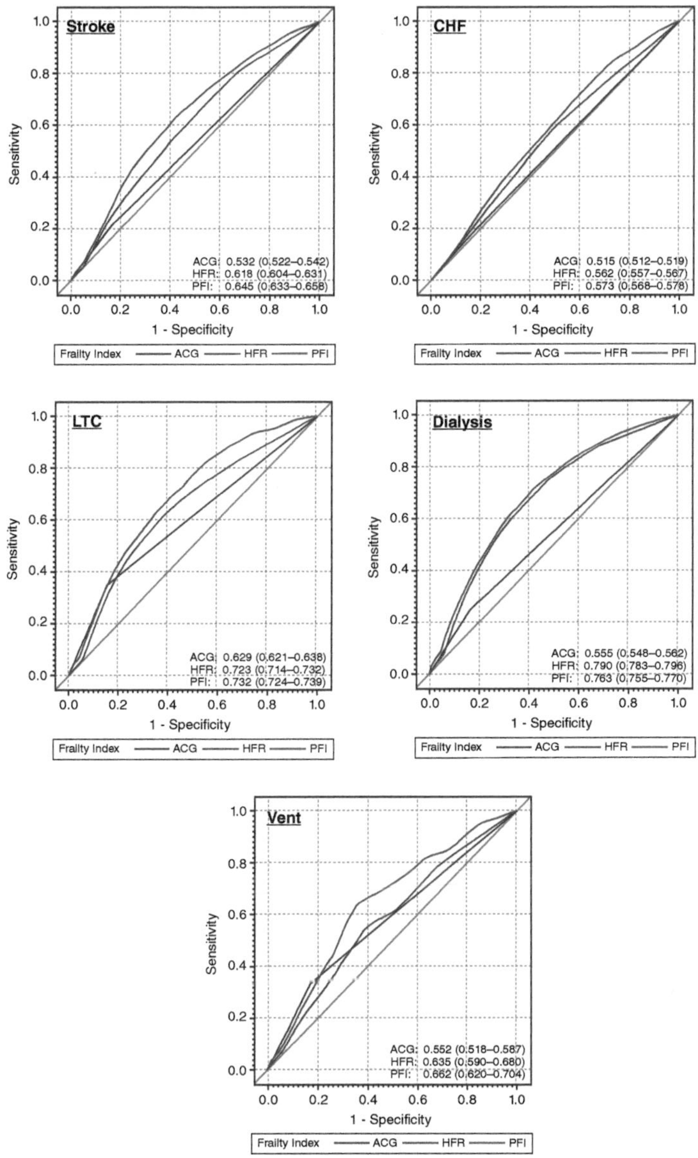

Fig. 37.4 Unadjusted receiver-operating characteristic curves for the prediction of individual PACE events according to each of the frailty instruments
The predictive accuracy on individual postoperative outcomes, in patients undergoing cardiac surgery, varies depending on the frailty instrument used. As highlighted by Sun et al. [7], this outcome-specific variability can assist clinicians in selecting the most suitable frailty screening tool that provides the most accurate outcome-specific risk assessment to patients
ACG Johns Hopkins adjusted clinical groups, *CHF* congestive heart failure, *HFR* hospital frailty risk score, *LTC* long-term care admission, *PACE* patient-defined adverse cardiovascular and non-cardiovascular events, *PFI* preoperative frailty index, *Vent* ventilator dependence
Reproduced with permission from the authors [7]

Time-Dependence

Moreover, the time-dependent nature of frailty tools on postoperative outcome predictions in cardiac surgery patients as recognized by Sun et al. [7] adds an additional layer of complexity to its assessment. Demonstrating time-varying ability of different frailty tools to estimate patient-centered outcomes (Fig. 37.5), the authors concluded that the choice of frailty instrument should be made according to a specific outcome and the desired follow-up duration [7].

Recognizing this time-dependent component is crucial in accurately capturing and monitoring changes in frailty status, enabling healthcare professionals to tailor interventions and optimize patient care accordingly.

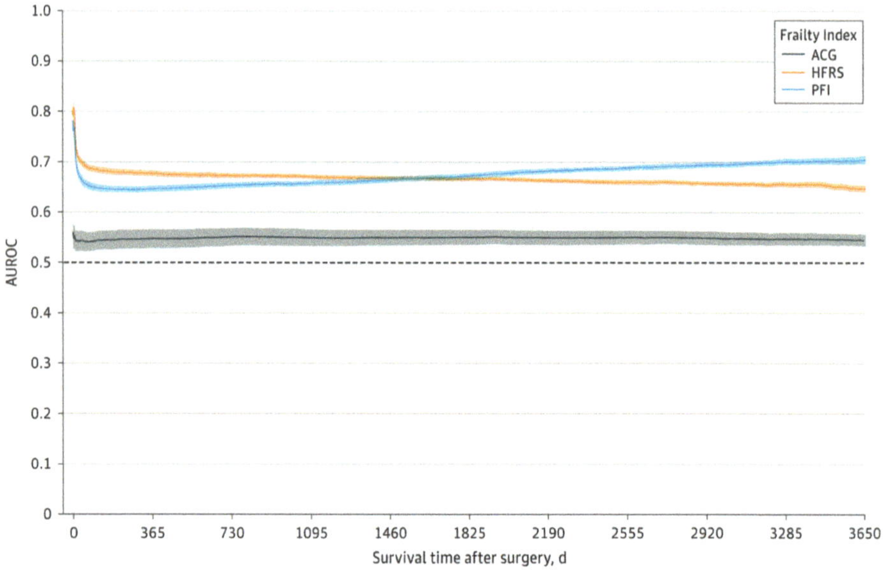

Fig. 37.5 Plot of unadjusted area under the receiver-operating characteristic curves over time for the estimation of patient-defined adverse cardiovascular and noncardiovascular events
Shaded areas represent 95% CI
Performance of different frailty instruments vary over time. The HFRS outperformed the PFI for the estimation of death up to 2 years after cardiac surgery (not depicted) and PACE up to 4 years, after which the PFI performed better as demonstrated above. This time-varying ability could be used to tailor the choice of frailty instrument according to a desired follow-up duration. The consistent poor long-term performance of the ACG indicator is likely attributed to its dichotomic nature*ACG* Johns Hopkins adjusted clinical groups, *AUROC* areas under the receiver-operating characteristic, *CI* confidence intervals, *d* days, *HFRS* hospital frailty risk score, *PACE* patient-defined adverse cardiovascular and noncardiovascular events, *PFI* preoperative frailty index
Reproduced with permission from the authors [7]

Future Directions

In an aging population, the number of frail older adults that undergo cardiac interventions is abound [7, 61, 97]. As such, it is important to focus on the early indicators of future age-related adverse events [45]. Recognizing the substantial impact of frailty on clinical outcomes in this patient demographic, there is a need for additional research to deepen our understanding of the most effective ways to incorporate frailty assessments into perioperative evaluations and optimization strategies. This integration should be done in a meaningful manner that ultimately enhances patient outcomes.

First and foremost, more studies comparing scales like the one conducted by Sun et al. [7] are advised. Since choice of frailty tool used can impact both the "composition" (i.e., different instruments capture different phenotypes) and prevalence of frailty detected (i.e., who is being diagnosed with frailty) [7, 45, 60, 85, 104], more scales and more clinical contexts need to be scrutinized [7, 113]. Without a "Gold Standard" definition to evaluate frailty, large outcome-based clinical trials cannot be completed.

Aforementioned, frailty is a dynamic condition rather than a permanent state [16, 114, 115], where individuals may transition between various stages. For instance, they may move from prefrailty to frailty [116], or even shift in and out of being classified as frail [16]. For this reason, it is recommended that most frailty assessments be done based on a patient's status 2 weeks prior to surgery [117]. Unfortunately, little is known about the epidemiology of these transitions, or the driving factors behind reversing frailty [115], highlighting a potential avenue for future research.

Irrespective of the tool used, the presence of frailty presents several opportunities for perioperative optimization. The identification of preoperative physical decline may allow a window of opportunity for exercise prehabilitation [118–120], and those with diagnoses of malnutrition can trigger nutritional supplementation [121]. Patients with prexisting dementia or cognitive dysfunction may benefit from programs such as the Hospital Elder Life Program to reduce the rates of delirium after surgery [122].

Prehabilitation as a New Frontier

There is extensive research data to suggest the presence of a significant progressive functional and physical decline in patients awaiting cardiac surgery [123]. Preoperative rehabilitation (or "prehabilitation") refers to a comprehensive home-based or inpatient program which aims to optimize outcomes in frail preoperative patients [124]. In a cardiac surgery setting, this concept refers to specific preventative measures and interventions to mitigate negative outcomes during the perioperative period [125, 126]. Prehabilitation is primarily composed of physical exercises (both aerobic and anerobic) but also often includes a multidisciplinary team approach with components of medical, psychological, lifestyle modification, and nutritional support. Frailty assessment is of utmost importance and plays a significant role in determining eligibility for prehabilitation [123–126]. Individuals who are motivated and awaiting an elective cardiac surgery that is several weeks or months away and are mild to moderately frail (i.e. a clinical frailty score of 4–6) would likely benefit from a prehabilitation program [127]. Geriatric syndromes such as falls, polypharmacy, cognitive impairment, and malnutrition are common with frailty [127] and could benefit from anesthesia and geriatric assessment for medical and physical optimization prior to surgery.

Conclusion

In conclusion, frailty represents a significant challenge in the field of cardiac surgery. Multidimensional frailty instruments offer a more comprehensive and robust approach to assessing frailty and should be considered the standard approach to assessing frailty in these patients. Additionally, understanding the time-dependent outcomes of frailty is crucial in capturing the dynamic nature of this condition. By recognizing and addressing these challenges, healthcare professionals can better identify frail patients, optimize care, outcomes and quality of life after cardiac surgery.

References

1. Max Roser EO-OaHR. Life expectancy. Our world in data. January 9th 2022, 2013
2. Divo MJ, Martinez CH, Mannino DM. Ageing and the epidemiology of multimorbidity. Eur Respir J. 2014;44(4):1055–68. https://doi.org/10.1183/09031936.00059814.
3. Ford ES, Capewell S. Proportion of the decline in cardiovascular mortality disease due to prevention versus treatment: public health versus clinical care. Annu Rev Public Health. 2011;32:5–22. https://doi.org/10.1146/annurev-publhealth-031210-101211.
4. Vos T, Lim SS, Abbafati C, et al. Global burden of 369 diseases and injuries in 204 countries and territories, 1990–2013; 2019: a systematic analysis for the global burden of disease study 2019. Lancet. 2020;396(10258):1204–22. https://doi.org/10.1016/S0140-6736(20)30925-9.
5. Ritchie H, Spooner F, Roser M. Causes of death. Our world in data; 2018.
6. Etzioni DA, Liu JH, Maggard MA, Ko CY. The aging population and its impact on the surgery workforce. Ann Surg. 2003;238(2):170–7. https://doi.org/10.1097/01.SLA.0000081085.98792.3d.
7. Sun LY, Jabagi H, Fang J, Lee DS. Comparison of multidimensional frailty instruments for estimation of long-term patient-centered outcomes after cardiac surgery. JAMA Netw Open. 2022;5(9):e2230959–9. https://doi.org/10.1001/jamanetworkopen.2022.30959.
8. Tran DTT, Tu JV, Dupuis JY, Eddeen AB, Sun LY. Association of frailty and long-term survival in patients undergoing coronary artery bypass grafting. J Am Heart Assoc. 2018;7(15):e009882. https://doi.org/10.1161/JAHA.118.009882.

9. Lee DH, Buth KJ, Martin B-J, Yip AM, Hirsch GM. Frail patients are at increased risk for mortality and prolonged institutional care after cardiac surgery. Circulation. 2010;121(8):973–8. https://doi.org/10.1161/CIRCULATIONAHA.108.841437.
10. Kim DH, Kim CA, Placide S, Lipsitz LA, Marcantonio ER. Preoperative frailty assessment and outcomes at 6 months or later in older adults undergoing cardiac surgical procedures: a systematic review. Ann Intern Med. 2016;165(9):650–60. https://doi.org/10.7326/m16-0652.
11. McIsaac DI, Fottinger A, Sucha E, McDonald B. Association of frailty with days alive at home after cardiac surgery: a population-based cohort study. Br J Anaesth. 2021;126(6):1103–10. https://doi.org/10.1016/j.bja.2021.02.011.
12. Rockwood K, Song X, MacKnight C, et al. A global clinical measure of fitness and frailty in elderly people. Can Med Assoc J. 2005;173(5):489–95. https://doi.org/10.1503/cmaj.050051.
13. O'Caoimh R, Sezgin D, O'Donovan MR, et al. Prevalence of frailty in 62 countries across the world: a systematic review and meta-analysis of population-level studies. Age Ageing. 2021;50(1):96–104. https://doi.org/10.1093/ageing/afaa219.
14. Turner G, Clegg A. Best practice guidelines for the management of frailty: a British geriatrics society, age UK and Royal College of general practitioners report. Age Ageing. 2014;43(6):744–7. https://doi.org/10.1093/ageing/afu138.
15. Mielke N, Schneider A, Huscher D, Ebert N, Schaeffner E. Gender differences in frailty transition and its prediction in community-dwelling old adults. Sci Rep. 2022;12(1):7341. https://doi.org/10.1038/s41598-022-11358-7.
16. Ofori-Asenso R, Chin KL, Mazidi M, et al. Global incidence of frailty and prefrailty among community-dwelling older adults: a systematic review and meta-analysis. JAMA Netw Open. 2019;2(8):e198398. https://doi.org/10.1001/jamanetworkopen.2019.8398.
17. Ritt M, Ritt JI, Sieber CC, Gaßmann KG. Comparing the predictive accuracy of frailty, comorbidity, and disability for mortality: a 1-year follow-up in patients hospitalized in geriatric wards. Clin Interv Aging. 2017;12:293–304. https://doi.org/10.2147/cia.S124342.
18. Fried LP, Ferrucci L, Darer J, Williamson JD, Anderson G. Untangling the concepts of disability, frailty, and comorbidity: implications for improved targeting and care. J Gerontol A Biol Sci Med Sci. 2004;59(3):255–63. https://doi.org/10.1093/gerona/59.3.m255.
19. Chen X, Mao G, Leng SX. Frailty syndrome: an overview. Clin Interv Aging. 2014;9:433–41. https://doi.org/10.2147/cia.S45300.
20. Cheng MH, Chang SF. Frailty as a risk factor for falls among community dwelling people: evidence from a meta-analysis. J Nurs Scholarsh. 2017;49(5):529–36. https://doi.org/10.1111/jnu.12322.
21. Persico I, Cesari M, Morandi A, et al. Frailty and delirium in older adults: a systematic review and meta-analysis of the literature. J Am Geriatr Soc. 2018;66(10):2022–30. https://doi.org/10.1111/jgs.15503.
22. Kojima G. Frailty as a predictor of nursing home placement among community-dwelling older adults: a systematic review and meta-analysis. J Geriatr Phys Ther. 2018;41(1):42–8. https://doi.org/10.1519/jpt.0000000000000097.
23. Kojima G, Iliffe S, Walters K. Frailty index as a predictor of mortality: a systematic review and meta-analysis. Age Ageing. 2018;47(2):193–200. https://doi.org/10.1093/ageing/afx162.
24. Dent E, Kowal P, Hoogendijk EO. Frailty measurement in research and clinical practice: a review. Eur J Intern Med. 2016;31:3–10. https://doi.org/10.1016/j.ejim.2016.03.007.
25. Collard RM, Boter H, Schoevers RA, Oude Voshaar RC. Prevalence of frailty in community-dwelling older persons: a systematic review. J Am Geriatr Soc. 2012;60(8):1487–92. https://doi.org/10.1111/j.1532-5415.2012.04054.x.
26. Lin H-S, Watts JN, Peel NM, Hubbard RE. Frailty and post-operative outcomes in older surgical patients: a systematic review. BMC Geriatr. 2016;16(1):157. https://doi.org/10.1186/s12877-016-0329-8.
27. McIsaac DI, Beaulé PE, Bryson GL, Van Walraven C. The impact of frailty on outcomes and healthcare resource usage after total joint arthroplasty: a population-based cohort study. Bone Joint J. 2016;98-b(6):799–805. https://doi.org/10.1302/0301-620x.98b6.37124.

28. Nieman CL, Pitman KT, Tufaro AP, Eisele DW, Frick KD, Gourin CG. The effect of frailty on short-term outcomes after head and neck cancer surgery. Laryngoscope. 2018;128(1):102–10. https://doi.org/10.1002/lary.26735.
29. Karam J, Tsiouris A, Shepard A, Velanovich V, Rubinfeld I. Simplified frailty index to predict adverse outcomes and mortality in vascular surgery patients. Ann Vasc Surg. 2013;27(7):904–8. https://doi.org/10.1016/j.avsg.2012.09.015.
30. Li Y, Pederson JL, Churchill TA, et al. Impact of frailty on outcomes after discharge in older surgical patients: a prospective cohort study. CMAJ. 2018;190(7):E184–e190. https://doi.org/10.1503/cmaj.161403.
31. Tsiouris A, Hammoud ZT, Velanovich V, Hodari A, Borgi J, Rubinfeld I. A modified frailty index to assess morbidity and mortality after lobectomy. J Surg Res. 2013;183(1):40–6. https://doi.org/10.1016/j.jss.2012.11.059.
32. Shinall MC Jr, Arya S, Youk A, et al. Association of preoperative patient frailty and operative stress with postoperative mortality. JAMA Surg. 2020;155(1):e194620. https://doi.org/10.1001/jamasurg.2019.4620.
33. Seib CD, Rochefort H, Chomsky-Higgins K, et al. Association of patient frailty with increased morbidity after common ambulatory general surgery operations. JAMA Surg. 2018;153(2):160–8. https://doi.org/10.1001/jamasurg.2017.4007.
34. Kojima G. Frailty as a predictor of emergency department utilization among community-dwelling older people: a systematic review and meta-analysis. J Am Med Dir Assoc. 2019;20(1):103–5. https://doi.org/10.1016/j.jamda.2018.10.004.
35. Bock J-O, König H-H, Brenner H, et al. Associations of frailty with health care costs—results of the ESTHER cohort study. BMC Health Serv Res. 2016;16(1):128. https://doi.org/10.1186/s12913-016-1360-3.
36. Gwyther H, Shaw R, Dauden E-AJ, et al. Understanding frailty: a qualitative study of European healthcare policy-makers' approaches to frailty screening and management. BMJ Open. 2018;8(1):e018653. https://doi.org/10.1136/bmjopen-2017-018653.
37. Lekan DA, Collins SK, Hayajneh AA. Definitions of frailty in qualitative research: a qualitative systematic review. J Aging Res. 2021;2021:6285058. https://doi.org/10.1155/2021/6285058.
38. Sobhani A, Fadayevatan R, Sharifi F, et al. The conceptual and practical definitions of frailty in older adults: a systematic review. J Diabetes Metab Disord. 2021;20(2):1975–2013. https://doi.org/10.1007/s40200-021-00897-x.
39. Rockwood K, Fox RA, Stolee P, Robertson D, Beattie BL. Frailty in elderly people: an evolving concept. CMAJ. 1994;150(4):489–95.
40. Van der Elst MCJ, Schoenmakers B, Op het Veld LPM, et al. Concordances and differences between a unidimensional and multidimensional assessment of frailty: a cross-sectional study. BMC Geriatr. 2019;19(1):346. https://doi.org/10.1186/s12877-019-1369-7.
41. Ambagtsheer RC, Beilby JJ, Visvanathan R, Dent E, Yu S, Braunack-Mayer AJ. Should we screen for frailty in primary care settings? A fresh perspective on the frailty evidence base: a narrative review. Prev Med. 2019;119:63–9. https://doi.org/10.1016/j.ypmed.2018.12.020.
42. Gobbens RJJ, Luijkx KG, Wijnen-Sponselee MT, Schols JMGA. In search of an integral conceptual definition of frailty: opinions of experts. J Am Med Dir Assoc. 2010;11(5):338–43. https://doi.org/10.1016/j.jamda.2009.09.015.
43. de Vries NM, Staal JB, van Ravensberg CD, Hobbelen JSM, Olde Rikkert MGM, Nijhuis-van der Sanden MWG. Outcome instruments to measure frailty: a systematic review. Ageing Res Rev. 2011;10(1):104–14. https://doi.org/10.1016/j.arr.2010.09.001.
44. Sternberg SA, Wershof Schwartz A, Karunananthan S, Bergman H, Mark CA. The identification of frailty: a systematic literature review. J Am Geriatr Soc. 2011;59(11):2129–38. https://doi.org/10.1111/j.1532-5415.2011.03597.x.
45. Roppolo M, Mulasso A, Gobbens RJ, Mosso CO, Rabaglietti E. A comparison between uni- and multidimensional frailty measures: prevalence, functional status, and relationships with disability. Clin Interv Aging. 2015;10:1669–78. https://doi.org/10.2147/cia.S92328.

46. Fried LP, Tangen CM, Walston J, et al. Frailty in older adults: evidence for a phenotype. J Gerontol A Biol Sci Med Sci. 2001;56(3):M146–56. https://doi.org/10.1093/gerona/56.3.m146.
47. Gobbens RJJ, van Assen MALM, Luijkx KG, Wijnen-Sponselee MT, Schols JMGA. The Tilburg frailty indicator: psychometric properties. J Am Med Dir Assoc. 2010;11(5):344–55. https://doi.org/10.1016/j.jamda.2009.11.003.
48. De Witte N, Gobbens R, De Donder L, et al. The comprehensive frailty assessment instrument: development, validity and reliability. Geriatr Nurs. 2013;34(4):274–81. https://doi.org/10.1016/j.gerinurse.2013.03.002.
49. Walston J, Hadley EC, Ferrucci L, et al. Research agenda for frailty in older adults: toward a better understanding of physiology and etiology: summary from the American Geriatrics Society/National Institute on Aging research conference on frailty in older adults. J Am Geriatr Soc. 2006;54(6):991–1001. https://doi.org/10.1111/j.1532-5415.2006.00745.x.
50. Gobbens RJ, Luijkx KG, Wijnen-Sponselee MT, Schols JM. Towards an integral conceptual model of frailty. J Nutr Health Aging. 2010;14(3):175–81. https://doi.org/10.1007/s12603-010-0045-6.
51. Markle-Reid M, Browne G. Conceptualizations of frailty in relation to older adults. J Adv Nurs. 2003;44(1):58–68. https://doi.org/10.1046/j.1365-2648.2003.02767.x.
52. Cigolle CT, Ofstedal MB, Tian Z, Blaum CS. Comparing models of frailty: the health and retirement study. J Am Geriatr Soc. 2009;57(5):830–9. https://doi.org/10.1111/j.1532-5415.2009.02225.x.
53. Ensrud KE, Ewing SK, Cawthon PM, et al. A comparison of frailty indexes for the prediction of falls, disability, fractures, and mortality in older men. J Am Geriatr Soc. 2009;57(3):492–8. https://doi.org/10.1111/j.1532-5415.2009.02137.x.
54. Ensrud KE, Ewing SK, Taylor BC, et al. Comparison of 2 frailty indexes for prediction of falls, disability, fractures, and death in older women. Arch Intern Med. 2008;168(4):382–9. https://doi.org/10.1001/archinternmed.2007.113.
55. Woo J, Leung J, Morley JE. Comparison of frailty indicators based on clinical phenotype and the multiple deficit approach in predicting mortality and physical limitation. J Am Geriatr Soc. 2012;60(8):1478–86. https://doi.org/10.1111/j.1532-5415.2012.04074.x.
56. Metzelthin SF, Daniëls R, van Rossum E, de Witte L, van den Heuvel WJ, Kempen GI. The psychometric properties of three self-report screening instruments for identifying frail older people in the community. BMC Public Health. 2010;10:176. https://doi.org/10.1186/1471-2458-10-176.
57. Pilotto A, Rengo F, Marchionni N, et al. Comparing the prognostic accuracy for all-cause mortality of frailty instruments: a multicentre 1-year follow-up in hospitalized older patients. PLoS One. 2012;7(1):e29090. https://doi.org/10.1371/journal.pone.0029090.
58. Hoogendijk EO, van der Horst HE, Deeg DJ, et al. The identification of frail older adults in primary care: comparing the accuracy of five simple instruments. Age Ageing. 2013;42(2):262–5. https://doi.org/10.1093/ageing/afs163.
59. Lytwyn J, Stammers AN, Kehler DS, et al. The impact of frailty on functional survival in patients 1 year after cardiac surgery. J Thorac Cardiovasc Surg. 2017;154(6):1990–9. https://doi.org/10.1016/j.jtcvs.2017.06.040.
60. Sündermann SH, Dademasch A, Seifert B, et al. Frailty is a predictor of short- and mid-term mortality after elective cardiac surgery independently of age†. Interact Cardiovasc Thorac Surg. 2014;18(5):580–5. https://doi.org/10.1093/icvts/ivu006.
61. Lee JA, Yanagawa B, An KR, et al. Frailty and pre-frailty in cardiac surgery: a systematic review and meta-analysis of 66,448 patients. J Cardiothorac Surg. 2021;16(1):184. https://doi.org/10.1186/s13019-021-01541-8.
62. Ad N, Holmes SD, Halpin L, Shuman DJ, Miller CE, Lamont D. The effects of frailty in patients undergoing elective cardiac surgery. J Card Surg. 2016;31(4):187–94. https://doi.org/10.1111/jocs.12699.

63. Dewan KC, Navale SM, Hirji SA, et al. The role of frailty in failure to rescue after cardiovascular surgery. Ann Thorac Surg. 2021;111(2):472–8. https://doi.org/10.1016/j.athoracsur.2020.06.065.
64. Jung P, Pereira MA, Hiebert B, et al. The impact of frailty on postoperative delirium in cardiac surgery patients. J Thorac Cardiovasc Surg. 2015;149(3):869–75. https://doi.org/10.1016/j.jtcvs.2014.10.118.
65. Tonelli CM, Ringhouse BJ, Bunn C, Luchette FA. The impact of the aging population on surgical diseases. Curr Geriatr Rep. 2021;10(1):21–31. https://doi.org/10.1007/s13670-020-00352-4.
66. Furukawa H, Tanemoto K. Frailty in cardiothoracic surgery: systematic review of the literature. Gen Thorac Cardiovasc Surg. 2015;63(8):425–33. https://doi.org/10.1007/s11748-015-0553-8.
67. Alexander KP, Newby LK, Cannon CP, et al. Acute coronary care in the elderly. Part I. Circulation. 2007;115(19):2549–69. https://doi.org/10.1161/CIRCULATIONAHA.107.182615.
68. Pegorari MS, Tavares DM. Factors associated with the frailty syndrome in elderly individuals living in the urban area. Rev Lat Am Enfermagem. 2014;22(5):874–82. https://doi.org/10.1590/0104-1169.0213.2493.
69. McManus DD, Nguyen HL, Saczynski JS, Tisminetzky M, Bourell P, Goldberg RJ. Multiple cardiovascular comorbidities and acute myocardial infarction: temporal trends (1990–2007) and impact on death rates at 30 days and 1 year. Clin Epidemiol. 2012;4:115–23. https://doi.org/10.2147/clep.S30883.
70. Vogeli C, Shields AE, Lee TA, et al. Multiple chronic conditions: prevalence, health consequences, and implications for quality, care management, and costs. J Gen Intern Med. 2007;22(Suppl 3):391–5. https://doi.org/10.1007/s11606-007-0322-1.
71. Uijen AA, van de Lisdonk EH. Multimorbidity in primary care: prevalence and trend over the last 20 years. Eur J Gen Pract. 2008;14(Suppl 1):28–32. https://doi.org/10.1080/13814780802436093.
72. Parekh AK, Barton MB. The challenge of multiple comorbidity for the US health care system. JAMA. 2010;303(13):1303–4. https://doi.org/10.1001/jama.2010.381.
73. Marengoni A, Rizzuto D, Wang HX, Winblad B, Fratiglioni L. Patterns of chronic multimorbidity in the elderly population. J Am Geriatr Soc. 2009;57(2):225–30. https://doi.org/10.1111/j.1532-5415.2008.02109.x.
74. Murad K, Kitzman DW. Frailty and multiple comorbidities in the elderly patient with heart failure: implications for management. Heart Fail Rev. 2012;17(4–5):581–8. https://doi.org/10.1007/s10741-011-9258-y.
75. Pálsson R, Patel UD. Cardiovascular complications of diabetic kidney disease. Adv Chronic Kidney Dis. 2014;21(3):273–80. https://doi.org/10.1053/j.ackd.2014.03.003.
76. Matsushita K, van der Velde M, Astor BC, et al. Association of estimated glomerular filtration rate and albuminuria with all-cause and cardiovascular mortality in general population cohorts: a collaborative meta-analysis. Lancet. 2010;375(9731):2073–81. https://doi.org/10.1016/s0140-6736(10)60674-5.
77. Sarnak MJ, Levey AS, Schoolwerth AC, et al. Kidney disease as a risk factor for development of cardiovascular disease: a statement from the American Heart Association councils on kidney in cardiovascular disease, high blood pressure research, clinical cardiology, and epidemiology and prevention. Circulation. 2003;108(17):2154–69. https://doi.org/10.1161/01.Cir.0000095676.90936.80.
78. Mikus E, Calvi S, Albertini A, et al. Impact of comorbidities on older patients undergoing open heart surgery. J Cardiovasc Med (Hagerstown). 2022;23(5):318–24. https://doi.org/10.2459/jcm.0000000000001296.
79. Clough RA, Leavitt BJ, Morton JR, et al. The effect of comorbid illness on mortality outcomes in cardiac surgery. Arch Surg. 2002;137(4):428–33. https://doi.org/10.1001/archsurg.137.4.428.

80. Boyd CM, Darer J, Boult C, Fried LP, Boult L, Wu AW. Clinical practice guidelines and quality of care for older patients with multiple comorbid diseases: implications for pay for performance. JAMA. 2005;294(6):716–24. https://doi.org/10.1001/jama.294.6.716.
81. Sachdev M, Sun JL, Tsiatis AA, Nelson CL, Mark DB, Jollis JG. The prognostic importance of comorbidity for mortality in patients with stable coronary artery disease. J Am Coll Cardiol. 2004;43(4):576–82. https://doi.org/10.1016/j.jacc.2003.10.031.
82. Yanagawa B, Graham MM, Afilalo J, Hassan A, Arora RC. Frailty as a risk predictor in cardiac surgery: beyond the eyeball test. J Thorac Cardiovasc Surg. 2018;156(1):172–6. https://doi.org/10.1016/j.jtcvs.2018.01.103.
83. Partridge JSL, Harari D, Dhesi JK. Frailty in the older surgical patient: a review. Age Ageing. 2012;41(2):142–7. https://doi.org/10.1093/ageing/afr182.
84. Afilalo J, Mottillo S, Eisenberg MJ, et al. Addition of frailty and disability to cardiac surgery risk scores identifies elderly patients at high risk of mortality or major morbidity. Circ Cardiovasc Qual Outcomes. 2012;5(2):222–8. https://doi.org/10.1161/CIRCOUTCOMES.111.963157.
85. Sündermann S, Dademasch A, Praetorius J, et al. Comprehensive assessment of frailty for elderly high-risk patients undergoing cardiac surgery. Eur J Cardiothorac Surg. 2011;39(1):33–7. https://doi.org/10.1016/j.ejcts.2010.04.013.
86. Nilsson J, Algotsson L, Höglund P, Lührs C, Brandt J. Comparison of 19 pre-operative risk stratification models in open-heart surgery. Eur Heart J. 2006;27(7):867–74. https://doi.org/10.1093/eurheartj/ehi720.
87. Granton J, Cheng D. Risk stratification models for cardiac surgery. Semin Cardiothorac Vasc Anesth. 2008;12(3):167–74. https://doi.org/10.1177/1089253208323681.
88. Hannan EL, Wu C, Bennett EV, et al. Risk stratification of in-hospital mortality for coronary artery bypass graft surgery. J Am Coll Cardiol. 2006;47(3):661–8. https://doi.org/10.1016/j.jacc.2005.10.057.
89. Nashef SAM, Roques F, Sharples LD, et al. EuroSCORE II. Eur J Cardiothorac Surg. 2012;41(4):734–45. https://doi.org/10.1093/ejcts/ezs043.
90. Shahian DM, Jacobs JP, Badhwar V, et al. The Society of Thoracic Surgeons 2018 adult cardiac surgery risk models: Part I—Background, design considerations, and model development. Ann Thorac Surg. 2018;105(5):1411–8. https://doi.org/10.1016/j.athoracsur.2018.03.002.
91. Ad N, Holmes SD, Patel J, Pritchard G, Shuman DJ, Halpin L. Comparison of EuroSCORE II, original EuroSCORE, and the Society of Thoracic Surgeons risk score in cardiac surgery patients. Ann Thorac Surg. 2016;102(2):573–9. https://doi.org/10.1016/j.athoracsur.2016.01.105.
92. Leontyev S, Walther T, Borger MA, et al. Aortic valve replacement in octogenarians: utility of risk stratification with EuroSCORE. Ann Thorac Surg. 2009;87(5):1440–5. https://doi.org/10.1016/j.athoracsur.2009.01.057.
93. Speziale G, Nasso G, Barattoni MC, et al. Operative and middle-term results of cardiac surgery in nonagenarians. Circulation. 2010;121(2):208–13. https://doi.org/10.1161/CIRCULATIONAHA.108.807065.
94. Sepehri A, Beggs T, Hassan A, et al. The impact of frailty on outcomes after cardiac surgery: a systematic review. J Thorac Cardiovasc Surg. 2014;148(6):3110–7. https://doi.org/10.1016/j.jtcvs.2014.07.087.
95. Green P, Woglom Abigail E, Genereux P, et al. The impact of frailty status on survival after transcatheter aortic valve replacement in older adults with severe aortic stenosis. JACC: Cardiovasc Intervent. 2012;5(9):974–81. https://doi.org/10.1016/j.jcin.2012.06.011.
96. Arenaza DP, Pepper J, Lees B, et al. Preoperative 6-minute walk test adds prognostic information to Euroscore in patients undergoing aortic valve replacement. Heart. 2010;96(2):113. https://doi.org/10.1136/hrt.2008.161174.
97. Sun LY, Spence SD, Benton S, et al. Age, not sex, modifies the effect of frailty on long-term outcomes after cardiac surgery. Ann Surg. 2022;275(4):800–6. https://doi.org/10.1097/sla.0000000000004060.

98. Friedrich I, Simm A, Kötting J, Thölen F, Fischer B, Silber RE. Cardiac surgery in the elderly patient. Dtsch Arztebl Int. 2009;106(25):416–22. https://doi.org/10.3238/arztebl.2009.0416.
99. Gogbashian A, Sedrakyan A, Treasure T. EuroSCORE: a systematic review of international performance. Eur J Cardiothorac Surg. 2004;25(5):695–700. https://doi.org/10.1016/j.ejcts.2004.02.022.
100. Dewey TM, Brown D, Ryan WH, Herbert MA, Prince SL, Mack MJ. Reliability of risk algorithms in predicting early and late operative outcomes in high-risk patients undergoing aortic valve replacement. J Thorac Cardiovasc Surg. 2008;135(1):180–7. https://doi.org/10.1016/j.jtcvs.2007.09.011.
101. Guida P, Mastro F, Scrascia G, Whitlock R, Paparella D. Performance of the European system for cardiac operative risk evaluation II: a meta-analysis of 22 studies involving 145,592 cardiac surgery procedures. J Thorac Cardiovasc Surg. 2014;148(6):3049–57. https://doi.org/10.1016/j.jtcvs.2014.07.039.
102. Wendt D, Osswald BR, Kayser K, et al. Society of thoracic surgeons score is superior to the EuroSCORE determining mortality in high risk patients undergoing isolated aortic valve replacement. Ann Thorac Surg. 2009;88(2):468–75. https://doi.org/10.1016/j.athoracsur.2009.04.059.
103. Marmelo F, Rocha V, Moreira-Gonçalves D. The impact of prehabilitation on post-surgical complications in patients undergoing non-urgent cardiovascular surgical intervention: systematic review and meta-analysis. Eur J Prev Cardiol. 2018;25(4):404–17. https://doi.org/10.1177/2047487317752373.
104. Aucoin SD, Hao M, Sohi R, et al. Accuracy and feasibility of clinically applied frailty instruments before surgery: a systematic review and meta-analysis. Anesthesiology. 2020;133(1):78–95. https://doi.org/10.1097/aln.0000000000003257.
105. Theou O, Brothers TD, Mitnitski A, Rockwood K. Operationalization of frailty using eight commonly used scales and comparison of their ability to predict all-cause mortality. J Am Geriatr Soc. 2013;61(9):1537–51. https://doi.org/10.1111/jgs.12420.
106. Rockwood K, Theou O. Using the clinical frailty scale in allocating scarce health care resources. Can Geriatr J. 2020;23(3):210–5. https://doi.org/10.5770/cgj.23.463.
107. Bandeen-Roche K, Xue QL, Ferrucci L, et al. Phenotype of frailty: characterization in the women's health and aging studies. J Gerontol A Biol Sci Med Sci. 2006;61(3):262–6. https://doi.org/10.1093/gerona/61.3.262.
108. Rockwood K, Mitnitski A. Frailty in relation to the accumulation of deficits. J Gerontol A Biol Sci Med Sci. 2007;62(7):722–7. https://doi.org/10.1093/gerona/62.7.722.
109. Searle SD, Mitnitski A, Gahbauer EA, Gill TM, Rockwood K. A standard procedure for creating a frailty index. BMC Geriatr. 2008;8(1):24. https://doi.org/10.1186/1471-2318-8-24.
110. Rolfson DB, Majumdar SR, Tsuyuki RT, Tahir A, Rockwood K. Validity and reliability of the Edmonton frail scale. Age Ageing. 2006;35(5):526–9. https://doi.org/10.1093/ageing/afl041.
111. McIsaac DI, MacDonald DB, Aucoin SD. Frailty for perioperative clinicians: a narrative review. Anesthe Analges. 2020;130(6):1450.
112. Rodríguez-Mañas L, Féart C, Mann G, et al. Searching for an operational definition of frailty: a Delphi method based consensus statement. The frailty operative definition-consensus conference project. J Gerontol: Ser A. 2012;68(1):62–7. https://doi.org/10.1093/gerona/gls119.
113. Peeler A, Moser C, Gleason KT, Davidson PM. Frailty as a predictor of postoperative outcomes in invasive cardiac surgery: a systematic review of literature. J Cardiovasc Nurs. 2022;37(3):231–47. https://doi.org/10.1097/jcn.0000000000000821.
114. Faller JW, Pereira DN, de Souza S, Nampo FK, Orlandi FS, Matumoto S. Instruments for the detection of frailty syndrome in older adults: a systematic review. PLoS One. 2019;14(4):e0216166. https://doi.org/10.1371/journal.pone.0216166.
115. Albert SM. The dynamics of frailty among older adults. JAMA Netw Open. 2019;2(8):e198438. https://doi.org/10.1001/jamanetworkopen.2019.8438.
116. Lang PO, Michel JP, Zekry D. Frailty syndrome: a transitional state in a dynamic process. Gerontology. 2009;55(5):539–49. https://doi.org/10.1159/000211949.

117. Haddad T, Mulpuru S, Salter I, et al. Development and evaluation of an evidence-based, theory-grounded online clinical frailty scale tutorial. Age Ageing. 2022;51(2) https://doi.org/10.1093/ageing/afab258.
118. Minnella EM, Awasthi R, Gillis C, et al. Patients with poor baseline walking capacity are most likely to improve their functional status with multimodal prehabilitation. Surgery. 2016;160(4):1070–9. https://doi.org/10.1016/j.surg.2016.05.036.
119. Mainini C, Rebelo PF, Bardelli R, et al. Perioperative physical exercise interventions for patients undergoing lung cancer surgery: what is the evidence? SAGE Open Med. 2016;4:2050312116673855. https://doi.org/10.1177/2050312116673855.
120. Theou O, Stathokostas L, Roland KP, et al. The effectiveness of exercise interventions for the management of frailty: a systematic review. J Aging Res. 2011;2011:569194. https://doi.org/10.4061/2011/569194.
121. Tobert CM, Hamilton-Reeves JM, Norian LA, et al. Emerging impact of malnutrition on surgical patients: literature review and potential implications for cystectomy in bladder cancer. J Urol. 2017;198(3):511–9. https://doi.org/10.1016/j.juro.2017.01.087.
122. Chen CC-H, Li H-C, Liang J-T, et al. Effect of a modified hospital elder life program on delirium and length of hospital stay in patients undergoing abdominal surgery: a cluster randomized clinical trial. JAMA Surg. 2017;152(9):827–34. https://doi.org/10.1001/jamasurg.2017.1083.
123. Waite I, Deshpande R, Baghai M, Massey T, Wendler O, Greenwood S. Home-based preoperative rehabilitation (prehab) to improve physical function and reduce hospital length of stay for frail patients undergoing coronary artery bypass graft and valve surgery. J Cardiothorac Surg. 2017;12(1):91. https://doi.org/10.1186/s13019-017-0655-8.
124. Molenaar CJL, Papen-Botterhuis NE, Herrle F, Slooter GD. Prehabilitation, making patients fit for surgery—a new frontier in perioperative care. Innov Surg Sci. 2019;4(4):132–8. https://doi.org/10.1515/iss-2019-0017.
125. McIsaac DI, Taljaard M, Bryson GL, et al. Frailty as a predictor of death or new disability after surgery: a prospective cohort study. Ann Surg. 2020;271(2):283–9. https://doi.org/10.1097/sla.0000000000002967.
126. McCann M, Stamp N, Ngui A, Litton E. Cardiac prehabilitation. J Cardiothorac Vasc Anesth. 2019;33(8):2255–65. https://doi.org/10.1053/j.jvca.2019.01.023.
127. Norris CM, Close JCT. Prehabilitation for the frailty syndrome: improving outcomes for our most vulnerable patients. Anesth Analg. 2020;130(6):1524–33. https://doi.org/10.1213/ane.0000000000004785.

Chapter 38
Perioperative Neurocognitive Disorders After Cardiac Surgery

Juan Pablo Espinosa-Leon, Andres de Lima, and Brian O'Gara

Abbreviations

3D-CAM	3-Minute Diagnostic Interview for the Confusion Assessment Method
ASA	American Society of Anesthesiologists
CABG	Coronary artery bypass grafting
CAM	Confusion Assessment Method
CAM-ICU	Confusion Assessment Method for the Intensive Care Unit
CAM-S	Confusion Assessment Method-Severity
CPB	Cardiopulmonary bypass
DNR	Delayed neurocognitive recovery
DSM-IIIR	Diagnostic and Statistical Manual for Mental Disorders, Third Edition, Revised
DSM-IV	Diagnostic and Statistical Manual for Mental Disorders, Fourth Edition
DSM-V	Diagnostic and Statistical Manual for Mental Disorders, Fifth Edition
HbA1c	Glycated hemoglobin
HELP	Hospital Elder Life Program
ICDSC	Intensive Care Delirium Screening Checklist
ICU	Intensive care unit
MAP	Mean arterial pressure
MCI	Mild cognitive impairment

J. P. Espinosa-Leon · B. O'Gara (✉)
Department of Anesthesia, Critical Care, and Pain Medicine, Beth Israel Deaconess Medical Center, Harvard Medical School, Boston, MA, USA
e-mail: jespino1@bidmc.harvard.edu; bpogara@bidmc.harvard.edu

A. de Lima
Department of Anesthesiology, Yale School of Medicine, New Haven, CT, USA
e-mail: andres.delimaarboleda@yale.edu

© The Author(s), under exclusive license to Springer Nature Switzerland AG 2024

J. Faintuch, S. Faintuch (eds.), *Recent Strategies in High Risk Surgery*,
https://doi.org/10.1007/978-3-031-56270-9_38

MMSE	Mini-Mental State Examination
MoCA	Montreal Cognitive Assessment
NCD	Neurocognitive disorder
NIRS	Near-infrared spectroscopy
PNCD	Postoperative neurocognitive disorder
PND	Perioperative neurocognitive disorder
POCD	Postoperative neurocognitive disorder
POD	Postoperative delirium
PODCAST Trial	Prevention of Delirium and Complications Associated with Surgical Treatments
RASS	Richmond Agitation Sedation Scale
SAVR	Surgical aortic valve replacement
TAVI	Transcatheter aortic valve implantation

Introduction

Cognitive impairment (CI) in hospitalized patients has been described using different terms, including delirium, acute confusional state, acute metabolic encephalopathy, and at least 30 others [1]. In the postoperative setting, the all-encompassing and now outdated term postoperative cognitive dysfunction, referred to as POCD, was used in the past. This phenomenon is defined as a new and possibly transient cognitive impairment after exposure to an anesthetic or after undergoing a surgical procedure [2]. Common manifestations include memory impairment, problems with intellectual tasks, and altered psychomotor dexterity, which can last up to 6 months and are often reversible.

Up to 40% of elderly adult patients and 30% of younger patients who undergo major noncardiac surgery will experience some form of cognitive impairment at hospital discharge [3]. Not surprisingly, 3 months after surgery the prevalence of cognitive dysfunction remains significantly higher in elderly patients, even when compared to age-matched controls. It is associated with a higher mortality risk 3 months and 1 year after surgery.

Diagnosis

Baseline and postoperative psychometric testing and the time frame in relation to surgery define the diagnosis. Commonly, a decline in >1 standard deviation in single or combined assessments, including the Trail Making Test, Rey Auditory Learning Test, Abbreviated Mental Test, Mini-Mental State Examination (MMSE), Montreal Cognitive Assessment (MoCA) tool, or Quick Mild Cognitive Impairment screen, is adopted as the diagnostic cutoff. The high variability and lack of uniformity is one of the main challenges in diagnosis.

Perioperative Neurocognitive Disorder

A multidisciplinary and international working group in 2018 recommended aligning the terminology used for postoperative cognitive changes with the diagnostic criteria of neurocognitive disorders used in the fifth edition of the *Diagnostic and Statistical Manual for Mental Disorders* (DSM-V) [4].

The term perioperative neurocognitive disorder (PND) serves to define any form of cognitive alteration identified in the perioperative period including prior to a surgical intervention. PNDs typically affect one or several domains of cognition, such as orientation, attention, perception, consciousness, and judgment [4–6]. Based on the timing of presentation and resolution, different terms have been proposed to designate this set of disorders.

Postoperative delirium (POD) describes acute and fluctuating disturbances in attention and awareness that develop shortly after surgery and last <7 days [7]. The symptoms are not explained by an underlying neurocognitive disorder or alterations to the patient's baseline arousal (i.e., coma). However, this definition is insufficient to describe some of the delirium-like alterations observed in the postoperative period, particularly those that develop or remain after days or weeks.

Delayed neurocognitive recovery (DNR) is diagnosed when the dysfunction persists after the expected duration of postoperative delirium but resolves within 30 days. Postoperative neurocognitive disorder, from here on referred to as PNCD, presents when the dysfunction is present after 30 days and resolves within the first 12 months.

Lastly, the term neurocognitive disorder (NCD) is used to describe any impairment that is present past the 1-year mark (see Fig. 38.1) [4]. Of note this last term is rather generic, indicating that it is often a permanent new level of cognition for the individual and does not stem from the surgical/anesthetic exposure.

These denominations are further classified as minor or major and the difference is established by objective testing such as the MMSE, MoCA, or Mini-Cog. Minor impairment corresponds to declines between 1 and 2 standard deviations below the

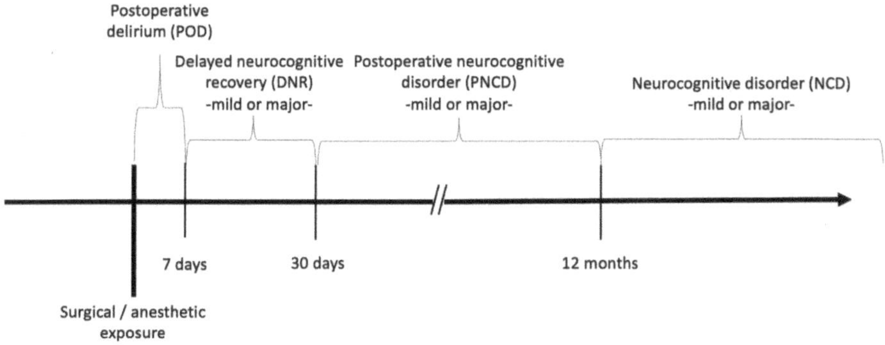

Fig. 38.1 Perioperative neurocognitive disorder (PND) nomenclature. Adapted from [4]. *DNR* delayed neurocognitive recovery, *NCD* neurocognitive disorder, *PNCD* postoperative neurocognitive disorder, *POD* postoperative delirium

general population, while major impairment points toward more serious impairment. Lastly, the implementation of this proposed nomenclature is derived from criteria established by DSM-V, which are based on three fundamental pillars: the decline must be noted subjectively (by a clinician, patient, or participant), measured objectively and compromising instrumental activities of daily living [4, 5].

Prevalence in Cardiac Surgery Patients

Postoperative Delirium (POD)

Individuals undergoing cardiac surgery seem to be subject to an elevated risk. This is likely due to a combination of different predisposing and precipitating factors seen in this population. A meta-analysis from 2021 by Chen and colleagues examined outcomes reported in 14 studies, including over 13,000 patients, and estimated a wide range of 4–55% prevalence of postoperative delirium (POD) after cardiac surgery [8]. In the first 3 days after transcatheter aortic valve implantation (TAVI), POD was present in up to 45% of patients [9]. A study in Norway with patients 80 years or older undergoing surgical aortic valve replacement (SAVR) or the TAVI registered delirium in 56% of cases [10]. Nevertheless also after noncardiac operations, in patients >60 years old with preoperative CI or dementia, a meta-analysis addressing over 196,000 individuals demonstrated elevated risk of delirium, 1-year mortality, discharge to assisted care, 30-day readmission, and postoperative complications when CI had been present. Previous dementia affected only the risk of 1-year mortality [11].

Other Perioperative NCDs

A meta-analysis of over 90,000 patients who underwent coronary artery bypass grafting (CABG) revealed, 1–4 months after surgery, a 28% prevalence of NCD, which diminished to 22% at 6–12 months [12]. A cohort from Duke University after the same procedure reported an incidence of cognitive decline of 53% at discharge, and although at 6 months the proportion had decreased to 24%, it was confirmed in not less than 42% of patients at 5 years [13]. These and other studies are summarized in Table 38.1.

Predisposing Factors for Postoperative Delirium

These encompass inherent characteristics that render individuals more prone to delirium; however, they alone are not causative. Precipitating factors elicit acute or transient disruptions in baseline brain functioning, triggering the onset of cognitive alterations. The interplay between these two underlies the clinical emergence of delirium and warrants a comprehensive understanding of enhanced clinical management [15].

Table 38.1 Association between cardiac surgery and postoperative cognitive outcomes

Sample size	Procedure	Outcome
16 studies, >62,000 patients	Cardiac surgery, meta-analysis [11]	Preoperative cognitive impairment[a]: 8.3 OR of POD
58 studies, >9600 patients	Cardiac surgery, meta-analysis [14]	DNR: 47.5% POCD: 30.2%
14 studies, >13,000 patients	Cardiac surgery, meta-analysis [8]	POD using several assessments[b] 4.1–54.9%
215 studies, >90,000 patients	Post-CABG, meta-analysis [12]	POD 1–7 days: 24% DNR: 1–4 months: 16%; 4–6 months: 19%; 6–12 months: 25% NCD: 1–3 years: 27%; 5–7 years: 7%
210 patients	Post-TAVI, prospective [9]	POD 1–3 days (CAM/CAM-ICU): transfemoral: 3–16%; transapical: 25–45%
143 patients	Aortic valve, SAVR vs. TAVI, prospective [10]	POD 1–5 days (CAM): SAVR: 66%, TAVI: 44%

CABG coronary artery bypass graft, *CAM* Confusion Assessment Method, *DNR* delayed neurocognitive recovery, *DRS* Delirium Rating Scale, *NCD* neurocognitive disorder, *OR* odds ratio, *POD* postoperative delirium, *SAVR* surgical aortic valve replacement, *TAVI* transcatheter aortic valve implantation

Neurologic tests used to define: [a]Preoperative cognitive impairment: MMSE, MoCA, Hasegawa Dementia Score, Stroop test, Clock-in-the-Box

[b]Postoperative delirium: DSI, DSM-IV or DSM-V, CAM or CAM-ICU, ICDSC

Multiplicity of Mechanisms

An umbrella review of meta-analyses addressing POCD identified 31 perioperative risk factors. The large number notwithstanding, only age and diabetes were ranked as suggestive evidence, other items being accorded weaker grades [2]. Other possibilities are not discarded, yet available studies are not sufficiently consistent up to now.

Age

Age over 65 years is considered a predisposing risk factor of POD, DNR, and PNCD following cardiac or noncardiac surgery. This association can be attributed to a higher burden of comorbidities, including neurovascular risk factors, and a relatively diminished baseline cognitive reserve [3, 8, 13].

Diabetes

Type 2 diabetic patients undergoing cardiac surgery are at higher risk of developing POD when compared to non-diabetic patients. The same is true for patients on preoperative oral hypoglycemic medications, and those with elevated fasting hyperglycemia and glycated hemoglobin (HbA1c), independent of a diagnosis of diabetes [16, 17]. Proposed mechanisms are related to increased neuroinflammation, altered cerebral neurotransmitter and glucose metabolism, and an overall impaired physiologic response to inflammatory stress [18].

Frailty

Reduced reserve and functionality across various organ systems, resulting in a compromised ability to manage daily activities and stressors, [19] is documented in approximately 30% of patients undergoing cardiac surgery. Unintentional weight loss, skeletal muscle weakness, easy exhaustion, low physical activity, and slow walking speed are the hallmarks of the condition. A relative risk of 18 for developing POD, compared to non-frail patients, recommends screening for frailty [20].

Baseline Cognitive Function, Neurocognitive Reserve, and Mental Health

Lower baseline cognitive function in patients undergoing cardiac surgery, defined by a Montreal Cognitive Assessment (MoCA) score below 26 or a Mini-Mental State Examination score under 25, seems to be associated with a greater risk of postoperative delirium [8, 13, 21]. The same has been shown to occur in patients with lower late-life cognitive reserve undergoing major noncardiac surgery [22]. In the cardiac surgery population, the presence of cognitive impairment prior to surgery is associated with an eightfold increased risk of postoperative delirium and a significantly prolonged length of stay in the intensive care unit and the hospital [11, 23]. In a similar fashion, there are reasons to believe that higher preoperative rates of depression, anxiety, and stress enhance the risk of PND [24, 25].

Protective or Insignificant Factors

High blood pressure, preoperative statin use, and obstructive sleep apnea have been found to either be protective or have an unclear association with PND [8, 17, 26].

Precipitating Factors for Postoperative Delirium

Cardiopulmonary Bypass

Cardiopulmonary bypass (CPB), along with cross-clamp times, can trigger a proinflammatory state and activation of the coagulation cascade. Aortic cannulation, aortotomy, or application of aortic cross-clamp is likely to precipitate postoperative infections, micro-embolic events, and a higher stroke burden. Hence, off-pump protocols have been proposed to support select cardiac surgeries such as CABG while limiting unnecessary exposure to CPB. A higher risk of POD in the first 24 h after surgery has been reported [27]. Moreover prolonged cardiopulmonary bypass can lead to increasing inflammation, ischemia, and ischemia-reperfusion phenomena, which are thought to contribute to neurological injury [28]. All this evidence notwithstanding, different long-term cognitive outcomes after heart surgery with and without CPB have not been recorded.

Surgical Approach

A reduction in inflammatory markers (particularly interleukin-6 and complement cascade) has been anticipated in patients undergoing CABG via a small anterolateral thoracotomy in comparison to a median sternotomy [29]. Minimally invasive techniques for CABG (a mini-thoracotomy and three thoracic ports for thoracoscopic access) have been associated with a significant reduction in POD rates (5–8%) compared to the previously reported values (over 50%) [13, 30, 31].

Cerebral Oxygenation

Maintenance of oxygen-metabolism balance at the neuronal tissue level is thought to be key in the prevention of postoperative cognitive impairment. The implementation of intraoperative algorithms guided by cerebral oxygenation targets using near-infrared spectroscopy (NIRS) has been advocated for early recognition of otherwise silent brain oxygenation imbalances. Despite conflicting evidence, various meta-analyses and randomized clinical trials assessing this intervention have shown a decrease in rates of POD and PNCD after cardiac surgery [32–36].

Temperature Management

Although still a highly controversial subject, recent literature suggests that hypothermia during CPB does not lead to improved neurocognitive outcomes [14]. Although some studies have demonstrated a benefit from hypothermic CPB in terms of neurologic protection, such as reduced incidence of stroke and PND, there is also an increase in perioperative myocardial damage [37].

In contrast, hyperthermia during CPB or postoperatively has been consistently demonstrated to have a negative effect over postoperative cognitive function and should be prevented [38, 39]. Current recommendations favor strict avoidance of hyperthermia (i.e., nasopharyngeal, tympanic, or arterial inflow temperature >37 °C). In cases in which hypothermia is induced, a slow rewarming rate toward normothermia is advised (<0.5 °C/min) [28, 37].

Intraoperative Blood Pressure Management

In patients undergoing CABG, targeting mean arterial pressures (MAPs) of 80–90 mmHg has been associated with a lower risk of POD and smaller postoperative decrease in scores on the Mini-Mental State Examination, when compared to lower MAPs of 60–70 mmHg [40]. According to some opinions, excursions in MAP that are above the range of cerebral autoregulation could also lead to a higher risk of developing delirium [41]. Yet the range of autoregulation in patients undergoing cardiac surgery is often unknown and hard to predict, more so when undergoing CPB [42]. Intraoperative impairments in autoregulation have been associated with the development of DNR at 10 days after surgery [43]. The best approach to management of MAP may be based on other surrogates for real-time perfusion, such as tissue oxygenation monitoring.

Sedation and Other Medications

Although the use of dexmedetomidine in the general intensive care unit (ICU) population has proven to increase days alive without delirium when compared to sedation with lorazepam infusion, [44] its effectiveness with contemporary sedatives other than lorazepam yields conflicting results [45, 46]. When used postoperatively, it failed to demonstrate any protective effect on POD and DNR [47]. The initiation of an infusion intraoperatively and continuation of such in the postoperative period reduced in POD in a clinical trial [46]. Another protocol that incorporated dexmedetomidine along with intravenous acetaminophen in the postoperative period significantly reduced delirium rates when compared to placebo or propofol infusion [48].

Lidocaine and Other Agents

Clear benefits for POD or PNCD have not been seen with lidocaine, magnesium, haloperidol, ziprasidone, or donepezil [16, 49–51].

Statins

Because statins have immunomodulatory, antithrombotic, and anti-inflammatory properties, they have been proposed as agents to reduce cognitive dysfunction after cardiac surgery. Nevertheless, current evidence in this field remains highly controversial [52–54].

Analgesia

The implementation of structured multimodal pain management regimens that include intravenous acetaminophen may reduce the incidence of delirium after cardiac surgery [48, 55]. This is likely a combination effect from adequate analgesia, reduced inflammation, and a decrease in opioid consumption. On the other hand, the Prevention of Delirium and Complications Associated with Surgical Treatments (PODCAST) trial evaluated the effects of a single dose of ketamine during induction of general anesthesia in major cardiac and noncardiac surgery patients. No differences in incidence of delirium compared to placebo occurred, whereas more postoperative hallucinations and nightmares were detected [56].

Table 38.2 Predisposing/precipitating risk factors for postoperative delirium

Predisposing	Precipitating
Age	Mechanical ventilation
Diabetes mellitus	Longer cross-clamp times
Frailty	ICU length of stay
Lower baseline cognitive function/neurocognitive reserve	Longer CPB times
Poor mental health	Hyperthermia during CPB
Fewer years of education	Cerebral hypoperfusion
	Inadequate analgesia

CPB cardiopulmonary bypass, *ICU* intensive care unit

Other Postoperative Drivers

Prolonged duration of postoperative mechanical ventilation and overall ICU length of stay have been associated with significantly increased risk of developing postoperative delirium [8]. Partly because improvement in delirium rates following cardiac surgery leads to improved neurocognitive outcomes, enhanced recovery pathways have been proposed to facilitate early extubation and mobilization in the acute postoperative period [30]. These and other mechanisms are briefly outlined in Table 38.2.

Pathophysiologic Mechanisms of Cognitive Dysfunction after Cardiac Surgery

Inflammation and Oxidative Stress

The relevance of oxidative stress has been extrapolated from post-cardiac arrest studies, where exposure to hyperoxia has been linked to worse neurological outcomes [57]. Yet prevention of hyperoxia and exposure to free oxygen radicals have not proven to have a significant impact on improving outcomes from a neurocognitive standpoint [28, 57–59].

Embolic Phenomena

The calcification burden present in the ascending aorta and aortic arch is incriminated with a higher risk of development of POD and PNCD. This supports the theory of how cognitive impairment after cardiac surgery is at least partially explained by both micro and macro embolic strokes, as previously discussed [28]. Heavier calcifications of the aorta and the carotid arteries could signal a higher risk.

Neurodegeneration

Levels of glial fibrillary acidic protein, a product of degradation from astrocyte filaments, have been demonstrated to be elevated in serum from patients following cardiac surgery. Higher serum concentrations of this protein after cardiac surgery have been associated with a significantly higher incidence of PNCD. For this reason, it has been proposed as a predictor of POD after cardiac surgery [27].

Diagnostic Tests

Confusion Assessment Method (CAM)

This instrument is helpful for nonpsychiatric clinicians to reliably assess delirium based on the *Diagnostic and Statistical Manual for Mental Disorders* (DSM-IIIR) criteria. The tool evaluates nine features of delirium, and diagnosis of delirium is made upon evaluation of four features: (1) acute onset and fluctuating course, (2) inattention, (3) disorganized thinking, and (4) altered level of consciousness. Features 1 and 2 must be present along with either 3 or 4. Besides being highly effective, it also demonstrates high concordance with other cognitive tests such as the MMSE.

Specialized versions are available such as the CAM for the Intensive Care Unit (CAM-ICU) for mechanically ventilated patients, the CAM-Severity (CAM-S) for scoring severity, and the 3-Minute Diagnostic Interview for the CAM (3D-CAM). Additionally it has been translated to over 10 languages.

3-Minute Diagnostic Interview for the Confusion Assessment Method (3D-CAM)

The 3d-CAM performs adequately in patients with dementia (sensitivity = 96%, specificity = 86%) and without dementia (sensitivity = 93%, specificity = 96%). Although originally validated in the general medicine inpatient population, it has also proven to be useful in the post-cardiac surgery population.

Table 38.3 The Richmond Agitation Sedation Scale (RASS)

Score	Term
+4	Combative
+3	Very agitated
+2	Agitated
+1	Restless
0	Alert and calm
−1	Drowsy[a]
−2	Light sedation[b]
−3	Moderate sedation[c]
−4	Deep sedation[d]
−5	Unarousable

Modified from [60]
[a]Sustained (>10 s) awakening
[a]Awakens <10 s
[c]Movement to voice (no eye contact)
[d]Movement to physical stimulation only

Confusion Assessment Method for the Intensive Care Unit

The CAM-ICU does not require verbal communication, and the initial step uses a validated level of consciousness scale, such as the Richmond Agitation Sedation Scale (RASS) (Table 38.3) to screen if the patient can be evaluated for delirium (i.e., RASS of ≥ -3). Next, the four criteria of delirium are evaluated. The patients can answer yes or no questions or follow simple commands by moving their head or fingers [57].

The CAM-ICU has high sensitivity, specificity, and interrater reliability. It is easy to use, requires minimal training, and appears to be equally effective across patients of different ages, those with dementia, and those with varying levels of illness severity, including the cardiac surgery population.

Montreal Cognitive Assessment (MoCA)

Designed for mild cognitive impairment (MCI), including participants with less than 12 years of education, the MoCA takes 10 min to perform and requires minimal training. The MoCA is better for detecting MCI than the MMSE, as it assesses the patient's executive functions, visuospatial processing, and language abilities in greater depth. Additionally, it includes more words, fewer learning trials, and a longer recall delay. The differences between healthy patients, those with MCI, and those with Alzheimer's disease are more pronounced with the MoCA than with the MMSE. Finally, the MoCA has high test-retest reliability, making it a valuable tool for tracking changes in cognitive performance over time [61].

Table 38.4 The Intensive Care Delirium Screening Checklist

1. Altered level of consciousness	Unable to score, 0 or 1
2. Inattention	Limited attention span = 1
3. Disorientation	Any evidence of disorientation = 1
4. Hallucination, delusion, or psychosis	Any of these = 1
5. Psychomotor agitation or retardation	Obvious hyperactivity or hypoactivity = 1
6. Inappropriate speech or mood	Any of these disturbances = 1
7. Sleep/wake cycle disturbance	Any positive finding = 1

Modified from [62]

A score of 4 or more suggests delirium; a higher score does not prove a more severe form of delirium; for instructions, kindly check lhsc.on.ca/media/8367/download, or the original Ref. [62]

Intensive Care Delirium Screening Checklist (ICDSC)

This simple tool, validated in cardiac surgery patients, targets the presence of eight different aspects of mentation that are graded by the evaluator as either "yes" or "no." A score of 4 or more positive answers is used to diagnose delirium. The Intensive Care Delirium Screening Checklist (ICDSC) also has the potential to diagnose subsyndromal delirium [60]. These and other tools [62] are depicted in Table 38.4.

Mini-Mental State Examination (MMSE)

The Mini-Mental State Examination (MMSE) is a widely used cognitive screening tool that was created in 1975. Unfortunately, its limited sensitivity in detecting mild cognitive impairment, and its reliance on language and cultural factors hinders application across different populations. Nonetheless, the MMSE has been employed as a screening tool to assess a patient's cognitive function and determine if further evaluation is needed [21].

Delirium Subtypes

Hypoactive delirium is the most prevalent type, and it is associated with worse clinical outcomes, including increased mortality and length of stay, more than hyperactive or mixed subtypes. However, it is more difficult to diagnose as patients have diminished levels of arousal, making participation in testing difficult. These patients typically demonstrate excessive somnolence, apathy, slow or decreased speech, and flat affect. This contrasts with hyperactive delirium, which typically presents with agitation and restlessness. Furthermore, patients with hypoactive delirium may be less likely to require pharmacologic or behavioral treatment than patients with hyperactive delirium. This has resulted in the underreporting of delirium, with an estimated 75% of missed cases of delirium being of the hypoactive subtype. Mixed delirium, as its name suggests, is characterized by shifts between the hypoactive and hyperactive states [63].

Clinical Outcomes

Cognitive decline at hospital discharge is among the factors with the strongest association with long-term cognitive decline up to 5 years after surgery even when controlling for other risk factors, such as older age and lower level of education [13]. Patients with significant PND after cardiac surgery tend to have higher rates of postoperative complications, longer lengths of stay in both the ICU and the hospital, and even increased mortality [11, 28, 64].

Reducing delirium rates has a significant effect on subsequent neurocognitive outcomes, which is mirrored in the context of cognitive impairment post-cardiac surgery, correlating with overall worse prognoses.

Association Between Cognitive Impairment and Quality of Life

Postoperative neurocognitive disorder can lead to a major functional and emotional burden on patients and their caregivers. Following cardiac surgery, the development of delirium is associated with a significant decline in quality of life within the first year. Patients who develop postoperative delirium are less likely to return to their preoperative cognitive baseline level after 6 months, compared to patients who do not develop delirium [21]. Furthermore, this population may exhibit higher prevalence of long-term deficits in memory and concentration and may require extended postoperative care and rehabilitation services, such as occupational and physical therapy, to improve their cognitive function and overall functional recovery [21, 64].

Prevention and Management

Both pharmacological and non-pharmacological prophylactic and therapeutic measures along with a multidisciplinary approach are advised, which include early involvement of a geriatric specialist, orientation protocols, perioperative sleep optimization, and appropriate nutrition [11].

Preoperative Screening

There have been recent calls by the American Society of Anesthesiologists (ASA) Perioperative Brain Health Initiative to incorporate routine baseline cognitive and delirium screening into the preoperative assessment [65].

Regional Anesthesia

The implementation of different regional anesthesia modalities, either pre- or postoperatively, has shown promise in reducing the occurrence of delirium. By improving pain management and decreasing exposure to systemic medications including opioids, regional analgesia contributes to a comprehensive approach in preventing postoperative delirium. However, more studies are necessary to establish its comparative efficacy in relation to other opioid-sparing techniques [66].

In the cardiac surgery population, there are important anatomic and technical considerations (i.e., need for heparinization during cardiopulmonary bypass) that interfere with the implementation of some techniques, such as neuraxial analgesia. Nevertheless, recent protocols incorporating thoracic epidural anesthesia may be effective in reducing POD [67–69].

Non-pharmacological Interventions

The Hospital Elder Life Program (HELP) is a care model that was established in 2000 with the primary goal of preventing functional and cognitive decline among older patients during their hospital stay. Patients are screened for six risk factors associated with delirium and if appropriate are managed by cognitive stimulation, early mobility, the use of sensory aids, and hydration in addition to avoidance of high-risk medications and restrictive interventions [70]. It has been proven effective in reducing the incidence of delirium and its associated complications, such as in-hospital falls. By preventing delirium, this initiative has been associated with a decrease in the length of hospital stays and lower rates of institutionalization, including those undergoing major surgery, but not specifically cardiac surgery.

Prehabilitation/Cognitive Training

Higher late-life cognitive reserve is associated with reduced incidence and severity of delirium [22]. Similarly, in older patients undergoing major noncardiac surgery, cognitive prehabilitation through brain exercise games targeting cognitive abilities such as problem-solving, attention, and memory reduced POD rates [71].

Despite clinical trials showing the feasibility of preoperative cognitive training in cardiac surgery patients, its validity and efficacy remain to be determined [72, 73].

References

1. Francis J, Kapoor WN. Delirium in hospitalized elderly. J Gen Intern Med. 1990;5:65–79.
2. Travica N, Lotfaliany M, Marriott A, Safavynia SA, Lane MM, Gray L, Veronese N, Berk M, Skvarc D, Aslam H, Gamage E, Formica M, Bishop K, Marx W. Peri-operative risk factors associated with post-operative cognitive dysfunction (POCD): an umbrella review of meta-analyses of observational studies. J Clin Med. 2023;12(4):1610.
3. Monk TG, Weldon BC, Garvan CW, et al. Predictors of cognitive dysfunction after major noncardiac surgery. Anesthesiology. 2008;108:18–30.

4. Evered L, Silbert B, Knopman DS, et al. Recommendations for the nomenclature of cognitive change associated with anaesthesia and surgery-2018. Br J Anaesth. 2018;121:1005–12.
5. Evered LA, Silbert BS. Postoperative cognitive dysfunction and noncardiac surgery. Anesth Analg. 2018;127:496–505.
6. Kotekar N, Shenkar A, Nagaraj R. Postoperative cognitive dysfunction—current preventive strategies. Clin Interv Aging. 2018;13:2267–73.
7. American Psychiatric Association. Diagnostic and statistical manual of mental disorders, 5th ed. 2013. psychiatry.org/psychiatrists/practice/dsm. Accessed 26 Feb 2024.
8. Chen H, Mo L, Hu H, et al. Risk factors of postoperative delirium after cardiac surgery: a meta-analysis. J Cardiothorac Surg. 2021;16:113.
9. Sharma V, Katznelson R, Horlick E, et al. Delirium after transcatheter aortic valve implantation via the femoral or apical route. Anaesthesia. 2016;71:901–7.
10. Eide LSP, Ranhoff AH, Fridlund B, et al. Readmissions and mortality in delirious versus non-delirious octogenarian patients after aortic valve therapy: a prospective cohort study. BMJ Open. 2016;6:e012683.
11. Au E, Thangathurai G, Saripella A, et al. Postoperative outcomes in elderly patients undergoing cardiac surgery with preoperative cognitive impairment: a systematic review and meta-analysis. Anesth Analg. 2023;136:1016–28.
12. Greaves D, Psaltis PJ, Ross TJ, et al. Cognitive outcomes following coronary artery bypass grafting: a systematic review and meta-analysis of 91,829 patients. Int J Cardiol. 2019;289:43–9.
13. Newman MF, Kirchner JL, Phillips-Bute B, et al. Longitudinal assessment of neurocognitive function after coronary-artery bypass surgery. N Engl J Med. 2001;344:395–402.
14. Linassi F, Maran E, De Laurenzis A, et al. Targeted temperature management in cardiac surgery: a systematic review and meta-analysis on postoperative cognitive outcomes. Br J Anaesth. 2022;128:11–25.
15. Marquetand J, Bode L, Fuchs S, et al. Predisposing and precipitating factors for delirium in the very old (≥80 years): a prospective cohort study of 3076 patients. Gerontology. 2021;67:599–607.
16. Mathew JP, Mackensen GB, Phillips-Bute B, et al. Randomized, double-blinded, placebo controlled study of neuroprotection with lidocaine in cardiac surgery. Stroke. 2009;40:880–7.
17. Galyfos GC, Geropapas GE, Sianou A, et al. Risk factors for postoperative delirium in patients undergoing vascular surgery. J Vasc Surg. 2017;66:937–46.
18. Adamis D, Treloar A, Martin FC, et al. APOE and cytokines as biological markers for recovery of prevalent delirium in elderly medical inpatients. Int J Geriatr Psychiatry. 2007;22:688–94.
19. Xue Q-L. The frailty syndrome: definition and natural history. Clin Geriatr Med. 2011;27:1–15.
20. Brown CH, Max L, LaFlam A, et al. The association between preoperative frailty and postoperative delirium after cardiac surgery. Anesth Analg. 2016;123:430–5.
21. Saczynski JS, Marcantonio ER, Quach L, et al. Cognitive trajectories after postoperative delirium. N Engl J Med. 2012;367:30–9.
22. Tow A, Holtzer R, Wang C, et al. Cognitive reserve and postoperative delirium in older adults. J Am Geriatr Soc. 2016;64:1341–6.
23. Chen L, Au E, Saripella A, et al. Postoperative outcomes in older surgical patients with preoperative cognitive impairment: a systematic review and meta-analysis. J Clin Anesth. 2022;80:110883.
24. Lin Y, Chen J, Wang Z. Meta-analysis of factors which influence delirium following cardiac surgery. J Card Surg. 2012;27:481–92.
25. Humphreys JM, Denson LA, Baker RA, Tully PJ. The importance of depression and alcohol use in coronary artery bypass graft surgery patients: risk factors for delirium and poorer quality of life. J Geriatr Cardiol JGC. 2016;13:51–7.
26. Rivas E, Shehata P, Bravo M, et al. Association between obstructive sleep apnea and atrial fibrillation and delirium after cardiac surgery. Sub-analysis of DECADE trial. J Clin Anesth. 2023;87:111109.

27. Nurcahyo WI, Hadisaputro S, Muttaqin Z, et al. Difference in GFAP levels in POCD and non-POCD patients after on pump CABG. Vasc Health Risk Manag. 2022;18:915–25.
28. Berger M, Terrando N, Smith SK, et al. Neurocognitive function after cardiac surgery: from phenotypes to mechanisms. Anesthesiology. 2018;129:829–51.
29. Gu YJ, Mariani MA, Boonstra PW, et al. Complement activation in coronary artery bypass grafting patients without cardiopulmonary bypass: the role of tissue injury by surgical incision. Chest. 1999;116:892–8.
30. Yilmaz A, Robic B, Starinieri P, et al. A new viewpoint on endoscopic CABG: technique description and clinical experience. J Cardiol. 2020;75:614–20.
31. Stessel B, Nijs K, Pelckmans C, et al. Neurological outcome after minimally invasive coronary artery bypass surgery (NOMICS): an observational prospective cohort study. PLoS One. 2020;15:e0242519.
32. Ortega-Loubon C, Herrera-Gómez F, Bernuy-Guevara C, et al. Near-infrared spectroscopy monitoring in cardiac and noncardiac surgery: pairwise and network meta-analyses. J Clin Med. 2019;8:2208.
33. Bennett SR, Smith N, Bennett MR. Cerebral oximetry in adult cardiac surgery to reduce the incidence of neurological impairment and hospital length-of-stay: a prospective, randomized, controlled trial. J Intensive Care Soc. 2022;23:109–16.
34. Zorrilla-Vaca A, Healy R, Grant MC, et al. Intraoperative cerebral oximetry-based management for optimizing perioperative outcomes: a meta-analysis of randomized controlled trials. Can J Anaesth. 2018;65:529–42.
35. Kara I, Erkin A, Saclı H, et al. The effects of near-infrared spectroscopy on the neurocognitive functions in the patients undergoing coronary artery bypass grafting with asymptomatic carotid artery disease: a randomized prospective study. Ann Thorac Cardiovasc Surg. 2015;21:544–50.
36. Colak Z, Borojevic M, Bogovic A, et al. Influence of intraoperative cerebral oximetry monitoring on neurocognitive function after coronary artery bypass surgery: a randomized, prospective study. Eur J Cardiothorac Surg. 2015;47:447–54.
37. Grigore AM, Murray CF, Ramakrishna H, Djaiani G. A core review of temperature regimens and neuroprotection during cardiopulmonary bypass: does rewarming rate matter? Anesth Analg. 2009;109:1741–51.
38. Grocott HP, Mackensen GB, Grigore AM, et al. Postoperative hyperthermia is associated with cognitive dysfunction after coronary artery bypass graft surgery. Stroke. 2002;33:537–41.
39. Grigore AM, Grocott HP, Mathew JP, et al. The rewarming rate and increased peak temperature alter neurocognitive outcome after cardiac surgery. Anesth Analg. 2002;94:4–10.
40. Siepe M, Pfeiffer T, Gieringer A, et al. Increased systemic perfusion pressure during cardiopulmonary bypass is associated with less early postoperative cognitive dysfunction and delirium. Eur J Cardiothorac Surg. 2011;40:200–7.
41. Hori D, Brown C, Ono M, et al. Arterial pressure above the upper cerebral autoregulation limit during cardiopulmonary bypass is associated with postoperative delirium. Br J Anaesth. 2014;113:1009–17.
42. Joshi B, Ono M, Brown C, et al. Predicting the limits of cerebral autoregulation during cardiopulmonary bypass. Anesth Analg. 2012;114:503–10.
43. Kumpaitiene B, Svagzdiene M, Sirvinskas E, et al. Cerebrovascular autoregulation impairments during cardiac surgery with cardiopulmonary bypass are related to postoperative cognitive deterioration: prospective observational study. Minerva Anestesiol. 2019;85:594–603.
44. Pandharipande PP, Pun BT, Herr DL, et al. Effect of sedation with dexmedetomidine vs lorazepam on acute brain dysfunction in mechanically ventilated patients: the MENDS randomized controlled trial. JAMA. 2007;298:2644–53.
45. Turan A, Duncan A, Leung S, et al. Dexmedetomidine for reduction of atrial fibrillation and delirium after cardiac surgery (DECADE): a randomised placebo-controlled trial. Lancet. 2020;396:177–85.

46. Likhvantsev VV, Landoni G, Grebenchikov OA, et al. Perioperative dexmedetomidine supplement decreases delirium incidence after adult cardiac surgery: a randomized, double-blind, controlled study. J Cardiothorac Vasc Anesth. 2021;35:449–57.
47. Li X, Yang J, Nie X-L, et al. Impact of dexmedetomidine on the incidence of delirium in elderly patients after cardiac surgery: a randomized controlled trial. PLoS One. 2017;12:e0170757.
48. Subramaniam B, Shankar P, Shaefi S, et al. Effect of intravenous acetaminophen vs placebo combined with propofol or dexmedetomidine on postoperative delirium among older patients following cardiac surgery: the DEXACET randomized clinical trial. JAMA. 2019;321:686–96.
49. Mathew JP, White WD, Schinderle DB, et al. Intraoperative magnesium administration does not improve neurocognitive function after cardiac surgery. Stroke. 2013;44:3407–13.
50. Girard TD, Exline MC, Carson SS, et al. Haloperidol and ziprasidone for treatment of delirium in critical illness. N Engl J Med. 2018;379:2506–16.
51. Doraiswamy PM, Babyak MA, Hennig T, et al. Donepezil for cognitive decline following coronary artery bypass surgery: a pilot randomized controlled trial. Psychopharmacol Bull. 2007;40:54–62.
52. Mariscalco G, Mariani S, Biancari F, Banach M. Effects of statins on delirium following cardiac surgery—evidence from literature. Psychiatr Pol. 2015;49:1359–70.
53. Vallabhajosyula S, Kanmanthareddy A, Erwin PJ, et al. Role of statins in delirium prevention in critical ill and cardiac surgery patients: a systematic review and meta-analysis. J Crit Care. 2017;37:189–96.
54. Lee D-S, Lee MY, Park C-M, et al. Preoperative statins are associated with a reduced risk of postoperative delirium following vascular surgery. PLoS One. 2018;13:e0192841.
55. Mamoun NF, Lin P, Zimmerman NM, et al. Intravenous acetaminophen analgesia after cardiac surgery: a randomized, blinded, controlled superiority trial. J Thorac Cardiovasc Surg. 2016;152:881–889.e1.
56. Avidan MS, Maybrier HR, Abdallah AB, et al. Intraoperative ketamine for prevention of postoperative delirium or pain after major surgery in older adults: an international, multicentre, double-blind, randomised clinical trial. Lancet. 2017;390:267–75.
57. Sessler CN, Gosnell MS, Grap MJ, Brophy GM, O'Neal PV, Keane KA, Tesoro EP, Elswick RK. The Richmond Agitation-Sedation Scale: validity and reliability in adult intensive care unit patients. Am J Respir Crit Care Med. 2002;166(10):1388–44.
58. Roberts BW, Kilgannon JH, Hunter BR, et al. Association between early hyperoxia exposure after resuscitation from cardiac arrest and neurological disability. Circulation. 2018;137:2114–24.
59. Shaefi S, Shankar P, Mueller AL, et al. Intraoperative oxygen concentration and neurocognition after cardiac surgery. Anesthesiology. 2021;134:189–201.
60. Nishimura K, Yokoyama K, Yamauchi N, et al. Sensitivity and specificity of the Confusion Assessment Method for the Intensive Care Unit (CAM-ICU) and the Intensive Care Delirium Screening Checklist (ICDSC) for detecting post-cardiac surgery delirium: a single-center study in Japan. Heart Lung J Crit Care. 2016;45:15–20.
61. Ciesielska N, Sokołowski R, Mazur E, et al. Is the Montreal Cognitive Assessment (MoCA) test better suited than the Mini-Mental State Examination (MMSE) in mild cognitive impairment (MCI) detection among people aged over 60? Meta-analysis. Psychiatr Pol. 2016;50:1039–52.
62. Bergeron N, Dubois MJ, Dumont M, Dial S, Skrobik Y. Intensive care delirium screening checklist: evaluation of a new screening tool. Intensive Care Med. 2001;27(5):859–64.
63. Krewulak KD, Stelfox HT, Leigh JP, et al. Incidence and prevalence of delirium subtypes in an adult ICU: a systematic review and meta-analysis. Crit Care Med. 2018;46:2029–35.
64. de la Varga-Martínez O, Gutiérrez-Bustillo R, Muñoz-Moreno MF, López-Herrero R, Gómez-Sánchez E, Tamayo E. Postoperative delirium: an independent risk factor for poorer quality of life with long-term cognitive and functional decline after cardiac surgery. J Clin Anesth. 2023;85:111030.
65. Deiner S, Fleisher LA, Leung JM, et al. Adherence to recommended practices for perioperative anesthesia care for older adults among US anesthesiologists: results from the ASA Committee

on Geriatric Anesthesia-Perioperative Brain Health Initiative ASA member survey. Perioper Med. 2020;9:6.
66. Peden CJ, Miller TR, Deiner SG, et al. Improving perioperative brain health: an expert consensus review of key actions for the perioperative care team. Br J Anaesth. 2021;126:423–32.
67. Fanelli A, Balzani E, Memtsoudis S, et al. Regional anesthesia techniques and postoperative delirium: systematic review and meta-analysis. Minerva Anestesiol. 2022;88:499–507.
68. Kasputytė G, Bukauskienė R, Širvinskas E, et al. Effects of combined and general anesthesia on cognitive functions for patients undergoing cardiac surgery under CPB. Heart Surg Forum. 2021;24:E593–7.
69. Chiew JK, Low CJW, Zeng K, et al. Thoracic epidural anesthesia in cardiac surgery: a systematic review, meta-analysis, and trial sequential analysis of randomized controlled trials. Anesth Analg. 2023;137:587–600.
70. Hshieh TT, Yang T, Gartaganis SL, et al. Hospital elder life program: systematic review and meta-analysis of effectiveness. Am J Geriatr Psychiatry. 2018;26:1015–33.
71. Humeidan ML, Reyes J-PC, Mavarez-Martinez A, et al. Effect of cognitive prehabilitation on the incidence of postoperative delirium among older adults undergoing major noncardiac surgery: the Neurobics Randomized Clinical Trial. JAMA Surg. 2021;156:148–56.
72. O'Gara BP, Mueller A, Gasangwa DVI, et al. Prevention of early postoperative decline: a randomized, controlled feasibility trial of perioperative cognitive training. Anesth Analg. 2020;130:586.
73. Butz M, Meyer R, Gerriets T, et al. Increasing preoperative cognitive reserve to prevent postoperative delirium and postoperative cognitive decline in cardiac surgical patients (INCORE): study protocol for a randomized clinical trial on cognitive training. Front Neurol. 2022;13:1040733.

Part X
End of Life Care and Other Ethical Challenges

Chapter 39
Palliative Surgery: When To and When Not To?

Jaewook Shin and Thomas J. Miner

Abbreviations

ACS	The American College of Surgeons
ES	Endoscopic stenting
GJ	Gastrojejunostomy
GOO	Gastric outlet obstruction
HJ	Hepaticojejunostomy
LBO	Large bowel obstruction
MBC	Metastatic breast cancer
MBO	Malignant bowel obstruction
SBR	Small bowel resection
SEMS	Self-expandable metallic stents
SUPPORT	The Study to Understand Prognoses and Preferences for Outcomes and Risks of Treatments

Introduction

The word "palliative" comes from a Latin word *palliat,* which means "cloaked"; as the root word suggests, palliative care aims to allay symptoms that cause pain and suffering when source control may not be plausible. The phrase "Palliative care" was first named in 1973 by Dr. Balfour Mount—the Canadian surgeon often credited as the father of palliative care in North America—to be used instead of "Hospice" which had a negative connotation [1]. While the term is of recent invention, the concept of palliative care dates back to early medicine when the focus, in the absence of effective

J. Shin · T. J. Miner (✉)
Department of Surgery, Rhode Island Hospital, Warren Alpert Medical School of Brown University, Providence, RI, USA
e-mail: jaewook_shin1@brown.edu; thomas.miner@brownphysicians.org

© The Author(s), under exclusive license to Springer Nature Switzerland AG 2024

J. Faintuch, S. Faintuch (eds.), *Recent Strategies in High Risk Surgery*,
https://doi.org/10.1007/978-3-031-56270-9_39

curative approaches, was primarily on alleviating pain and suffering. It is only a modern conception that achieving a cure is of sole importance—enabled by unprecedented technological advances in medical, surgical, and critical care therapies—as caring for patient's comfort has been relatively de-emphasized.

Importantly, surgeons have been at the forefront of these early medical initiatives that focused on palliative care. Not only did patient presentations that warranted palliative considerations often involve surgical emergencies such as obstruction, bleeding, and perforation, [2] but there also was a dire need for relief of pain and suffering. A handful of landmark operations began with an intent to palliate rather than cure, many of them in the field of surgical oncology. For instance, the Halstead radical mastectomy was first used in 1882 to ease pain caused by locally advanced and ulcerating breast cancers. Over time, it also showed some success in curing breast cancer, rendering it a gold standard for breast cancer treatment until the mid-1970s [3]. Theodor Billroth performed the first successful gastrectomy for obstructing cancer of the pylorus, thereby enabling a more peaceful end-of-life without incessant vomiting. The Whipple procedure also began as a palliative operation as it relieves pain and duodenal and biliary obstruction. Aside from oncology, coronary artery bypass grafting was also originally used to palliate angina pectoris then found to have survival benefits, so did valvular operations. Even organ transplantation may be considered inherently palliative rather than solely curative, as transplanted state provides long-term respite rather than immediate cure for organ failures given the ramifications of immunosuppression [4].

Despite the rich history of surgeon involvement in palliative care, many surgeons are insufficiently prepared to provide palliative care. Many reasons can be surmised, including cursory surgical training in palliative care, inadequate quantity and quality of peer-reviewed studies [5], and not enough coverage or depth of the topic in surgical textbooks [6]. Consequently, comprehensive end-of-life care for dying patients has also been sub-standard [7] while open conversations regarding death and dying have been standard-of-care [8] as death became more accepted as a natural fact of life [9]. Surgeons are often confronted with difficult patient encounters marked by medical, surgical, and social complexity where death and dying are realities especially in high-risk patients. Thus, the decision to pursue palliative operations and procedures entail appreciation of multidisciplinary treatment options and technical attentions weighing risks and benefits which then must be clearly and compassionately communicated to patients and families.

Given the inherent challenges that surgeons at all levels of training must face daily, we propose a primer for bedside assistance and decisions for the busy surgeon caring for high-risk patients needing palliative surgery. The definition and evolution of palliative surgery including early prospective studies and types of palliative surgery will be presented. Practical applications based on recent literature supporting more appropriate new outcome measures, improving communication and decision-making, and enhancing resident education will follow. The Palliative Triangle and Best Case/Worst Case framework will be discussed as models of communication, a quintessential component of palliative surgery. Finally, patient selection will be discussed in detail. This chapter will help each surgeon consider, learn, and decide "when to" and "when not to" perform palliative surgery with a foundational understanding that the crux of surgical palliative care lies in a dynamic relationship connecting patient, family, and surgeon.

Palliative Surgery—Where It Came From

Definition of Palliative Surgery

Palliative care has been characterized in various realms. For instance, the World Health Organization defines as "the total active care of patients whose disease is not responsive to curative treatment. Control of pain, of other symptoms, and of psychological, social, and spiritual problems, is paramount. The goal of palliative care is achievement of the best quality of life for patients and their families" [10]. Of note, this definition emphasizes that palliative care is a "total" (i.e. biopsychosocial-spiritual) and "active" (i.e. not passively waiting for death) care model that aims to achieve symptom control when source control is not plausible and care for patient and family when cure is not plausible. Surgical palliative care has been sub-defined as initial evaluation and local control of disease, followed by control of discharge, hemorrhage, and pain, and ending with reconstruction and rehabilitation [11].

While different definitions may provide unique views that facilitate overall understanding, imprecise characterizations of palliative care have also conflated the role of surgery and its indications and outcomes in patients, especially with advanced cancer [12, 13]. Unlike traditional curative therapies, surgical palliative therapies cannot be defined by the type of operation (e.g. the same surgery can be used to achieve a distinct purpose in different patients) or the extent of disease (e.g. gross margin analysis may be irrelevant to the goal of the surgery)—the key difference lies in the *intent* of care and *individualized* care. Thus, surgical palliation or palliative surgery is best defined as an operation or procedure deliberately performed with the primary intention of improving *quality of life* or relieving *symptoms* in a patient with incurable disease such as advanced malignancy. And improving quality of life may mean addressing the underlying etiology such as obstruction, bleeding, or perforation and symptoms may include pain, nausea, vomiting, anorexia, or jaundice. Similarly, the effectiveness of palliative surgery is best defined by the duration of patient-acknowledged symptom resolution, rather than the duration of overall survival [14, 15].

Evolution of Palliative Surgery

Prior to the inception of dedicated research in palliative surgery was a social milieu characterized by right-to-die movement and the state of Oregon-sanctioned physician-assisted euthanasia in the mid-1990s. As medical technology (i.e. ventilators, dialysis, transplant) grew at an unprecedented pace, some Americans with formerly fatal illnesses regained their productive lives while others merely experienced prolonged dying and suffering. Many were struck with fear of losing control of their lives in the face of a critical illness and dying a slow, painful, and impersonal death [16]. In light of this, a group of physicians, ethicists, and others conducted a controlled trial called The Study to Understand Prognoses and Preferences for Outcomes and Risks of Treatments (SUPPORT) in 1995. The objective was to improve end-of-life decision-making, thereby reducing the frequency of prolonged death on a mechanical ventilator. Unfortunately, the trial showed 50% of physicians did not know their patients' goals of care at the end-of-life and 40% of patients suffered potentially treatable pain before they died. Given that increased opportunities for patient-physician communication alone were insufficient to change outcomes, the trial called for a larger societal commitment and systemic implementations to improve end-of-life decision-making [17].

Around the same time, the American College of Surgeons (ACS) had also begun to wrestle with end-of-life issues in the form of a symposium on physician-assisted suicide held in 1997. Such considerations, along with the SUPPORT trial, vividly revealed that surgeons were inadequately equipped to manage even the rudimentary components of end-of-life care such as communication, pain control, and the scope of appropriate life-prolonging measures. Since then, conscious efforts to incorporate palliative care in the college has led to a symposium and a task force dedicated to surgical palliative care and the official ACS statement of principles of palliative care in 2005 [18].

As surgical palliative care began to surface in the public sphere, dedicated research efforts also ensued—more specifically, first by showing that there is a paucity of reliable, reproducible, and global data in palliative surgery research to guide decision-making. Miner et al. [16] identified 348 articles published between 1990 and 1996 on the surgical palliation of cancer and reviewed keywords pertinent to practicing good palliative care. The study found that more than 70% of the available literature on surgical palliation were retrospective in nature in contrast with abundant prospective multicenter trials available on cancer cures. Even the few prospective studies were limited by small sample sizes and lack of representation of common cancer operations. In addition, much of the discussion was regarding increased survival rather than important palliative concepts such as patient's psychosocial wellbeing, functional status, and feelings. While some palliative concepts describing benefits (e.g. quality of life, pain control) were discussed, the extent was minimal compared to risks (e.g. morbidity and mortality, physiologic response). Overall, the study demonstrated a need for robust prospective research delineating reliable measures that uniquely define a good palliative operation and can aid in decision-making.

Miner et al. [19] enrolled 26 patients at Walter Reed Army Medical Center between 1997 and 1999 requiring palliative surgery then followed to characterize their course. Although less than half of patients experienced improved outcomes (e.g. quality of life, pain), the study represented a first attempt at obtaining prospective data on palliative surgical patients based on patient-centered outcome measures and also the first to propose a critical palliative triangle that aids palliative surgical decision-making.

This pilot study was followed by a larger prospective endeavor in palliative surgery. Miner et al. [20] prospectively followed 823 patients at Memorial Sloan

Kettering Cancer Center from 2002 to 2003 who underwent 1022 palliative procedures to obtain data required to facilitate evidence-based palliative surgical decision-making. The results showed symptom resolution or improvement was seen in 80% of patients within 30 days though 50% required further intervention within 2 months of the index operation for new or recurrent symptoms. In addition, operative morbidity (40%) and mortality (10%) were not insignificant. The study also highlighted that poor palliative outcomes were associated with poor performance status, poor nutrition, and weight loss. In light of the morbidity and mortality seen in palliative surgery, Miner et al. [21] then explored the role of preemptive palliative surgery on palliative outcomes. Among 107 patients who underwent anticipatory surgery, 84% experienced prevention of anticipated symptom and greater overall survival (309 days versus 181 days) than symptomatic patients who underwent surgery, while morbidity and mortality were similar. This suggested that preemptive palliative surgery may yield beneficial palliative outcomes in highly select cases.

Types of Palliative Surgery

As the field of palliative surgery evolved, research on palliative surgery also expanded to include various types of operations and procedures. We will discuss available data for palliative surgery for each disease entity, such as malignant obstructions and specific advanced cancers, and then provide a brief "when to" and "when not to" recommendations. For the purpose of clarity, "palliative operations" will be used to describe invasive interventions taking place in the operating room and palliative procedures will refer to minimally invasive approaches excluding operations, usually taking place at the bedside, gastroenterology or interventional radiology suite. Specifically, "when to" or "when not to" recommendations will pertain to performing palliative operations, such as gastrojejunostomy, colostomy, and hepaticojejunostomy. Thus, palliative procedures (i.e. endoscopic stents, transhepatic biliary drainage) will remain as options when palliative operations are not indicated. Of note, these recommendations are by no means comprehensive and may not capture the complex nuance of shared decision-making in palliative surgery—they are included to help summarize the current literature to aid our decision-making. As always, communication with the patient and family must be at the center. Also, general evaluation of each patient's fitness for surgery (i.e. nutritional and functional status, comorbidity, age) is phrased as "able to undergo general anesthesia and invasive surgery" and will be discussed more in detail in the "Patient Selection" section.

Malignant Gastric Outlet Obstruction

Gastric outlet obstruction (GOO) can be caused by advanced malignancies of the upper gastrointestinal tract, such as gastric, periampullary, and biliary/pancreatic cancer. Given the likely unresectable nature of the underlying malignancy and limited length of survival around 3–6 months, GOO often necessitates palliative approaches to alleviate symptoms and improve quality of life. Surgical options include open and laparoscopic gastrojejunostomy (GJ), and nonsurgical option is endoscopic stenting (ES). Both GJ and ES relieve obstructive symptoms and facilitate oral eating, thereby improving quality of life—7.6 days versus 3.1 days until resuming oral intake, respectively [22]. While laparoscopic approach is less invasive, research shows no or inconclusive difference in morbidity and mortality, operating time, or analgesia. GJ has a higher rate of immediate complications, including postoperative issues and delayed gastric emptying, while ES has a higher rate of late complications, such as bleeding and perforation [23]. GJ also provides more durable relief of symptoms than ES which can migrate and re-obstruct—in a retrospective review of 113 patients with GOO, median patency duration for ES was 125 days, significantly shorter than 282 days for GJ [24].

When to perform GJ—able to undergo general anesthesia and invasive surgery, willing to be inpatient for 1–2 weeks, expected survival longer than 2 months [25], unwilling to accept risk of repeat procedures associated with limited durability of ES.

When not to perform GJ—unable to undergo general anesthesia or invasive surgery, prefers outpatient procedure, expected survival is shorter, thus may benefit from ES with an understanding that it may only provide limited durability, limited symptom severity.

Malignant Small Bowel Obstruction

Malignant bowel obstruction (MBO) is a common pre-terminal condition for patients with advanced gastrointestinal and ovarian cancer. Nonoperative management includes octreotide and corticosteroids in addition to standard nasogastric decompression, pain control, and antiemetics. Consideration of palliative surgery for MBO is challenging due to a lack of high-quality data. In general, surgical palliation can yield more success for patients with intraluminal or localized tumors compared to peritoneal carcinomatosis. A systematic review of 17 studies with outcomes after palliative surgery for MBO secondary to peritoneal carcinomatosis revealed high morbidity and mortality, frequent readmissions and re-obstructions with prolonged hospitalizations without much survival benefit—palliative outcome measures such as quality of life and symptom relief were not reported. Notably, patients with carcinomatosis may only have weeks or months to live, thus likely to avoid any invasive operations near the end-of-life [26]. For patients with intraluminal or localized tumors, bypass, small bowel resection (SBR), or ostomy may be performed with caution taken to avoid proximal ostomy to prevent high output. In addition, patients with ascites and under active chemotherapy bear higher risk [27].

When to perform bypass, SBR, or ileostomy—able to undergo general anesthesia and invasive surgery, intraluminal or localized tumors, adequate distal unaffected bowel for ostomy.

When not to perform bypass, SBR, or ileostomy—unable to undergo general anesthesia or invasive surgery, diffuse peritoneal carcinomatosis/obstructing lesions, patients with ascites or under active chemotherapy.

Malignant Large Bowel Obstruction

Large bowel obstruction (LBO) can be a serious complication of advanced, incurable colorectal, ovarian, or prostate cancer and distant metastases. If left untreated, necrotic colon can lead to septic shock and death. Standard palliative surgery includes Hartmann's operation and loop colostomy. Given high mortality and morbidity and the negative impact of colostomy on quality of life, self-expandable metallic stents (SEMS) have been developed. One meta-analysis of 13 randomized controlled trials or case control studies with 837 patients revealed SEMS group had lower clinical success of relieving obstructive symptoms than surgery (93.1% versus 99.8%) but with shorter length of stay, time to initiate chemotherapy, and lower rate of 30-day mortality [28].

When to perform colectomy or colostomy—able to undergo general anesthesia and invasive surgery, right-sided LBO, most left-sided LBO unless SEMS preferred, if patient amenable to colostomy.

When not to perform colectomy or colostomy—unable to undergo general anesthesia or invasive surgery, may use SEMS in select left-sided LBO for shorter length of stay, and not amenable to colostomy.

Advanced Esophageal Cancer

The palliation of esophageal cancer is complicated. Operative indications are limited due to high preoperative mortality and complications; thus, endoscopic interventions are generally pursued. However, endoscopic stents also pose considerable risks. A retrospective review of 46 patients who underwent self-expanded drug-coated stents for palliation of dysphagia due to esophageal cancer was performed. The study revealed life-threatening complications in 9% of all patients and 17% with complications such as stent migration, tracheoesophageal fistula, and aspiration [29]. This suggests that while stenting remains an option for palliation, clear expectations should be communicated.

When to perform esophagectomy—limited operative indications.

When not to perform esophagectomy—most cases of palliation utilize endoscopic stents though with risks.

Advanced Pancreatic Cancer

Palliative surgical consideration for pancreatic cancer is important since only 20% of patients are suitable for a curative resection and are often asymptomatic, thus discovered late. Specifically, obstructive jaundice and duodenal obstruction can be palliated with surgery. This section will focus on obstructive jaundice as duodenal obstruction is treated similarly as GOO discussed above.

Surgical option for obstructive jaundice is a biliary-enteric bypass including Roux-en-Y hepaticojejunosotomy (HJ). It is indicated when unresectable disease is found during laparotomy. Open, laparoscopic, and robotic venues can be utilized—no definite differences in outcome have been studied but the robotic system offers improved visualization and ergonomics. Otherwise, endoscopic biliary stent remains a favored palliative intervention given it is minimally invasive, highly feasible in over 90% of patients, and yields lower length of stay while having similar mortality and readmission rates as surgical bypass. It may, however, be associated with higher reintervention and obstructive complication rates. If stent placement is unsuccessful or not feasible, then transhepatic biliary drainage can be pursued though it may need routine catheter changes and can lead to malfunctions [30].

When to perform HJ—able to undergo general anesthesia and invasive surgery, unresectable disease found during laparotomy, endoscopic or percutaneous palliation not feasible.

When not to perform HJ—unable to undergo general anesthesia and invasive surgery, shorter life expectancy, preference for minimally invasive procedure such as stent and drains.

Advanced Gastric Cancer

While the survival benefit of palliative resection for incurable gastric cancer has been purported, this argument is limited because the appropriate outcome measure for palliative surgery should primarily be symptom relief and quality of life [31]. One study showed the importance of clarifying "noncurative gastric resection" as with palliative intent and non-palliative, as the reported survival benefit of gastrectomy may falsely encourage the practice of invasive operations which in fact may not have palliative intent or benefits [12]. Ever since, further evidence for gastrojejunostomy and endoscopic stent have been published with favorable results.

When to perform gastrectomy—limited indications for palliative gastrectomy (particularly total gastrectomy), symptomatic bleeding requiring control, longer than anticipated with palliative radiation.

When not to perform gastrectomy—availability of gastrojejunostomy or stent.

Metastatic Breast Cancer

Despite the advances in systemic therapy, patients with metastatic breast cancer (MBC) may still develop symptoms, including neurologic, thoracic, and musculoskeletal. However, there is a lack of guidelines for pursuing palliative surgery for symptom relief of different systems. Morrogh et al. [32] identified 91 patients from a prospective database who underwent 109 palliative operations or procedures for symptom control. Most common interventions were craniotomy, open reduction and internal fixation, and thoracostomy tube. The study showed that a composite group of palliative interventions provided 30-day symptom improvement in 91% of patients and ongoing palliation for the duration of life in 70% of patients. This was associated with 20% morbidity rate but most were minor and was not associated with compromised palliation, suggesting the reasonable benefit of palliation for symptom control in MBC.

Soft Tissue Malignancy

Soft tissue lesions can represent locoregional progression or distant metastasis and cause pain, odor, ulceration, bleeding, and disfiguration. Blakely et al. [33] identified 31 patients in a prospective database who received palliative soft tissue resections. Tumor types included melanoma, squamous cell carcinoma, sarcoma, among others. The results showed 90% of patients stating the decision was "worth it" and 80% with symptom improvement within 30 days also with low morbidity and mortality. This suggests that palliative surgery for local control of advanced soft tissue malignancy can provide symptom relief and improved quality of life.

Palliative Surgery—Where It Is Headed

As discussed, surgical palliative care has made notable progress including early prospective studies and growth in data for various types of palliative surgery. Studies show that palliative care interventions for surgical patients improve advance care planning without increasing mortality and reduce healthcare utilization. However, integration of palliative care principles into current surgical culture has been challenging, in part due to major gaps in the current evidence. Lilley et al. [34] have identified three priorities for research on surgical palliative care: measuring patient-centered outcomes, communication and decision-making, and delivery of palliative care to surgical patients. We will explore relevant literature that will aid surgeons in making palliative surgical decisions with patients and families.

Outcome Measures

The outcomes of palliative surgery ought to be measured by symptom control and quality of life rather than survival, need for reintervention, and morbidity of surgery, which are appropriate outcomes for non-palliative operations but still used in the majority of palliative research. Below are scoring systems for the two outcome measures [35]:

Symptom control

- The Edmonton Symptom Assessment Scale

- Visual Analogue Scale/Numerical Rating Scale
- Short-Form McGill Pain Questionnaire

Quality of life

- McGill Quality of Life Questionnaire
- Quality of Life at End of Life
- Quality of Dying and Death Questionnaire

Unfortunately, symptom control and quality of life are inherently limited since patient's disease will likely still progress. Thus, novel outcome measures have been explored. Cohen et al. [36] reported the usefulness of asking, "Was it worth it?", in a retrospective review of a longitudinal palliative surgery database at an academic tertiary-care center. All 180 patients who underwent palliative-intent operations for advanced cancer from 2003 to 2022 were identified. The study showed that patients who answered "Not worth it" were more likely to have advanced age over 65, lack of family engagement, and need for re-operation, thus suggesting that "Was it worth it?" is a patient-centered and practical metric that can complement the existing outcome measures for palliative surgical patients.

Communication and Decision-Making

As discussed, the early prospective studies, recent data on various types of palliative surgery and novel outcome measures contribute immensely to building foundational knowledge on surgical palliative care and evidence-based practice. However, translation to daily clinical environment requires communication of highest standards. Here we present two models of communication well-known in palliative surgical community—the Palliative Triangle and Best Case/Worst Case—and other helpful tools to facilitate communication.

The Palliative Triangle

The idea of the Palliative Triangle initially stemmed from the aforementioned prospective study by Miner et al. [19]. Despite showing less than expected improvement in symptoms and quality of life, the study demonstrated a close interaction and overall satisfaction between the patient, family, and surgeon throughout the palliative treatment. Functional Assessment of Cancer Therapy-G data—an objective measure that scores each patient's physical, functional, social, and emotional wellbeing along with relationship with doctor—showed high scores in the preoperative period and maintained until death. In addition, Miner et al. [20] also showed superior patient selection in encounters where surgeons were experienced in shared decision-making with patients and families. The Palliative Triangle was also evaluated as a tool for careful patient selection. Miner et al. [37] assessed 227 patients symptomatic from incurable cancer identified from comprehensive prospective palliative surgery database at Rhode Island Hospital from 2004 to 2009. Importantly, 1 or 2 meetings between patient, family, and surgeon lasting 60–90 min took place before making a decision for palliative surgery and the use of the Palliative Triangle was confirmed with each attending surgeon. Overall, more than 90% of patients reported symptom improvement or resolution, and palliative operations were associated with lower 30-day postoperative morbidity (20.1%) and mortality (3.9%) than previously published results, showing the promising value of the Palliative Triangle.

The key to the Palliative Triangle (Fig. 39.1) is a *dynamic* relationship between the patient, family, and surgeon *throughout* the palliative phase of the treatment—*dynamic* because the relationship must withstand the lability of patient's state and curveballs and *throughout* because the relationship must be sustained despite difficulties and roadblocks. In the beginning, there needs to be a clear definition of goals of each patient's treatment, in accordance with the *intent* and *individualized* nature of palliative surgery. Then, through the dynamics of the triangle, each patient's values and meaning of life, available social and emotional support, and current medical and surgical alternatives would be shared and weighed. Ideally, the strengthened triangle will also help mediate patient's and/or family's at times unrealistic expectations. Each participant of the Triangle is expected to fulfill his or her unique obligation, as all three progress toward the collective picture of hope formed by the dynamic relationship (Fig. 39.2).

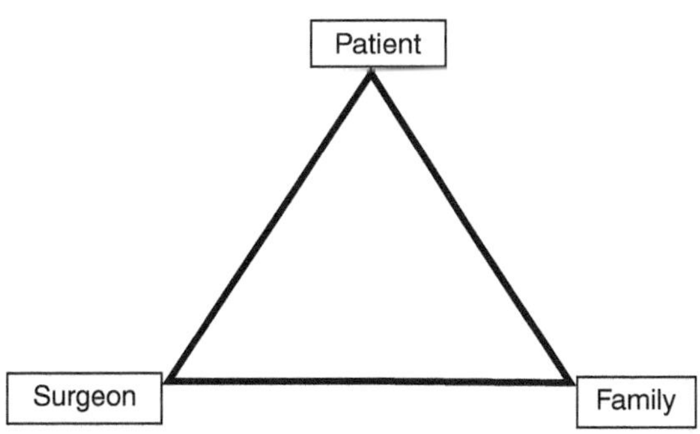

Fig. 39.1 An ideal palliative triangle in which equal interactions between the patient, family, and surgeon guide individualized decision for palliative surgery. [From Miner TJ, Jaques DP & Shriver CD (2002). A prospective evaluation of patients undergoing surgery for the palliation of an advanced malignancy. Annals of Surgical Oncology, 9(7), 696–703; permission obtained.]

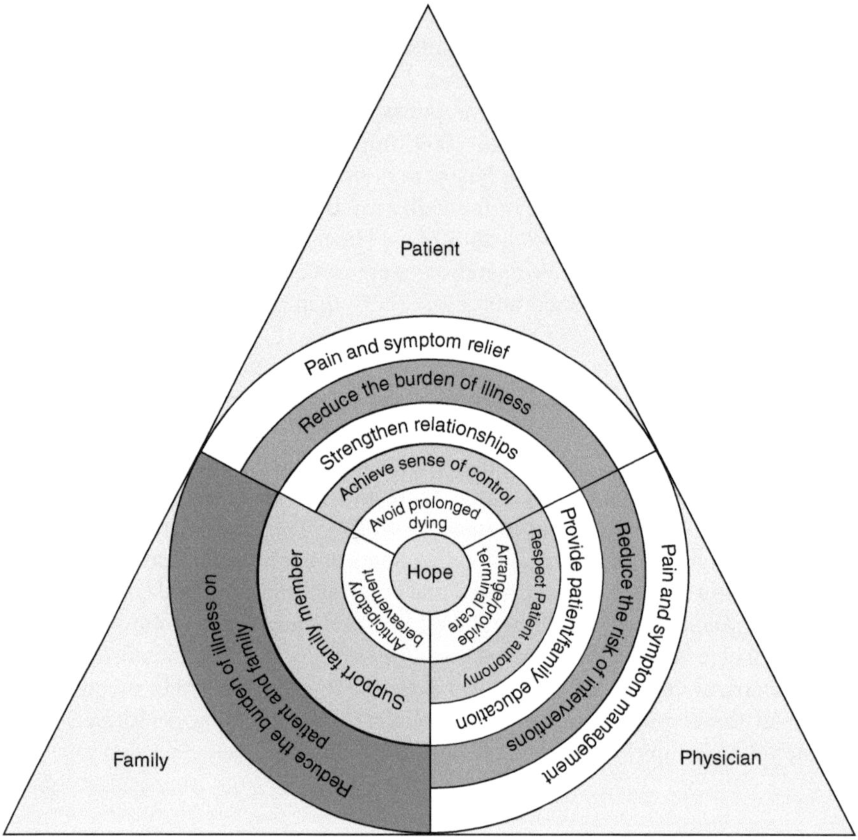

Fig. 39.2 The palliative triangle. The hope for patient-specific goals is progressively achieved as each participant fulfills unique roles and effective communication takes place. (From Thomay AA, Jaques DP, Miner TJ. Surgical palliation: getting back to our roots. Surg Clin North Am 2009; 89:33; permission obtained)

Best Case/Worst Case

Schwarze et al. [38] provides a helpful and practical communication tool called Best Case/Worst Case. This was designed to aid patient, family, and surgeon in better communicating a clinical context in which the surgery is to take place and impact patient's life. This is to prevent scenarios where only bare statistics detached from the clinical context is provided during informed consent, failing to paint an accurate picture of postoperative scenarios based on which patient can make the decision to undergo surgery. For instance, consider a case of a frail elderly patient with ischemic cardiomyopathy and chronic obstructive pulmonary disease. She is found to have a symptomatic thoracic aortic aneurysm in the emergency department and consents to an emergent surgery. The informed consent was performed by providing risks, benefits, and alternatives. Patient ends up in the

ICU with mechanical ventilator and family shares that patient would not have wanted any life-prolonging measures. There was a miscommunication between the surgeon and patient in the definition of the best and worst case—surgeon's idea of the best case was prolonged intensive care unit stay and at best discharge to the nursing home while the patient's values and goals in life discorded. With the Best Case/Worst Case framework, a clearer communication of expectations could have occurred and have led to peaceful transition to hospice without a morbid operation that scarred the family and went against patient's wishes. Practically, surgeon would begin by presenting the best and worst cases for each scenario—surgery and palliative care—augmented by a visual aid (Fig. 39.3), followed by exploring patient's values and goals of care with family, then proceeding to shared decision-making.

This Best Case/Worst Case model was also evaluated in a prospective study that examined its impact on the quality of communication by surgeons. Taylor et al. [39] conducted a 2-h training session regarding the Best Case/Worst Case communication framework to 25 surgeons at a tertiary-care hospital in Madison, Wisconsin, from 2014 to 2015. They engaged in decision-making conversations with 32 patients with acute non-emergent surgical issues and their family members and each conversation was scored using OPTION 5, an observer measure of shared decision-making, then compared pre- and post-training. Not only did the scores improve, but the surgeons also demonstrated a shift in the focus of communication from isolated surgical problem to a contextualized discussion about outcomes, alternatives, and integration of patient preference and recommendation. The promising result coupled with its applicability makes Best Case/Worst Case framework an attractive model for palliative surgical decision-making.

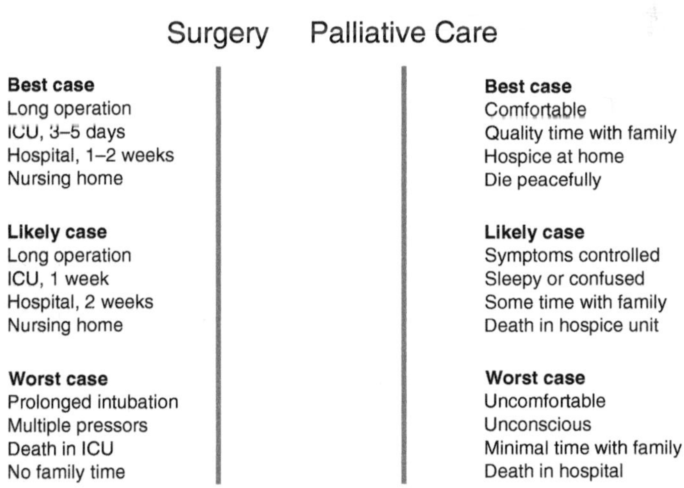

Fig. 39.3 The best case/worst case visual aid. [Adapted from Taylor LJ, Nabozny MJ, Steffens NM, et al. (2017). A framework to improve surgeon communication in high-stakes surgical decision. JAMA Surgery 2017; 152(6): 531–8.]

Helpful Tools

Other helpful tools for guiding communication include the CLASS protocol of Buckman and the SPIKES protocol [14, 40].

The CLASS protocol stands for context, listening, acknowledgment, strategy, and summary (Fig. 39.4) and is a methodical way to frame a conversation with patients and families regarding palliative procedures. As always, quintessential to the success of this method is empathy and relationship.

The SPIKES protocol is a variant of the CLASS protocol and can be used when delivering bad news or managing a high-stress situation during a family meeting. The components are setting, patient's perception, invitation, knowledge, emotions, and strategy/summary (Fig. 39.5).

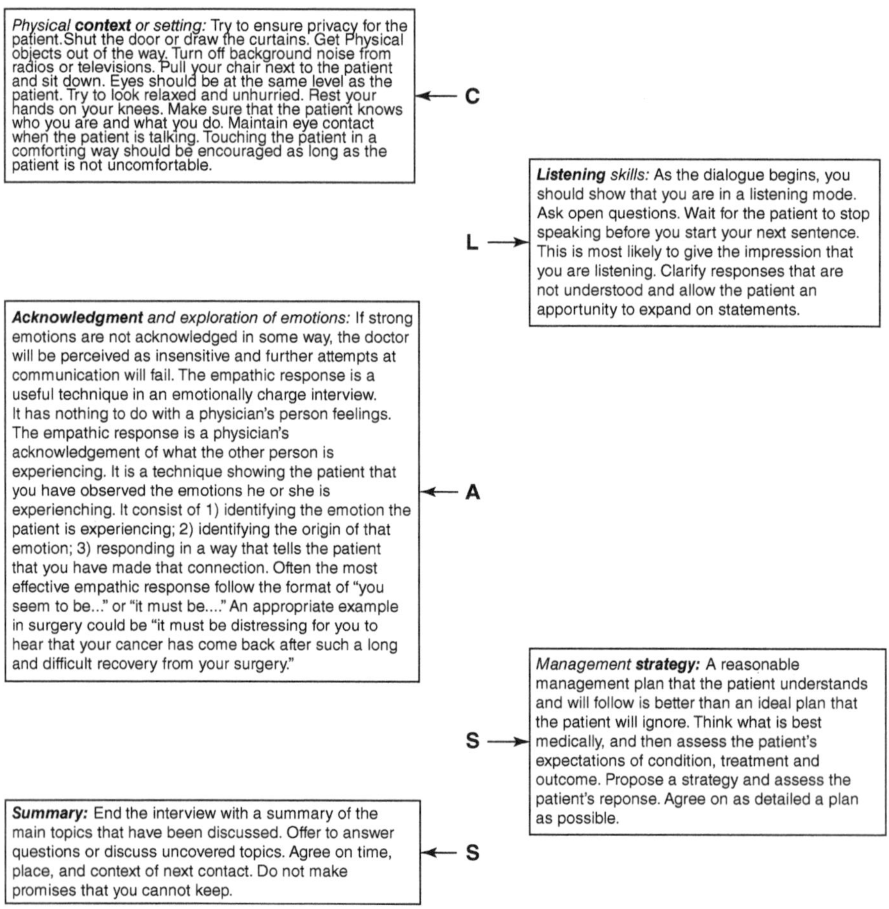

Fig. 39.4 The CLASS protocol, a methodical framework to base a surgical palliative conversation with patient and family. Examples of practical implementation are provided. [From Miner TJ (2012). Communication as a Core Skill of Palliative Surgical Care. Anesthesiology Clin, 30, 47–58; permission obtained)

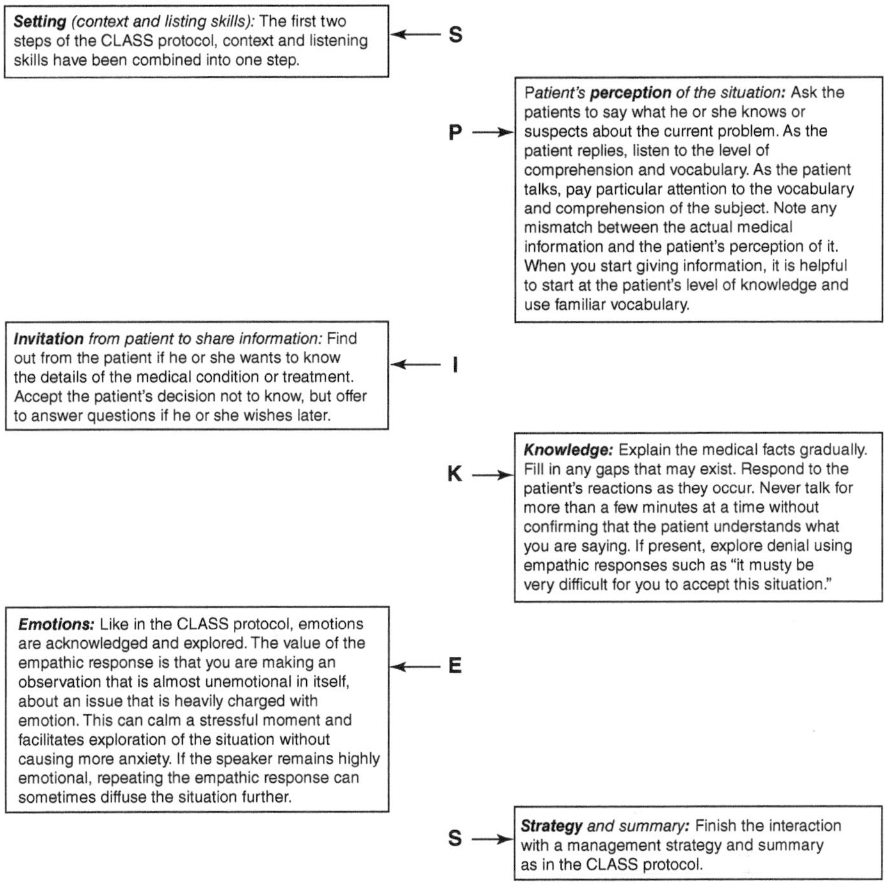

Fig. 39.5 The SPIKES protocol, a variant of the CLASS protocol. May be used for relieving a high-stress situation and/or breaking bad news. Examples of practical implementation are provided. [From Miner TJ (2012). Communication as a Core Skill of Palliative Surgical Care. Anesthesiology Clin, 30, 47–58; permission obtained]

Delivery of Palliative Care to Surgical Patients

In this section, we explore two proposed ways to enhance delivery and integration of palliative care to surgical patients: palliative care education during surgical training and interdisciplinary collaboration with palliative care service.

Education

To find an efficient way to teach busy surgical residents, Klaristenfeld et al. [41] presented a pilot curriculum at Brown University in surgical palliative care consisting of three 1-h sessions of group discussion, role playing, and instruction in clinical decision-making. Total of 47 surgical residents participated and showed marked improvement in comfort level in palliative discussions. All residents confirmed that palliative care is a valuable skill for surgeons, and 92% had used the curriculum content in clinical environment by the third month with 85% sharing that this was sufficient training. Such need and desire for a formal surgical palliative care curriculum were reaffirmed in another survey of surgery residents and faculty at a different tertiary center which showed only half of residents felt comfortable leading a palliative discussion and 90% of faculty agreed that more training is needed for chief residents [42]. As a solution, Surgery Residency Program at Brown University has implemented scheduled palliative care sessions within weekly educational conferences facilitated by palliative care faculty. In addition, there has been an increasing interest within surgical community in Hospice and Palliative Care board certification, as evidenced by the establishment of Surgical Palliative Care society in 2021 and more than 80 double-boarded surgeons who have shown satisfaction in the formal palliative care training in positively impacting their surgical patient care [43].

Consultation to Palliative Care Service

While it is paramount that surgeons learn palliative care skillsets, prompt and opportune consultation of inpatient palliative care service have also shown promising results. Early evidence showed that high-quality palliative care does not increase mortality in the intensive care unit and even may prolong life [44]. Recent data found that early palliative care consultation was associated with shorter length of stay, reduced ventilator days and number of invasive procedures, and lower healthcare costs in trauma patients [45, 46]. This suggests that early interdisciplinary collaboration can enhance surgical palliative care.

When To and When Not To?

Patient Selection

In determining "when to" and "when not to," patient selection remains the single most important factor in effective surgical palliation [2]. This entails identifying a subset of patients who will achieve the greatest benefit (i.e. relief of symptoms, improved quality of life, those who will deem it "worth it") at the lowest cost possible (i.e. treatment toxicity such as morbidity and mortality from surgery, duration of treatment including length of hospital stay and reintervention, and healthcare utilization) for the longest possible duration of palliation that can be achieved with the palliative surgery. This decision-making process is represented in Fig. 39.6 [47].

As discussed throughout the chapter, it is important to use symptom control [48] and quality of life as a primary measure of palliative surgical benefit instead of traditional measures of morbidity, mortality, and survival. Scoring systems developed for each component were also discussed in the "Outcome measures" section. Of

$$\uparrow \text{Value} = \frac{\uparrow \text{Benefit}\left(\text{Relief of symptoms, Improved quality of life}\right)}{\downarrow \text{Cost}\left(\text{Treatment toxicity, Duration of treatment, Resource utilization}\right)} \times \text{Anticipated duration of palliation}$$

Fig. 39.6 Value of palliative surgery can be represented as benefit divided by cost multiplied by anticipated duration of palliation. [From Cohen JT, Miner TJ (2019). Patient selection in palliative surgery: Defining value. Journal of Surgical Oncology. 120:35–44. permission obtained]

note, recent data also show that ability to rise from chair and need for re-operation are associated with patients who experience long-term survival after palliative surgery, which highlight the need for selecting for patients with these factors for greater symptom control [49].

A variety of biochemical and functional patient factors have been studied to be associated with the cost of palliative surgery, including morbidity and mortality. These include history of 10 or more lb. weight loss, anemia (hemoglobin <10.5), hypoalbuminemia (<3.5), elevated C-reactive protein, elevated creatinine, leukocytosis, neutrophil to lymphocyte ratio, National Cancer Institute fatigue scale of 1 or greater, and Eastern Cooperative Oncology Group score of 2 or greater. Some systems that provide composite scores for these factors to better predict palliative surgical cost have been developed, such as Palliative Index, UC Davis Nomogram, Glasgow Prognostic Score, and LENT score [47, 50].

Conclusion

While patient selection is the single most important factor in palliative surgery, surgeons cannot solely rely on the above scoring systems, biochemical and functional factors. Not only do these measures have inherent limitations, but they also may mislead each surgeon to reduce the complex nature of surgical palliative care into a set of formula. Ultimately, the shared decision-making for "when to" and "when not to" recommend palliative surgery should be a collectively determined individualized process—collectively determined within the Palliative Triangle by establishing strong rapport with both family and patient and individualized by taking each patient's unique value system, comorbidity, and disease process and contextualizing within the available evidence.

In this chapter, we have defined palliative surgery as a deliberately performed operation or procedure with the primary intention of improving *quality of life* or relieving *symptoms* in a patient with incurable disease and provided an overview of what entails a decision-making process for "when to" and "when not to" recommend palliative surgery. In doing so, we have traced the history and evolution of palliative surgery from an obscure field mostly reliant on personal experiences and anecdotes to a promising and growing area with increasingly robust research and rising interest. We discussed the available evidence for each type of palliative surgery, ongoing and future directions of surgical palliative care including improving outcome measures and education, and appropriately selecting patients to maximize benefit and minimize cost for the longest duration of palliation. Most importantly, we have established that practicing surgical palliative care is built upon the dynamic relationship of patient, family, and surgeon who will walk with each other toward patient- and family-specific picture of hope—one that is realistic and comforting, one that will motivate all involved persons to move forward in the face of an incurable ailment, all of which must be championed in the practice of palliative surgery.

References

1. McCahill LE, Dunn GP, Mosenthal AC, et al. Palliation as a core surgical principle: part 1. J Am Coll Surg. 2004;199(1):149–60.
2. Thomay AA, Jaques DP, Miner TJ. Surgical palliation: getting back to our roots. Surg Clin N Am. 2009;89(1):27–41.
3. Halstead WJ. The results of radical operations for the cure of cancer of the breast. Ann Surg. 1907;46:1–27.
4. Dunn GP, Johnson AG. Surgical palliative care. Oxford University Press; 2004. p. 5.
5. Miner TJ, Tavaf-Motamen H, Shriver CD, et al. An evaluation of surgical palliation based on patient outcome data. Am J Surg. 1999;177:150–4.
6. Easson AM, Crosby JA, Librach SL. Discussion of death and dying in surgical textbooks. Am J Surg. 2001;182:34–9.
7. Lynn J. Learning of care for people with chronic illness facing the end of life. JAMA. 2000;284:2508–11.
8. Figg WD, Smith EK, Price DK, et al. Disclosing a diagnosis of cancer: where and how does it occur? J Clin Oncol. 2010;28:3630–5.
9. McCue JD. The naturalness of dying. JAMA. 1995;273:1039–43.
10. World Health Organization. Cancer pain relief and palliative cure: report of a WHO expert committee (technical report series No. 804). Geneva: World Health Organization; 1990. p. 11.
11. Ball ABS, Baum M, Breach NM, Shepherd JH, Shearer J, Thomas JM, et al. Surgical palliation. In: Doyle D, Hanks GWC, MacDonald N, editors. Oxford textbook of palliative medicine. 3rd ed. Oxford: Oxford University Press; 1998. p. 282–4.
12. Miner TJ, Jaques DP, Karpeh MS, et al. Defining non-curative gastric resections by palliative intent. J Am Coll Surg. 2004;198:1013–21.
13. McCahill LE, Krouse RS, Chu DZ, et al. Decision making in palliative surgery. J Am Coll Surg. 2002;195:411–22.
14. Miner TJ. Communication as a core skill of palliative surgical care surgical palliation palliative triangle communication skills. Anesthesiol Clin. 2012;30:47–58.
15. Miner TJ. Palliative surgery for advanced cancer: lessons learned in patient selection and outcome assessment. Am J Clin Oncol. 2005;28:411–4.
16. Miner TJ, Jaques DP, Tavaf-Motamen H, et al. Decision making on surgical palliation based on patient outcome data. Am J Surg. 1999;177(2):150.
17. Connors AF, Dawson NV, Desbiens NA, et al. A controlled trial to improve care for seriously ill hospitalized patients: the study to understand prognoses and preferences for outcomes and risks of treatments (SUPPORT). JAMA. 1995;274(20):1591–8.
18. Dunn GP. Surgery, palliative care, and the American College of Surgeons. Ann Palliat Med. 2015;4(1):5–9.

19. Miner TJ, Jaques DP, Shriver CD. A prospective evaluation of patients undergoing surgery for the palliation of an advanced malignancy. Ann Surg Oncol. 2002;9(7):696–703.
20. Miner TJ, Brennan M, et al. A prospective, symptom related, outcomes analysis of 1022 palliative procedures for advanced cancer. Ann Surg. 2004;240:719–27.
21. Miner TJ, Jaques PP. The role of preemptive palliation in advanced cancer. Ann Surg Oncol. 2006;5:173s.
22. Upchurch E, Ragusa M, Cirocchi R. Stent placement versus surgical palliation for adults with malignant gastric outlet obstruction. Cochrane Database Syst Rev. 2018;5:CD012506.
23. Potz BA, Miner TJ. Surgical palliation of gastric outlet obstruction in advanced malignancy. World J Gastrointest Surg. 2016;8(8):545.
24. Kim SW, Lim C-H, Kim JS, et al. Long-term outcome of palliative therapy for gastric outlet obstruction caused by unresectable gastric cancer in patients with good performance status: endoscopic stenting versus surgery. Gastrointest Endosc. 2013;78(1):55–62.
25. Jeurnink SM, Steyerberg EW, van Hooft JE, et al. Surgical gastrojejunostomy or endoscopic stent placement for the palliation of malignant gastric outlet obstruction (SUSTENT study): a multicenter randomized trial. Gastrointest Endosc. 2010;71:490–9.
26. Paul Olson TJ, Pinkerton C, Brasel KJ, Schwarze ML. Palliative surgery for malignant bowel obstruction from carcinomatosis. JAMA Surg. 2014;149(4):383–92.
27. Ripamonti CI, Easson AM, Gerdes H. Management of malignant bowel obstruction. Eur J Cancer. 2008;44(8):1105–15.
28. Zhao XD. Palliative treatment for incurable malignant colorectal obstructions: a meta-analysis. World J Gastroenterol. 2013;19(33):5565–74.
29. Kujawski K, Stasiak M, Rysz J. The evaluation of esophageal stenting complications in palliative treatment of dysphagia related to esophageal cancer. MedSciMon. 2012;18(5):CR323–9.
30. Ciambella CC, Beard RE, Miner TJ. Current role of palliative interventions in advanced pancreatic cancer. World J Gastrointest Surg. 2018;10(7):75.
31. Blakely AM, Miner TJ. Surgical considerations in the treatment of gastric cancer. Gastroenterol Clin N Am. 2013;42(2):337–57.
32. Morrogh M, Miner TJ, Park A, Jenckes A, Gonen M, Seidman A, et al. A prospective evaluation of the durability of palliative interventions for patients with metastatic breast cancer. Cancer. 2010;116(14):3338–47.
33. Blakely AM, McPhillips J, Miner TJ. Surgical palliation for malignant disease requiring locoregional control. Ann Palliat Med. 2015;4(2):48–53.
34. Lilley EJ, Cooper Z, Schwarze ML, Mosenthal AC. Palliative care in surgery: defining the research priorities. Ann Surg. 2018;267(1):66–72.
35. Louie AD, Miner TJ. Palliative surgery and the surgeon's role in the palliative care team: a review. Ann Palliat Med. 2022;11(2):907–17.
36. Cohen JT, Beard RE, Cioffi WG, Miner TJ. Was it worth it? Critical evaluation of a novel outcomes measure in oncologic palliative surgery. J Am Coll Surg. 2023;236(6):1156–62.
37. Miner TJ, Cohen JT, Charpentier K, et al. The palliative triangle: improved patient selection and outcomes associated with palliative operations. JAMA. 2011;146(5):517–23.
38. Schwarze ML, Kehler JM, Campbell TC. Navigating high risk procedures with more than just a street map. J Palliat Med. 2015;16(10):1169–71.
39. Taylor LJ, Nabozny MJ, Steffens NM, et al. A framework to improve surgeon communication in high-stakes surgical decision. JAMA Surg. 2017;152(6):531–8.
40. Buckman R. Communication skills in palliative care: a practical guide. Neurol Clin. 2001;19:989–1004.
41. Klaristenfeld DD, Harrington DT, Miner TJ. Teaching palliative care and end-of-life issues: a core curriculum for surgical residents. Ann Surg Oncol. 2007;14(6):1801–6.
42. Bonanno AM, Kiraly LN, Siegel TR, Brasel KM, et al. Surgical palliative care training in general surgery residency: an educational needs assessment. Am J Surg. 2019;217:928–31.
43. Bassette E, Salyer C, et al. Hospice and palliative medicine fellowship after surgical training: a roadmap to the future of surgical palliative care. J Surg Ed. 2002;79(5):1177–87.

44. Mosenthal AC, et al. Integrating palliative care in the surgical and trauma intensive care unit: a report from the Improving Palliative Care in the Intensive Care Unit (IPAL-ICU) project advisory board and the center to advance palliative care. Crit Care Med. 2012;40(4):1199–206.
45. Spencer AL, Miller PR, et al. Timing is everything: early versus late palliative care consults in trauma. J Trauma Acute Care Surg. 2023;94(5):652–8.
46. Spencer AL, Nunn AM, et al. The value of compassion: healthcare savings of palliative care consults in trauma. Injury. 2023;54:249–55.
47. Cohen JT, Miner TJ. Patient selection in palliative surgery: defining value. J Surg Oncol. 2019;120:35–44.
48. Miner TJ, Jaques DP, Paty PB, Guillem JG, Wong WD. Symptom control in patients with locally recurrent rectal cancer. Ann Surg Oncol. 2003;10(1):72–9.
49. Cohen JT, Fallon EA, Charpentier KP, Cioffi WG, Miner TJ. Improving the value of palliative surgery by optimizing patient selection: the role of long-term survival on high impact palliative intent operations. Am J Surg. 2021;221(5):1018–23.
50. Cohen JT, Miner TJ. Chapter 14: Principles, assessment, and evaluation for palliative surgery. In: Dunn G, Mosenthal A, editors. Surgical palliative care. Oxford Press; 2019.

Chapter 40
How Should Surgical Palliative Success Be Defined?

Karishma Mistry, Allie Stover, and Sabha Ganai

Introduction

Palliative care is defined as specialized medical care that aims to provide relief from pain and offers support in conjunction with treatment plans to help patients who are suffering from serious, life altering illnesses to live as actively as possible until death [1]. It offers a range of care from general supportive to end-of-life treatment plans. Palliative care focuses on the patient and understanding their goals to ultimately improve quality of life for the duration of life available. Considering the patient's diagnosis, treatment needs, family goals, and desired quality of life, palliative care involves care coordination in the decision-making process to construct an individualized and dynamic plan.

Surgical palliation involves multiple elements and intents: surgery with palliative intent and surgery with curative intent. Surgery with palliative intent includes doing a surgical procedure with an outcome that hopes to improve the patients' quality of life, whether that be symptom resolvement or easier self-management. Surgery with curative intent is done with the hopes of prolonging the lifespan and quality of life. Choosing surgery as a treatment option for palliative care is one that also comes with the difficult task of prognostication. Whether that be because of the uncertainty

K. Mistry
Creighton University, Omaha, NE, USA

A. Stover (✉)
University of North Dakota School of Medicine and Health Sciences, Grand Forks, ND, USA
e-mail: allie.stover@und.edu

S. Ganai (✉)
University of North Dakota School of Medicine and Health Sciences, Grand Forks, ND, USA

Sanford Fargo Medical Center, Fargo, ND, USA
e-mail: Sabha.ganai@sanfordhealth.org

© The Author(s), under exclusive license to Springer Nature Switzerland AG 2024

J. Faintuch, S. Faintuch (eds.), *Recent Strategies in High Risk Surgery*,
https://doi.org/10.1007/978-3-031-56270-9_40

or the wide margins for error, weighing risks and benefits is a large part when picking a surgical option. While every surgery has a level of uncertainty and has the potential for adverse outcomes, the decision to pursue a surgical option for palliative care comes with a greater degree of risk [2]. Pursuing a surgical treatment route may not seem to be the best option as it would not necessarily prolong life span, but it may be effective at improving the patient's quality of life, even if for a short time span. On the other hand, surgery may prove detrimental and provide no benefit to the patient, or worse, result in an escalation of symptoms. However, a literature review of palliative surgical intervention from 1994 to 2014 suggests that palliation options, despite higher risk, have the capacity to improve advance care planning and reduce healthcare utilization, without increasing mortality. Palliative care decision making involves finding a balance between physician duty of nonmaleficence and patient autonomy. Nonmaleficence is often prioritized as physicians come with the intention of trying to protect rather than make worse if given a choice. This paternalistic attribute is tough to push aside even when the patient is ready to take risk for even the smallest of benefits.

When assessing for a palliative consult, there are many aspects of a patient's care that need to be considered. For example, the patient's diagnosis and life expectancy play an important role in determining what treatment options are even feasible given their stability, but the patient's desired treatment goals may be just as, if not more, important, and may contradict the suggested treatment recommendations given their disease status. Palliative care may be offered for patients that have a serious or chronic illness, a declining ability to complete activities of daily life, personal or family distress, the need for ongoing long-term treatment, and many others. Calling for a palliative care consult can cause distress and anxiety for the patient, family, and care team as it requires an existential conversation about goals of care for the duration of life left available and in some cases, whether undergoing a surgery is the best palliative option.

Risks and Benefits of Palliative Surgery

With any surgery comes both risk and uncertainty, and this is especially important to take into consideration for palliative surgery where there are many other factors that come into play such as disease progression, prognosis, prior interventions, frailty, co-morbidities, and overall stability. Previous studies have found that palliative surgery indeed has higher risk than nonpalliative surgeries in terms of morbidity and mortality [3]. In a prospective study of 1022 palliative procedures, morbidity rate was determined to be around 29%, while mortality rate was around 11% at 30 days post-surgery [4]. This is significantly higher than the estimated 12% morbidity and 2% mortality rate of general surgical procedures on the general population [5]. Morbidity and mortality rates are higher in patients with malignancy, even with minimally invasive, relatively benign procedures. In a study examining the differences in risk of PEG tube placement, patients with a diagnosed malignancy were associated with an in-hospital mortality rate of 20% due to the PEG tube placement procedure compared to the overall mortality rate of 0.2% of this procedure [6]. However, reporting the quantity of days post-palliative surgery alone does not attest to the patient experience and therefore falls short of measuring meaningful patient outcomes such as functional independence, pain reduction, appetite, and days spent at home.

While palliative surgery comes with substantial risks, it also has the potential to provide many benefits. A surgical option can offer pain relief, improved functional status, better symptom management, and increased emotional support [7]. When implicated and available, surgery should always be discussed as a potential treatment option for the patient. There have been many cases of success in palliative surgeries showing a variety of benefits. In a retrospective review study of 193 patients with malignant bowel obstruction who opted for surgical treatment, 91% were able to consume a solid diet post-recovery. This may not sound like a significant outcome in comparison to the typical goals of surgery, but food provides major quality of life enhancement for many people. Additionally, these patients experienced less pain, nausea, vomiting, and skin erosions [8]. In the aforementioned study of 1022 advanced cancer patients who underwent palliative surgery, 80% of patients had improvement or resolution of symptoms such as GI obstruction, neurological symptoms, pain, and/or dyspnea within 30 days [4]. Similarly, in another study, patients with cervical spine metastases experienced reduced need for pain relief medication post-surgical decompression and stabilization, also reporting an improvement of neurological deficits [9].

While palliative surgery has shown to be a beneficial option for many, the question remains: What if the surgery does not achieve the desired result, but makes things worse? One prospective study of 26 patients with advanced malignancy reports that even though 54% of its patient population did not achieve their desired surgical outcome, post-operative physical and emotional well-being were significantly improved [6]. However, positive outcomes may not occur for every patient that elects palliative surgical care, regardless of whether their main surgical goal was achieved or not. Thus, it is important for the surgeon to do some method of benefit versus cost analysis for all patients, especially palliative ones.

Patient Selection

Although there is supporting evidence that palliative surgery can improve quality of life for patients in various ways, patient selection plays a significant role in maximizing outcomes. In the case of palliative surgical intervention, traditional factors used to gauge surgical candidacy are of limited use because curing disease and overall survival is no longer the definition of success. For example, tumor staging is an important criterion for "curative" surgical candidacy in cancer patients. However, in a prospective study on 31 cancer patients with soft tissue metastases, palliative surgical resection provided durable symptom relief and improved quality of life, regardless of the extent of tumor invasion [10]. Still, the value of surgery for a patient may be more objectively defined as the ratio of benefit to cost for the patient. Some of the possible benefits could include improved quality of life, relief of symptoms, duration of symptom relief, and days spent at home; costs may include things like treatment-related adverse effects or toxicity, the duration of the treatment, and resources utilized such as ventilators, skilled-nursing facilities, and intensive care admission.

In the case of palliative care, psychosocial factors are of primary consideration in predicting patient benefit. This can be a difficult evaluation for physicians as a balance must be struck between improving quality of life for patients while still considering the biological logistics of surgical efficacy. The palliative triangle can be a helpful tool in managing the relationship between physician(s), patient, and the patient's family by portraying the role that potential treatment outcomes may play for all parties involved in the patient's care (Fig. 40.1). At the center of the triangle is hope, which can ideally be achieved for all patients regardless of disease prognosis.

Despite psychosocial factors being at the core of palliative care decision making, overall patient health status inevitably plays a role in patient selection. Patient health

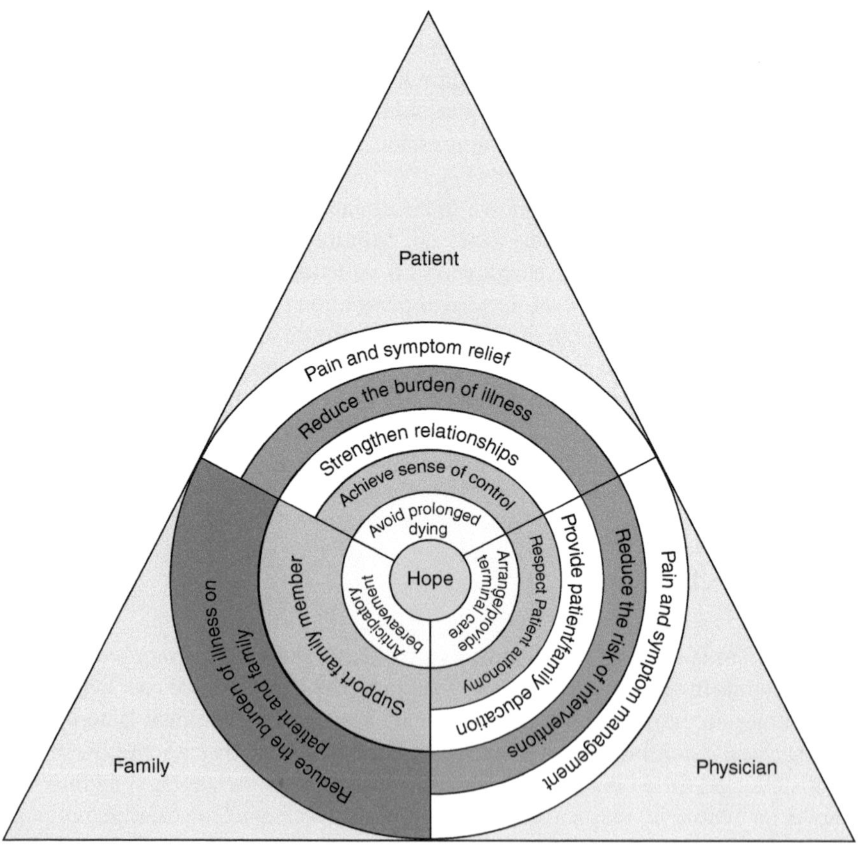

Fig. 40.1 Palliative care triangle

characteristics that would make one a favorable surgical candidate depend highly on the disease at hand. For example, one study found that the presence of ascites and palpable masses were poor prognostic factors for patients undergoing surgery for malignant bowel obstruction [11]. Additionally, primary tumor site has been shown to play a significant role in post-operative survival, with esophageal, pancreatic, and stomach cancer having a worse prognosis (Hirabayashi). However, there are certain measures of prognosis that are not necessarily disease-specific that can be used as parameters for considering palliative surgical candidacy.

The "get up and go" test is a sensitive marker for frailty done by having the patient simply stand up on their own from a seated position in a chair. It is similar to grip strength and the presence of sarcopenia in its ability to measure frailty and therefore poor surgical prognosis, but it doesn't require any special equipment, making it an easy test to be applied in various clinical environments. One study found the "get up and go" test to be associated with over an 11-month average survival for palliative cancer patients [6]. This is in line with previous studies that have found pretreatment neurological status such as fatigue and ambulatory function to be significant prognostic factors in predicting palliative surgical candidacy [12, 13]. Additionally, a study done by Blakely et al. found elevated CRP to be associated with worse outcomes following elective palliative surgery in cancer patients, regardless of disease progression, baseline functional status, or type of malignancy [14]. Patient selection for surgical palliative candidacy can also be supplemented with screening indices such as the Glasgow Prognostic Score, the Palliative Index, the UC Davis Nomogram, and the LENT score. Though there are mixed reports on the individual efficacy of these in predicting patient prognosis, they can be used collectively to strengthen prognostic accuracy [6]. Another study done using the best case/worse case framework showed a significant increase in surgeon communication and shared decision making with family members. Using the best case/worse case framework, surgeons were able to clearly present a choice between treatments, describe a range of post-operative trajectories including functional decline, and involve patients and families in deliberation. This helped family members understand the choices, the range of outcomes, and take part in a shared and informed decision [15].

Ultimately there will always be risks and benefits with surgery, regardless of whether surgery is performed for palliative or curative intent. Whichever one the patient decides to weigh more heavily on is ultimately their decision when potential outcomes are discussed openly and thoroughly with their physician. Though a benefit-to-cost analysis is a difficult task for surgeons in such a risky patient population, it allows for a more appropriate discussion about the capacity that surgery has to support patient goals and guides clinical decision making. For example, in those patients with a better prognosis, a more invasive, but durable, surgical procedure may be opted for to provide longer symptom relief. It is important for providers to remember that palliative surgery is not intended to cure the underlying condition but rather to provide relief from symptoms and improvement in patient quality of life. Even when outcomes of palliative surgical care seem bleak from a medical standpoint, physicians ought to respect patient autonomy when informed consent is given, because extending poor quality of life is not necessarily better than shortening the quantity of life.

Quality Versus Quantity

The overriding battle in palliative care is the choice between the physician's duty to uphold a balance between nonmaleficence and beneficence versus respecting patient autonomy. While conducting a palliative surgical procedure could help improve the patient's quality of life, it could also prove detrimental for the patient's ongoing treatment or length of survival. Therefore, the conflict of determining whether to pursue nonmaleficence or patient autonomy arises.

Patient autonomy and physician duty to avoid harm are two important principles that guide decision making. Patient autonomy refers to the right of a patient to make their own decisions about their healthcare, based on their values, beliefs, and preferences [16]. Physician duty, on the other hand, refers to the responsibility of a physician to act in the best interest of their patients and provide care that meets the highest standards of medical practice [17]. Physician duties promoting nonmaleficence and beneficence have been the core of medicine for decades; however, there has been a shift in the last few years from the traditional "paternalistic" practice of medicine to an emphasis on "patient-centered care". This framework shifts the focus from telling the patient what to do to facilitating shared decision making with the patient based on their goals and values. It means the physician is no longer the dictator of patient healthcare but rather an expert that is involved in the discussion and present for advice, guidance, and most importantly, information. The Institute of Medicine identifies this as being "responsive to individual patient preferences, needs, and values" [18]. In palliative care, physicians often find themselves deciding whether to support the patients' preferences or doing what is considered to be the highest standard of medical practice. One way to find a balance between the two is by prioritizing the principle of informed consent.

Informed consent involves providing patients with all the information they need to make an informed decision about their care. This includes information about all the potential risks, benefits, and the capacity of each treatment option that is not skewed by physician opinion [19]. The goal with informed consent is that the patient may then make an educated decision regarding their medical care that best serves their goals and values in life, which are highly specific to and vary for each individual. If the patient decides the risks and outcomes of a surgical intervention are worth the potential benefits, then it is their choice to take those risks. While a surgeon may not agree with the treatment choice, if they are willing and able to complete the surgery, it is the best treatment route to be taken. By providing patients with information about their options, providers can respect autonomy while also fulfilling their duty to act in the patient's best interest.

Communication in Palliative Surgery Discussions

Counseling on palliative surgery has unique complexities for a variety of reasons. While surgical palliation does not exclusively occur at the end-of-life, patients approaching an end-of-life trajectory often harbor an ever-changing disease status. This makes it difficult to plan surgical intervention as patients may be stable 1 day and considered sufficient candidates for surgery and then decline drastically within the days before surgery. Second, patients must be counseled on the capacity and limitations of surgical interventions and the short- and long-term effects that surgery may have on their quality of life, which are not always easy to predict, especially in such an unstable patient population. Though surgery is an unmatched treatment option in the sense that it can provide immediate relief of symptoms, patients may not fully understand the stress that it puts the body through, which is often compounded by pre-existing immunosuppression, hematologic instability, and/or neurological insufficiencies. Because of this, other healthcare professionals are often involved in the conversation of palliative care goals, creating another dimension of complexity in navigating the decision to undergo surgery for both the patient and the surgeon. Other healthcare providers involved in the discussion that are more familiar with palliative care may be less likely to support a surgical route which can dampen surgeons' willingness to provide surgery, create patient anxiety, and prolong decision making. Not surprisingly, one study found that surgical rescue culture and surgeon responsibility to provide excellent care are most often cited as barriers to practicing palliative surgical care [20].

One way to help reduce surgeon hesitancy while simultaneously improving patient satisfaction is by clarifying, prior to surgery, the extent of intervention that they are willing to undergo post-operatively should complications arise. This should be discussed with all palliative surgical candidates as even those with pre-existing advanced directives may want to temporarily halt such directives in the immediate post-operative period; alternatively, those without an advanced directive may want to limit invasive, burdensome life-supporting therapy following surgery should it be necessary. This is a great way to avoid post-operative interpersonal conflict and to help the surgeon feel more comfortable in proceeding with riskier levels of care. Additionally, the patient's desired outcome of and expectations for the surgery should continuously be discussed, as providing a high value operation does not guarantee a positive impact if symptoms being palliated do not significantly interfere with the patient's life or if the operation cannot support their goals. Interestingly, one study found that many patients rate trusting their doctor and being treated the way they want as "very important" priorities, representing the importance of perceived control which has been demonstrated to be associated with improved psychosocial well-being in breast cancer patients [21].

Measuring Treatment Outcomes

Measuring outcomes of palliative surgical care is unique in that the typical standards for surgical success, such as disease prevention or cure and life prolongment, are not valued as heavily. For this reason, the data on how to measure palliative surgical success is scarce and the peri-operative and long-term outcomes of palliative surgery have not been clearly defined. Improving and optimizing quality of life while allowing for patients to have a good death is the main goal of palliative surgery. Therefore, systems to identify the effects that surgical care has on the quality of life are more heavily relied upon. These include indices such as the McGill Quality of Life Questionnaire (MQDL), Quality of Life at the End of Life (QUAL-E), Quality of Dying and Death Questionnaire (QODD), and the Physical and Functional Wellbeing Subscales of the Functional Assessment of Cancer Therapy-General (FACT-G). However, these continue to be a challenge in accurately measuring palliative surgical success as they fail to take into account the trauma of surgery and the burden of recovering from surgery. The Euro QoL Five Dimension (EQ-5d) and European Organization for Research and Treatment of Cancer (EOTC) Quality of Life Questionnaire (QLQ-STO22) are both quality of life assessments specific for post-palliation surgery. Unfortunately, quality of life improvements in this specific patient population are often masked by the characteristics of their disease, even though clinically evident improvements may be present [6]. Interestingly, in a study by Blakely et al. when a group of palliative surgical patients were simply asked, "Was it worth it?", after their procedure, around 88% of them agreed that it was [10]. Though this may not give us a detailed evaluation on their quality of life status, it gives us important insight into the patient's experience of symptom management and perception of care, which is ultimately what matters most.

Aside from patient questionnaires, there are other measures of quality of life that can be considered. For example, the majority of patients would prefer to die in the comfort of their own home. This is important to consider as surgery often requires time spent recovering in the hospital which can be prolonged, especially in vulnerable patients, taking away from time at home and potentially dying at home if there are significant complications. In a study done on palliative surgical intervention for malignant bowel obstruction, approximately ¼ of patients spent their remaining time in the hospital [11]. For this reason, measuring complication rates can be beneficial, as they often require longer hospitalization and greater risk for readmission [22]. In a review done on 70 cancer patients that underwent palliative surgical resection, 26% had major complications—the most common being infection and bleeding [22]. Length of survival post-surgery is an outcome that is commonly measured in palliative surgical studies but ought to be less relevant when considering surgical candidacy as quality, not length, of life is what matters. In support of this, one study found that there was no significant difference between the top quartile and the bottom three quartiles of patient survival when asked if the operation was "worth it" [21].

References

1. Palliative Care in Cancer. National Care Institute. (2023). https://www.cancer.gov/about-cancer/advancedcancer/care-choices/palliative-care-fact-sheet.
2. Ghaferi AA, Birkmeyer JD, Dimick JB. Complications, failure to rescue, and mortality with major inpatient surgery in Medicare patients. JAMA. 2009;302(14):1572–9. https://doi.org/10.1001/jama.2009.1461.
3. Bateni SB, Meyers FJ, Bold RJ, Canter RJ. Current perioperative outcomes for patients with disseminated cancer. J Surg Res. 2015;197(1):118–25. https://doi.org/10.1016/j.jss.2015.03.063.

4. Miner TJ, Brennan MF, Jaques DP. A prospective, symptom related, outcomes analysis of 1022 palliative procedures for advanced cancer. Ann Surg. 2004;240:719–26.
5. Mullen MG, Michaels AD, Mehaffey JH, et al. Risk associated with complications and mortality after urgent surgery vs elective and emergency surgery: implications for defining "quality" and reporting outcomes for urgent surgery. JAMA Surg. 2017;152(8):768–74. https://doi.org/10.1001/jamasurg.2017.0918.
6. Cohen JT, Miner TJ. Patient selection in palliative surgery: defining value. J Surg Oncol. 2019;120:35–44.
7. World Health Organization. (2023). Palliative care. World Health Organization. https://www.who.int/healthtopics/palliative-care.
8. Maeda Y, Shinohara T, Katayama T, et al. A laparoscopic approach is associated with a decreased incidence of SSI in patients undergoing palliative surgery for malignant bowel obstruction. Int J Surg. 2017;42:90–4.
9. Rao J, Tiruchelvarayan R, Lee L. Palliative surgery for cervical spine metastasis. Singap Med J. 2014;55:569–73.
10. Blakely AM, McPhillips J, Miner TJ. Surgical palliation for malignant disease requiring locoregional control. Ann Palliat Med. 2015;4(2):48–53. https://doi.org/10.3978/j.issn.2224-5820.2015.04.03.
11. Paul Olson TJ, Pinkerton C, Brasel KJ, Schwarze ML. Palliative surgery for malignant bowel obstruction from carcinomatosis: a systematic review. JAMA Surg. 2014;149(4):383–92. https://doi.org/10.1001/jamasurg.2013.4059.
12. Hirabayashi H, Ebara S, Kinoshita T, et al. Clinical outcome and survival after palliative surgery for spinal metastases: palliative surgery in spinal metastases. Cancer. 2003;97(2):476–84. https://doi.org/10.1002/cncr.11039.
13. Ilyas M, Sivaswamy L, Asano E, Sood S, Zidan M, Chugani H. Seizure control following palliative resective surgery for intractable epilepsy-a pilot study. Pediatric neurology. 2014;51(3):330–5. https://doi.org/10.1016/j.pediatrneurol.2014.05.005.
14. Blakely AM, Heffernan DS, McPhillips J, Cioffi WG, Miner TJ. Elevated C-reactive protein as a predictor of patient outcomes following palliative surgery. J Surg Oncol. 2014;110(6):651–5. https://doi.org/10.1002/jso.23682.
15. Taylor LJ, Nabozny MJ, Steffens NM, et al. A framework to improve surgeon communication in high-stakes surgical decisions: best case/worst case. JAMA Surg. 2017;152(6):531–8. https://doi.org/10.1001/jamasurg.2016.5674.
16. Code of Medical Ethics. American Medical Association n.d. https://code-medical-ethics.ama-assn.org/.
17. Barry MJ, Edgman-Levitan S. Shared decision making—the pinnacle of patient-centered care. N Engl J Med. 2012;366:780–1. https://doi.org/10.1056/NEJMp1109283.
18. Institute of Medicine. Crossing the quality chasm: a new health system for the 21st century. National Academy Press; 2001.
19. Beauchamp TL, Childress JF. Principles of biomedical ethics. New York: Oxford University Press; 2001.
20. Lilley EJ, Cooper Z, Schwarze ML, Mosenthal AC. Palliative care in surgery: defining the research priorities. Ann Surg. 2018;267(1):66–72. https://doi.org/10.1097/SLA.0000000000002253.
21. Cohen JT, Fallon EA, Charpentier KP, Cioffi WG, Miner TJ. Improving the value of palliative surgery by optimizing patient selection: the role of long-term survival on high impact palliative intent operations. Am J Surg. 2021;221(5):1018–23. https://doi.org/10.1016/j.amjsurg.2020.08.034.
22. Thalji SZ, Tsai S, Gamblin TC, et al. Outcomes of palliative-intent surgery in retroperitoneal sarcoma-results from the US sarcoma collaborative. J Surg Oncol. 2020;121(7):1140–7. https://doi.org/10.1002/jso.25890.

Part XI
Supplementary Material

Chapter 41
Colorectal Surgery in Critically Unwell Patients

Ashwin Subramaniam, Robert Wengritzky, and Vladimir Bolshinsky

Introduction

With reductions in mortality rates from cardiovascular diseases, there has been a significant expansion in the number of older people in the Western world in the last 20 years. As a consequence, many people over the age of 75 years are undergoing surgery [1–3]. As people age, they are more likely to develop medical comorbidities [4], which may increase the risk of postoperative complications and poorer outcomes [5]. Some older people may be vulnerable to the risk of poor outcomes over and above the risk explained by age or comorbidities. The heightened susceptibility referred to as frailty indicates a diminished physiological capacity to withstand stressors [6]. Although age and frailty predict poor functional outcomes [7], there is an increasing use of critical care services in older people [8]. Older people will continue to undergo surgical procedures at ever-increasing rates and are likely to experience excess morbidity and mortality. While this may be supported by

A. Subramaniam (✉)
Department of Intensive Care Medicine, Dandenong Hospital, Monash Health, Dandenong, VIC, Australia

Department of Intensive Care Medicine, Peninsula Health, Frankston, VIC, Australia

Peninsula Clinical School, Monash University, Frankston, VIC, Australia

Australian and New Zealand Intensive Care Research Centre, Department of Epidemiology and Preventive Medicine, Monash University, Melbourne, VIC, Australia

Department of Intensive Care, The Bays Healthcare, Mornington, VIC, Australia
e-mail: ashwin.subramaniam@monash.edu

R. Wengritzky
Department of Anaesthesia, Peninsula Health, Frankston, VIC, Australia

V. Bolshinsky
Department of Surgery, Peninsula Health, Frankston, VIC, Australia

© The Author(s), under exclusive license to Springer Nature Switzerland AG 2024

J. Faintuch, S. Faintuch (eds.), *Recent Strategies in High Risk Surgery*,
https://doi.org/10.1007/978-3-031-56270-9_41

complex models surrounding frailty, homeostatic failure, and multiple morbidity [9], new knowledge is emerging that frailty is a better predictor of mortality and morbidity than chronological age and comorbidity indices [10–12]. The prevalence of frailty in older people aged ≥65 years hospitalized for surgery and critical illness ranges between 19 and 62% [13]. The assessment of preoperative frailty in older adults admitted to hospitals is becoming more common as a part of their risk evaluation [14, 15]. The impact of frailty on outcomes following planned surgery is progressively being explored within hospital settings [12, 14, 16–19] and population-based studies [20, 21]. Frail people who undergo surgery are more frequently associated with increased mortality [19], especially after emergency surgery [22], greater intensive care unit (ICU) readmission rates [15], longer hospital length of stay [12, 13, 23], hospital readmission rates [24], increased postoperative delirium [18], and other complications [23, 24]. Moreover, these frail people have a significantly lower chance of getting back to their usual residence with functional independence and are more likely to have a poorer quality of life if they survive the surgery and its complications [5, 12, 13, 15, 24–29]. The 1-year healthcare costs for such people were higher compared with costs for those who were not frail [22]. This association of frailty with poor surgical outcomes appears to be independent of critical illness severity [15, 30], suggesting that opportunities may exist to modify preoperative frailty and improve postoperative outcomes. Creating patient-centered multidisciplinary collaborative services to offer care for older individuals undergoing elective surgery must be considered [31].

Colorectal cancer is the fourth most frequently diagnosed cancer worldwide with over 1.8 million new cases diagnosed in 2018 [32]. It is the second leading cause of cancer death in industrialized countries [33]. The incidence of colorectal cancer is strongly related to age and is largely diagnosed in older people when comorbidities and frailty are common. Furthermore, the existence of frailty and concurrent medical conditions have been identified as significant prognostic indicators for the survival of patients with colorectal cancer [34]. The outcomes of surgical procedures are frequently assessed according to whether the surgery is elective or emergent [5].

Assessing critically ill or deteriorating patients who require colorectal surgical interventions may be perplexing. In addition to physiological instability resulting from an acute illness, patients frequently contend with various pre-existing health conditions and functional limitations before the illness, all of which are crucial factors to weigh when assessing the risk-to-benefit ratio of surgical intervention. Achieving technical surgical success for critically ill patients does not always translate into functional survival. While some older patients die early in the postoperative period, many may develop prolonged critical illness, which may increase the likelihood of mortality further down the track or result in disability. The assessment of preoperative frailty in older adults admitted to hospitals is becoming more common as a part of their risk evaluation [14, 15]. Simple frailty assessment may be a trigger to adopt pathways to avoid poor clinical and functional outcomes in either setting [31]. Therefore, when stratifying risk and evaluating the appropriateness of surgery, it is important to consider not only the patient's immediate physiology and the risks associated with the surgical procedure, but also the impact of their existing comorbidities, the values they hold, and their expectations regarding the quality of life.

Preoperative Assessment

Evaluating critically ill patients in the ICU before surgery differs from assessing patients scheduled for elective procedures. Emergency management and stabilization of abdominal surgical patients typically involve two main approaches: (1) stabilizing the patient in the ICU before surgery and (2) providing ICU care after surgical stabilization. In certain situations, simultaneous assessment, resuscitation, and prompt surgical intervention may be necessary. It is crucial to implement an assessment system that prioritizes tasks, avoids oversights, and allows for the immediate implementation of life-saving measures and definitive management.

Baseline Examination

It is essential to focus on the patient's clinical presentation, integrating information from clinical history, monitors, and diagnostic tests. Clinical examination of hemodynamically unstable patients provides timely, low-risk, and potentially useful diagnostic and prognostic information. Vital signs are often the first method of clinical assessment in evaluating for hemodynamic instability. While postural changes in heart rate may indicate hypovolemia [35], changes in heart rate or respiratory rate alone are neither sensitive nor specific for diagnosing hemodynamic instability [36]. Mean arterial pressure (MAP) >65 mmHg, 0.5 mL/kg/h urine output [37], and capillary return time of <4.5 s combined with warm extremities [38] are advised for preliminary stabilization. The combined history and physical examination allow obtaining a diagnosis in 70–80% of the population [39].

Assessment of Hemodynamics and Organ System Failures

Central venous access devices (CVAD) and pulmonary artery catheters (PAC) are invasive and often inaccurate [40]. New algorithms for indirect measurements are available for cardiac output (CO), intravascular volume status, responsiveness to intravenous fluid administration, and tissue perfusion. Specifically for volume status and fluid responsiveness, pulse pressure variation (PPV) [41–44] and stroke volume variation (SVV) [45, 46] as well as ultrasonography of the vena cava and lung [47, 48] have been recommended. An intra-arterial catheter is used, and subjects need to be in normal sinus rhythm and mechanically ventilated [46]. In the absence of a PAC, an upper body CVAD and maintaining central venous oxygen saturation of >65% is a poor surrogate measure of optimal tissue oxygenation [49, 50]. CO can be estimated by arterial waveform, thoracic bioimpedance and bioreactance, aortic Doppler, and point-of-care echocardiography [51, 52]. Arterial pulse waveform analysis requires an arterial catheter [52, 53]. Their performance compared with standard echocardiography or PAC-determined CO is variable [54, 55]. Near-infrared spectroscopy is also a variable related to CO at tissue level (oxygen delivery and utilization) [56, 57].

Assessment of an Intubated Patient

Endotracheal tube position (~21–23 cm at the lips) and ventilator settings [ventilator mode, respiratory rate, tidal volume, fraction of inspired oxygen, positive end-expiratory pressure (PEEP), flow rates, and peak and plateau pressures] are essential observations. A patient with severe respiratory failure and poor pulmonary system compliance needing emergency surgery may not tolerate laparoscopic procedures and may require open laparotomy. Readiness to wean the patient off the ventilator should also be repeatedly evaluated. Abdominal examination should never be overlooked or minimized including signs of tenderness, distention, bowel sounds, and inspection of surgical incisional sites or wounds for erythema or other signs of infection or perforation, for example, purulent, enteric, or bilious drainage; its output volumes; and color. Suspicion of abdominal hypertension or compartment syndrome may warrant intraabdominal pressure measurements. Nutritional and metabolic needs can be vital in the face of prolonged derangements such as intestinal obstruction or fistulas. In all circumstances, bowel output should be daily recorded. In an adult ICU, light levels of sedation are recommended, and daily interruptions can reduce the amount of time on a ventilator and the ICU stay [58]. Sedation and pain can be documented by the Richmond Agitation-Sedation Scale (RASS) [59] and Wong-Baker FACES Pain Rating Scale [60]. Delirium can occur in nearly 60–80% of mechanically ventilated patients and is associated with increased mortality in the ICU and long-term cognitive impairment [61]. The Confusion Assessment Method for the ICU (CAM-ICU) is recommended [62].

Surgical Assessment and Oncologic Implications

The surgical assessment of clinically unwell patients poses multifactorial challenges. Most patients can be divided into two groups. Patients can require surgical involvement due to a clear diagnosis that necessitates operative intervention, typically a form of source control. Alternatively, patients may require surgical involvement in the form of a diagnostic laparotomy due to time-critical deterioration and an absence of a clear diagnosis. Interventions such as endoscopy or interventional radiology should always be considered but only adopted if the success of such projected interventions is comparable to operative management, particularly as all intervention on compromised patients is time critical. When faced with a critically unwell patient in the ICU, the decision for the surgeon to decline operative intervention, both psychologically and philosophically, is more challenging than proceeding with intervention.

Therefore, it is imperative to remain objective. A thorough understanding of the past surgical history, including endoscopic intervention, is imperative. A comprehensive physical exam, always including turning the patient to perform a digital rectal exam is essential. Awareness of an active malignancy, particularly with systemic disease, is also important. An increased understanding of the patient's condition, including the analysis of radiological and biochemical investigations, helps gauge surgical risk. Several surgical risk calculators such as the American College of Surgeons National Surgical Quality Improvement Program (ACS-NSQIP) Surgical risk calculator can aid in the prognostication of surgical risk in critically unwell patients [63].

Preoperative Optimization

In seriously unwell patients, optimization should be addressed in an ABCDE approach: patent airway, breathing with supplemental oxygenation if required, hemodynamic status with eventual multi-lumen CVAD and arterial line for blood pressure monitoring, metabolic status, and analgesia. Maintaining euvolemia, with fluid resuscitation consistent with the presentation, preoperatively is essential. In critically ill patients, a balanced crystalloid solution is favored over normal saline, to avoid a high sodium and chloride load [64]. Hypotension is associated with various unfavorable outcomes, including increased mortality, longer hospitalization, all-cause morbidity, acute kidney injury (AKI), myocardial injury, postoperative congestive heart failure, stroke, postoperative cognitive decline, and postoperative delirium [65]. It is essential to fluid status and commencing vasoactive agents, if required, to maintain a MAP of >65 mmHg. Targeting a higher MAP may be required for patients with hypertension [65]. There is no benefit to transfusing packed red cells to aim for a hemoglobin value of >100 g/L in most situations. A hemoglobin level between 70 and 90 g/L is sufficient unless modified by certain comorbidities or acute illnesses [66–68]. Iron infusion is not recommended in critically ill patients requiring emergency surgery [66].

Nephrotoxic medications should be reviewed and ceased where possible, especially in the shocked patient. Alternative routes of drug administration should be considered for certain essential medications (anti-epileptics, treatment for Parkinson's disease, etc.) if enteral absorption of medications is questionable or difficult due to the surgical pathology. This should be done in consultation with the relevant specialty and the pharmacist involved for alternative options in the perioperative period [68]. Medications with a narrow therapeutic window should be monitored due to the effect that acute illness or drug interactions may have on metabolism and clearance.

Checking biochemistry and having a blood group and hold ready is important. Biomarkers such as raised antinatriuretic peptide and C-reactive protein (CRP), and low eGFR (<45 mL/min) predict postoperative adverse cardiac events [69]. Preoperative elevated CRP is associated with a higher incidence of postoperative delirium [70], suggesting that a pre-inflammatory state and enhanced inflammatory response to surgery are likely pathophysiologic mechanisms of delirium [70].

The American Society of Anesthesiology physical status (ASA-PS) score is associated with postoperative outcomes [71, 72]. Consideration of the patients' right heart disease requires a multidisciplinary approach, given the high risk associated with right heart failure and general anesthesia. Any patient with ASA-PS scores of 4E or higher is best managed in large, tertiary institutions with specialized anesthetist care available.

Mechanical and pharmacologic thromboprophylaxis should be given to critically unwell patients undergoing major abdominal surgery who are not at high risk for bleeding complications [73]. Coagulopathic and therapeutically anticoagulated patients may require specialty input.

Risk Stratification Tools

The APACHE score is probably the most adopted worldwide, even though it is rather complex for general surgical use. Also, the almost obligatory ASA-PS is deemed subjective by some [74–76]. The accuracy of estimation by different tools depends on the selected outcome, such as death, prolonged hospitalization, major cardiac events, respiratory failure, acute kidney injury, postoperative nausea, and vomiting, for both planned and emergency surgeries [74, 77, 78]. For example, the Lee Revised Cardiac Risk Index (RCRI) is a commonly used generic tool [79]. Surgery-specific ColoRectal Physiological and Operative Severity Score for the enUmeration of Mortality and morbidity (CR-POSSUM) is also an abridged and easy tool [76]. Given that laparoscopic colorectal surgery has become increasingly widespread the need for a model which can predict individual causes of morbidity such as anastomotic leak is crucial to allow meaningful comparisons of patient outcomes with different surgical techniques and between different centers. Sophisticated "artificial intelligence" systems leveraging "big data" are also available to facilitate the real-time integration of physiological and laboratory data, dynamically adjusting risk predictions [74] for outcomes such as death, unplanned ICU admission, or the need for Rapid Response Team (RRT) intervention [80]. This may form the basis of automated staff escalations [81]. While possessing reasonable predictive accuracy, risk scoring systems, however, do have limitations due to their inherent simplicity, adjustments in treatment protocols over time, and variations in populations or institutions [74]. Furthermore, its accuracy for use for individual patients is imperfect [77].

Factors Predicting Patient Outcome

The perioperative patient outcome is predominantly determined by factors such as age, functional status (physical fitness), comorbidities such as cardiorespiratory disease and diabetes, abnormalities of biomarkers such as hemoglobin (Hb), albumin and renal function, and inflammatory markers [74]. Recently, the importance of considering patient frailty as a factor in predicting outcomes in the perioperative setting has been recognized [74]. Screening for frailty and conducting a thorough preoperative multidisciplinary assessment can facilitate appropriate patient selection for surgery and proactively optimize the health status of frail older individuals to prevent adverse outcomes [31]. Interventions aimed at preoperative optimization of an older frail person are single but are usually multiple [31]. Furthermore, identifying frailty in the elective setting may allow targeted resource-driven comprehensive assessment and planning in a high-risk group to facilitate the best outcome for an older person.

The interventions in such people may be preoperative, intraoperative (including anesthetic choices), and postoperative [82]. Basic principles involve enhancing physical resilience, proactively optimizing medical factors (such as cardiorespiratory status, anemia, biochemistry, and metabolic status), evaluating pharmacological management, especially regarding medications that could contribute to postoperative delirium, and addressing social and psychological aspects that may influence recovery [83]. Prehabilitation encourages healthy behaviors through the needs-based prescription of preoperative exercise programs, nutrition optimization, and psychological interventions in elective surgical settings. All these facilitate improved functional capacity and resilience, therefore, potentially offsetting postoperative complications [84–86]. The prehabilitation exercise programs can vary significantly by type (cardiovascular vs. resistance training of extremities), site (total body exercise vs. muscle or joint specific), intensity, duration, and frequency (sessions per week) [84].

Prehabilitation enhanced postoperative clinical outcomes in those undergoing elective major abdominal surgery [87]. But the effectiveness of such programs in the setting of frailty and elective surgery is yet to be extensively investigated. An added challenge with prehabilitation is whether the exercise program needs supervision in the community, which leads to queries about resources, logistics, and financial impact in effectively running such programs. Furthermore, older frail people may have pre-existing chronic inflammation or suffer trauma that hinders their capacity to build reserve [88] which may limit the benefits of prehabilitation. Some evidence suggests that structured multicomponent programs such as a combination of enhancement of respiratory and general fitness with moderate aerobic exercise and resistance training, smoking cessation, nutritional counseling with protein supplementation to treat malnutrition, and relaxation techniques in older people in elective surgical settings [89–91] were associated with clinically meaningful changes (improved 6-minute walk test distance) in postoperative functional capacity [90]. In another observational study, patients aged 65 years and over undergoing elective abdominal surgery and receiving the modified multicomponent nurse-led intervention (Hospital Elder Life Program) were less likely to be frail on discharge compared with matched controls [89]. Prehabilitation along with rationalizing pharmacological approaches, addressing anemia and other biochemical/metabolic abnormalities, and refining cardiorespiratory status may improve outcomes, including post-discharge function and caregiver burden [92].

Goals of Care

It is crucial to acknowledge that the objectives of a frail elderly individual in the later stages of life may conflict with current standards of optimal surgical care. As a result, many individuals in this demographic may undergo treatments that do not align with their values and life goals. Older frail hospitalized patients who have timely goals of care (GOC) documentation had approximately a threefold increase in hospital mortality than older non-frail patients [93]. Although the study was in patients hospitalized for medical reasons, this may be relevant for patients undergoing colorectal cancer surgery, who are generally older and frailer. Consequently, shared decision-making must be adopted to align the person's goals with the choice of surgical interventions in the presence of frailty. Timely GOC will achieve a better quality of care toward their end-of-life in such patients and, therefore, avoid burdensome and unnecessary treatment [93]. Adopting the Best Case/Worst Case [94] framework will endorse shared decision-making and aid surgeons in structuring treatment conversations to obtain the best outcome for the patient and their family [95, 96].

Intraoperative Anesthetic Management

Induction Strategy

Intravascular volume, cardiac output, oxygen delivery, and broad-spectrum antibiotics should be reviewed whenever required [97]. A three-lead ECG, oxygen saturation, end-tidal CO_2, temperature, and depth of anesthesia are traditionally monitored. Minimally invasive cardiac output monitoring may also be beneficial in some services including transthoracic echocardiography [51, 52]. Vasoactive agents can be considered after optimal intravascular volume; however, it is important to avoid occult splanchnic hypovolemia and hypoperfusion. Sometimes, this may not be possible if the patient's condition is critical, which means that fluid resuscitation and vasoactive agents need to be administered concurrently [98]. Preoxygenation is crucial to minimize hypoxemia. Rapid sequence induction (RSI) must be considered to secure the airway quickly and minimize pulmonary aspiration risks. RSI is classically performed with a predetermined dose of induction agent, suxamethonium, and the addition of cricoid pressure to reduce this risk. RSI is often modified by administering opioids and titration of induction agents to better manage hemodynamic situations and by using rocuronium (instead of suxamethonium) in patients with renal failure and hyperkalemia. Intubation adjuncts such as a gum elastic bougie, video laryngoscopes, and fiberoptic laryngoscopes should be immediately available [97]. Neuraxial techniques for severe COPD could reduce respiratory complications [99–101]. It is important to consider coagulopathy and the risk of infections when using regional anesthesia techniques [102, 103].

Maintenance Strategy

Total intravenous anesthesia (TIVA) is still controversial compared to inhalational anesthesia [104]. A peripheral nerve stimulator should be used throughout the procedure to guide the maintenance of muscle relaxation. Maintain normothermia with the help of forced-air warming and by administering warm fluids and blood products. IV lignocaine (lidocaine) could be useful as an opioid/ketamine-sparing agent [105].

Mechanical Ventilation

There is a modest survival advantage, faster recovery, and shorter hospital stays with laparoscopic colectomy [106–111]. However, the intraperitoneal pressure from CO_2 insufflation can potentially cause respiratory distress by increased intraperitoneal CO_2 absorption and by opposing the diaphragmatic descent [112]. Respiratory mechanics are further compromised by the head-down Trendelenburg position during laparoscopic colectomy [113–115]. Tidal volumes of 6 mL/kg, aiming for plateau pressures <30 cmH_2O, and addition of PEEP as little as 5 cmH_2O should target a PaO_2 >62 mmHg and $PaCO_2$ <60 mmHg in intermediate-risk and high-risk patients [112, 116–119].

Intraoperative Fluid Management

Esophageal Doppler-guided fluid management has demonstrated advantages in addressing euvolemia [120]; however it is not readily available. Utilizing a restrictive fluid therapy, characterized by a zero-balance approach that replaces only the fluid lost during surgery, aims to prevent fluid overload [121]. However, acute kidney injury (AKI) and the necessity for renal replacement therapy could ensue [122]. It is, therefore, recommended to adopt a moderately liberal (aiming for 1–2 L positive) or goal-directed approach to intraoperative fluid management [122, 123].

Temperature Regulation and Management of Coagulopathy

Hypothermia more frequently occurs when surgical procedures go beyond 2 h, especially in older frail adults with lower adiposity, and in those with comorbid illnesses [124, 125]. Hypothermia leads to a reversible impairment of platelet aggregation by reducing the release of thromboxane A3 [126, 127]. Additionally, hypothermia diminishes enzyme activity in the coagulation cascade, thereby reducing the formation of blood clots. This effect may contribute to coagulopathy, increase the risk of adverse cardiac events, and decrease resistance to surgical wound infections [128]. Major bleeding features hemodynamic instability, a requirement for blood transfusion, and emergency endoscopic, angiographic, or surgical intervention to control the bleeding. Following colorectal surgery, it occurs in 0.5–4.2% [129–131]. Blood transfusions and correction of any underlying coagulopathy could be sufficient. Surgical intervention should be considered for patients who are unstable or do not respond to conservative measures [131]. A 1:1:1 ratio of plasma, packed red blood cells, and platelets is advised for severe bleeding [132]. Perioperative point-of-care coagulation tests (POCCT) such as **T**hrombo**E**lasto**G**raphy (TEG) and **RO**tational **T**hrombo**E**lasto**M**etry (ROTEM) should be considered, conducted to differentiate mechanisms such as thrombocytopenia or low fibrinogen levels [133].

Factors Preventing Extubation in the Operating Room

Older, male sex, higher body mass index, Desflurane anesthesia, and prolonged anesthesia time can all contribute to delayed extubation time [104]. COPD or other medical conditions could also interfere with success. In doubt, patients are returned to the ICU intubated and mechanically ventilated, where they can be safely extubated in due course.

Intraoperative Surgical Management

Surgical Decision-Making Before Incision

When considering operative intervention for critically unwell patients, the surgeon's focus is on implementing damage control principles. The primary objective is to achieve source control while minimizing potential complications associated with the intervention. Preoperative communication with the staff emphasizes the availability of equipment and streamlining operative steps to reach this goal. Adhering to standard algorithms for all cases helps reduce variability and, consequently, minimizes errors. While traditional wisdom suggests that a laparotomy is the optimal operative approach, advancements in medical technology and surgical techniques have made minimally invasive approaches effective in achieving source control in certain situations. Examples include laparoscopic total colectomy for toxic megacolon [134], colonoscopic decompression for acute colonic pseudo-obstruction, and the use of stents in the setting of a malignant large bowel obstruction [135] as a bridge to surgery [136].

Surgical Decision-Making During Surgery

An experienced surgeon should possess the ability to foresee the required technical steps of the operation in advance. This Foresight allows the surgeon to maintain focus and responsiveness to patient factors while working within the depths of the operative cavity. Subtle changes in tissue quality resulting from factors such as malnutrition, bleeding, sepsis, and tissue edema may require the surgeon to make adjustments to the surgical technique [137]. A liberal use of fecal diversion also reduces postoperative complications.

Postoperative Care

General Supportive Care in ICU

Typical issues in this population are sepsis, effective circulating volume, metabolic acidosis, compartment pressure–volume relationships, mean arterial pressure in the context of bleeding, work of breathing, hypoxia, hypercapnia, and mechanical ventilation. Underlying troubles may concern anastomotic leak, hemorrhage, atelectasis, pain, delirium, acute kidney injury (AKI), sepsis, venous thromboembolic events, and antibiotic management [138]. Early mobilization of a hemodynamic stable patient is recommended to reduce venous thromboembolism (VTE) [139–141]. However, ensure that the patient has adequate pain relief before mobilization [142, 143]. Nutritional status and hyperglycemia require attention [144]. Checklists like FAST-HUG or FAST-HUGS-BID mnemonics identify the key aspects in the supportive care of critically ill patients admitted to ICU [138, 145–147].

Postoperative Acute Pain Management

Systemic opioids and ketamine are often employed. Lignocaine has been extensively used; however, its benefits are seriously questioned [148]. Single-shot transverse abdominis plane (TAP) block or the addition of bilateral TAP catheters with continuous local anesthetic infusion may be considered [149, 150].

Mechanical Ventilation Postoperatively

Acute respiratory failure (often due to sepsis), compromised lung function (such as postoperative atelectasis or ventilator-associated pneumonia), or difficult breathing, particularly if related to frailty and muscle weakness, are not uncommon in this population. In addition, general inhalation anesthetic agents can induce hypoxic pulmonary vasoconstriction, while IV narcotics blunt the hypoxemic and hypercapnic ventilatory drive. This can cause a significant reduction in the vital capacity following abdominal surgery. Administering peri-extubation bronchodilators may be beneficial. Extubating high-risk patients directly onto non-invasive ventilation may reduce their work of breathing and gas trapping, as well as the need for reintubation [151].

Postoperative Fluid Management

After major surgery blood is redirected away from "non-vital" organs like the intestine, skin, and muscles to ensure perfusion to critical organs such as the heart, brain, and kidneys. However, an excess of salt and water can have adverse effects on anastomotic integrity, including ileus and other postoperative complications [152]. The current protocols recommend moderately liberal fluid administration rather than a restrictive regimen up to 24 h after surgery [122]. Fluid replacement should be continued until normovolemia is achieved, and subsequently, a maintenance period should be initiated [153], which accounts for 30–60 mL/h of balanced crystalloids. Algorithms driven by systolic (stroke) volume variation or pulse wave variation, and Doppler ultrasound to maintain even fluid balance to ensure adequate perfusion, should be considered where possible [154].

Inotropes and Vasopressor Agents

Noradrenaline (norepinephrine) or adrenaline (epinephrine) are usually considered first-line drugs [155–157]. Dopamine is associated with arrhythmias [156]. Steroids should be considered in patients with refractory shock, particularly hydrocortisone (IV 200 mg daily), which is safe and without an increased risk of complications [158]. There is a threefold increase in anastomotic leaks with prolonged exposure to vasopressors due to splanchnic vasoconstriction, deterioration of microcirculation, and local hypoxia [159]. These are independent of clinical/surgical status or hypotension [160]. Nevertheless, perioperative vasopressors are significantly associated with reduced postoperative complications and hospital length of stay [161].

Antimicrobial Therapy

High-quality evidence suggests that broad-spectrum antibiotics covering aerobic and anaerobic bacteria administered before colorectal surgery reduce surgical site infection risk by as much as 75% [162]. In cases where sepsis is suspected, antibiotics should be initiated urgently, regardless of the timing of surgery [68]. A 4–5-day antibiotic course is required for intraabdominal sepsis that has had adequate source control [163]. Postoperative pneumonia (hospital-acquired pneumonia [HAP] and ventilator-associated pneumonia [VAP]) is sometimes caused by resistant organisms, and the antibiotic duration is dependent on clinical, radiologic, and laboratory parameters, notably in frail patients [163]. The duration of antibiotics for *Clostridioides difficile* infection is usually 10 days, depending on the response to therapy and clinical course.

Postoperative Adverse Events

Almost 95% of those who undergo laparoscopic surgery develop adhesions, a major cause of small bowel obstruction (SBO). The open is not less prone, be it elective or emergency surgery, along with other mechanisms [164]. Ileus is similarly frequent, characterized by bowel distension, vomiting, and delay in oral feeding that can be associated with increased postoperative pain [165]. Longer surgical duration, increased bowel manipulation, delayed enteral nutrition/nasogastric tube placement, intraabdominal inflammation, and postoperative complications are some of the triggers of ileus. Prophylactic suggestions encompass minimally invasive surgical techniques and avoiding prolonged opiate prescriptions [166].

Surgical Wound Infection

Nosocomial surgical wound infections are classically linked to malnutrition, diabetes mellitus, immunosuppression, age >60 years, ASA-PS score >2, fecal contamination, prolonged hospitalization before surgery, and extensive surgical procedures [167]. The prevalence range is wide, depending on predisposing factors (1.2–26%), with 14% mean mortality [49]. These infections are classified as superficial, deep, or organ-space infections. Source control, broad-spectrum antibiotics, and hemodynamic support, as appropriate and the main lines of managing surgical wound infections.

Dehiscence of the abdominal wall: Abdominal wall dehiscence happens uncommonly (0.4–3.5%); however it is associated with high mortality (up to 45%) and morbidity (prolonged hospitalizations and nosocomial infections). Emergency reoperation is often necessary [168].

Anastomotic Leakage

Between 3 and 19% are affected, and about 10% of the patients die as a result [169]. Local and systemic manifestations tend to occur, from evident peritonism to dehydration and electrolyte imbalance, depending on the drainage origin, trajectory, volume, and composition. Management includes endoscopic or colonoscopic maneuvers in cases of proximal (esophagus, stomach) or distal lesions (left colon, rectum), along with general therapy (fluids, nutritional and metabolic support, antibiotics, octreotide).

Cardiovascular Complications

About 5% of patients develop acute myocardial infarction, with almost 75% suffering it within the first 48 postoperative hours. Nearly two-thirds of the affected patients do not have clinical signs; it is, therefore, essential to proactively measure cardiac enzymes in individuals at high risk and/or with a history of ischemic events [170]. The 30-day mortality rate is 11% [170].

Atrial fibrillation occurs in 8% of all non-cardiac surgical patients postoperatively. Catecholamine stress resulting from tissue trauma and pain, hypovolemia or atrial stretch, hypoxia (leading to pulmonary vasoconstriction), and electrolyte disturbances may be implicated. The hemodynamic effects are often subtle, but the loss of atrial kick compromises the stroke volume by 25% and results in pulmonary arterial hypertension, tachycardia, and increased myocardial work. While many patients experiencing postoperative atrial fibrillation episodes are asymptomatic and tolerate it well, individuals with pre-existing arterial hypertension or diastolic dysfunction may become hemodynamically unstable [170].

Postoperative heart failure can result from an acute ischemic cardiac event. Additional contributing factors may include inadequate fluid management and/or volume overload, acute kidney injury, sepsis, acute lung injury, and diastolic dysfunction [170, 171]. Postoperative organ dysfunction significantly modifies the surgical trajectory, recovery, and mortality from colorectal surgery. A recent study has found that factors such as older age (≥65 years), male sex, emergency surgery, rising social deprivation, congestive cardiac failure, and diabetes mellitus are associated with an increased likelihood of requiring organ support during the perioperative period [172]. Nearly 10% receive postoperative organ support, and this was associated with a nearly tenfold in-hospital mortality (3% vs. 28%, respectively) [172]. Unfortunately, from the social, financial, and ethical point of view, the potential need for advanced postoperative organ support such as extracorporeal membrane oxygenation is not routinely discussed with patients undergoing colorectal surgery during their preoperative consultation [172].

Postoperative Respiratory Complications (PRCs)

PRCs range between 3 and 7.9% [173, 174]. Reintubation, acute respiratory failure, pulmonary edema, pneumonia, and atelectasis are the most common causes of PRCs [153], and this is associated with increased hospitalization, in-hospital mortality, loss of independence, and higher healthcare costs [153, 175–177]. Frail older patients are more susceptible to PRCs [178, 179]. Postoperative respiratory failure is multifactorial and is linked to an approximately tenfold increase in perioperative 30-day mortality in patients undergoing abdominal surgery [175]. Preoperative risk stratification (as discussed earlier), with an individualized patient-centered treatment plan along with intraoperative (laparoscopic surgical technique [180] lung-protection ventilation) or postoperative pathways (low-dose opioid administration, restrictive fluid administration, inhaled anesthetic agents, and extubating patients in reversed Trendelenburg position and early mobilization), was associated with lower incidences of PRCs [153, 181, 182].

Acute Kidney Injury

Acute kidney injury and/or acute renal failure manifest in 7% of all patients in the postoperative period. About 6% of these patients will require renal replacement measures, and these patients have a high mortality rate (50–70%) [183].

Delirium and Cognitive Impairment

Postoperative delirium is common, notably among the elderly. In some series more than a third of the patients admitted to the ICU after surgery develop delirium; however, it is often underestimated [184, 185]. Delirium is associated with considerable morbidity and occasional mortality, such as prolongation hospitalization, higher need for re-hospitalization, and loss of independence requiring admissions to residential aged care facilities [186].

Recognizing Futility and End-of-Life Care

It is important to address the inappropriateness of continued care when there are no prospects of a meaningful outcome [187]. Recognizing futility and delivering timely comfort-oriented care not only is crucial for preserving the dignity of patients but also serves to minimize moral distress among healthcare professionals and families. Surgery to facilitate palliation should not be dismissed. This is commonly considered in patients with advanced malignancy and consequent bowel obstruction. Palliative endoscopic stenting for left-sided large bowel obstruction has been progressively adopted. It must be noted that stenting is most successful for (intrinsic) malignant obstruction [188] and is optimal for patients with a limited life expectancy. Proximal diversion should be considered for patients with a large bowel obstruction due to extrinsic compression of a frozen abdomen or advanced peritoneal disease. A proximal jejunostomy, while subjecting the patient to the consequence of a high output stoma, with insufficient bowel length to maintain oral nutrition, will nevertheless free the patient from nasogastric decompression, avoid vomiting, and enable comfort-based oral intake.

Post ICU Care

Long-term cognitive, psychiatric, and physical disabilities after prolonged critical illness are becoming more frequent particularly in the elderly, as patients survive their initial insult. This phenomenon is now recognized as post-intensive care syndrome [189], with diminished quality of life, much suffering, and major costs for both patients and their families. A multidisciplinary team approach is advised, which may include intensivists, neuropsychiatrists, physiotherapists, and respiratory therapists.

Timing of Stomal Revision and Other Complementary Procedures

The danger period for a surgical takeback is from 12 days to 12 weeks following an index laparotomy [137]. The inflammatory adhesions, edematous and fragile tissues, along with the temporary closure of the peritoneal cavity elevate the risk of bleeding and the inadvertent occurrence of bowel injuries, with the potential development of enteric fistulae and sepsis. Importantly, there is a low likelihood of clearly defining anatomy and achieving effective source control in such conditions. Delaying reoperation or replacing it with interventional radiology or endoscopic maneuvers, if appropriate, can prevent many troubles.

Funding No funding sources to declare.

Conflicts of Interest All authors declare no support from any organization for the submitted work, and no competing interests with regard to the submitted work.

References

1. Bufalari A, Ferri M, Cao P, Cirocchi R, Bisacci R, Moggi L. Surgical care in octogenarians. Br J Surg. 1996;83(12):1783–7. https://www.ncbi.nlm.nih.gov/pubmed/9038570.
2. Hamel MB, Henderson WG, Khuri SF, Daley J. Surgical outcomes for patients aged 80 and older: morbidity and mortality from major noncardiac surgery. J Am Geriatr Soc. 2005;53(3):424–9. https://doi.org/10.1111/j.1532-5415.2005.53159.x.

3. Polanczyk CA, Marcantonio E, Goldman L, et al. Impact of age on perioperative complications and length of stay in patients undergoing noncardiac surgery. Ann Intern Med. 2001;134(8):637–43. https://www.ncbi.nlm.nih.gov/pubmed/11304103.
4. Davis JW, Chung R, Juarez DT. Prevalence of comorbid conditions with aging among patients with diabetes and cardiovascular disease. Hawaii Med J. 2011;70(10):209–13. https://www.ncbi.nlm.nih.gov/pubmed/22162595.
5. Tang B, Green C, Yeoh AC, Husain F, Subramaniam A. Post-operative outcomes in older patients: a single-centre observational study. ANZ J Surg. 2018;88(5):421–7. https://doi.org/10.1111/ans.14433.
6. Clegg A, Young J, Iliffe S, Rikkert MO, Rockwood K. Frailty in elderly people. Lancet. 2013;381(9868):752–62. https://doi.org/10.1016/S0140-6736(12)62167-9.
7. Fisher C, Karalapillai DK, Bailey M, Glassford NG, Bellomo R, Jones D. Predicting intensive care and hospital outcome with the Dalhousie clinical frailty scale: a pilot assessment. Anaesth Intensive Care. 2015;43(3):361–8. https://www.ncbi.nlm.nih.gov/pubmed/25943611.
8. Nguyen YL, Angus DC, Boumendil A, Guidet B. The challenge of admitting the very elderly to intensive care. Ann Intensive Care. 2011;1(1):29. https://doi.org/10.1186/2110-5820-1-29.
9. Gordon AL, Evans BJ, Dhesi J. The physician's role in perioperative management of older patients undergoing surgery. Clin Med (Lond). 2017;17(4):357–9. https://doi.org/10.7861/clinmedicine.17-4-357.
10. Rockwood K, Song X, MacKnight C, et al. A global clinical measure of fitness and frailty in elderly people. CMAJ. 2005;173(5):489–95. https://doi.org/10.1503/cmaj.050051.
11. Song X, Mitnitski A, Rockwood K. Prevalence and 10-year outcomes of frailty in older adults in relation to deficit accumulation. J Am Geriatr Soc. 2010;58(4):681–7. https://doi.org/10.1111/j.1532-5415.2010.02764.x.
12. Makary MA, Segev DL, Pronovost PJ, et al. Frailty as a predictor of surgical outcomes in older patients. J Am Coll Surg. 2010;210(6):901–8. https://doi.org/10.1016/j.jamcollsurg.2010.01.028.
13. Darvall JN, Gregorevic KJ, Story DA, Hubbard RE, Lim WK. Frailty indexes in perioperative and critical care: a systematic review. Arch Gerontol Geriatr. 2018;79:88–96. https://doi.org/10.1016/j.archger.2018.08.006.
14. Beggs T, Sepehri A, Szwajcer A, Tangri N, Arora RC. Frailty and perioperative outcomes: a narrative review. Can J Anaesth. 2015;62(2):143–57. https://doi.org/10.1007/s12630-014-0273-z.
15. Bagshaw SM, Stelfox HT, McDermid RC, et al. Association between frailty and short- and long-term outcomes among critically ill patients: a multicentre prospective cohort study. CMAJ. 2014;186(2):E95–102. https://doi.org/10.1503/cmaj.130639.
16. Afilalo J, Eisenberg MJ, Morin JF, et al. Gait speed as an incremental predictor of mortality and major morbidity in elderly patients undergoing cardiac surgery. J Am Coll Cardiol. 2010;56(20):1668–76. https://doi.org/10.1016/j.jacc.2010.06.039.
17. Bagshaw SM, Webb SA, Delaney A, et al. Very old patients admitted to intensive care in Australia and New Zealand: a multi-centre cohort analysis. Crit Care. 2009;13(2):R45. https://doi.org/10.1186/cc7768.
18. Pol RA, van Leeuwen BL, Visser L, et al. Standardised frailty indicator as predictor for post-operative delirium after vascular surgery: a prospective cohort study. Eur J Vasc Endovasc Surg. 2011;42(6):824–30. https://doi.org/10.1016/j.ejvs.2011.07.006.
19. Sundermann S, Dademasch A, Praetorius J, et al. Comprehensive assessment of frailty for elderly high-risk patients undergoing cardiac surgery. Eur J Cardiothorac Surg. 2011;39(1):33–7. https://doi.org/10.1016/j.ejcts.2010.04.013.
20. McIsaac DI, Bryson GL, van Walraven C. Association of frailty and 1-year postoperative mortality following major elective noncardiac surgery: a population-based cohort study. JAMA Surg. 2016;151(6):538–45. https://doi.org/10.1001/jamasurg.2015.5085.
21. McIsaac DI, Beaule PE, Bryson GL, Van Walraven C. The impact of frailty on outcomes and healthcare resource usage after total joint arthroplasty: a population-based cohort study. Bone Jt J. 2016;98-B(6):799–805. https://doi.org/10.1302/0301-620X.98B6.37124.

22. Zampieri FG, Iwashyna TJ, Viglianti EM, et al. Association of frailty with short-term outcomes, organ support and resource use in critically ill patients. Intensive Care Med. 2018;44(9):1512–20. https://doi.org/10.1007/s00134-018-5342-2.
23. Hewitt J, Long S, Carter B, Bach S, McCarthy K, Clegg A. The prevalence of frailty and its association with clinical outcomes in general surgery: a systematic review and meta-analysis. Age Ageing. 2018;47(6):793–800. https://doi.org/10.1093/ageing/afy110.
24. Panayi AC, Orkaby AR, Sakthivel D, et al. Impact of frailty on outcomes in surgical patients: a systematic review and meta-analysis. Am J Surg. 2018;218:393. https://doi.org/10.1016/j.amjsurg.2018.11.020.
25. Robinson TN, Wallace JI, Wu DS, et al. Accumulated frailty characteristics predict postoperative discharge institutionalization in the geriatric patient. J Am Coll Surg. 2011;213(1):37–42. https://doi.org/10.1016/j.jamcollsurg.2011.01.056.
26. Brummel NE, Bell SP, Girard TD, et al. Frailty and subsequent disability and mortality among patients with critical illness. Am J Respir Crit Care Med. 2017;196(1):64–72. https://doi.org/10.1164/rccm.201605-0939OC.
27. Bagshaw SM, Stelfox HT, Johnson JA, et al. Long-term association between frailty and health-related quality of life among survivors of critical illness: a prospective multicenter cohort study. Crit Care Med. 2015;43(5):973–82. https://doi.org/10.1097/ccm.0000000000000860.
28. Dasgupta M, Rolfson DB, Stolee P, Borrie MJ, Speechley M. Frailty is associated with postoperative complications in older adults with medical problems. Arch Gerontol Geriatr. 2009;48(1):78–83. https://doi.org/10.1016/j.archger.2007.10.007.
29. Lin HS, Watts JN, Peel NM, Hubbard RE. Frailty and post-operative outcomes in older surgical patients: a systematic review. BMC Geriatr. 2016;16(1):157. https://doi.org/10.1186/s12877-016-0329-8.
30. Le Maguet P, Roquilly A, Lasocki S, et al. Prevalence and impact of frailty on mortality in elderly ICU patients: a prospective, multicenter, observational study. Intensive Care Med. 2014;40(5):674–82. https://doi.org/10.1007/s00134-014-3253-4.
31. Subramaniam A, Tiruvoipati R, Lodge M, Moran C, Srikanth V. Frailty in the older person undergoing elective surgery: a trigger for enhanced multidisciplinary management—a narrative review. ANZ J Surg. 2020;90(3):222–9. https://doi.org/10.1111/ans.15633.
32. Bray F, Ferlay J, Soerjomataram I, Siegel RL, Torre LA, Jemal A. Global cancer statistics 2018: GLOBOCAN estimates of incidence and mortality worldwide for 36 cancers in 185 countries. CA Cancer J Clin. 2018;68(6):394–424. https://doi.org/10.3322/caac.21492.
33. Siegel RL, Miller KD, Jemal A. Cancer statistics, 2016. CA Cancer J Clin. 2016;66(1):7–30. https://doi.org/10.3322/caac.21332.
34. Boakye D, Rillmann B, Walter V, Jansen L, Hoffmeister M, Brenner H. Impact of comorbidity and frailty on prognosis in colorectal cancer patients: a systematic review and meta-analysis. Cancer Treat Rev. 2018;64:30–9. https://doi.org/10.1016/j.ctrv.2018.02.003.
35. McGee S, Abernethy WB 3rd, Simel DL. The rational clinical examination. Is this patient hypovolemic? JAMA. 1999;281(11):1022–9. https://doi.org/10.1001/jama.281.11.1022.
36. Sevransky J. Clinical assessment of hemodynamically unstable patients. Curr Opin Crit Care. 2009;15(3):234–8. https://doi.org/10.1097/MCC.0b013e32832b70e5.
37. Dellinger RP, Levy MM, Carlet JM, et al. Surviving sepsis campaign: international guidelines for management of severe sepsis and septic shock: 2008. Crit Care Med. 2008;36(1):296–327. https://doi.org/10.1097/01.CCM.0000298158.12101.41.
38. Lima A, Jansen TC, van Bommel J, Ince C, Bakker J. The prognostic value of the subjective assessment of peripheral perfusion in critically ill patients. Crit Care Med. 2009;37(3):934–8. https://doi.org/10.1097/CCM.0b013e31819869db.
39. Sandler G. The importance of the history in the medical clinic and the cost of unnecessary tests. Am Heart J. 1980;100(6 Pt 1):928–31. https://doi.org/10.1016/0002-8703(80)90076-9.
40. Marik PE, Baram M, Vahid B. Does central venous pressure predict fluid responsiveness? A systematic review of the literature and the tale of seven mares. Chest. 2008;134(1):172–8. https://doi.org/10.1378/chest.07-2331.

41. Michard F, Teboul JL. Predicting fluid responsiveness in ICU patients: a critical analysis of the evidence. Chest. 2002;121(6):2000–8. https://doi.org/10.1378/chest.121.6.2000.
42. Michard F, Lopes MR, Auler JO Jr. Pulse pressure variation: beyond the fluid management of patients with shock. Crit Care. 2007;11(3):131. https://doi.org/10.1186/cc5905.
43. Michard F, Boussat S, Chemla D, et al. Relation between respiratory changes in arterial pulse pressure and fluid responsiveness in septic patients with acute circulatory failure. Am J Respir Crit Care Med. 2000;162(1):134–8. https://doi.org/10.1164/ajrccm.162.1.9903035.
44. Marik PE, Cavallazzi R, Vasu T, Hirani A. Dynamic changes in arterial waveform derived variables and fluid responsiveness in mechanically ventilated patients: a systematic review of the literature. Crit Care Med. 2009;37(9):2642–7. https://doi.org/10.1097/CCM.0b013e3181a590da.
45. Biais M, Nouette-Gaulain K, Cottenceau V, Revel P, Sztark F. Uncalibrated pulse contour-derived stroke volume variation predicts fluid responsiveness in mechanically ventilated patients undergoing liver transplantation. Br J Anaesth. 2008;101(6):761–8. https://doi.org/10.1093/bja/aen277.
46. Pinsky MR. Functional haemodynamic monitoring. Curr Opin Crit Care. 2014;20(3):288–93. https://doi.org/10.1097/MCC.0000000000000090.
47. Marik PE, Monnet X, Teboul JL. Hemodynamic parameters to guide fluid therapy. Ann Intensive Care. 2011;1(1):1. https://doi.org/10.1186/2110-5820-1-1.
48. Rudski LG, Lai WW, Afilalo J, et al. Guidelines for the echocardiographic assessment of the right heart in adults: a report from the American Society of Echocardiography endorsed by the European Association of Echocardiography, a registered branch of the European Society of Cardiology, and the Canadian Society of Echocardiography. J Am Soc Echocardiogr. 2010;23(7):685–713. https://doi.org/10.1016/j.echo.2010.05.010.
49. van Beest P, Wietasch G, Scheeren T, Spronk P, Kuiper M. Clinical review: use of venous oxygen saturations as a goal—a yet unfinished puzzle. Crit Care. 2011;15(5):232. https://doi.org/10.1186/cc10351.
50. Nebout S, Pirracchio R. Should we monitor $ScVO_2$ in critically ill patients? Cardiol Res Pract. 2012;2012:370697. https://doi.org/10.1155/2012/370697.
51. Marik PE, Baram M. Noninvasive hemodynamic monitoring in the intensive care unit. Crit Care Clin. 2007;23(3):383–400. https://doi.org/10.1016/j.ccc.2007.05.002.
52. Marik PE. Noninvasive cardiac output monitors: a state-of the-art review. J Cardiothorac Vasc Anesth. 2013;27(1):121–34. https://doi.org/10.1053/j.jvca.2012.03.022.
53. De Backer D, Marx G, Tan A, et al. Arterial pressure-based cardiac output monitoring: a multicenter validation of the third-generation software in septic patients. Intensive Care Med. 2011;37(2):233–40. https://doi.org/10.1007/s00134-010-2098-8.
54. Noritomi DT, Vieira ML, Mohovic T, et al. Echocardiography for hemodynamic evaluation in the intensive care unit. Shock. 2010;34(Suppl 1):59–62. https://doi.org/10.1097/SHK.0b013e3181e7e8ed.
55. De Backer D. Ultrasonic evaluation of the heart. Curr Opin Crit Care. 2014;20(3):309–14. https://doi.org/10.1097/MCC.0000000000000094.
56. Creteur J, Carollo T, Soldati G, Buchele G, De Backer D, Vincent JL. The prognostic value of muscle StO_2 in septic patients. Intensive Care Med. 2007;33(9):1549–56. https://doi.org/10.1007/s00134-007-0739-3.
57. Masip J, Mesquida J, Luengo C, et al. Near-infrared spectroscopy StO_2 monitoring to assess the therapeutic effect of drotrecogin alfa (activated) on microcirculation in patients with severe sepsis or septic shock. Ann Intensive Care. 2013;3(1):30. https://doi.org/10.1186/2110-5820-3-30.
58. Girard TD, Kress JP, Fuchs BD, et al. Efficacy and safety of a paired sedation and ventilator weaning protocol for mechanically ventilated patients in intensive care (awakening and breathing controlled trial): a randomised controlled trial. Lancet. 2008;371(9607):126–34. https://doi.org/10.1016/S0140-6736(08)60105-1.

59. Sessler CN, Gosnell MS, Grap MJ, et al. The Richmond agitation-sedation scale: validity and reliability in adult intensive care unit patients. Am J Respir Crit Care Med. 2002;166(10):1338–44. https://doi.org/10.1164/rccm.2107138.
60. W-BF F. Wong-Baker FACES® Pain Rating Scale. http://www.WongBakerFACES.org.
61. Barr J, Fraser GL, Puntillo K, et al. Clinical practice guidelines for the management of pain, agitation, and delirium in adult patients in the intensive care unit. Crit Care Med. 2013;41(1):263–306. https://doi.org/10.1097/CCM.0b013e3182783b72.
62. Ely EW, Margolin R, Francis J, et al. Evaluation of delirium in critically ill patients: validation of the confusion assessment method for the intensive care unit (CAM-ICU). Crit Care Med. 2001;29(7):1370–9. https://doi.org/10.1097/00003246-200107000-00012.
63. Bilimoria KY, Liu Y, Paruch JL, et al. Development and evaluation of the universal ACS NSQIP surgical risk calculator: a decision aid and informed consent tool for patients and surgeons. J Am Coll Surg. 2013;217(5):833–42.e1. https://doi.org/10.1016/j.jamcollsurg.2013.07.385.
64. Semler MW, Self WH, Rice TW. Balanced crystalloids versus saline in critically ill adults. N Engl J Med. 2018;378(20):1951. https://doi.org/10.1056/NEJMc1804294.
65. Meng L, Yu W, Wang T, Zhang L, Heerdt PM, Gelb AW. Blood pressure targets in perioperative care. Hypertension. 2018;72(4):806–17. https://doi.org/10.1161/HYPERTENSIONAHA.118.11688.
66. Retter A, Wyncoll D, Pearse R, et al. Guidelines on the management of anaemia and red cell transfusion in adult critically ill patients. Br J Haematol. 2013;160(4):445–64. https://doi.org/10.1111/bjh.12143.
67. Munoz M, Acheson AG, Auerbach M, et al. International consensus statement on the perioperative management of anaemia and iron deficiency. Anaesthesia. 2017;72(2):233–47. https://doi.org/10.1111/anae.13773.
68. Poulton T, Murray D, National Emergency Laparotomy Audit Project Team. Pre-optimisation of patients undergoing emergency laparotomy: a review of best practice. Anaesthesia. 2019;74(Suppl 1):100–7. https://doi.org/10.1111/anae.14514.
69. James S, Jhanji S, Smith A, O'Brien G, Fitzgibbon M, Pearse RM. Comparison of the prognostic accuracy of scoring systems, cardiopulmonary exercise testing, and plasma biomarkers: a single-centre observational pilot study. Br J Anaesth. 2014;112(3):491–7. https://doi.org/10.1093/bja/aet346.
70. Dillon ST, Vasunilashorn SM, Ngo L, et al. Higher C-reactive protein levels predict postoperative delirium in older patients undergoing major elective surgery: a longitudinal nested case-control study. Biol Psychiatry. 2017;81(2):145–53. https://doi.org/10.1016/j.biopsych.2016.03.2098.
71. Wolters U, Wolf T, Stutzer H, Schroder T. ASA classification and perioperative variables as predictors of postoperative outcome. Br J Anaesth. 1996;77(2):217–22. https://doi.org/10.1093/bja/77.2.217.
72. Sankar A, Johnson SR, Beattie WS, Tait G, Wijeysundera DN. Reliability of the American Society of Anesthesiologists physical status scale in clinical practice. Br J Anaesth. 2014;113(3):424–32. https://doi.org/10.1093/bja/aeu100.
73. Patel SV, Liberman SA, Burgess PL, et al. The American Society of Colon and Rectal Surgeons clinical practice guidelines for the reduction of venous thromboembolic disease in colorectal surgery. Dis Colon Rectum. 2023;66(9):1162–73. https://doi.org/10.1097/dcr.0000000000002975.
74. Ajitsaria P, Eissa SZ, Kerridge RK. Risk assessment. Curr Anesthesiol Rep. 2018;8(1):1–8. https://doi.org/10.1007/s40140-018-0246-9.
75. Koo CY, Hyder JA, Wanderer JP, Eikermann M, Ramachandran SK. A meta-analysis of the predictive accuracy of postoperative mortality using the American Society of Anesthesiologists' physical status classification system. World J Surg. 2015;39(1):88–103. https://doi.org/10.1007/s00268-014-2783-9.
76. Leung E, McArdle K, Wong LS. Risk-adjusted scoring systems in colorectal surgery. Int J Surg. 2011;9(2):130–5. https://doi.org/10.1016/j.ijsu.2010.10.016.

77. Moonesinghe SR, Mythen MG, Das P, Rowan KM, Grocott MP. Risk stratification tools for predicting morbidity and mortality in adult patients undergoing major surgery: qualitative systematic review. Anesthesiology. 2013;119(4):959–81. https://doi.org/10.1097/ALN.0b013e3182a4e94d.
78. Oliver CM, Walker E, Giannaris S, Grocott MP, Moonesinghe SR. Risk assessment tools validated for patients undergoing emergency laparotomy: a systematic review. Br J Anaesth. 2015;115(6):849–60. https://doi.org/10.1093/bja/aev350.
79. Lee TH, Marcantonio ER, Mangione CM, et al. Derivation and prospective validation of a simple index for prediction of cardiac risk of major noncardiac surgery. Circulation. 1999;100(10):1043–9. https://doi.org/10.1161/01.cir.100.10.1043.
80. Churpek MM, Yuen TC, Winslow C, et al. Multicenter development and validation of a risk stratification tool for ward patients. Am J Respir Crit Care Med. 2014;190(6):649–55. https://doi.org/10.1164/rccm.201406-1022OC.
81. Kollef MH, Chen Y, Heard K, et al. A randomized trial of real-time automated clinical deterioration alerts sent to a rapid response team. J Hosp Med. 2014;9(7):424–9. https://doi.org/10.1002/jhm.2193.
82. Anaya DA, Johanning J, Spector SA, et al. Summary of the panel session at the 38th Annual Surgical Symposium of the Association of VA Surgeons: what is the big deal about frailty? JAMA Surg. 2014;149(11):1191–7. https://doi.org/10.1001/jamasurg.2014.2064.
83. Partridge J, Sbai M, Dhesi J. Proactive care of older people undergoing surgery. Aging Clin Exp Res. 2018;30(3):253–7. https://doi.org/10.1007/s40520-017-0879-4.
84. Santa Mina D, Clarke H, Ritvo P, et al. Effect of total-body prehabilitation on postoperative outcomes: a systematic review and meta-analysis. Physiotherapy. 2014;100(3):196–207. https://doi.org/10.1016/j.physio.2013.08.008.
85. Woodard F. Prehabilitation for people with cancer. BMJ. 2019;366:I5120.
86. Whittle J, Wischmeyer PE, Grocott MPW, Miller TE. Surgical prehabilitation: nutrition and exercise. Anesthesiol Clin. 2018;36(4):567–80. https://doi.org/10.1016/j.anclin.2018.07.013.
87. Barberan-Garcia A, Ubre M, Roca J, et al. Personalised prehabilitation in high-risk patients undergoing elective major abdominal surgery: a randomized blinded controlled trial. Ann Surg. 2018;267(1):50–6. https://doi.org/10.1097/SLA.0000000000002293.
88. Van Epps P, Oswald D, Higgins PA, et al. Frailty has a stronger association with inflammation than age in older veterans. Immun Ageing. 2016;13:27. https://doi.org/10.1186/s12979-016-0082-z.
89. Chen CC, Chen CN, Lai IR, Huang GH, Saczynski JS, Inouye SK. Effects of a modified hospital elder life program on frailty in individuals undergoing major elective abdominal surgery. J Am Geriatr Soc. 2014;62(2):261–8. https://doi.org/10.1111/jgs.12651.
90. Gillis C, Li C, Lee L, et al. Prehabilitation versus rehabilitation: a randomized control trial in patients undergoing colorectal resection for cancer. Anesthesiology. 2014;121(5):937–47. https://doi.org/10.1097/ALN.0000000000000393.
91. Mazzola M, Bertoglio C, Boniardi M, et al. Frailty in major oncologic surgery of upper gastrointestinal tract: how to improve postoperative outcomes. Eur J Surg Oncol. 2017;43(8):1566–71. https://doi.org/10.1016/j.ejso.2017.06.006.
92. Bakker FC, Persoon A, Bredie SJH, et al. The CareWell in hospital program to improve the quality of care for frail elderly inpatients: results of a before–after study with focus on surgical patients. Am J Surg. 2014;208(5):735–46. https://doi.org/10.1016/j.amjsurg.2014.04.009.
93. Subramaniam A, Tiruvoipati R, Green C, et al. Frailty status, timely goals of care documentation and clinical outcomes in older hospitalised medical patients. Intern Med J. 2020;51:2078. https://doi.org/10.1111/imj.15032.
94. Schwarze ML, Brasel KJ, Mosenthal AC. Beyond 30-day mortality: aligning surgical quality with outcomes that patients value. JAMA Surg. 2014;149(7):631–2. https://doi.org/10.1001/jamasurg.2013.5143.
95. Taylor LJ, Nabozny MJ, Steffens NM, et al. A framework to improve surgeon communication in high-stakes surgical decisions: best case/worst case. JAMA Surg. 2017;152(6):531–8. https://doi.org/10.1001/jamasurg.2016.5674.

96. Schwarze ML, Kehler JM, Campbell TC. Navigating high risk procedures with more than just a street map. J Palliat Med. 2013;16(10):1169–71. https://doi.org/10.1089/jpm.2013.0221.
97. Peden C, Scott MJ. Anesthesia for emergency abdominal surgery. Anesthesiol Clin. 2015;33(1):209–21. https://doi.org/10.1016/j.anclin.2014.11.012.
98. Levy MM, Artigas A, Phillips GS, et al. Outcomes of the surviving sepsis campaign in intensive care units in the USA and Europe: a prospective cohort study. Lancet Infect Dis. 2012;12(12):919–24. https://doi.org/10.1016/S1473-3099(12)70239-6.
99. Neuman MD, Silber JH, Elkassabany NM, Ludwig JM, Fleisher LA. Comparative effectiveness of regional versus general anesthesia for hip fracture surgery in adults. Anesthesiology. 2012;117(1):72–92. https://doi.org/10.1097/ALN.0b013e3182545e7c.
100. Rigg JR, Jamrozik K, Myles PS, et al. Epidural anaesthesia and analgesia and outcome of major surgery: a randomised trial. Lancet. 2002;359(9314):1276–82. https://doi.org/10.1016/S0140-6736(02)08266-1.
101. van Lier F, van der Geest PJ, Hoeks SE, et al. Epidural analgesia is associated with improved health outcomes of surgical patients with chronic obstructive pulmonary disease. Anesthesiology. 2011;115(2):315–21. https://doi.org/10.1097/ALN.0b013e318224cc5c.
102. Baldini G, Fawcett WJ. Anesthesia for colorectal surgery. Anesthesiol Clin. 2015;33(1):93–123. https://doi.org/10.1016/j.anclin.2014.11.007.
103. Working Party, Association of Anaesthetists of Great Britain & Ireland, Obstetric Anaesthetists' Association, Regional Anaesthesia UK. Regional anaesthesia and patients with abnormalities of coagulation: the Association of Anaesthetists of Great Britain and Ireland the Obstetric Anaesthetists' Association regional Anaesthesia UK. Anaesthesia. 2013;68(9):966–72. https://doi.org/10.1111/anae.12359.
104. Lai HC, Chan SM, Lu CH, Wong CS, Cherng CH, Wu ZF. Planning for operating room efficiency and faster anesthesia wake-up time in open major upper abdominal surgery. Medicine (Baltimore). 2017;96(7):e6148. https://doi.org/10.1097/MD.0000000000006148.
105. Dunn LK, Durieux ME. Perioperative use of intravenous lidocaine. Anesthesiology. 2017;126(4):729–37. https://doi.org/10.1097/ALN.0000000000001527.
106. Clinical Outcomes of Surgical Therapy Study Group, Nelson H, Sargent DJ, et al. A comparison of laparoscopically assisted and open colectomy for colon cancer. N Engl J Med. 2004;350(20):2050–9. https://doi.org/10.1056/NEJMoa032651.
107. Colon Cancer Laparoscopic or Open Resection Study Group, Buunen M, Veldkamp R, et al. Survival after laparoscopic surgery versus open surgery for colon cancer: long-term outcome of a randomised clinical trial. Lancet Oncol. 2009;10(1):44–52. https://doi.org/10.1016/S1470-2045(08)70310-3.
108. Lacy AM, Garcia-Valdecasas JC, Delgado S, et al. Laparoscopy-assisted colectomy versus open colectomy for treatment of non-metastatic colon cancer: a randomised trial. Lancet. 2002;359(9325):2224–9. https://doi.org/10.1016/S0140-6736(02)09290-5.
109. Kennedy RH, Francis EA, Wharton R, et al. Multicenter randomized controlled trial of conventional versus laparoscopic surgery for colorectal cancer within an enhanced recovery programme: EnROL. J Clin Oncol. 2014;32(17):1804–11. https://doi.org/10.1200/JCO.2013.54.3694.
110. Bonjer HJ, Hop WC, Nelson H, et al. Laparoscopically assisted vs open colectomy for colon cancer: a meta-analysis. Arch Surg. 2007;142(3):298–303. https://doi.org/10.1001/archsurg.142.3.298.
111. Jackson TD, Kaplan GG, Arena G, Page JH, Rogers SO Jr. Laparoscopic versus open resection for colorectal cancer: a metaanalysis of oncologic outcomes. J Am Coll Surg. 2007;204(3):439–46. https://doi.org/10.1016/j.jamcollsurg.2006.12.008.
112. Choi S, Yang SY, Choi GJ, Kim BG, Kang H. Comparison of pressure- and volume-controlled ventilation during laparoscopic colectomy in patients with colorectal cancer. Sci Rep. 2019;9(1):17007. https://doi.org/10.1038/s41598-019-53503-9.
113. Sharma KC, Brandstetter RD, Brensilver JM, Jung LD. Cardiopulmonary physiology and pathophysiology as a consequence of laparoscopic surgery. Chest. 1996;110(3):810–5. https://doi.org/10.1378/chest.110.3.810.

114. Rauh R, Hemmerling TM, Rist M, Jacobi KE. Influence of pneumoperitoneum and patient positioning on respiratory system compliance. J Clin Anesth. 2001;13(5):361–5. https://doi.org/10.1016/s0952-8180(01)00286-0.
115. Grabowski JE, Talamini MA. Physiological effects of pneumoperitoneum. J Gastrointest Surg. 2009;13(5):1009–16. https://doi.org/10.1007/s11605-008-0662-0.
116. Futier E, Constantin JM, Paugam-Burtz C, et al. A trial of intraoperative low-tidal-volume ventilation in abdominal surgery. N Engl J Med. 2013;369(5):428–37. https://doi.org/10.1056/NEJMoa1301082.
117. Lam SM, Lau AC, Chan KK. Intraoperative low-tidal-volume ventilation. N Engl J Med. 2013;369(19):1861–2. https://doi.org/10.1056/NEJMc1311316.
118. Futier E, Jaber S. Lung-protective ventilation in abdominal surgery. Curr Opin Crit Care. 2014;20(4):426–30. https://doi.org/10.1097/MCC.0000000000000121.
119. Futier E, Godet T, Millot A, Constantin JM, Jaber S. Mechanical ventilation in abdominal surgery. Ann Fr Anesth Reanim. 2014;33(7–8):472–5. https://doi.org/10.1016/j.annfar.2014.07.007.
120. Wakeling HG, McFall MR, Jenkins CS, et al. Intraoperative oesophageal Doppler guided fluid management shortens postoperative hospital stay after major bowel surgery. Br J Anaesth. 2005;95(5):634–42. https://doi.org/10.1093/bja/aei223.
121. Brandstrup B. Fluid therapy for the surgical patient. Best Pract Res Clin Anaesthesiol. 2006;20(2):265–83. https://doi.org/10.1016/j.bpa.2005.10.007.
122. Myles PS, Bellomo R, Corcoran T, et al. Restrictive versus liberal fluid therapy for major abdominal surgery. N Engl J Med. 2018;378(24):2263–74. https://doi.org/10.1056/NEJMoa1801601.
123. Miller TE, Pearse RM. Perioperative fluid management: moving toward more answers than questions—a commentary on the RELIEF study. Perioper Med. 2019;8(1):2. https://doi.org/10.1186/s13741-019-0113-3.
124. Lenhardt R, Marker E, Goll V, et al. Mild intraoperative hypothermia prolongs postanesthetic recovery. Anesthesiology. 1997;87(6):1318–23. https://doi.org/10.1097/00000542-199712000-00009.
125. Kurz A, Sessler DI, Narzt E, Lenhardt R, Lackner F. Morphometric influences on intraoperative core temperature changes. Anesth Analg. 1995;80(3):562–7. https://doi.org/10.1097/00000539-199503000-00023.
126. Valeri CR, Khabbaz K, Khuri SF, et al. Effect of skin temperature on platelet function in patients undergoing extracorporeal bypass. J Thorac Cardiovasc Surg. 1992;104(1):108–16. https://www.ncbi.nlm.nih.gov/pubmed/1614195.
127. Wolberg AS, Meng ZH, Monroe DM 3rd, Hoffman M. A systematic evaluation of the effect of temperature on coagulation enzyme activity and platelet function. J Trauma. 2004;56(6):1221–8. https://doi.org/10.1097/01.ta.0000064328.97941.fc.
128. Kurz A, Sessler DI, Lenhardt R. Perioperative normothermia to reduce the incidence of surgical-wound infection and shorten hospitalization. Study of wound infection and temperature group. N Engl J Med. 1996;334(19):1209–15. https://doi.org/10.1056/NEJM199605093341901.
129. Cirocco WC, Golub RW. Endoscopic treatment of postoperative hemorrhage from a stapled colorectal anastomosis. Am Surg. 1995;61(5):460–3. https://www.ncbi.nlm.nih.gov/pubmed/7733557.
130. Malik AH, East JE, Buchanan GN, Kennedy RH. Endoscopic haemostasis of staple-line haemorrhage following colorectal resection. Color Dis. 2008;10(6):616–8. https://doi.org/10.1111/j.1463-1318.2007.01459.x.
131. Martinez-Serrano MA, Pares D, Pera M, et al. Management of lower gastrointestinal bleeding after colorectal resection and stapled anastomosis. Tech Coloproctol. 2009;13(1):49–53. https://doi.org/10.1007/s10151-009-0458-6.
132. Borgman MA, Spinella PC, Perkins JG, et al. The ratio of blood products transfused affects mortality in patients receiving massive transfusions at a combat support hospital. J Trauma. 2007;63(4):805–13. https://doi.org/10.1097/TA.0b013e3181271ba3.

133. Srivastava A, Kelleher A. Point-of-care coagulation testing. Contin Educ Anaesth Crit Care Pain. 2012;13(1):12–6. https://doi.org/10.1093/bjaceaccp/mks049.
134. Stocchi L. Laparoscopic surgery for ulcerative colitis. Clin Colon Rectal Surg. 2010;23(4):248–58. https://doi.org/10.1055/s-0030-1268251.
135. Arthur T, Burgess A. Acute colonic pseudo-obstruction. Clin Colon Rectal Surg. 2022;35(3):221–6. https://doi.org/10.1055/s-0041-1740044.
136. Arezzo A, Passera R, Lo Secco G, et al. Stent as bridge to surgery for left-sided malignant colonic obstruction reduces adverse events and stoma rate compared with emergency surgery: results of a systematic review and meta-analysis of randomized controlled trials. Gastrointest Endosc. 2017;86(3):416–26. https://doi.org/10.1016/j.gie.2017.03.1542.
137. Lundy M, Ashburn JH. Management of the hostile abdomen. Clin Colon Rectal Surg. 2022;35(3):169–76. https://doi.org/10.1055/s-0041-1740043.
138. Nair AS, Naik VM, Rayani BK. FAST HUGS BID: modified mnemonic for surgical patient. Indian J Crit Care Med. 2017;21(10):713–4. https://doi.org/10.4103/ijccm.IJCCM_289_17.
139. van der Leeden M, Huijsmans R, Geleijn E, et al. Early enforced mobilisation following surgery for gastrointestinal cancer: feasibility and outcomes. Physiotherapy. 2016;102(1):103–10. https://doi.org/10.1016/j.physio.2015.03.3722.
140. Schaller SJ, Anstey M, Blobner M, et al. Early, goal-directed mobilisation in the surgical intensive care unit: a randomised controlled trial. Lancet. 2016;388(10052):1377–88. https://doi.org/10.1016/S0140-6736(16)31637-3.
141. Lipshutz AK, Gropper MA. Acquired neuromuscular weakness and early mobilization in the intensive care unit. Anesthesiology. 2013;118(1):202–15. https://doi.org/10.1097/ALN.0b013e31826be693.
142. Bartlett MA, Mauck KF, Stephenson CR, Ganesh R, Daniels PR. Perioperative venous thromboembolism prophylaxis. Mayo Clin Proc. 2020;95(12):2775–98. https://doi.org/10.1016/j.mayocp.2020.06.015.
143. Subramaniam A, Wengritzky R, Skinner S, Shekar K. Colorectal surgery in critically unwell patients: a multidisciplinary approach. Clin Colon Rectal Surg. 2022;35(3):244–60. https://doi.org/10.1055/s-0041-1740045.
144. Thompson RE, Broussard EK, Flum DR, Wisse BE. Perioperative glycemic control during colorectal surgery. Curr Diab Rep. 2016;16(3):32. (In eng). https://doi.org/10.1007/s11892-016-0722-x.
145. Vincent JL. Give your patient a fast hug (at least) once a day. Crit Care Med. 2005;33(6):1225–9. https://doi.org/10.1097/01.ccm.0000165962.16682.46.
146. Vincent WR 3rd, Hatton KW. Critically ill patients need "FAST HUGS BID" (an updated mnemonic). Crit Care Med. 2009;37(7):2326–7.; (author reply 2327). https://doi.org/10.1097/CCM.0b013e3181aabc29.
147. Papadimos TJ, Hensley SJ, Duggan JM, et al. Implementation of the "FASTHUG" concept decreases the incidence of ventilator-associated pneumonia in a surgical intensive care unit. Patient Saf Surg. 2008;2:3. https://doi.org/10.1186/1754-9493-2-3.
148. Weibel S, Jelting Y, Pace NL, et al. Continuous intravenous perioperative lidocaine infusion for postoperative pain and recovery in adults. Cochrane Database Syst Rev. 2018;6:CD009642. https://doi.org/10.1002/14651858.CD009642.pub3.
149. Abdallah FW, Chan VW, Brull R. Transversus abdominis plane block: a systematic review. Reg Anesth Pain Med. 2012;37(2):193–209. https://doi.org/10.1097/AAP.0b013e3182429531.
150. Johns N, O'Neill S, Ventham NT, Barron F, Brady RR, Daniel T. Clinical effectiveness of transversus abdominis plane (TAP) block in abdominal surgery: a systematic review and meta-analysis. Color Dis. 2012;14(10):e635–42. https://doi.org/10.1111/j.1463-1318.2012.03104.x.
151. Lumb A, Biercamp C. Chronic obstructive pulmonary disease and anaesthesia. Contin Educ Anaesth Crit Care Pain. 2013;14(1):1–5. https://doi.org/10.1093/bjaceaccp/mkt023.
152. Lobo DN, Bostock KA, Neal KR, Perkins AC, Rowlands BJ, Allison SP. Effect of salt and water balance on recovery of gastrointestinal function after elective colonic resection:

a randomised controlled trial. Lancet. 2002;359(9320):1812–8. https://doi.org/10.1016/S0140-6736(02)08711-1.
153. Ruscic KJ, Grabitz SD, Rudolph MI, Eikermann M. Prevention of respiratory complications of the surgical patient: actionable plan for continued process improvement. Curr Opin Anaesthesiol. 2017;30(3):399–408. https://doi.org/10.1097/ACO.0000000000000465.
154. Scheeren TW, Wiesenack C, Gerlach H, Marx G. Goal-directed intraoperative fluid therapy guided by stroke volume and its variation in high-risk surgical patients: a prospective randomized multicentre study. J Clin Monit Comput. 2013;27(3):225–33. https://doi.org/10.1007/s10877-013-9461-6.
155. Annane D, Vignon P, Renault A, et al. Norepinephrine plus dobutamine versus epinephrine alone for management of septic shock: a randomised trial. Lancet. 2007;370(9588):676–84. https://doi.org/10.1016/S0140-6736(07)61344-0.
156. De Backer D, Biston P, Devriendt J, et al. Comparison of dopamine and norepinephrine in the treatment of shock. N Engl J Med. 2010;362(9):779–89. https://doi.org/10.1056/NEJMoa0907118.
157. Myburgh JA, Higgins A, Jovanovska A, et al. A comparison of epinephrine and norepinephrine in critically ill patients. Intensive Care Med. 2008;34(12):2226–34. https://doi.org/10.1007/s00134-008-1219-0.
158. Venkatesh B, Finfer S, Cohen J, et al. Adjunctive glucocorticoid therapy in patients with septic shock. N Engl J Med. 2018;378(9):797–808. https://doi.org/10.1056/NEJMoa1705835.
159. Adanir T, Nazli O, Kara C, et al. The relationship between vasopressor dose and anastomotic leak in colon surgery: an experimental trial. Int J Surg. 2010;8(3):221–4. https://doi.org/10.1016/j.ijsu.2010.01.004.
160. Zakrison T, Nascimento BA Jr, Tremblay LN, Kiss A, Rizoli SB. Perioperative vasopressors are associated with an increased risk of gastrointestinal anastomotic leakage. World J Surg. 2007;31(8):1627–34. https://doi.org/10.1007/s00268-007-9113-4.
161. Deng C, Bellomo R, Myles P. Systematic review and meta-analysis of the perioperative use of vasoactive drugs on postoperative outcomes after major abdominal surgery. Br J Anaesth. 2020;124(5):513–24. https://doi.org/10.1016/j.bja.2020.01.021.
162. Nelson RL, Gladman E, Barbateskovic M. Antimicrobial prophylaxis for colorectal surgery. Cochrane Database Syst Rev. 2014;5:CD001181. https://doi.org/10.1002/14651858.CD001181.pub4.
163. Solomkin JS, Mazuski JE, Bradley JS, et al. Diagnosis and management of complicated intra-abdominal infection in adults and children: guidelines by the surgical infection society and the Infectious Diseases Society of America. Surg Infect. 2010;11(1):79–109. https://doi.org/10.1089/sur.2009.9930.
164. Pak H, Maghsoudi LH, Soltanian A, Gholami F. Surgical complications in colorectal cancer patients. Ann Med Surg (Lond). 2020;55:13–8. https://doi.org/10.1016/j.amsu.2020.04.024.
165. Delaney CP, Marcello PW, Sonoda T, Wise P, Bauer J, Techner L. Gastrointestinal recovery after laparoscopic colectomy: results of a prospective, observational, multicenter study. Surg Endosc. 2010;24(3):653–61. https://doi.org/10.1007/s00464-009-0652-7.
166. Debarros M, Steele SR. Perioperative protocols in colorectal surgery. Clin Colon Rectal Surg. 2013;26(3):139–45. https://doi.org/10.1055/s-0033-1351128.
167. Platell C, Hall JC. The prevention of wound infection in patients undergoing colorectal surgery. J Hosp Infect. 2001;49(4):233–8. https://doi.org/10.1053/jhin.2001.1061.
168. Lawson EH, Hall BL, Ko CY. Risk factors for superficial vs deep/organ-space surgical site infections: implications for quality improvement initiatives. JAMA Surg. 2013;148(9):849–58. https://doi.org/10.1001/jamasurg.2013.2925.
169. Komen N, Dijk JW, Lalmahomed Z, et al. After-hours colorectal surgery: a risk factor for anastomotic leakage. Int J Color Dis. 2009;24(7):789–95. https://doi.org/10.1007/s00384-009-0692-4.
170. Devereaux PJ, Xavier D, Pogue J, et al. Characteristics and short-term prognosis of perioperative myocardial infarction in patients undergoing noncardiac surgery: a cohort

study. Ann Intern Med. 2011;154(8):523–8. https://doi.org/10.7326/0003-4819-154-8-201104190-00003.
171. Gupta H, Gupta PK, Fang X, et al. Development and validation of a risk calculator predicting postoperative respiratory failure. Chest. 2011;140(5):1207–15. https://doi.org/10.1378/chest.11-0466.
172. Dale CD, McLoone P, Sloan B, et al. Critical care provision after colorectal cancer surgery. BMC Anesthesiol. 2016;16(1):94. https://doi.org/10.1186/s12871-016-0243-9.
173. Mazo V, Sabate S, Canet J, et al. Prospective external validation of a predictive score for postoperative pulmonary complications. Anesthesiology. 2014;121(2):219–31. https://doi.org/10.1097/ALN.0000000000000334.
174. Johnson RG, Arozullah AM, Neumayer L, Henderson WG, Hosokawa P, Khuri SF. Multivariable predictors of postoperative respiratory failure after general and vascular surgery: results from the patient safety in surgery study. J Am Coll Surg. 2007;204(6):1188–98. https://doi.org/10.1016/j.jamcollsurg.2007.02.070.
175. Kim M, Brady JE, Li G. Interaction effects of acute kidney injury, acute respiratory failure, and sepsis on 30-day postoperative mortality in patients undergoing high-risk intraabdominal general surgical procedures. Anesth Analg. 2015;121(6):1536–46. https://doi.org/10.1213/ANE.0000000000000915.
176. Davis PJ, Bailey JG, Molinari M, Hayden J, Johnson PM. The impact of nonelective abdominal surgery on the residential status of older adult patients. Ann Surg. 2016;263(2):274–9. https://doi.org/10.1097/SLA.0000000000001126.
177. Bailey JG, Davis PJ, Levy AR, Molinari M, Johnson PM. The impact of adverse events on health care costs for older adults undergoing nonelective abdominal surgery. Can J Surg. 2016;59(3):172–9. https://doi.org/10.1503/cjs.013915.
178. Goeteyn J, Evans LA, De Cleyn S, et al. Frailty as a predictor of mortality in the elderly emergency general surgery patient. Acta Chir Belg. 2017;117(6):370–5. https://doi.org/10.1080/00015458.2017.1337339.
179. Mueller N, Murthy S, Tainter CR, et al. Can sarcopenia quantified by ultrasound of the rectus Femoris muscle predict adverse outcome of surgical intensive care unit patients as well as frailty? A prospective, observational cohort study. Ann Surg. 2016;264(6):1116–24. https://doi.org/10.1097/SLA.0000000000001546.
180. Fuks D, Cauchy F, Fteriche S, et al. Laparoscopy decreases pulmonary complications in patients undergoing major liver resection: a propensity score analysis. Ann Surg. 2016;263(2):353–61. https://doi.org/10.1097/SLA.0000000000001140.
181. Corcoran T, Rhodes JE, Clarke S, Myles PS, Ho KM. Perioperative fluid management strategies in major surgery: a stratified meta-analysis. Anesth Analg. 2012;114(3):640–51. https://doi.org/10.1213/ANE.0b013e318240d6eb.
182. Thacker JK, Mountford WK, Ernst FR, Krukas MR, Mythen MM. Perioperative fluid utilization variability and association with outcomes: considerations for enhanced recovery efforts in sample US surgical populations. Ann Surg. 2016;263(3):502–10. https://doi.org/10.1097/SLA.0000000000001402.
183. Dennen P, Douglas IS, Anderson R. Acute kidney injury in the intensive care unit: an update and primer for the intensivist. Crit Care Med. 2010;38(1):261–75. https://doi.org/10.1097/CCM.0b013e3181bfb0b5.
184. McDaniel M, Brudney C. Postoperative delirium: etiology and management. Curr Opin Crit Care. 2012;18(4):372–6. https://doi.org/10.1097/MCC.0b013e3283557211.
185. Collins N, Blanchard MR, Tookman A, Sampson EL. Detection of delirium in the acute hospital. Age Ageing. 2010;39(1):131–5. https://doi.org/10.1093/ageing/afp201.
186. Witlox J, Eurelings LS, de Jonghe JF, Kalisvaart KJ, Eikelenboom P, van Gool WA. Delirium in elderly patients and the risk of postdischarge mortality, institutionalization, and dementia: a meta-analysis. JAMA. 2010;304(4):443–51. https://doi.org/10.1001/jama.2010.1013.
187. Grant SB, Modi PK, Singer EA. Futility and the care of surgical patients: ethical dilemmas. World J Surg. 2014;38(7):1631–7. https://doi.org/10.1007/s00268-014-2592-1.

188. Bayraktar B, Ozemir IA, Kefeli U, et al. Colorectal stenting for palliation and as a bridge to surgery: a 5-year follow-up study. World J Gastroenterol. 2015;21(31):9373–9. https://doi.org/10.3748/wjg.v21.i31.9373.
189. Rawal G, Yadav S, Kumar R. Post-intensive care syndrome: an overview. J Transl Int Med. 2017;5(2):90–2. https://doi.org/10.1515/jtim-2016-0016.

Chapter 42
Useful Tables and Internet Sites

Joel Faintuch, Jacob J. Faintuch, and Asher Mishaly

See Tables 42.1, 42.2, 42.3, 42.4, 42.5, 42.6, 42.7, 42.8 and 42.9.

Table 42.1 Official sites of major international surgical societies

iss-sic.com	International Society of Surgery
icsglobal.org	International College of Surgeons
theifsc.org	International Federation of Surgical Colleges
theiaas.net	International Association for Ambulatory Surgery
Isakos.com	International Society of Arthroscopy, Knee Surgery and Orthopaedic Sports Medicine
miectis.org	Minimal Invasive Extracorporeal Technologies International Society
wscts.net	World Society of Cardiovascular and Thoracic Surgeons
wses.org	World Society of Emergency Surgery
surgonc.org	Society of Surgical Oncology

J. Faintuch (✉)
Department of Gastroenterology, São Paulo University Medical School, Sao Paulo, Brazil
e-mail: j.faintuch@hc.fm.usp.br

J. J. Faintuch
Department of Internal Medicine, Clinicas Hospital, Sao Paulo University Medical School, Sao Paulo, Brazil
e-mail: Jacob.Faintuch@hc.fm.usp.br

A. Mishaly
Internal medicine private practice, São Paulo, SP, Brazil

© The Author(s), under exclusive license to Springer Nature Switzerland AG 2024

J. Faintuch, S. Faintuch (eds.), *Recent Strategies in High Risk Surgery*,
https://doi.org/10.1007/978-3-031-56270-9_42

Table 42.2 Sites and educational material (guidelines, videos, apps) from surgical societies

ifso.com	International Federation for the Surgery of Obesity
facs.org	American College of Surgeons
asmbs.org	American Society of Bariatric and Metabolic Surgery
Fascrs.org	American Society of Colon and Rectal Surgeons
aast.org	American Association for the Surgery of Trauma
aaos.org	American Academy of Orthopaedic Surgeons
sts.org	Society of Thoracic Surgeons
erassociety.org	Enhanced Recovery after Surgery Society (ERAS guidelines)
sccm.org	Guidelines and bundles from Surviving Sepsis Campaign, as well as general critical care (Society of Critical Care Medicine)
surgonc.org/resources/guidelines/	Guidelines on surgical oncology
guidelinecentral.com	Guidelines on multiple conditions from official medical societies along with commercial and sponsored information

Table 42.3 Surgical videos and technical instructions

websurg.com	Educational material from IRCAD (Institut de recherche contre les cancers de l'appareil digestif, Strasburg, France)
csurgeries.com	Journal for surgical vídeos
medprofvideos.mayoclinic.org	Educational resources supplied by Mayo Clinic (USA)
aofoundation.org	Authoritative source for handling of bone fractures (American Orthopedic Foundation)
touchsurgery.com	Videos and apps (associated with Medtronic), one of the most complete and accessed sites
youtube.com/@sccm	Videos on sepsis, fluid overload and many other topics (Society of Critical Medicine)
criticalcarepractitioner.co.uk/videos	Critical care videos from the Critical Care Practitioner (UK)
aorn.org/education/education-for-facilities/periop-nursing-video-library	Educational videos from the Association of Perioperative Registered Nurses
upmc.com/services/south-central-pa/orthopaedics/patients/post-op	Videos on physical and occupational therapy for orthopaedic (and general) patients
mayoclinic.org/medical-professionals/trauma/videos	Trauma videos from Mayo Clinic/USA
surgery.ucsd.edu/divisions/trauma-burn/training/videos/index.html	Videos on trauma, surgical critical care and burns from University of California San Diego

Apps for cellphones and tablets occasionally available, with or without subscription

Table 42.4 General medical sites (including surgical conditions)

webmd.com	Diagnosis and treatment of many diseases, including surgical conditions
uptodate.com	Medical information site of publisher Wolters Kluwer
dynamed.com	EBSCO industries site encompassing about 40 specialties
medtube.net	A vast site of videos and professional resources
mdcalc.com	Online calculation of scores, equations and prognostic indexes
nice.org.uk	Recommendations from the National Institute for Health and Care Excellence (UK)

Some sites demand registration and/or subscription for use as well as for app download

Table 42.5 Instant calculation of prognosis and severity indexes by mdcalc

mdcalc.com/calc/1868	APACHE II (Acute physiology and chronic health evaluation)
mdcalc.com/calc/10024	ASA score (American Society of Anesthesiologists)
mdcalc.com/calc/691	SOFA (sequential organ failure assessment)
mdcalc.com/calc/2654	Quick SOFA
mdcalc.com/calc/3927	POSSUM (Physiological and Operative Severity Score for the enUmeration of mortality and morbidity)
mdcalc.com/calc/64	Glasgow coma score
mdcalc.com/calc/4044	SAPS II (simplified acute physiology score)
mdcalc.com/calc/10179	Euroscore II (cardiac operative risk)

The site encompasses dozens of other scores with potential surgical interest

Table 42.6 Instant calculation of scores at other sites

riskcalculator.facs.org/RiskCalculator	NSQIP (American College of Surgeons) universal surgical risk calculator
riskprediction.org.uk/index-pp.php	P-POSSUM (Portsmouth-POSSUM)
thecalculator.co/health/MODS-score-for-multiple-organ-failure-Calculator-1106.html	MODS (multiple organ dysfunction score)
mdapp.co/trauma-injury-severity-score-triss-calculator-277	Trauma injury severity score

Table 42.7 Surgery, complications and general management of diabetic patients

cdc.gov/diabetes	Guidelines from the Centers for Disease Control and Prevention (USA)
who.int/health-topics/diabetes	Data from the World Health Organization
joslin.org	Official site of Joslin Clinic (Harvard)
niddk.nih.gov/health-information/diabetes	Recommendations of the National Institutes of Health (USA)
professional.diabetes.org/content-page/practice-guidelines-resources	Resources from the American Diabetes Association
idf.org/e-library/guidelines/165-idf-dar-practical-guidelines-2021.html	Directives from the International Diabetes Federation
diabetes.org.uk/professionals/position-statements-reports/specialist-care-for-children-and-adults-and-complications/management-of-adults-with-diabetes-undergoing-surgery-and-elective-procedures-improving-standards	Surgery guidelines from the British Diabetic Association

Table 42.8 Surgical safety checklist

Before induction of anaesthesia—(with at least nurse and anaesthetist)
Has the patient confirmed his/her identity, site, procedure and consent?
☐ Yes
Is the site marked?
☐ Yes
☐ Not applicable
Is the anaesthesia machine and medication check complete?
☐ Yes
Is the pulse oximeter on the patient and functioning?
☐ Yes
Does the patient have a:
Known allergy?
☐ No
☐ Yes

Table 42.8 (continued)

Difficult airway or aspiration risk?
☐ No
☐ Yes, and equipment/assistance available
Risk of >500 mL blood loss (7 mL/kg in children)?
☐ No
☐ Yes, and two IVs/central access and fluids planned
☐ Confirm all team members have introduced themselves by name and role
☐ Confirm the patient's name, procedure and where the incision will be made
Has antibiotic prophylaxis been given within the last 60 min?
☐ Yes
☐ Not applicable
Anticipated critical events
To surgeon
☐ What are the critical or non-routine steps?
☐ How long will the case take?
☐ What is the anticipated blood loss?
To anaesthetist
☐ Are there any patient-specific concerns?
To nursing team
☐ Has sterility (including indicator results) been confirmed?
☐ Are there equipment issues or any concerns?
Is essential imaging displayed?
☐ Yes
☐ Not applicable
Nurse verbally confirms
☐ The name of the procedure
☐ Completion of instrument, sponge and needle counts
☐ Specimen labelling (read specimen labels aloud, including patient name)
To surgeon, anaesthetist and nurse
☐ What are the key concerns for recovery and management of this patient?

This checklist is not intended to be comprehensive. Additions and modifications to fit local practice are encouraged. Revised 1/2009—© WHO, 2009
Useful surgical recommendations from the World Health Organization
Reproduction rights granted by the WHO Permissions Team Request 391824 on March 10, 2023
Reproduced from: Implementation Manual—WHO Surgical Safety Checklist 2009—ISBN 978 92 4159859 0 © World Health Organization 2009; Available at who.int/iris/bitstream/handle/10665/44186/9789241598590_eng.pdf?

Table 42.9 Summary of core topics, research questions and recommendations for the prevention of surgical site infection

Topic	Research questions	Recommendations	Strength	Quality of evidence
Preoperative measures				
Preoperative bathing	1. Is preoperative bathing using an antimicrobial soap more effective in reducing the incidence of SSI in surgical patients compared to bathing with plain soap? 2. Is preoperative bathing with CHG-impregnated cloths more effective in reducing the incidence of SSI in surgical patients compared to bathing with antimicrobial soap?	It is good clinical practice for patients to bathe or shower prior to surgery		
		The panel suggests that either plain soap or an antimicrobial soap may be used for this purpose	Conditional	Moderate
		The panel decided not to formulate a recommendation on the use of CHG-impregnated cloths for the purpose of reducing SSI due to the very low quality of evidence		
Decolonization with mupirocin ointment with or without CHG body wash for the prevention of *Staphylococcus aureus* infection in nasal carriers	Is mupirocin nasal ointment in combination with or without CHG body wash effective in reducing the number of *S. aureus* infections in nasal carriers undergoing surgery?	The panel recommends that patients undergoing cardiothoracic and orthopaedic surgery with known nasal carriage of *S. aureus* should receive perioperative intranasal applications of mupirocin 2% ointment with or without a combination of CHG body wash	Strong	Moderate
		The panel suggests considering to treat also patients with known nasal carriage of *S. aureus* undergoing other types of surgery with perioperative intranasal applications of mupirocin 2% ointment with or without a combination of CHG body wash	Conditional	Moderate

Table 42.9 (continued)

Topic	Research questions	Recommendations	Strength	Quality of evidence
Screening of ESBL colonization and the impact on antibiotic prophylaxis	1. Should SAP be modified in high (>10%) ESBL prevalence areas? 2. Should SAP be modified in patients who are colonized with or a carrier of ESBL? 3. Should patients be screened for ESBL prior to surgery?	The panel decided not to formulate a recommendation due to the lack of evidence	NA	NA
Optimal timing for preoperative SAP	How does the timing of SAP administration impact on the risk of SSI, and what is the precise optimal timing?	The panel recommends that SAP should be administered prior to the surgical incision when indicated (depending on the type of operation)	Strong	Low
		The panel recommends the administration of SAP within 120 min before incision, while considering the half-life of the antibiotic	Strong	Moderate
Mechanical bowel preparation and the use of oral antibiotics	Is mechanical bowel preparation combined with or without oral antibiotics effective for the prevention of SSI in colorectal surgery?	The panel suggests that preoperative oral antibiotics combined with mechanical bowel preparation should be used to reduce the risk of SSI in adult patients undergoing elective colorectal surgery	Conditional	Moderate
		The panel recommends that mechanical bowel preparation alone (without the administration of oral antibiotics) should **not** be used for the purpose of reducing SSI in adult patients undergoing elective colorectal surgery	Strong	Moderate

(continued)

Table 42.9 (continued)

Topic	Research questions	Recommendations	Strength	Quality of evidence
Hair removal	1. Does hair removal affect the incidence of SSI? 2. What method and timing of hair removal are associated with the reduction of SSI?	The panel recommends that in patients undergoing any surgical procedure, hair should either **not** be removed or, if absolutely necessary, be removed only with a clipper. Shaving is strongly discouraged at all times, whether preoperatively or in the operating room	Strong	Moderate
Surgical site preparation	Should alcohol-based antiseptic solutions or aqueous solutions be used for skin preparation in surgical patients, and, more specifically, should CHG or PVP-I solutions be used?	The panel recommends alcohol-based antiseptic solutions based on CHG for surgical site skin preparation in patients undergoing surgical procedures	Strong	Low to moderate
Antimicrobial skin sealants	Should antimicrobial sealants (in addition to standard surgical site skin preparation) be used in surgical patients for the prevention of SSI compared to standard surgical site skin preparation only?	The panel suggests that antimicrobial sealants should **not** be used after surgical site skin preparation for the purpose of reducing SSI	Conditional	Very low
Surgical hand preparation	1. What is the most effective type of product for surgical hand preparation to prevent SSI? 2. What are the most effective technique and ideal duration for surgical hand preparation?	The panel recommends that surgical hand preparation should be performed by either scrubbing with a suitable antimicrobial soap and water or using a suitable alcohol-based handrub before donning sterile gloves	Strong	Moderate

Table 42.9 (continued)

Topic	Research questions	Recommendations	Strength	Quality of evidence
Preoperative and/or intraoperative measures				
Enhanced nutritional support	In surgical patients, should enhanced nutritional support be used for the prevention of SSI?	The panel suggests considering the administration of oral or enteral multiple nutrient-enhanced nutritional formulas for the purpose of preventing SSI in underweight patients who undergo major surgical operations	Conditional	Very low
Perioperative discontinuation of immunosuppressive agents	Should immunosuppressive agents be discontinued perioperatively, and does this affect the incidence of SSI?	The panel suggests not to discontinue immunosuppressive medication prior to surgery for the purpose of preventing SSI	Conditional	Very low
Perioperative oxygenation	How safe and effective is the perioperative use of an increased fraction of inspired oxygen in reducing the risk of SSI?	The panel suggests that adult patients undergoing general anaesthesia with tracheal intubation for surgical procedures should receive an 80% fraction of inspired oxygen intraoperatively and, if feasible, in the immediate postoperative period for 2–6 h to reduce the risk of SSI	Conditional	Moderate
Maintaining normal body temperature (normothermia)	Should systemic body warming vs. no warming be used for the prevention of SSI in surgical patients?	The panel suggests the use of warming devices in the operating room and during the surgical procedure for patient body warming with the purpose of reducing SSI	Conditional	Moderate

(continued)

Table 42.9 (continued)

Topic	Research questions	Recommendations	Strength	Quality of evidence
Use of protocols for intensive perioperative blood glucose control	1. Do protocols aiming to maintain optimal perioperative blood glucose levels reduce the risk of SSI? 2. What are the optimal perioperative glucose target levels in diabetic and non-diabetic patients?	The panel suggests the use of protocols for intensive perioperative blood glucose control for both diabetic and non-diabetic adult patients undergoing surgical procedures to reduce the risk of SSI	Conditional	Low
		The panel decided not to formulate a recommendation on this topic due to the lack of evidence to answer question 2		
Maintenance of adequate circulating volume control/ normovolaemia	Does the use of specific fluid management strategies during surgery affect the incidence of SSI?	The panel suggests the use of goal-directed fluid therapy intraoperatively to reduce the risk of SSI	Conditional	Low
Drapes and gowns	1. Is there a difference in SSI rates depending on the use of disposable non-woven drapes and gowns or reusable woven drapes and gowns? 1.1. Is there a difference in SSI rates depending on the use of disposable non-woven or reusable woven drapes? 1.2. Is there a difference in SSI rates depending on the use of disposable non-woven or reusable woven gowns?	The panel suggests that either sterile, disposable non-woven or sterile, reusable woven drapes and gowns can be used during surgical operations for the purpose of preventing SSI No specific evidence was retrieved to answer questions 1.1 and 1.2	Conditional	Moderate to very low
	2. Does the use of disposable, adhesive, incise drapes reduce the risk of SSI?	The panel suggests **not** to use plastic adhesive incise drapes with or without antimicrobial properties for the purpose of preventing SSI	Conditional	Low to very low

Table 42.9 (continued)

Topic	Research questions	Recommendations	Strength	Quality of evidence
Wound protector devices	Does the use of wound protector devices reduce the rate of SSI in open abdominal surgery?	The panel suggests considering the use of wound protector devices in clean-contaminated, contaminated and dirty abdominal surgical procedures for the purpose of reducing the rate of SSI	Conditional	Very low
Incisional wound irrigation	Does intraoperative wound irrigation reduce the risk of SSI?	The panel considered that there is insufficient evidence to recommend for or against saline irrigation of incisional wounds before closure for the purpose of preventing SSI	NA	NA
		The panel suggests considering the use of irrigation of the incisional wound with an aqueous PVP-I solution before closure for the purpose of preventing SSI, particularly in clean and clean-contaminated wounds	Conditional	Low
		The panel suggests that antibiotic incisional wound irrigation should **not** be used for the purpose of preventing SSI	Conditional	Low
Prophylactic negative pressure wound therapy	Does prophylactic negative pressure wound therapy reduce the rate of SSI compared to the use of conventional dressings?	The panel suggests the use of prophylactic negative pressure wound therapy in adult patients on primarily closed surgical incisions in high-risk wounds for the purpose of the prevention of SSI, while taking resources into account	Conditional	Low

(continued)

Table 42.9 (continued)

Topic	Research questions	Recommendations	Strength	Quality of evidence
Use of surgical gloves	1. When is double-gloving recommended? 2. What are the criteria for changing gloves during an operation? 3. What type of gloves should be used?	The panel decided not to formulate a recommendation due to the lack of evidence to assess whether double-gloving or a change of gloves during the operation or the use of specific types of gloves are more effective in reducing the risk of SSI	NA	NA
Changing of surgical instruments	At the time of wound closure, is there a difference in SSI when instruments are changed for fascial, subcutaneous and skin closure using a new set of sterile instruments?	The panel decided not to formulate a recommendation on this topic due to the lack of evidence	NA	NA
Antimicrobial-coated sutures	Are antimicrobial-coated sutures effective to prevent SSI? If yes, when and how should they be used?	The panel suggests the use of triclosan-coated sutures for the purpose of reducing the risk of SSI, independent of the type of surgery	Conditional	Moderate
Laminar flow ventilation systems in the context of OR ventilation	1. Is the use of laminar air flow in the OR associated with the reduction of overall or deep SSI?	The panel suggests that laminar airflow ventilation systems should **not** be used to reduce the risk of SSI for patients undergoing total arthroplasty surgery	Conditional	Low to very low
	2. Does the use of fans or cooling devices increase SSIs? 3. Is natural ventilation an acceptable alternative to mechanical ventilation?	The panel decided not to formulate a recommendation on these topics due to the lack of evidence to answer questions 2 and 3	NA	NA

Table 42.9 (continued)

Topic	Research questions	Recommendations	Strength	Quality of evidence
Postoperative measures				
SAP prolongation	Does continued postoperative SAP reduce the risk of SSI compared with preoperative and (if necessary) intraoperative prophylaxis only?	The panel recommends **against** the prolongation of SAP after completion of the operation for the purpose of preventing SSI	Strong	Moderate
Advanced dressings	In surgical patients, should advanced dressings vs. standard sterile wound dressings be used for the prevention of SSI?	The panel suggests **not** using any type of advanced dressing over a standard dressing on primarily closed surgical wounds for the purpose of preventing SSI	Conditional	Low
Antimicrobial prophylaxis in the presence of a drain and optimal timing for wound drain removal	1. In the presence of drains, does prolonged antibiotic prophylaxis prevent SSI?	The panel suggests that preoperative antibiotic prophylaxis should **not** be continued in the presence of a wound drain for the purpose of preventing SSI	Conditional	Low
	2. When using drains, how long should they be kept in place to minimize SSI as a complication?	The panel suggests removing the wound drain when clinically indicated. No evidence was found to allow making a recommendation on the optimal timing of wound drain removal for the purpose of preventing SSI	Conditional	Very low

Reproduced from: Global guidelines for the prevention of surgical site infection, second edition ISBN 978-92-4-155047-5 © World Health Organization 2018; Available at who.int/iris/handle/10665/277399

Index

© The Editor(s) (if applicable) and The Author(s), under exclusive license to Springer Nature Switzerland AG 2024
J. Faintuch, S. Faintuch (eds.), *Recent Strategies in High Risk Surgery*,
https://doi.org/10.1007/978-3-031-56270-9

B

D

E

N

O

SPRINGER NATURE

GPSR Compliance

The European Union's (EU) General Product Safety Regulation (GPSR) is a set of rules that requires consumer products to be safe and our obligations to ensure this.

If you have any concerns about our products, you can contact us on ProductSafety@springernature.com

In case Publisher is established outside the EU, the EU authorized representative is:

Springer Nature Customer Service Center GmbH
Europaplatz 3
69115 Heidelberg, Germany

FSC
www.fsc.org
MIX
Papier | Fördert
gute Waldnutzung
FSC® C083411

Kolibri 360 GmbH
Ferdinand-Jühlke-Straße 7
99095 Erfurt, Deutschland
produktsicherheit@kolibri360.de